Otto G. Bier   Wilmar Dias da Silva
Dietrich Götze   Ivan Mota

Fundamentals of Immunology

With 164 Figures

Springer-Verlag New York Heidelberg Berlin

Dr. Otto G. Bier
Laboratório Especial de Imunologia Aplicada
Instituto Butantan, São Paulo, SP., Brazil

Dr. Wilmar Dias da Silva
Instituto de Biociências, Departamento de Microbiologia e Imunologia
Cidade Universitária, São Paulo, SP., Brazil
Formerly Center for Blood Research, Boston, MA,USA

Dr. med. habil. Dietrich Götze
University of Munich, Medical School, Munich, FRG
and Max-Planck-Institut für Biologie, Tübingen, FRG
Formerly Associate Professor of Immunology
The Wistar Institute – The University of Pennsylvania
Philadelphia, PA, USA

Dr. Ivan Mota
Centro de Imunologia da OMS/OPS, Instituto Butantan
CP. 65, São Paulo, SP., Brazil

Library of Congress Cataloging in Publication Data
Main entry under title:

Fundamentals of immunology.

  Bibliography: p.
  Includes indexes.
  1. Immunology. I. Bier, Otto, 1906–
[DNLM: 1. Immunity. QW 504 F981]
QR181.F85   616.07′9   81-1112   AACR2

ISBN 0-387-90529-4 Springer-Verlag New York Heidelberg Berlin
ISBN 3-540-90529-4 Springer-Verlag Berlin Heidelberg New York

Typesetting, printing, and bookbinding by Universitätsdruckerei Brühl, Giessen

2120/3130–54321

Preface

This textbook of basic and clinical immunology has been written primarily for medical and biology students who are receiving their first introduction to this fascinating field. Although we have presumed some knowledge of basic biology (particularly physiology and biochemistry), our primary intent has not been to cover in depth the latest research findings. Rather, we have sought to lay a firm foundation for subsequent reading in the laboratory and clinical sciences: internal medicine, pediatrics, microbiology, serology, physiology, cell biology, and genetics. Hence the first part of the text presents the various components of basic immunology, while the second shows how these elements interact under both normal physiologic and pathologic conditions.

To facilitate comprehension of the relationship between basic and clinical immunology, we have introduced cross-references throughout the book. A glossary of important terms has also been included. Selected references are provided with each chapter to guide the student to additional information on topics of special interest.

Throughout the book we have attempted to convey to new students of immunology some of the excitement which the subject has long held for us. If we have succeeded, the task of writing will have been worthwhile.

December 1980

OTTO G. BIER
WILMAR DIAS DA SILVA
DIETRICH GÖTZE
IVAN MOTA

Contents

Chapter 1   Tissue and Cells of the Immune System

IVAN MOTA

Contents

Histology and Histogenesis of Lymphoid Tissue

Lymphoid tissue is constructed of fibrillar reticulum whose networks contain free cells. This fibrillar reticulum is composed of reticular fibers, reticular cells, and fixed macrophages that are integral to the reticuloendothelial system. The majority of free cells are lymphocytes in different stages of differentiation; including free macrophages and plasma cells. Two types of lymphoid tissues are recognized – loose lymphoid tissue in which reticulum cells predominate, and dense lymphoid tissue in which lymph cells predominate. The dense lymphoid tissue is capable of organizing nodular formations that constitute nodular lymphoid tissue.

Lymph and Lymph Vessels

Lymph vessels originate in tissue as extremely fine lymph capillaries that communicate with each other and then anastomose, forming networks. These capillaries are of varying diameter and develop into the major lymphatic vessels. Their walls are composed of a layer of endothelial cells, outwardly surrounded by a loose reticular fibrous lattice. Lymphatic capillaries, unlike blood capillaries, do not possess basement membranes. This fact is probably responsible for the capacity exhibited by lymphatic capillaries to absorb macromolecules present in interstitial liquid and in inflammatory exudates. Lymph results from interstitial liquid that passes through the walls of lymphatic capillaries and is directed via these capillaries to the lymph nodes. The passage of lymph through the interstices of the meshwork of these organs allows intimate contact between substances or particles borne in the lymph and the macrophages, as well as immunologically competent cells of these organs. At the same time, the lymph receives cells originating from the lymph nodes. After passage through these organs, the lymph of the entire organism finally is delivered to venous circulation through the thoracic lymphatic ducts.

Primary and Secondary Lymphoid Organs

Lymphoid tissue is found concentrated in the lymphoid organs, which are divided functionally into primary and secondary organs. During phylogenetic evolution and embryogenesis, the first lymphoid organs to appear are the thymus and the bursa of Fabricius, together with the first lymphocytes. These organs are thus termed the primary lymphoid organs. From an embryologic point of view, the primary lymphoid organs are distinguished from other lymphoid structures by their points of origin – points at which there exists a direct contact between the ectoderm and the endoderm. This fact suggests that such areas may have special inductive properties in relation to those lymphoid elements that are formed in these organs.

The spleen, the lymph nodes, and the other lymphoid aggregates of the vertebrates whose lymphoid populations are dependent upon primary organs, constitute the secondary lymphoid organs. Lymphoid tissue appears first in the thymus and in the bursa of Fabricius, and only later in the other lymphoid organs. The thymus maintains a pure epithelial structure until the end of the second month of intrauterine life in man, when for the first time cells appear bearing lymphoid characteristics. In the bursa of Fabricius, which is found only in birds, the first lymphocytes appear on the fifteenth embryonic day. The abundance of lymphocytes in the thymus and bursa of Fabricius contrasts with the scarcity of these cells in the spleen, in the lymph nodes, in Peyer's patches, and in the serum during the embryonic stage of life. Lymphopoiesis becomes evident in these organs only after birth, possibly due to antigenic stimulus. In fact, animals born in sterile environments, despite having well-developed thymuses, possess poorly developed secondary lymphoid organs. In birds the development of secondary lymphoid organs is also accelerated by antigenic stimulus. However, this response of secondary organs to antigenic stimuli proceeds only in the presence of the thymus,

thymectomized animals being incapable of such response. All these observations are compatible with the notion that most lymphocytes are differentiated in the thymus and in the bursa of Fabricius (or its equivalent in mammals), then migrate through the lymphatic circulation to the secondary lymphoid organs, where they localize and proliferate under antigenic stimulus.

Origin of the Lymphoid Cells of the Primary Lymphoid Organs

The origin of lymphocytes present in lymphoid organs has been extensively debated. Some have contended that these cells originated by differentiation of the embryonic epithelial reticulum of these organs, whereas others have held that lymphocytes of these organs were derived from undifferentiated mesenchymal cells that invaded the epithelial structures at an early stage. Although initially it was accepted that the lymphocytes of the thymus originated from the epithelium of the organ, more recent experiments with parabiosis and transfer of cells with labeled chromosomes to irradiated animals demonstrated that immature cells resembling hemocytoblasts migrate early to the blastema of the thymus and to the bursa of Fabricius, where they differentiate under the influence of the epithelium of these organs. The cells that migrate to these organs originate in the embryo, from the blood islands of the vitelline sac and from hematopoietic tissue of the liver and, in the adult, from the bone marrow.

Studies of regeneration of destroyed lymphoid tissue by transfusion of cells of diverse origins have shown that cells present in the bone marrow are responsible for the regeneration of lymphoid tissue. The morphology of this cell in the adult is not known. Thus, the repopulation of the primary lymphoid organs appears to depend upon undifferentiated cells that normally originate in the bone marrow and that either migrate to the thymus, where they differentiate and are transformed into immature T cells under the influence of the hormones produced by the epithelium of the organ, or mature in the bone marrow, are transformed into B cells, and migrate to the lymphatic system. It is thought that the cells that migrate from the bone marrow to the thymus are already specifically preconditioned to differentiate into T cells. Apparently, the cells of the bone marrow destined to be transformed into T cells have receptors for thymopoietine whereas the cells destined to differentiated into B cells do not. Once localized in the primary lymphoid organs, these cells, under the influence of their environment, differentiate, proliferate, and migrate to the secondary lymphoid organs where they complete their differentiation, acquiring new functional characteristics and transforming into immunocompetent cells (Fig. 1.1).

Functional Properties of Primary Lymphoid Organs. The lymphoid cells of the primary organs are characterized by an intense proliferative activity that is independent of antigenic stimuli. For this reason, the mitotic activity of lymphoid populations of these organs is high even in the fetus and in animals born in aseptic conditions. This situation contrasts with that existing in secondary lymphoid organs, in which lymphopoiesis is practically nil in the fetus and even in the newborn, and continues as such in animals born and maintained in sterile environments. Furthermore, the cellular alterations that occur in secondary lymphoid organs in response to antigenic stimulus normally do not occur in primary lymphoid organs subjected to a stimulus of the same type. This,

Fig. 1.1. Origin and differentiation of the lymphoid cells in the primary lymphoid organs

however, does not signify that the lymphoid cells of these organs are not modified in response to determined situations of antigenic stimulus. For example, thymic suppressor cells (i.e., cells capable of specifically inhibiting the production of the antibody) can be obtained from the thymuses of hyperimmunized animals. The ablation of the primary lymphoid organs, if performed before they have an opportunity to promote the development of secondary lymphoid organs, prejudices the specific immunologic functions of the latter.

Immunologic Dichotomy of the Lymphoid System

In birds, there is a distinct dichotomy between the production of cells capable of evolving into antibody-producing cells – a process dependent on the bursa of Fabricius – and the production of cells capable of evolving into sensitized cells, which is a thymus-dependent process. Thus, bursectomized chicken do not exhibit primary or secondary responses (i.e., do not respond with formation of antibodies) after either a first or a second antigenic stimulus. However, cellular responses that depend upon the production of sensitized cells (e.g., the rejection of grafts) proceed normally because the development of cellular immunity depends upon the thymus. Removal of the thymus in birds, if performed just after hatching, leaves the immunoglobulin-producing system intact but seriously affects development of cellular immunity. In mammals, also, thymectomy diminishes the reactions of cellular immunity but has less impact on the antibody system. This finding indicates that a system corresponding to the bursa of Fabricius, i.e., one that regulates the development of antibody-producing cells, must develop in mammals. Certain syndromes of immunologic deficiency encountered in the clinic mimic, in man, the experimental surgical ablation of lymphoid organs in laboratory animals. In DiGeorge's syndrome, in which there is agenesis of the thymus, the cellular immunologic reactions are deficient, whereas the

production of antibodies is practically normal. With other syndromes not associated with thymus anomalies, the opposite is true: One observes hypogammaglobulinemia, whereas the cellular immune reactions are normal. These clinical observations permit the deduction that in man there exists a thymus-dependent system that regulates the cell-based immunologic reactions, and another system whose function is similar to that of the bursa of Fabricius in birds, the components of which are unknown, and which regulates production of antibodies.

Cells of the Immune System

Several types of cells participate in the defense system of organisms. In adults, they almost all originate, multiply and mature in the bone marrow, and are found in the mature stages in the blood, in which they either stay or from where they migrate into the tissue. The different cell types are: Polymorphonuclear cells (PMN) or granulocytes, the least specifically reacting cells in a defense reaction but able to phagocytose; they form the first line of defense against intruders. The monocytes, endowed with the capacity of phagocytosis, processing, and presenting antigenic material in a manner recognizable by specific immune cells, and able to bind specifically reacting receptors, forming the second line of immunity. The lymphocytes, the immune cells *sensu strictu*, endowed with the capacity to recognize as well as react specifically with foreign (antigenic) material via specific receptors. A fourth lineage of cell assumes only a peripheral role in the immune system but nevertheless an important one: the thrombocytes or platelets.

Polymorphonuclear Cells

Metchnikoff, the great Russian zoologist, was the first to recognize a group of cells which played a major role in the defense of the organism against a great variety of extraneous invaders. Metchnikoff named the white cells of the blood microphages (now known as polymorphonuclear cells), believing them to be concerned solely with the defense of the organism against small microorganisms, i.e., bacteria, and designated as macrophages certain cells in the tissues because they phagocytozed large preys like parasites and other cells. The distinction is now known to be erroneous, since both cell types are capable of phagocytozing large and small particles.

The polymorphonuclear leukocytes constitute about 60%–70% of the total circulating leukocytes and are subdivided into three types, based on staining characteristics (Wright or Giemsa type stain): (1) neutrophils possess granules that do not stain intensively when viewed under the light microscope; (2) eosinophils have granules that stain a bright orange-red; and (3) basophils having granules that stain a dark blue-black.

Fig. 1.2. Stages of granulocytopoesis. Left: bone marrow; middle: blood; right: tissue. *1* Myeloblast, *2* Promyelocyte, *3,4* Myelocyte, *5* Metamyelocyte, *6* Band, and *7–9* Segmented granulocyte. (Reproduced with permission from M. Bessis, 1977)

The normal range of total polymorphonuclear leukocytes is between 4,000 and 8,000 per mm³ of blood; the vast majority (>90%) consist of the neutrophilic series.

All three lineages derive from a common pluripotent stem cell in the bone marrow (of adults) under the influence of granulopoietin probably identical to the "colony stimulating factor" (CSF); CSF has been partially characterized in serum and urine as a glycoprotein with a molecular weight of approximately 45,000. The earliest morphologically distinct *neutrophil* precursor is the myeloblast (Fig. 1.2), which has a large nucleus and very little cytoplasm. Granules begin to appear in the next, or promyelocyte stage and are very obvious in the myelo-

cytes; because of their histochemical staining characteristics, the granules are referred to as azurophilic. They arise from the concave side of the Golgi-apparatus, are relatively large in size, and are electron dense. They contain acid hydrolases, lysozyme, myeloperoxidase, neutral proteases, cationic proteins with bactericidal activity and NADPH-oxidase.

As the cells continue to develop, the beginning of segmentation of the nucleus occurs in the metamyelocyte stage. At this stage, secondary or specific granules appear, which are smaller and less dense than azurophilic granules. The specific granules contain alkaline phosphatase, lysozyme, lactoferrin, and collagenase.

Fig. 1.3. Polymorphonuclear cells and monocyte. **A** Neutrophil PMN (band form); *1, 5,* neutrophilic granules; *2,* microtubules; *3,* glycogen particles; *4,* azurophilic granules; *6,* contractile vacuole. **B** Eosinophil; **C** Basophil; **D** Monocyte; *1–5* stages of digestion of phagocytized lymphocytes. (Reproduced with permission from M. Bessis, 1977)

The band form and the mature neutrophil arise from the metamyelocyte stage and enter the circulation from the bone marrow (Fig. 1.3 A). The mature cells are virtually devoid of mitochondria. There is a large reserve of granulocyte precursors in the bone marrow; the complete maturation process requires approximately 9–11 days. Once in the circulation, however, the half-life of the mature neutrophil in the blood is only 6–8 h. This gives rise to an estimated neutrophil turnover of approximately 126 billion cells per day in a normal 70-kg individual. The largest number of granulocytes seem to be lost from the blood through the gastrointestinal tract. Granulocytes also pass from the blood vessels into the tissue, attracted by bacterial and other chemotactic substances, and die there quite rapidly. The death can occur by fragmentation or the cells may be phagocytized and rapidly digested by macrophages.

Neutrophils have a well developed capacity for locomotion when they are attached to a solid surface (endothelia). They extend a clear cytoplasmatic projection (protopod) in the direction of locomotion, while the opposite end of the cell (uropod) is attached to the support by a number of filaments (Fig. 1.4). They easily adhere to surfaces, migrate into the tissue by diapedesis, and are able to phagocytoze microorganisms but also cells and inorganic substances of considerable size (erythrocytes, leukocytes, crystals).

Maturation of *eosinophils* parallels that of neutrophils, except that large eosinophilic granules take the place of neutrophilic granules in the myelocyte, in which the production of the secondary, specific granules starts. The granules are formed at the Golgi-complex in the same fashion as those of the neutrophils. Very recent findings suggest that the differentiation and maturation of eosinophils might be under control of their "own CSF", distinct from neutrophil CSF. The granules contain acid phosphatase, glycuronidase, cathepsin, ribonuclease, arylsulphatase, and other enzymes. Peroxidase is present but different from the myeloperoxidase of neutrophils. The eosine granules contain phospholipids as well as basic proteins (Fig. 1.3 B).

The mature eosinophils possess more and larger mitochondria than neutrophils, and their Golgi-apparatus is well developed. They have numerous glycogen particles.

The fate of eosinophils is unknown; some of them are phagocytized, others are probably eliminated through the intestinal tract and the lungs. The eosinophils respond to the same chemotactic stimuli as neutrophils, but particularly to soluble bacterial factors and

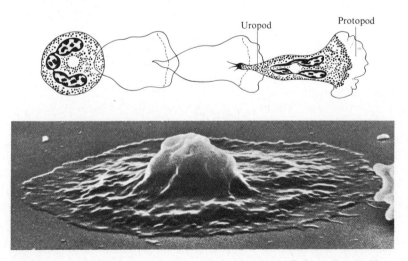

Fig. 1.4. Locomotion and spreading of a polymorphonuclear cell. (Reproduced with permission from M. Bessis, 1977)

antigen-antibody-complexes. They play a particular role in allergies and helminthic infections (see Chap. 11, p. 326).

The maturation of *basophils* runs a course very similar to the one of neutrophils and eosinophils, except that metachromatic granules are produced. The earliest identifiable granules are formed in the Golgi complex during the promyelocyte stage and contain abundant glycogen deposits in their cytoplasm. The mature basophil has numerous large and opaque granules masking the nucleus (Fig. 1.3 C). The granules contain acid mucopolysaccharides, histamine, and heparin in large quantities, and numerous enzymes, e.g. dehydrogenases, diaphorase, histidin-carboxylase, and peroxidases. The movement of basophils is ameboid and is similar to the movement of eosinophils though less active. The basophils have little phagocytic capability. They possess on their surface receptors for IgG and IgE as well as C 3 b. Nothing is known about life span and death.

Mast Cells

Mast cells are mononuclear cells which contain metachromatically stained granulations (Fig. 1.5 A). Their origin is not known, but they are thought to be related to lymphocytes. They are rarely seen in the blood, but distributed throughout the connective tissue, particularly in the vicinity of blood and lymphatic vessels and peripheral nerves. They may be especially abundant near epithelial surfaces exposed to environmental antigens such as those of the respiratory and gastrointestinal tract and the skin. Mast cells are long-lived cells that apparently may either differentiate *in situ* or undergo mitotic divisions as morphologically mature cells; apparently, intestinal mast cells can differentiate *in situ* from cells resembling lymphoblasts. There are some indications that mast cells represent a heterogeneous population of cells. Two subpopulations are distinguished by morphological, biochemical, and functional criteria: connective tissue mast cells and mucosal mast cells. The latter do not contain heparin in their granules (see below).

In stained smears, they have a diameter of 10–25 µm and they are usually round. The nucleus is oval and stains uniformly. The cytoplasm is pale and contains a mixture of violet to red-purple granules. The granules contain sulfated mucopolysaccharides, heparin, histamine, peptides with eosinophil chemotactic activity, prostaglandins, platelet-activating factor (PAF), kallikreins cationic chymase, slow-reacting substances of anaphylaxis (SRS-A), and a large number of enzymes; they do not contain myeloperoxidase. In rodents, mastocytes contain large amounts of biologically active amines (serotonin, dopamine).

The cells are capable of ameboid movement and of phagocytosis. They possess on their surface receptors for IgG, IgE, and the complement fragments C 3 a and C 5 a (anaphylatoxins). Toluidin blue in very low concentrations can be used as a vital dye to stain the mastocyte granules an intensive red-orange. Mastocytes perform their physiological function by releasing their granules extracellularly. Various substances can lead to the degranulation, among them: ACTH (adrenocorticotrope hormone), dextran, certain venoms, vitamin A, protamine sulfate, antigens to which the body responds, and antigen-antibody complexes, particularly those containing IgE antibodies. Degranulation liberates histamine, heparin, hyaluronic acid, and different enzymes. It produces local edema and permits fixation and activation of certain toxins.

Monocytes

The monocyte lineage comprises a variety of phagocytic cells, related by origin and function, which include the blood monocyte, alveolar (lung) macrophages, peritoneal macrophages, Kupffer cells in the liver, free and fixed macrophages of the bone marrow (osteoclasts) and lymphatic tissue, and histiocytes in tissues. It is generally believed that all of these cells are derived from bone marrow monoblasts and promonocytes, that they enter the blood stream as monocytes, and later the tissue to develop into macrophages.

The precursor cell of the monocyte in the bone marrow is unknown, but most probably, it derives from a stem cell common with granulocytes and thrombocytes. Monocytes vary considerably in size, i.e., from 20 to 40 μm in diameter, they have a large, usually kidney-shaped nucleus. The chromatin appears pale and has lace-like or reticular appearance without compact chromatin blocks. The cytoplasm is ample, greyish-blue and has fine azurophilic granulations. Cytoplasmic vacuoles are quite common (Fig. 1.3 D).

Monocytes stay in the circulation between 15 and 30 h, after which they leave the blood randomly and regardless of age, by diapedesis, after they have become adherent. In sites of inflammation, they accumulate very rapidly. The daily monocyte turnover is approximately 7×10^6 cells per hour per kg body weight.

The life span of macrophages is long and can attain 75 days and more. The death of monocytes and histiocytes proceeds in an unknown manner, but it is known that the cells when damaged and particularly after intense phagocytosis can, in turn, be phagocytized by other macrophages.

Monocytes adhere very well to solid surfaces, have a locomotion similar, though more slow, to the one of PMN, possess a quite marked sensitivity for chemotactic stimuli, and are very actively phagocytic. They may ingest a variety of cells, including protozoa, bacilli, viruses as well as antigen-antibody complexes, and a variety of inorganic substances (carbon, silica, asbestos, a. o.). They are endowed with receptors for immunoglobulins (Fc receptors) and complement components (C3b receptor) (see Chap. 5).

Lymphocytes

The lymphocytic lineage consists of a succession of cells which, starting with the committed stem cell, leads to the production of the small lymphocyte. Morphologically, it comprises the lymphoblast, the large lymphocyte, and the small lymphocyte (Fig. 1.5 B and C). In stained blood smears (Wright or Giemsa staining), lymphoblasts (15–20 μm in size) have a round or oval nucleus. The cytoplasm is sharply delineated, scanty, and basophilic. Large lymphocytes (9–15 μm in size) have a large nucleus, usually eccentric, the cytoplasm is scant, moderately basophil, or a light blue, and contains azurophilic granules (lysosomes). Small lymphocytes (6–9 μm in size) have a round, indented nucleus, and scanty cytoplasm often barely visible.

The maturation and differentiation of lymphocytes diverges at the stage of pre-lymphoblasts or lymphoblasts into two sublineages, which are not distinguishable by morphological criteria: part of the lymphocytes differentiates in the thymus (thymus-derived, or T lymphocytes), the other part in the bone marrow (bone-marrow, or B lymphocytes).

In the mouse embryo, lymphocytes originate in the fetal liver on about the eleventh day of gestation. These large basophilic blast-like cells gradually accumulate by migration into the thymus and begin to proliferate. Ultrastructurally, these basophilic cells are large and have the typical morphology of lymphoblasts, with copious dense cytoplasm filled with ribosomes but relatively few other organelles and a large nucleus that contains prominent nucleoli. The proliferation of these cells results in the production of typical small thymic cortical lymphocytes. By other than morphological studies, the intrathymic small lymphocytes can be subdivided into two populations: a major group accounts for about 90% of the total; they are small, dense, and short lived, located predominantly in the cortex, and express the TL antigen, high levels of Thy-1 antigen but low levels of H-2 antigens (these antigens are cell-surface markers which can be detected by serological methods and are explained in more detail in forthcoming chapters), and are cortisone sensitive. The minor population which appears to be the functionally ac-

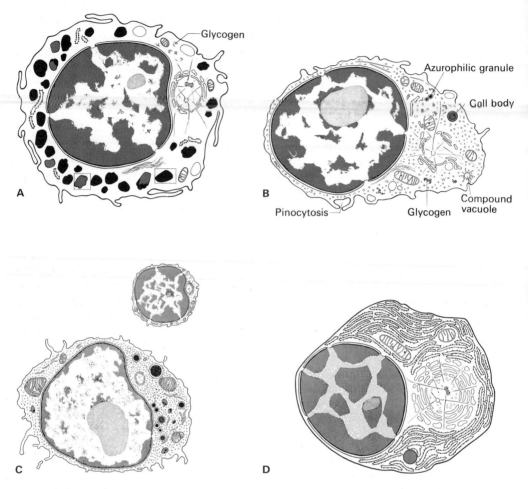

Fig. 1.5 A–D. Lymphocytes and mastocytes. **A** Mastocyte. **B** Lymphoblast. **C** Small lymphocytes with indentation of the nucleus caused by the centrosome and a transformed lymphocyte. **D** Plasmocyte (Reproduced with permission from M. Bessis, 1977)

tive group, is also composed of small lymphocytes, though they are generally larger and less dense than the major group. This minor population, located mainly in the thymic medulla, is cortisone resistant and differs antigenically in being TL negative and expressing high levels of H-2 antigens but low levels of Thy-1 antigen.

The high rate of intrathymic mitotic activity and the differentiation of the stem cells are independent of antigenic stimuli and are probably under some as yet poorly understood thymic epithelial cell influence. There

are indications that the induction of mitotic activity is in some way due to close contact between lymphocytes and cortical epithelial cells.

Once they leave the thymus, the thymus-derived, or T lymphocytes (virgin cells) can react with antigens and undergo a second stage of differentiation and proliferation to form the functional population of T lymphocytes. In this cycle, the cells transform into large blast-like "activated" T lymphoblasts, part of them divide, and then revert to small lymphocytes with differentiated (and committed) functions, i.e., cytotoxic, helper, suppressor T lymphocytes, or memory lymphocytes thereof.

In the mouse fetus, B lymphocytes arise in the liver at about 14 days of gestation (in adults in the bone marrow); these cells are larger than normal B lymphocytes, they divide rapidly and synthesize small amounts of monomeric IgM. These cells, called pre-B cells, contain cytoplasmic IgM but do not bear on their external surface the stable immunoglobulin receptors which characterize B lymphocytes. Pre-B cells lack most of the surface components characteristic of the majority of mature B lymphocytes: functional surface antibody receptors, Fc-receptors for IgG, and receptors for C 3, a complement component. It is also unlikely that pre-B cells will be found to express surface receptors for T helper factors (see Chap. 6). The absence of these functional receptors serves to protect them from influences exerted by contact with antigens, antigen-antibody complexes, and activated C 3. In this stage, clonal diversification has occured, i.e., selective expression of immunoglobulin genes present either on the paternal or on the maternal chromosomes, selective expression of either kappa (κ) or lambda (λ) light chains, and expression of different sets of genes encoding light- and heavy-chain variable regions (V_L and V_H). The expression of V gene products in pre-B cells implies that the genetic translocation event (see Chap. 4) has occured by this stage of differentiation. By this time, each small pre-B cell is ready to become an sIgM$^+$ B lymphocyte, its antibody specificity is determined.

Expression of sIgM (secrete IgM) antibodies signals the onset of B lymphocyte differentiation. The gradual acquisition of receptors for activated C 3 and IgG and of other classes of surface Ig appears.

Within a given clone of B lymphocytes, all cells are committed to the synthesis of antibodies of identical specificity, but some members become genetically programmed to convert from IgM antibody synthesis to synthesis of IgG, IgA, or IgE antibodies. At this stage, B lymphocytes express sIgD in addition to either IgM, IgA, or IgE. After mature sIgD$^+$ B lymphocytes are triggered by antigens (or mitogens), sIgD expression is rapidly reduced to low or undetectable levels (Fig. 1.6).

When B cells with all of these receptors are stimulated by the appropriate antigens and T helper cells, they may respond with division giving rise to memory B lymphocytes and with further differentiation into mature plasma cells. Thus memory cells are generated by antigen-driven expansion of B cell clones.

Contrary to red blood cells and platelets (see below) whose entire functional life takes place in the blood, and unlike mature granulocytes, which leave the blood vessels without entering them again, lymphocytes leave the circulation and return to it many times in the course of their life. They leave the blood stream predominantly in the lymphoid spaces of the tissue, are taken up by the lymphatics, and after traversing one or more lymph nodes return to the blood stream by way of the thoracic duct.

The life span is believed to be 10–20 days for nonstimulated lymphocytes; committed lymphocytes may live several months or even years.

The peripheral blood of man contains about 3,000 lymphocytes per mm^3, 70%–80% are T lymphocytes and 15%–20% are B lymphocytes, the rest being difficult to classify. About 85% of the lymphocytes in thoracic duct are T lymphocytes, about 80% in lymph nodes, and about 35% of the lymphocytes of the spleen are T cells.

Plasma cells are the final stage of fully differentiated B lymphocytes. They are usually oval, the nucleus is almost always situated at one pole. The arrangement of the chromatin is characteristic: the chromocenters form seven to nine large blocks of approximately polygonal outline, resembling a tortoise shell or a "cartwheel" picture. In stained smear preparations, the cytoplasma is intensely basophilic and its ultramarine colour identifies them immediately (Fig. 1.5 D).

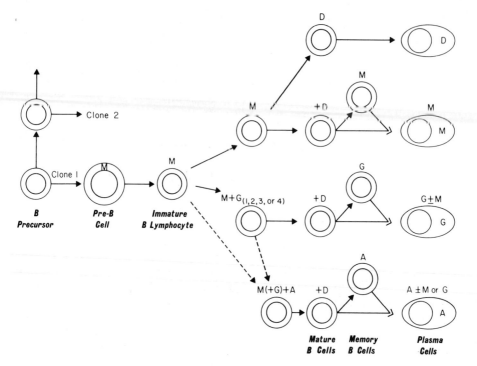

Fig. 1.6. Model illustrating some of the different stages in differentiation of a B cell clone. It outlines the present view of the intraclonal generation of immunoglobulin class or isotype diversity. The pivotal cell type in the switch is the immature surface IgM$^+$ lymphocyte which may mature to express other Ig classes. Each of the cell types depicted in this diagram represents multiple cells. For example, each maturing sIgM$^+$ cell that begins to express IgG makes only one of the four IgG subclasses (see Chap. 4). Thus there are multiple sublines of B cells within the clone which are capable of differentiation into mature plasma cells secreting the various subclasses of IgG antibodies. Two pathways leading from sIgM$^+$ to sIgA$^+$ expression are indicated by arrows since the available evidence suggests that both may be possible. sIgD is a late expression on all of the B cell sublines and, except for the subline of IgD producing cells, is lost after antigen or mitogen stimulation. (Reproduced with permission from Cooper et al., 1979)

Under normal conditions, they are rarely found in the blood. Lymph nodes and particularly their medullary cords are rich in plasmocytes, they are also present in the spleen, bone marrow, and the intestine. Plasma cells develop from stimulated B lymphocytes within 2–3 days and probably die within a few days.

Thrombocytes

Thrombocytes, or platelets, are non-nucleated cells liberated into the circulation from megakaryocytes in the bone marrow. Thrombocytic cells are derived from a committed stem cell susceptible to the action of thrombopoietin and, in turn, derived from a pluripotential cell. In contrast to other cell lineages in which multiplication (amplification) is accomplished by the successive duplication of DNA accompanied by cell division (see Fig. 1.2), megakaryocytes multiply their DNA (about four-times) without cytoplasmic division. Amplification thus consists of polyploidization of the cell. The cells enlarge during amplification but maturation takes place almost exclusively after amplification is completed (Fig. 1.7). Maturation includes lobulation of the nucleus, increase in cytoplasm, appearance of granules, and later, of platelet territories. Four stages of maturation can be distinguished: basophilic, granular and, platelet-producing megakaryocytes, and platelets. The total maturation

Fig. 1.7. Different stages of thrombopoesis. *1* Basophilic megakaryocytes (amplification = polyploidization 2 N to 32 N); *2* granular megakaryocyte; *3* platelet-forming megakaryocyte and liberation of platelets; *4* platelets in the circulation. Maturation starts after amplification has been completed. (Reproduced with permission from M. Bessis, 1977)

time is estimated to be 34 h. A 32 N mega-karyocyte produces approximately 4,000 platelets.

Platelets measure 2–5 μm in diameter, they contain microtubules, microfilaments, granules, vacuoles, canaliculi, mitochondria, and inclusions (glycogen).

The granules are of several types: azurophilic granules, the content of which is still being debated. Dense granules are storage sites of serotonin (5-hydroxytryptamine) which is made by the enterochromaffin cells of the intestine and picked up by the circulating platelets from the plasma. The dense granules also contain calcium and nucleotides. Catalase has been identified in perioxisomes which are also small vesicles. Platelets secrete all of these substances as well as platelet factor 4 and fibrinogen during the "release" reaction (see below).

Platelets play a role in adhesion and aggregation. They are capable of endocytosis. Various stimuli, e.g. contact to foreign surfaces, but also thrombin, proteolytic enzymes, bacterial endotoxin, and collagen, can trigger the release of their granules.

Immunologic Activity
of the Primary Lymphoid Organs

Thymus

The thymus is located in the thorax immediately behind the upper portion of the breastbone (sternum). Its two lobes are enveloped by a thin capsule of connective tissue that emits prolongations or septula that penetrate the organ and divide it into incomplete overlapping lobes. The peripheral part of each lobe, the cortex, is composed of dense lymphoid tissue, whereas the central portion or medulla is loosely arranged lymphoid tissue. The lobes may be considered a three-dimensional mesh of epithelial cells in whose networks are found lymphoid cells. These are much more numerous in the cortex than in the medulla. In the thymus, the lymphoid tissues do not form nodules as in other structures of this tissue. In the medulla are found Hassal's corpuscles, structures typical of this organ, formed by a central part containing concentric layers of epithelial cells (Fig. 1.8). The origin and nature of these corpuscles are unknown. The capillaries and small vessels of the thymus possess special structural features, including a thick basement membrane and an enveloping layer of epithelial cells, that is also supported by a basement membrane. Even though the epithelial membrane is not totally continuous, it acts as a barrier that impedes, but does not totally prevent, the passage of macromolecules present in the blood into the interior of the parenchyma and consequently into contact with the lymphocytes of the organ. The thymus does not possess lymphatic circulation – only efferent lymphatics that pass through the septula and upon leaving the organ lead to the lymph nodes of the mediastinum.

Fig. 1.8. Photomicrograph of human thymus, showing Hassal's corpuscles. (Courtesy of LC Junqueira and J Carneiro, Instituto de Ciências Biomédicas, Universidade de São Paulo)

Mitotic Activity of Lymphocytes of the Thymus. The intensity of production of lymphocytes in the thymus is much greater than that of the other lymphoid organs of the organism. It has been calculated that in the mouse 1 mg of thymic tissue produces approximately 1 million lymphocytes per day. The number of mitoses in this organ is five to ten times that in the lymph nodes or in the Peyer's patches. This mitotic activity is greater in the neonate, thereafter diminishing with age. The majority of the mitoses occur in the cortex, mitoses being rare in the medulla.

The proliferative activity of lymphoid cells of the thymus has been studied through the injection of tritiated thymidine. After a single dose of this substance, only labeled large lymphocytes appear initially; later labeled small lymphocytes appear in increasing numbers. The accumulation of labeled lymphocytes is, as would be expected, much greater in the thymus than in the other lymphoid structures. When observed over a period of time, the augmentation in the percentage of labeled lymphocytes follows a linear distribution. Since 50% of the lymphocytes are labeled within 2 days, the population of lymphocytes in the organ must therefore be substituted every 4 days. However, since the percentage of labeled cells present 4 days after the injection of tritiated thymidine is only 95%, it may be deduced that the remaining 5% must have a greater life span. Since the size of the thymus remains constant for periods in excess of 4 days, this rapid production of cells must be offset by a loss of equal magnitude, either through the destruction or the migration of these cells.

Destiny of Lymphocytes of the Thymus. The possibility that lymphocytes migrate from the thymus to other lymphoid organs was initially suggested by the observation of histologic preparations of this organ, which suggested diapedesis of these cells to the inside of the vessels. Furthermore, large numbers of lymphocytes were found in blood collected from the veins of this organ. In subsequent studies, tritiated thymidine was injected directly into the thymus in quantities adjusted so as to label just the cells of that organ. Later observations of histologic sections taken from other organs indicated that cells labeled with thymidine had migrated to the lymph nodes and to the spleen. However, the number of migrated cells was always small. The same results were obtained when mice thymectomized just after birth were subjected to thymic grafts from syngeneic newborn donor mice whose cells contained labeled chromosomes. In this case also, only a small number of donor cells were discovered in the lymph nodes and spleen of the recipient. These results, which indicate that only a small proportion of the thymic lymphocytes migrate to other lymphoid organs, imply that the great majoritiy of lymphocytes generated in this organ is destroyed in situ.

Effect of Thymectomy. Until 1961, when for the first time the effect of thymectomy was studied in newborn animals, numerous attempts to illuminate the functions of the thymus failed. Only then was it observed that removal of this organ in the first hours after birth resulted in noticeable diminution in the development and function of lymphoid tissue (Fig. 1.9). Thus, within 2–3 months following thymectomy, the quantity of circulating lymphocytes diminishes – particularly the small lymphocytes – and the lymphoid organs exhibit a significant reduction in volume. For example, the number of lymphocytes that may be drained from the thoracic duct of the rat in a 48-h period, though normally in the range of 100 million, falls to just 3 or 4 million following thymectomy. The intensity of these effects varies, however, with the degree of development of the lymphoid organs at birth – the less developed, the greater the effects of the thymectomy. In the mouse and in the rat, the organ must be removed no later than 48 h after birth, for after the third postnatal day, the effects of the thymectomy approximate those obtained in the adult, where only a slight depression in the number of lymphocytes occurs. Apparently, once stimulated by the functioning of the thymus, the secondary lymphoid organs under normal conditions become relatively self-sufficient. The thymus is the first lymphoid organ to appear during embryogenesis, whereas the spleen and the lymph nodes develop as lymphoid organs only later from cells that migrate from the thymus and the bone marrow to these organs.

In the lymphoid organs, the diminution in the lymphoid population induced by thymectomy occurs selectively in certain areas. For example, there is an accentuated diminution of lymphocytes in the paracortical areas of the lymph nodes (see section "Lymph Nodes" in this chapter) and in the periarterial sheaths of the spleen and of the diffuse lymphoid tissue of the Peyer's patches. Accordingly, such regions are termed *thymus dependent*. These are the areas through which the small lymphocytes circulate in their path from the blood to the lymph. As we have seen in the discussion of lymphocytes, all the experimental evidence favors the idea that the majority of circulating small lymphocytes constitutes a class of cells whose development depends upon the normal functioning of the thymus. On the

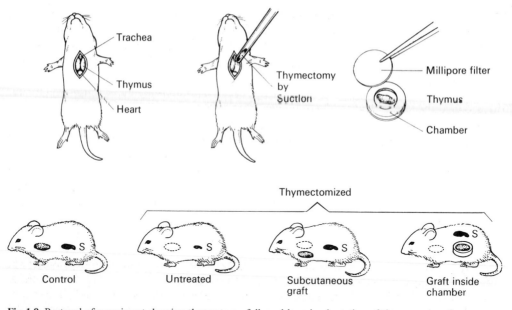

Fig. 1.9. Protocol of experiment showing thymectomy followed by reimplantation of the organ in a free state or enclosed within a Millipore chamber. The Millipore chamber permits the passage of macromolecules but not of cells. The experiments, performed with newborn mice, demonstrate that the presence of the thymus, even in conditions that make migration of cells to other organs impossible, permits the development of immunologic functions that are prejudiced by thymectomy. The development of the lymphoid organs is indicated by the size of the spleen (*S*) (Adapted from Levey RH (1964) The thymus hormone. Sc American 211:66)

other hand, the lymphoid nodules, the germinal centers of the spleen, and the lymph nodes are not altered by thymectomy, being composed of *thymus-independent* cells (B lymphocytes). The number of plasma cells present in these organs and in the connective tissue also ordinarily remains unaffected after thymectomy.

Importance of the Thymus in the Production of Antibodies. As we have seen, in animals thymectomized shortly after birth there is a cessation in the development of cellular immunity. Animals in this condition do not demonstrate delayed hypersensitivity or rejection of grafts; humoral immunity – reflected in the level of immunoglobulins and in the production of antibodies in response to various antigens – is normal. However, an exception is observed with certain antigens, such as sheep erythrocytes, which regularly suffer a reduction in immunogenic capacity in thymectomized mice. Antigens whose immunogenic capacity is impaired with respect to a specific species of thymectomized animals, are termed thymus-dependent antigens. The depression and restoration of the humoral response to these antigens, particularly to sheep erythrocytes in mice, became a model for the study of the immunologic functions of the thymus. Experiments suggest that the humoral response to these antigens requires the interaction of thymus-dependent cells with thymus-independent cells (see discussion of cooperation between T lymphocytes and B lymphocytes, Chaps. 2 and 6). This conclusion is based upon experiments in which mice incapable of forming antibodies against sheep erythrocytes after neonatal thymectomy evidence a restoration in the ability to produce antibodies after reimplantation of their thymus. An interaction between cells of the thymus and cells that are precursors of cells that form antibodies was first demonstrated by injecting thymectomized and irradiated mice with sheep erythrocytes mixed with cells of the thymus, the bone marrow, or of both. The humoral response of the mice injected with both types of cells always exceeded the sum of the responses induced by each of the individual cell types.

The interaction between thymus-dependent cells and thymus-independent cell precursors of antibodies does not contradict the fact that humoral responses are fundamentally thymus-independent. As we have seen, the cells that synthesize antibodies (B lymphocytes) develop independently of the thymus, generally speaking, whereas the cells responsible for the cell-based immune reaction require the thymus in order to develop immunologic competence. Nevertheless, both cell systems – T and B lymphocytes must work together in order to mount a mature, humoral immune response. This collaboration is discussed in greater detail elsewhere (see Chaps. 2 and 6).

Functions of the Thymus in the Adult. In man, the thymus continues to grow after birth and attains its maximum size at about 15 years of age, after which it slowly involutes. In the mouse, the organ continues to grow for 2 months after birth. Despite this, a thymectomy performed a few days after birth does not cause the dramatic effects produced when performed immediately after birth. Ordinarily, thymectomy in the adult produces only a slight drop in the number of lymphocytes and in the weight of the lymphoid organs. T lymphocytes represent long-lived cells that make up part of the pool of circulating lymphocytes; as a result, the effects of thymectomy appear only after a lengthy period of months in the mouse and of years in man. Accordingly, the thymectomized adults ordinarily do not sicken, but apparently remain in normal health. However, under certain conditions, harmful effects may be observed in the thymectomized adult. Thus, animals sublethally irradiated, in which a dramatic reduction in hematocytopoiesis occurs, do survive – recovering their immunologic activity within 2–3 weeks. Yet when the animal has been thymectomized prior to irradiation, it does not then fully recover its immunologic activity.

Apparently, despite total regeneration of the bone marrow, undifferentiated cells, which normally migrate to the thymus, do not, in the absence of this organ, develop into mature lymphoid cells. This indicates that the thymus is necessary in the adult to compensate for attrition in the population of lymphocytes already immunologically differentiated. This attrition, which occurs slowly under normal conditions, may occur rapidly in exceptional circumstances. It should be noted that thymectomized adult mice, when observed for many months, reveal what is frequently verifiable as a noticeable diminution in their immune responses.

Effects of Thymic Grafts in Thymectomized Animals. Animals that are immunologically deficient due to thymectomy regain their immunologic functions upon receipt of a grafted thymus. The grafted organ functions the same even if it is allogeneic or if its lymphoid cells have been destroyed by irradiation. Regeneration of the grafted thymus occurs slowly; 1 or 2 days after the graft is performed, the transplanted organ consists of a necrotic central mass and a peripheral area of live tissue consisting of lymphoid and reticular cells. The central necrosis results from nutritional deficiency due to lack of circulation. The cells in the peripheral area remain viable, receiving nutrients locally available through diffusion of tissue fluid. From the third day on, the mitotic activity of the surviving tissue increases, and within 5–6 days the typical structure of the organ is regenerated, with its lobules and cortical and medullary areas totally regenerated.

It was thought initially that the transplanted thymus, once regenerated, dispatched its own cells to the secondary lymphoid organs, thus repopulating them. However, analysis of the contribution of the recipient of the engrafted thymus to the process of regeneration revealed that events transpire differently. Animals whose cells contained chromosomal markers were recipients of the grafts. It was shown that, although initially the cells that proliferated in the transplanted organ had originated exclusively in the donor, beginning with the third week, the proliferating population of the graft consisted of cells from the recipient. Moreover, the lymphoid cells that then appeared in the secondary lymphoid organs also originated from the recipient. When the lymphoid cells of the engrafted thymus were destroyed previously by irradiation, the initial phase of regeneration by donor cells failed to occur, but the graft functioned and the animal nevertheless recuperated immunologically. If, however, the recipient animal also had been irradiated previously, the graft endured only as an epithelial structure without ever becoming lymphoid in character.

Origin and Differentiation of Lymphocytes of the Thymus. Results of experiments that restore immunologic function in thymectomized animals, achieved through the engrafting of another thymus, are completely compatible with the notion that lymphoid cells do not originate from the epithelium of that organ. Rather, they originate from cells that migrate to this organ through the circulation. It now appears definitely established that during the embryonic stage undifferentiated cells migrate from the yolk sac and from the liver (centers of myeloid hematopoiesis in the embryo) to the thymus. There, in contact with the epithelium of the organ, they proliferate and differentiate both functionally and structurally, acquire new antigens in their membranes, such as the TL and Thy-1 (theta, θ) antigens of mice.
The TL antigen is present only on the thymocytes and on thymus leukemia cells. The Thy-1 antigen is present on thymocytes and on the surfaces of lymphocytes originating from the thymus. The TL antigen is lost when the thymocytes leave the thymus. The Thy-1 antigen may thus serve as a marker for lymphocytes originating in the thymus but appearing in other lymphoid organs. Undifferentiated cells appear in the thymus of mice around the 11th day of embryonic life, at which point they still do not bear Thy-1 or TL antigens on their surfaces. About 8 days after this, these cells take on

the aspect of lymphoid cells, from which point they have these antigens on their surfaces. Cell populations undergoing mitosis and lymphocytes are sensitive to radiation; thus, the hematopoietic cells of animals subjected to a lethal dose of X-rays are destroyed, including the lymphoid cells of the thymus. Lethally irradiated animals can be saved by transfusion of cells taken from the bone marrow of normal syngeneic donors. In such cases, not only the bone marrow is repopulated, but also the lymphoid cells of the thymus and the secondary lymphoid organs. Under the same conditions, other transfused lymphoid cells – whether obtained from the lymph, from the lymph nodes, or from the thymus – failed to repopulate. Myeloid cells of the donor proliferate initially in the bone marrow and the thymus and appear only later in the lymph nodes. Identical results were obtained through experiments involving transplantation of the thymus in which cells of this organ were rendered identifiable through chromosome markers. In this case, although the regeneration of the lymphoid population of the transplanted thymus initially takes place at the expense of its own cells, within a few days its cells are totally replaced with cells from the bone marrow of the recipient. If, however, the marrow of the recipient was previously destroyed by irradiation, repopulation of this organ does not proceed beyond the first few days, in which case repopulation of the organ occurs at the expense of its own cells. These experiments demonstrate (1) that the lymphoid population of the thymus originates from cells that migrate from the bone marrow to this organ and (2) that the lymphoid cells present in the thymus have a minimal capacity for autoregeneration.
It is recognized that the undifferentiated cells of the marrow acquire immunologic specificity while they remain in the thymus, i.e., they become capable of recognizing a specific antigen. However, they are not transformed into immunologically competent cells. These affirmations are made to explain (1) the fact that contact by the thymus

Table 1.1. Active substances produced by the thymus

Designation	Composition	Mol Wt	Biologic Activity
Thymosine fraction	Protein	1,000–15,000	Lymphocytopoiesis + differentiation of T cells
Thymosin α_1	Protein	3,108	Induction of expression of Ly-1,2,3 phenotype and T-cell helper functions
Thymopoietine I	Protein	5,562	Induction of the appearance of specific antigens of the T cells + inhibition of neuromuscular transmission
Serum thymic factor (STF)	Polypeptide	857	Induction of specific antigens of T cells in vitro; induction of positive Thy-1 cells in nude mice
Thymic humoral factor (THF)	Polypeptide	3,000	Restoration of immunologic competence in vivo and in vitro

cells of the newborn with a determined antigen renders the animal specifically tolerant only to this antigen; and (2) that the lymphocytes of the thymus do not react immunologically either when stimulated locally or when inoculated into newborn mice of another strain (such a reaction would result in the graft-versus-host rejection syndrome). It is possible that a small number of the lymphocytes of the thymus are immunologically competent cells, but it is not known whether these cells differentiate in situ or whether they make up part of the pool of circulating lymphocytes in transit through the thymus.

Hormonal Activity of the Thymus. For many decades, numerous unfruitful attempts were made to demonstrate a hormonal function in the thymus. The subsequent demonstration of the effects of neonatal thymectomy and the observations that these effects could be eliminated by grafts of thymus enclosed in millipore chambers impermeable to cells, have renewed interest in the probable hormonal activity of the thymus and its influence in immunologic phenomena. This renewed interest resulted in the isolation of numerous substances from thymus extracts, some of which are listed in Table 1.1.

It is possible that some of the activities now attributed to different substances will subsequently be established as due to the same substance. Thymopoietine is an extremely active substance that induces the differentiation into thymocytes (immature T cells) of the immature cells of the bone marrow that

migrate to the thymus. The addition of thymopoietine in vitro to mouse bone marrow or spleen cultures produces the appearance of cells with surface antigens typical of the T lymphocytes. Studies that culminated in the isolation of this substance resulted from investigations into the pathogenesis of myasthenia gravis, a disease characterized by symptoms of muscular weakness due to a defect in the mechanism of neuromuscular transmission, frequently in association with pathologic alterations of the thymus. The idea that the central cause of the disease might be autoimmune thymitis gave rise to a series of experiments that culminated in the isolation of two polypeptides (thymopoietine I and II) that are slightly different physicochemically but that behave functionally as the same substance. The thymopoietines apparently are produced by the epithelial cells of the thymus. In addition to inducing the differentiation of the cells originating in the bone marrow into T cells, they also impede the transmission of the neuromuscular impulse. Their neuromuscular effect appears only 18 h after the first injection of the hormone (in mice). The primary effect of thymopoetine is the transformation of "stem cells" into immature T cells. Evidence suggests that adenosine 3′,5′-phosphate (cyclic AMP) is the intracellular mediator of the differentiation of prothymocytes and that the response of the prothymocytes can be induced or facilitated by substances that augment the intracellular level of cyclic AMP.

In addition to the active substances extracted from the thymus that are listed in Table 1.1, one other active polypeptide has been obtained from the thymus and from other tissues. It differs from the other active substances isolated from the thymus in several ways: (1) it is found in other tissues, (2) it does not affect neuromuscular transmission, and (3) it is capable of inducing the differentiation of both T-cell precursors and B-cells. In recognition of its presence in diverse tissues, this hormone has been termed "ubiquitine."

Wasting Disease. Animals thymectomized just after birth contract a disease characterized by weakness, discontinued growth, lethargy, bristling hair, loss of weight, periorbital edema, diarrhea, and death

within a few weeks. This syndrome closely resembles runt disease, provoked by the graft-versus-host reaction, which occurs when mice are neonatally inoculated with allogeneic lymphoid cells. The cause of this syndrome is not well understood. However, the fact that wasting disease is prevented by treatment with constant doses of broad-spectrum antibiotics or by maintenance of the thymectomized animals in sterile environments suggests that this syndrome is in some manner caused by multiple infections.

Bursa of Fabricius

Encountered in birds and located near the cloaca, this organ is structurally similar to the thymus (Fig. 1.10). In the chick, this or-

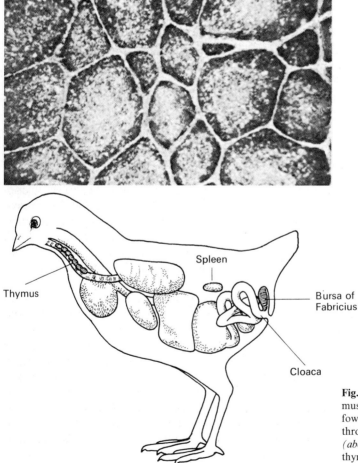

Fig. 1.10. Localization of the thymus and bursa of Fabricius in fowl. Photomicrograph of section through the bursa of Fabricius (*above*). Note similarity to the thymus

gan appears on the tenth day of incubation as a diverticulum of the cloaca that originates from a region where there is intimate contact of the ectoderm with the endoderm. The organ is composed of numerous epithelial folds whose lamina propria contain numerous isolated groupings of dense lymphoid tissue that resolve into structures similar to the lobules of the thymus. At the time of hatching, the lobules are distinguishable into cortical and medullary zones. Extirpation of the bursa of Fabricius, or bursectomy, when performed immediately after hatching, produces a diminution or even complete absence of the germinal centers and of plasma cells of the secondary lymphoid organs, accompanied by a considerable diminution in the formation of antibodies. However, the thymus and the thymus-dependent areas of the lymphoid organs are not altered, nor are the cell-based immunologic reactions affected. There thus exists in birds a clear dichotomy of the immunologic functions, which are governed either by the thymus or by the bursa of Fabricius. A structure equivalent to the bursa of Fabricius is unknown in mammals. Although the appendix, Peyer's patches, and the tonsils have been suggested as organs capable of exercising the functions of the bursa in mammals, there is lack of definitive experimental data supporting these contentions.

Immunologic Activity of the Secondary Lymphoid Organs

Lymph Node System

The secondary lymphoid organs are complex structures that possess mixed populations composed of thymus-dependent and bursa-dependent cells (thymus-independent in mammals). These cells occupy selectively determined areas in these organs. The terms thymus-dependent and thymus-independent merely signify that for their formation, these cellular zones are dependent upon the thymus. Once located in the secondary lymphoid organs, these cells do not depend for their functioning upon the thymus or the bursa of Fabricius (in birds). This explains why a normal immunologic response is obtained in animals thymectomized or bursectomized upon reaching adulthood (that is, after the secondary lymphoid organs have been populated by cells that have been conditioned by the primary lymphoid organs).

Lymphoid Nodules. The lymphoid nodules are irregular spherical formations of dense lymphoid tissue that measure 0.2 mm–1 mm in diameter. They are not permanent structures and may appear and disappear in a determined location. In neonates and in animals born in sterile environments, the nodules are scarce or even absent, which indicates that their presence may depend upon the existence of local antigenic stimuli. They exist isolated in the connective tissue of numerous organs (particularly in the lamina propria of the digestive tract, in the upper respiratory tract, and the urinary system), and are always present in normal secondary lymphoid organs, where they are usually termed "lymph follicles". They frequently exhibit a clearer central region called a germinal center, in which cells of an immature aspect appear, sometimes in intense proliferative activity. A single dose of tritiated thymidine results in a great number of labeled cells in these structures. Most of these cells are immature lymphocytes in differentiation, among which are found free macrophages and a network of dendritic reticular cells. The role of these lymphoid nodules in the immune response is discussed in conjunction with that of the lymph nodes.

Lymph Nodes. The lymph nodes are ovoid or reniform formations that measure from 1 mm to several centimeters in length and appear along the routes of the lymphatic vessels. On one border of a lymph node, there is a depression, or a hilus, where blood vessels enter and exit, and where the efferent lymphatics exit (Fig. 1.11). The afferent lymphatics enter the organ through diverse points along the border opposite the hilus. The lymph nodes are enveloped in a capsule

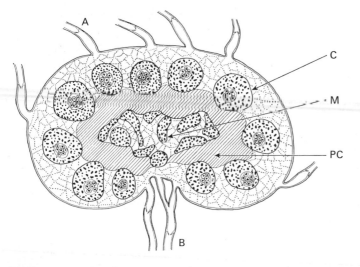

Fig. 1.11. Schematic structure of lymph node *A*, afferent lymphatics; *B*, efferent lymphatics; *C*, cortical region with lymphoid nodules exhibiting germinal center; *PC*, paracortical region; *M*, medullary zone with medullary cords and sinuses. The cortical and medullary regions are thymus-independent, whereas the paracortical region is thymus-dependent

of dense connective tissue and are composed of a delicate web of reticular fibers that support reticular cells and fixed macrophages. In the networks of this web, there are two lymphocytes populations: the thymus-dependent and thymus-independent.

Lymphoid tissue is distributed in the organ in three distinct regions that are recognizable as containing specific structures, but whose limits are imprecise: (1) There is a superficial, peripheral area termed the cortical region. The lymphocytes of this region are grouped in rounded or oval formations constituting the primary nodules or lymphoid follicles. In the central portions of the lymphoid follicles, germinal centers appear frequently that are rich in immature cells in the process of proliferation, in dendritic reticular cells, and in fixed macrophages. This region is thymus-independent and as such is not affected by thymectomy. (2) There is a central or medullary region in which dense lymphoid tissue is distributed in irregular formations that appear as trabeculae or threads, between which run the medullary sinuses. This region also is thymus-independent. (3) There is an intermediate zone called the paracortical region, situated imprecisely between the cortical and medullary zones. Situated under and between the follicles, it is composed of irregular masses of dense lymphoid tissue (Fig. 1.12). This region, also called the diffuse cortical area, hypertrophies considerably after antigenic stimuli that induce delayed hypersensitivity reactions. The lymphocytes of this region disappear after thymectomy and for this reason are considered thymus-dependent.

All formations of dense lymphoid tissue are permeated by loose lymphoid tissue constituting the subcapsular, perifollicular, and medullary sinuses through which the lymph travels in the direction of the efferent lymphatics. It is important to remember that all of the dense lymphoid tissue of the lymph node and of the lymphatic sinuses is continuous. The latter are not composed of vacant spaces separated by membranes; rather, they are an open meshwork of reticular tissue that constitutes the stroma of the organ. The lymph that enters the subcapsular sinus continues through the interfollicular sinuses and, upon passing through the medullary sinuses, reaches the efferent lymphatics. In this fashion, contact is facilitated between the foreign particles of the lymph and the macrophages of the reticulum. It should be remembered that the retention capacity of the lymph nodes for foreign particles is greatly augmented during inflammatory processes.

Postcapillary Venules. Once it had been verified that the great majority of lymphocytes

Afferent
lymphatics

Ag   Ag

Postcapillary
venule

←Postcapillary
venule

— Vein

— Artery

Efferent
lymphatic

● T lymphocyte

◉ B lymphocyte

Macrophage

Dendritic cell

Fig. 1.12. Localization of the T and B lymphocytes in the lymph nodes. The thymus-dependent (*TD*) region is in *white;* the *shaded* area shows the thymus-independent (*TI*) regions. In the *TD* region, the majority of the cells are conditioned to react to the antigen with the production of sensitized cells; in the *TI* regions, the majority of the cells are antibody-forming cells when they come in contact with antigens. The T lymphocytes circulate constantly, passing from the postcapillary venule to the lymphatic parenchyma, where they enter into contact with the dendritic cells and the B lymphocytes. In passing through the lymph nodes, the T lymphocytes localize preferentially in the paracortical region (in *white*), from which they reach the medullary sinuses and gain access to the lymphatic circulation (Adapted from Cradock CG et al. (1971) Lymphocytes and the immune response. New Engl Med 285:378)

reaching the systemic circulation returned to the lymph, attention was focused upon tracing the return path of these cells, i.e., a precise determination of the structures through which the lymphocytes passed in penetrating the lymphatic circulation. Rats were inoculated with lymphocytes labeled with tritium (^{3}H) and were killed a few hours later. Autoradiographic examination of their organs indicated that the lymphocytes leave the blood through the so-called postcapillary venules (called Schulze venules in man), situated in the paracortical region of the lymph nodes. The venules are characterized by narrow central cavities constricted by an endothelium of cuboid cells, through which lymphocytes pass in their migration from the blood to the paracortical region of the lymph nodes (Fig. 1.13). Apparently, the passage of the lymphocytes through the endothelial cells is due to the presence of polysaccharides in the lymphocyte membranes for which specific receptors exist on the endothelial cells. Autoradiographs of lymph nodes reveal numerous labeled lymphocytes migrating through the endothelial cells of these venules. These lymphocytes are concentrated in the paracortical zone of the organ and later are encountered in the lymphatic sinuses, through which they return to the lymphatic circulation together with newly formed lymphocytes.

Lymphoid Follicles. These are represented fundamentally by groupings of lymphocytes and dendritic reticular cells that possess long cytoplasmic extremities, numerous and contorted, which form veritable labyrinths in

Fig. 1.13. Electron micrograph of postcapillary venule. Lymphocytes are observed within the cytoplasm of the cuboid epithelial cells (L_1 and L_2) and within the lumen of the vessel (L_3). Modified from Nossal GJV, Ada GL (1971) Antigens, lymphoid cells and the immune response. Academic Press, New York

which lymphocytes move about. Antigens are retained for long periods among these prolongations. Unlike the medullary macrophages, these cells do not phagocytize the antigens, but maintain them on their surfaces. Two types of follicles may be distinguished – primary follicles, which do not possess germinal centers, and secondary follicles, which possess a germinal center surrounded by a mantle of small lymphocytes in stained histological sections. Germinal centers appear as a light area in the internal portion of the follicle; they are composed of proliferating immature cells and, frequently, macrophages containing nuclear inclusions that apparently result from the phagocytosis of lymphocytes in degeneration. The germinal center appears in response to antigenic stimuli, and its development is a function of the intensity of such stimuli. Germfree animals possess follicles without germinal centers, which, after administration of an antigenic stimulus, reduce their proliferative activity and resume the appearance of primary follicles, which in this case frequently contain elevated quantities of macrophages with nuclear inclusions.

Antigen-Induced Cellular Alterations in Lymphatic Organs. The cellular alterations that occur with a humoral reaction and cellular immunity are caused by antigen recognition, transformation of blasts, and proliferation of lymphocytic cells, particularly in the lymph nodes and spleen.

Early histologic changes consist primarily of an increase in T cells in the paracortical areas around the postcapillary venules in the lymph nodes and in the periarterial sheath in the spleen. Only later do plasmablasts appear in the lymph nodes and in the red pulp of the spleen. In most cases, antigens induce a mixed immune response with cellular modifications in both thymus-dependent and thymus-independent areas. Some antigens preferably give rise to cell alterations in only one area. Thus, pneumococcal polysaccharides cause changes only in thymus-independent areas, whereas, for example, oxazolam induces changes in thymus-dependent areas.

Antigenic stimulation can result in a humoral reaction, with production of antibodies, or in a cellular hypersensitivity reaction, with production of sensitized cells. These reactions differ according to whether they are a primary or a secondary response. At the beginning of a primary reaction, the antigen is encountered in numerous macrophages in the medullary region and possibly later in a small but significant quantity of dendritic reticular cells of the germinal centers. When labeled antigen is used, it is notable that although the antigen present in the macrophages diminishes rapidly, that attached to the dendritic reticular cells persists for many weeks. Four to five days after contact with the antigen, moderate proliferations of immature cells can be observed that, because of the difficulty in foreseeing their future proliferation, are designated immunoblasts. These cells appear principally in the medullary chords and rarely inside the lymphatic nodules. Most of these cells give origin to plasmablasts and plasma cells. In the primary response, the germinal centers usually exhibit discrete alterations, revealing minimal hypertrophy in the late phase (sixth day) of the response. However, these alterations can be more intense when the antigen used is highly immunogenic. After a second contact with the same antigen, i.e., in the secondary response, the immunoblasts appear not only in the medullary chords but also in the germinal follicles, which greatly increase in size. In the secondary response, the intervention of the germinal centers is much more accentuated and the plasma cells appear much more rapidly and in greater number than in the primary response. Moreover, the antigen is encountered not only in the macrophages of the medulla but also in a large portion of the dendritic reticular cells of the germinal centers, thereby coming in close contact with the lymphocytes. It is recognized that these cells represent a mechanism for retention of antigens that is particularly efficient in the secondary response. This situation, particularly due to the mobility of the lymphocytes, augments the contact of these cells with the antigens present in the dendritic macrophages. It is possible that the antigens remain on the surfaces of the dendritic reticular cells in the form of antigen-antibody complexes. The activity of the germinal centers results in the production of a large number of cells that differentiate into plasma cells or lymphocytes. A large number of these cells migrate to the medullary region, from which some of them reach the circulation. When an antigen is introduced into an organism for the first time, it induces not only the production of plasma cells but also a considerable increase in the number of cells capable of recognizing it. These recognition lymphocytes, which appear to originate in the germinal centers, are termed memory cells and are responsible for the secondary response.

When the antigen is applied in order to excite a response of the delayed type, the alterations of the lymph nodes, which also become evident from the fourth day, consist of the appearance of numerous immunoblasts in the paracortical region. The percentage of these cells in this region, which under normal conditions is about 1%, rises to 8%–10%. Subsequently, these cells differentiate into lymphocytes. In this type of response, plasmablasts do not appear, nor do the nodules become involved.

The hypertrophied areas of the paracortical region sometimes assume a nodular appearance and are thus termed paracortical nodules. One characteristic peculiarity of this type of response is the obstruction of the medullary sinuses by agglomerations of small lymphocytes that disappear as soon as the reaction begins to diminish. The sinuses apparently represent the exit routes for lymphocytes from the paracortical region; these become temporarily obstructed by the great numbers of cells produced under these conditions. Often, there is simultaneous activation of the germinal center and the paracortical area of the lymph nodes, so that a picture arises of simultaneously occurring reactions of the immediate and delayed types.

Spleen

Histology. The spleen constitutes the major accumulation of lymphoid tissue interposed in the systemic circulation. Examination of sections of this organ reveals white-gray, rounded nodules dispersed in a dark red mass called the red pulp. The white-gray nodules are composed of dense lymphoid tissue (Fig. 1.14) termed white pulp. The capsula of the organ, formed of dense lymphoid tissue, emits trabeculae that divide the parenchyma or splenic pulp into incomplete compartments. Through these trabeculae run arteries that, upon attaining a diameter of 200 μm, penetrate the parenchyma of the

organ where they are immediately enclosed in a sheath of dense lymphoid tissue. This tissue expands at certain points, forming lymphatic nodules or splenic follicles (Malpighian bodies). In this fashion, the white pulp becomes divided into a periarterial sheath of lymphoid tissue and into lymphoid nodules. The latter, together with the adjacent lymphoid tissues, constitute the thymus-independent zone of the organ, whereas the periarterial lymphoid tissue represents a thymus-dependent zone. The relations between the thymus-dependent and thymus-independent zones of the white pulp are schematized in Fig. 1.15. The red pulp is made up of splenic cords and venous sinuses. The splenic cords are composed of cytofibrillar reticulum, itself composed of reticular fibers, reticular cells, and fixed macrophages, in whose meshes are found formed elements of the blood along with free macrophages and plasma cells. Among the cords appear venous sinuses, which are capillaries of irregular diameter coated with intensely phagocytic cells. Although these cells voraciously phagocytoze carbon particles, they phagocytoze only inefficiently numerous protein antigens. The spleen differs from the lymph nodes in that it is not involved in lymphatic circulation, in its erythrocatheretic function, and – in certain spe-

Capsule

Follicle
(white pulp)

Trabecula   red pulp

Fig. 1.14. Photomicrograph of the spleen showing the white pulp and the red pulp. Also seen are the capsula and a trabecula

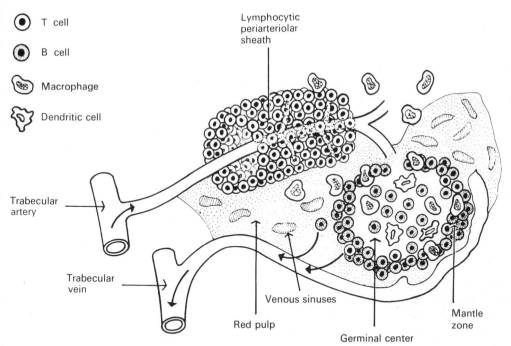

T cell

B cell

Macrophage

Dendritic cell

Lymphocytic
periarteriolar
sheath

Trabecular
artery

Trabecular
vein

Venous sinuses

Red pulp

Germinal center

Mantle
zone

Fig. 1.15. Thymus-dependent (*TD*) and thymus-independent (*TI*) regions of the spleen. The lymphocytic periarteriolar sheath constitutes a *TD* region whereas the lymphoid follicles and adjacent lymphoid tissue represent the *TI* zone (Adapted from Cradock CG et al. (1971) Lymphocytes and the immune system. New Engl Med 285:378)

cies – in its possession of myelopoietic capabilities. On the other hand, a series of splenic structures in this organ is similar to those of the lymph nodes: the lymphoid follicles, the lymphoid tissue of the periarterial sheath, which corresponds to the paracortical lymphoid tissue of the lymph nodes, and the cords of the red pulp, which correspond to the medullary cords of the lymph nodes. In addition, the spleen possesses an anatomic structure apparently without equivalent in the lymph nodes – the marginal sinuses. These structures result from anastomoses of the terminal capillaries of the white pulp, which are situated immediately inside the marginal zone (thus far, the marginal sinus has been described only in the rat). Common to many species, including the human, this structure consists of loose lymphoid tissue that possesses long, ramified prolongations constituting a network of mesh containing a small number of lymphocytes and macrophages. The limits between the marginal

zone and the red pulp are not well defined. The relation between these splenic structures is shown in Fig. 1.16. The marginal zone is important immunologically, since it is the region where many of the antigens carried in the blood are retained. Radioactive protein antigens, after injection, are rapidly encountered along the surfaces of the cytoplasmic prolongations of the reticular cells of this region and only later in the interior of the lymphoid follicles.

Antigen-Induced Modifications of the Spleen. The cellular alterations of the spleen after antigen stimulus are similar to those that occur in the lymph nodes. One to four days after intravenous injection of antigen, immunoblasts appear in the white pulp, localizing in the periphery of the periarterial sheath and in the marginal zone. These cells proliferate and differentiate, originating a large number of plasmablasts and plasma cells, many of which invade the red pulp.

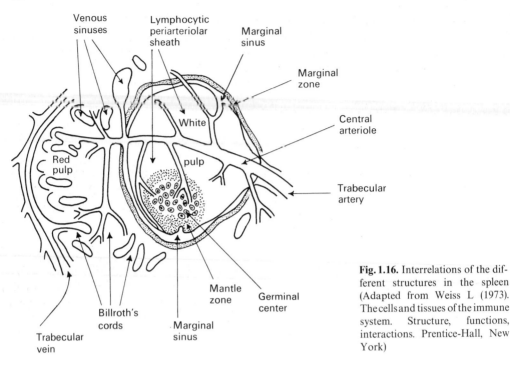

Fig. 1.16. Interrelations of the different structures in the spleen (Adapted from Weiss L (1973). The cells and tissues of the immune system. Structure, functions, interactions. Prentice-Hall, New York)

Some of these cells also appear in the lymphoid follicles of the white pulp. After 5–6 days, the plasma cells rapidly disappear; it is supposed that they move from this organ into the blood. In the secondary reaction, there is, in addition to these alterations, intense proliferative activity in the lymphoid follicles, resulting in the presence of numerous plasma cells situated in the periphery of the follicles and principally in the red pulp.

Other Lymphoid Structures

Agglomerations of lymphoid nodules appear along the respiratory and digestive systems in close association with the epithelium of the region. In man, these organs are represented by the palatine, lingual, and pharyngeal tonsils, whose lymphoid tissue is associated with the epithelial crypts of these structures; by Peyer's patches, agglomerations of lymphoid nodules localized in the wall of the small intestine; and by the appendix vermiformis, whose follicles form dense agglomerations in the submucosa of the organ. The lymphoid follicles of these structures behave as thymus-independent zones whereas the interfollicular tissue corresponds to the thymus-dependent paracortical zones of the lymph nodes. The alterations induced by antigens are similar to those induced by the lymph nodes.

In addition to blast transformation and proliferation, there is an accumulation of lymphocytes in lymphatic tissue following antigenic stimulation. If ^{51}Cr-labeled lymphocytes are injected intravenously or intraperitoneally into antigen-stimulated syngeneic mice, the lymphocytes are found in the spleen; after subcutaneous administration or after transplantation of nonsyngeneic skin, they are found in the lymph nodes. This aggregation of lymphocytes occurs within 1 h following intravenous injection and reaches a maximum after an additional 24 h. During the following 48 h, this aggregation dissolves again. The increase of lymphocytes in the lymphatic organs increases the possibility for contact between the antigen-coated dendritic cells and the antigen-sensitive cells. The mechanism of lymphocyte accumulation is unknown. Thymus-dependent soluble mediators may play a role.

Localization of the Antigen in the Lymphoid Organs

Knowledge regarding the localization of antigens in the tissues has resulted from the injection of fluorescent antigens or of antigens labeled with radioactive isotopes (particularly ^{3}H, ^{131}I, and ^{125}I) into the organism, followed by the study of sections or smears of lymphoid organs through fluorescence microscopy or autoradiography.

The entrance of antigens into the internal medium of an organism appears to constitute a threat to its integrity even for the most primitive forms of life. This perhaps is the explanation for the phylogenic observation that the means for the elimination of foreign substances that penetrate an organism have appeared well before the capacity developed to produce antibodies. In fact, most antigens that penetrate the organism are eliminated without having a chance to activate the immune system. Possibly for this reason, the locations in which antigens have been detected after introduction into an organism do not always represent the region where immunologic reactivity occurs. Actually, it is usual to observe antibody-producing cells in areas of lymphoid tissue that are practically free from concentrations of antigens; conversely, concentrations of antigens may occur in areas where antibody-forming cells do not exist.

It is now accepted as certain that the first event that stimulates an organism to demonstrate its immunologic potential is the encounter of the antigen with antibodies existing on the surfaces of immunologically competent cells. Where and how the antigens enter into contact with these cells depends upon the manner in which they gain entrance into the organism. Generally, antigens that penetrate the epithelia move to the lymph nodes that drain the region, where they localize in the macrophages of the medullary region and in the dendritic cells of the lymphoid follicles; antigens that penetrate directly into the blood circulation are captured principally by the cells of the marginal zone and dendritic cells of the spleen. When the antigen is injected subcutaneously, it reaches the satellite lymph node through the afferent lymphatic vessels, enters into the marginal sinus, and is encountered about 3 min after injection in the medullary sinuses. Within 5 min, it is encountered in the macrophages of the medullary cords. One to two hours later, the antigen concentration in the medullary region reaches its peak; the antigen may disappear within days or may persist for months, depending upon the nature and the quantity of the antigen. In the medullary sinuses as well as in the medullary cords, macrophages containing antigen are occasionally found enclosed in a layer of lymphocytes.

Although this discovery has been interpreted as functionally significant (passage of information regarding the nature of the antigen from the macrophage to the lymphocyte), this interpretation is speculative. The localization of antigen in the dendritic cells of the lymphoid follicles occurs later than in the medullary macrophages and is really only significant in the secondary response or in animals previously injected with antibodies specific for the antigen in question. In this respect, it is important to consider the observation that the localization of antigens in animals born and kept in sterile environments is minimal. In immunized animals, the antigen combined with the antibody penetrates rapidly into the cortex, and within 15 min after injection is encountered among the lymphocytes of the superficial region of the lymphoid follicles. Autoradiographs of lymph nodes 1 h after injection of antigen into immunized animals frequently reveals a crown of antigens in the perifollicular regions (Fig. 1.17). Subsequently, the antigen is encountered within the secondary follicles and, more diffusely, in the primary follicles. In the dendritic cells, the antigen becomes localized on the surfaces of its cyto-

Fig. 1.17. Autoradiograph of lymph node taken 1 h after injection of radioactive antigen. Note location of the antigen in the follicles. Photograph by courtesy of A Szenberg, WHO, Geneva

plasmic prolongations. Thus, the function of the dendritic cells appears to be that of concentrating the antigen in a locale that is strategically favorable to the establishment of contact with immunocompetent cells.

In the spleen, the antigen is encountered initially in the marginal zone, associated with the cytoplasmic prolongations of reticular cells found therein. Autoradiographs of spleens of animals killed at different intervals following injection of antigen appear to indicate a continuous flow of antigen from the marginal zone to the white pulp, where the antigen is retained in the follicles for long periods. For many antigens, the lymphoid follicles represent the only site of retention in this organ, whereas the marginal zone appears to be an important region for a transitory concentration of antigen. The localization of antigens in the other lymphoid structures is similar to that described for the lymph nodes.

Phylogenic and Ontogenic Development of Immunologic Capacity

Knowledge of the phylogeny of the immune response is still scanty. Some invertebrates such as the annelids and, perhaps, the tunicates may have an immune response, albeit primitive (such as rejection of grafts, which in these invertebrates requires a considerably longer period of time than in the vertebrates). These animals do not possess a thymus, and the cells present in cellular infiltrate in the graft area are purely histiocytic in character. There are as yet no data that suggest the production of humoral antibodies by any species of invertebrate. The first species to exhibit immunologic activity, including both humoral and cellular responses, is found among the agnates. The hagfish and the lamprey are capable of rejecting grafts and of responding with production of antibodies when stimulated with particulate or soluble antigens. The antibodies produced, however, appear to be of a single class, similar to IgM in vertebrates. Little if anything is known regarding the cellular mechanism of the immune response in this species – save merely the fact that adult specimens examined have neither a thymus nor lymphoid aggregates. It should be noted, however, that cells similar to lymphocytes, present in the peripheral blood of hagfish immunized with sheep erythrocytes, exhibit specific immunofluorescence when incubated together with antigen; possibly, these cells are totally or partially responsible for the production of antibodies. In more highly developed vertebrates, such as sharks and rays, there is already a central lymphatic sys-

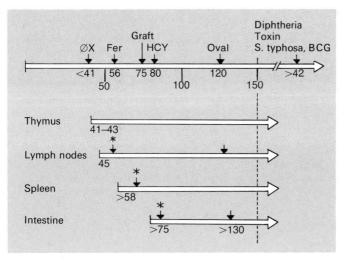

Fig. 1.18. Comparison of the appearance of the immune response and the development of the lymphoid system in the sheep. The *numbers* represent the elapsed time of gestation. Ø, bacteriophage; *Fer*, ferritin; *HCY*, hemocyanin; and *Oval*, ovalbumin. From Silverstein AM, Prendergast RA (1971) The maturation of lymphoid tissue structure and function in ontogeny. In: Lindahl-Kiessling K, Ada GL, Hanna MJ, Jr (eds) Morphological and functional aspects of immunity. Plenum, New York

tem in the form of a thymus-primordium, lymphoid cell follicles in the spleen, and circulating lymphocytes; however, lymph nodes are still absent. In these animals – which also have the capability to reject grafts and to exhibit distinct humoral responses – the antibodies produced are still predominantly of the IgM type. In the teleosts, two different classes of antibodies appear for the first time – IgG and IgM. The pulmonate fish of Australia appears to be the first vertebrate with two well-defined classes of immunoglobulins. The amphibians also exhibit two well-defined classes of antibodies and, although they possess no lymph nodes, they have lymphatic agglomerates responsible for the production of antibodies. The highest point in the evolution of the immune response is attained by birds and mammals – as evidenced by the appearance of at least five classes of antibodies that are functionally and antigenically different.

During ontogenesis, the capacity of the developing vertebrate to exhibit an immunologic response coincides, generally speaking, with the appearance of the thymus and the first lymphocytes. In tadpoles, for example, the capacity to reject skin grafts is established only when the first lymphocytes ap-

pear; in the opossum, the capacity for the production of antibodies appears simultaneously with the first lymphocytes. In sheep, the capacity to respond to antigenic stimulus appears gradually during embryogenesis – apparently as a series of isolated occurrences (Fig. 1.18). As shown, from the 75th day of gestation, the fetus is capable of rejecting grafts, whereas the capacity to respond with the formation of antibodies against bacteriophages can be induced after 41 days of gestation, against ferritin after 56 days, against hemocyanin after 80 days, and against ovalbumin after 120 days of gestation (in sheep the period of gestation is 150 days). It is interesting to compare these data with the development of lymphoid tissue in this species. The first lymphocytes are seen in the rudiments of the thymus from the 41 st day of gestation and later in the lymph nodes (45 th day), in the spleen (58 th day), and in Peyer's patches (130 th day).

References

Baum SJ, Ledney GD (eds) (1979) Experimental Hematology Today, 1979. Springer-Verlag, New York-Heidelberg

Bessis M (1977) Blood Smears Reinterpreted. Springer-Verlag, New York-Heidelberg

Cooper MD, Lawton AR, Preud'homme JL, Selig-
mann M (1979) Primary Antibody Deficiencies. In:
Cooper MD, Lawton AR, Miescher PA, Müller-
Eberhard HJ (eds) Immune Deficiency. Springer-
Verlag, New York-Heidelberg

DeChatelet LR (1979) Phagocytosis by human neutrophils. In: Gadebusch HH (ed) Phagocytes and cellular immunity. CRC Press, Boca Raton, Florida

Friedman H (1975) Thymus factors in immunity. New
York Academy of Science, New York

Low TLK, Goldstein AL (1980) Thymosin and other
thymic hormones and their synthetic analogues. In:
Immunostimulation, Chedid L, Miescher PA,
Mueller-Eberhard HJ (eds). Springer-Verlag, Hei-
delberg-New York, pp. 129–146

Moretta L, Webb SR, Grossi CE, Lydyard PM, Cooper MD (1977) Functional analysis of two human
T cell subpopulations: Help and suppression of
B cell responses by T cells bearing receptors for IgM
(T_M) and IgG(T_G). J Exp Med 146:184

Owen JJ (1971) The origins and development of lymphocyte populations. Ontogeny of acquired immunity. Excerpta Media, Amsterdam

Sprent J (1977) Recirculating lymphocytes. In: Mar-
chalonis JJ (ed) The Lymphocyte, part I. Dekker,
New York

Walford RL (1974) The immunologic theory of aging:
current status. Fed Proc 33:2020

Chapter 2   Activity of Immune Cells

Ivan Mota

Contents

Lymphocytes

Lymphocytes originate from an undifferentiated cell and, through a series of divisions and differentiations, transform as follows: lymphoblasts → prolymphocytes → large lymphocytes → small lymphocytes. It is estimated that 6–9 mitoses occur during this process. The lymphocyte precursor cells exist in the liver and in the bone marrow in the fetus, but only in the bone marrow in the adult. In the intrauterine state as well as in adults, these cells migrate from the bone marrow to the thymus and other lymphoid organs where they proliferate and produce the lymphoid cell populations of these organs.

Usually, the cells are resting. In vitro, however, they are extremely mobile, with a particular tendency to slide about the surfaces of other cells, including macrophages. The small lymphocytes were for many years defined solely in negative terms, or as cells with little cytoplasm, containing few organelles, and were considered terminal cells. However, even some of the early researchers, such as Maximow, considered the lymphocyte a cell endowed with great capacity for differentiation – a totipotential cell. Since then, numerous experimental data have definitively demonstrated that small lymphocytes are not terminal cells; although they are represented morphologically by a homogeneous population, functionally, they represent an extremely heterogeneous population. Moreover, there are significant variations in size (6–12 μm), in the density of components (separable into at least four fractions of different densities), in longevity (several days to years), and, most importantly, in function. Some lymphocytes are precursors of plasma cells, others of sensitized cells responsible for the rejection of grafts and for delayed hypersensitivity reactions, whereas still others act as memory cells or committed lymphocytes. Furthermore, small lymphocytes of the thymus potentially differ from cells of the same type present in the other organs.

Migration of Lymphocytes. Together, lymphocytes represent nearly 1% of total body weight and are distributed among the so-called lymphoid organs, represented in mammals by the thymus, peripheral lymphoid organs (spleen, lymph nodes, and lymphoid aggregates), and by the pool of circulating lymphocytes. In the lymphoid organs, lymphocytes do not constitute a static population; on the contrary, they recirculate actively, passing through the blood and through the lymph – eventually to return to the lymphoid compartments (Fig. 2.1). The cellular migratory currents thus produced (Fig. 2.2) have been established by experiments involving transfusion of labeled lymphocytes to normal or irradiated recipient animals. It is recognized, moreover, that cells from the bone marrow migrate to the secondary lymphoid organs, with some of these cells passing first through the thymus, where they multiply and differentiate, acquiring special properties.

These migratory currents constitute what Yoffey called the fourth circulation. The lymphocytes present in the blood and lymphatic circulation represent cells in transit among diverse organs. The existence of these migratory patterns of lymphocytes explains why immunologic reactions always acquire a systemic character; in other words,

why contact of the antigen with a restricted part of an organism produces a generalized immunologic response. The migratory patterns of lymphocytes are schematized in Fig. 2.2.

Ecotaxis. If an animal is repopulated with labeled T and B lymphocytes, the T and B cells localize in the regions which gave them their origin, e.g., thymus lymphocytes in thymus-dependent regions, marrow lym-

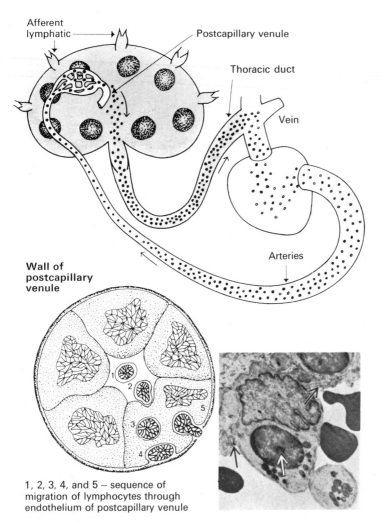

Afferent
lymphatic
Postcapillary venule
Thoracic duct
Vein
Arteries
Wall of postcapillary venule

1, 2, 3, 4, and 5 — sequence of migration of lymphocytes through endothelium of postcapillary venule

Fig. 2.1. Path followed by the lymphocyte in passing from the lymph node to the lymph, thence to the blood, and then returning to the lymph node. The electron photomicrograph *(lower right)* shows a lymphocyte *(white arrow)* passing through the endothelium of the postcapillary vein. At the junction of the two cells, intact endothelia are indicated by the *black arrows*. (Modified from Gowans, 1971)

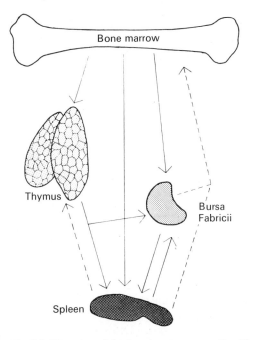

Fig. 2.2. Migration of the lymphocytes among the different lymphoid compartments. The *broken lines* indicate less certain migratory pathways

phocytes in thymus-independent areas, and spleen lymphocytes, which consist of T and B cells, in both areas. This capacity of the lymphocytes to recognize the appropriate original area of the lymphatic organ is called ecotaxis (Gr. *oikos*, house; *taxis*, movement). Ecotaxis is a phenomenon probably related to the presence of specific recognition structures on the membrane of the cell in question.

Long-lived and Short-lived Lymphocytes. Experiments concerning the incorporation and persistence of thymidine labeling have demonstrated the existence of two populations of lymphocytes – one consisting of long-lived cells and one of short-lived cells. The first experiments on this subject were performed by injecting compounds containing radioactive phosphorus into patients, then following over time the radioactivity of the circulating lymphocytes. Using this method, it has been calculated that approximately 80% of lymphocytes have an average life span of 100–200 days. In later experiments, the percentage of labeled lymphocytes after either fleeting or prolonged contact with tritiated thymidine was determined by means of autoradiography. In both humans and various laboratory animals, it was soon verified that the majority of lymphocytes are of the long-lived sort, for only a small number of these became radioactive after short contact with thymidine. In the rat, for example, after continuous injection of thymidine over a 12-h period, only 1% of the small lymphocytes of the thoracic duct exhibited radioactivity. In other experiments in which the organism remained in contact with tritiated thymidine for up to 200 days in order to guarantee that all recently formed cells became radioactive, only 10% of the small lymphocytes of the blood had not been labeled. This means that 10% of the cells had been formed before the thymidine was administered – about 7 months earlier. Autoradiographic studies indicated that the percentage of long-lived lymphocytes in the different lymphoid sectors of the rat varies widely – 90% in the thoracic duct, 66% in the peripheral blood, 75% in the lymph nodes, and 25% in the spleen. In humans, there is evidence that some small lymphocytes survive without division for about 10 years. This finding was possible because of observations on lymphocytes obtained from patients subjected to X-ray therapy approximately 10 years earlier. When mitosis was induced in these lymphocytes by the addition of phytohemagglutinin in vitro, chromosomal alterations incompatible with the survival of postmitotic cells were observed. This finding led to the conclusion that the observed mitoses were the first undergone by these lymphocytes since the moment the patients had last been irradiated – about 10 years earlier. It is now known that both types of lymphocyte populations (T and B) possess long-lived cells.

Immunocompetence of Lymphocytes. The technique of draining lymph from the thoracic duct was used to demonstrate that small lymphocytes function as immunologically competent cells. Animals thus treated were unable to respond to a primary antigenic stimulus with the production of antibodies – even to antigens extremely immunogenic to the control animals. However, the capacity to respond to these stimuli was rapidly restored by inoculation of small lymphocytes obtained from syngeneic animals. Moreover, lymphocytes obtained from an immunized animal and injected into a normal syngeneic recipient transferred to the latter the capacity to mount a secondary response. In other experiments, the specificity of the immunologic response transferred by the lymphocytes was demonstrated by the injection of small lymphocytes taken from animals tolerant to sheep erythrocytes. Under such conditions, the recipient animal demonstrated incapacity to react to the sheep erythrocytes, yet responded normally to other immunogenic stimuli.

The small lymphocytes also include cells responsible for the rejection of grafts and for delayed hypersensitivity reactions, since these also are restored by transfusion of small lymphocytes. In all these experiments, special methods were utilized that made it possible to obtain cellular suspensions extremely rich in small lymphocytes. One particularly recommended technique that permits collection of a practically pure sample of small lymphocytes consists of draining lymph from the thoracic duct and incubating it at 37° C for 24 h with light shaking. This procedure destroys large and medium-sized lymphocytes, leaving just the small lymphocytes. However, the lymph obtained after 4–5 days of continuous drainage of the thoracic duct contains almost exclusively large and medium-sized lymphocytes that, unlike small lymphocytes, are incapable of restoring immunologic capacity to animals deprived of their small lymphocytes.

Memory Cells. The immunologic memory is specific and long-lasting and results from the first contact of immunologically competent cells with the antigen. This contact leads to an increase in such lymphocytes, which carry on their membranes a receptor specific for the antigen. As shown in the experiments reproduced in Fig. 2.3, the small lymphocytes are responsible for immunologic memory. Because both B and T cells have antigen specificity, both types of cells are capable of expressing immunologic memory. The following experiments have proved the existence of T and B memory cells:

1. *The production of antibodies* against a protein–hapten complex depends on the cooperation of carrier-specific T cells with hapten-specific B cells (see below). The first contact with the carrier protein (through which the formation of carrier-specific T cells is induced) enhances the formation of hapten-specific antibodies, when the body is subsequently stimulated with the protein–hapten conjugate. These results are indicative of the presence of T memory cells.

2. *Lymphocytes treated with anti-Thy-1 serum* (Thy-1-antigen, formerly θ antigen, is specific for T cells (p. 39) whereby almost all T cells are destroyed, and lose the capability to transmit a secondary response in vivo as well as in vitro.

3. *Lymphocytes treated with an anti-B-cell serum* lose the capacity to transmit passively a secondary antibody response. The addition of B cells to this cell population restores this capacity.

The induction of memory cells is dose-dependent. T memory cells appear quickly following a small dose of antigen; B cells appear slowly and only after a relatively large dose of antigen. It is thought that B memory cells originate in the germinal center.

Thymus-Dependent and Thymus-Independent Lymphocytes. Extensive data obtained from experiments with laboratory animals, particularly mice, suggest that in mammals, cells obtained from the bone marrow mature into two populations of lymphocytes, the T lymphocytes and B lymphocytes. Both populations circulate, yet they pass through different areas within the lymphoid organs. After leaving the thymus, the T lymphocytes enter the paracortical areas of the lymph nodes and the periarterial sheaths of the lymphoid follicles of the spleen. From these

Experiment I

Rat A receives a primary dose
of antigen X

One year later, his small lymphocytes
are removed by drainage
of the thoracic duct

Rat B, previously
irradiated, is inoculated
with the small lymphocytes

Injection of antigen X
into animal B induces
a secondary response

Experiment II

Small lymphocytes are obtained
from rats that have received
a primary dose of antigen Y

The small lymphocytes are placed
in contact with antigen Y in vitro and later
inoculated into irradiated mice

Three days later, histologic observation
of the spleens of the mice reveals rat plasma
cells producing antibodies against the Y
antigen

Fig. 2.3. Experiment showing the existence of immunologic memory cells among small lymphocytes

organs, the T lymphocytes pass via the blood through the efferent lymphatics and possibly also through the blood vessels of the spleen, thereupon to return again to the lymphoid compartments. One characteristic of the T lymphocyte is the ability, upon contact with antigen, to form a "blast", from which the small, sensitized lymphocytes originate. These lymphocytes are responsible for hypersensitivity reactions and for the rejection of grafts. The T lymphocytes do not produce antibodies in the classic sense – that of molecules of immunoglobulin being secreted in the serum. However, they probably possess antigen-recognizing receptors on their surfaces. The thymus is considered a source of T lymphocytes uncontaminated with B lymphocytes. When T lymphocytes of the thymus are injected into previously irradiated recipient animals, a portion of these cells migrate to the spleen where they acquire new characteristics, the most notable of which is a greater efficiency in collaborating with the B lymphocytes in the immune response.

Adult thymectomized mice, lethally irradiated and then protected through transfusion of bone marrow cells, possess a lymphoid population composed almost exclusively of B lymphocytes. The life cycle of B lymphocytes is not well understood. It is recognized that these cells also originate from cells proceeding from the marrow that may be influenced in some extrathymic lymphoid compartment – perhaps in the germinal centers of the lymph nodes. Actually, the immature cells present in these centers divide frequently and are unaffected by thymectomy. It is possible that they represent those B lymphocytes that, once stimulated by antigen, yield antibody-producing cells. The possible origins and destinies of this type of lymphocyte are schematized in Fig. 2.4.

T Lymphocytes

The importance of lymphocytes derived from the thymus (T lymphocytes) in the genesis of immunologic competence has only been recognized in the last few years because T lymphocytes are involved only indirectly in the formation of antibodies – therefore their activities can be analyzed only by complex methods involving analysis of the function of the cells rather than simple measurement of antibody quantities. Even so, description of the functions of the lymphoid system is impossible without an adequate comprehension of the function of T lymphocytes.

The thymus lymphocytes originate from primordial cells (stem cells) present in the fetal liver and, later on, also in the bone marrow. These cells migrate to the interior of the thymus and, probably under hormonal influences, enter into a process of differentiative proliferation. The thymus is imperme-

Fig. 2.4. Origin and destiny of T and B lymphocytes

able to the majority of the blood cells, and the mechanism by which the stem cells are admitted to the thymus is unknown.

Stem cells initially transform into large pyroninophilic blasts in the cortex of the thymus and undergo a series of divisions during which the size of the cells diminishes and they acquire the morphology of lymphocytes. These are different lymphocytes, called thymocytes, which possess on their cell membrane alloantigens that are not found on stem cells or on B lymphocytes. These alloantigens are termed Thy-1 (formerly theta), Tla, Gv-1, Ly-1, Ly-2, Ly-3, and Ly-5. Moreover, the thymocytes also differ from mature T lymphocytes, which are formed in the medulla of the thymus. For example, when compared with T lymphocytes, the thymocytes bear less histocompatibility antigens on their surface and are more sensitive to destruction by corticosteroids and radiation than T lymphocytes. During maturation the T lymphocytes lose the Tla antigens, lose some Thy-1 antigens, and gain histocompatibility antigens, acquiring the membrane conformation typical of the recirculating T lymphocytes.

There is evidence that the thymic environment is not indispensable for the differentiation of stem cells into thymocytes. Thus, when a suspension of peripheral cells, e.g. spleen cells, from athymic mice (mutant mice congenitally without thymuses) is exposed in vitro to hormonal substances extracted from the thymus (thymopoitin), it is possible to detect the rapid appearance of cells expressing the alloantigens Tla and Thy-1, typically expressed by thymocytes. More significantly, these antigens can be expressed even in the absence of thymopoitin, when the cells are exposed to mitogens such as concanavalin A or even endotoxins. Under normal conditions, obviously, this differentiation occurs in the thymus, but these observations are important in that they indicate that the stem cells can be stimulated to differentiate in the absence of the thymus.

With maturation completed, the T lymphocytes leave the thymus for the circulation where they remain for very long periods, stopping for various intervals in the "thymus-dependent" areas of the spleen, the lymph nodes, and other lymphoid structures. Large concentrations of T lymphocytes are encountered in the lymph of the thoracic duct and in the blood; they are more abundant in the lymph nodes than in the spleen and are relatively rare in the bone marrow.

Upon contact with antigen, the T lymphocytes undergo a second cycle of differentiation and develop to distinct subgroups characterized by functional and phenotypic markers: cells which are able to positively cooperate with B lymphocytes and other subsets of T lymphocytes, T helper cells; cells that are able to cooperate negatively with the former, T suppressor cells; and cells that are able to lyse by direct contact without the help of antibodies other cells, cytotoxic or cytolytic T lymphocytes.

T Helper Cells. One observation that clearly demonstrated the necessity of cellular cooperation for mounting an antibody response to antigens is the carrier specificity phenomenon. Numerous experimental data have shown that the immune response against proteins conjugated with haptens (delayed hypersensitivity, secondary response to haptens) exhibit varying but significant degrees of specificity, linked to the carrier protein. This specificity initially was attributed to partial specificity of the cell receptors for the antigenic determinants of the carrier protein. This interpretation, however, is insufficient to explain several essential characteristics of the humoral response against the hapten: (1) A humoral response against the hapten requires that the carrier protein be immunogenic; nonimmunogenic substances serve poorly or not at all as carrier for haptens. (2) An optimum immunologic response against the hapten requires a "challenge" with the original immunogen. (3) The induction of tolerance to the carrier protein results in a partial or total suppression of the response to a hapten conjugated to the same protein.

Because the specificity of the antibody encountered in the serum reflects the specificity of the immunoglobulin of the cells that are precursors of the antibody-forming cells, these observations suggested the existence of an additional mechanism in the overall mechanism for recognition of the carrier molecule. This interpretation is supported by verification that interaction between lymphoid cells specific for the hapten and lymphoid cells specific for the carrier protein is necessary for the production of an immune response against the hapten. Two models in vivo have been used to demonstrate the necessity for two cell types in the induction of carrier protein specificity: (1) the antihapten adoptive response after transfer of cells that have been in contact with the hapten or with the carrier protein, in irradiated recipients; and (2) preimmunization or supplementary immunization with the unconjugated carrier protein to augment the primary response to the hapten. Even before direct evidence was found for the existence of cellular cooperation in the response to carrier proteins, there were various observations that, seen in retrospect, indicated the existence of this phenomenon. One such indication was the observation of genetic differences in the capacity of certain animals to exhibit an immune response to different antigenic determinants.

The phenomenon of carrier protein specificity was initially observed in two cases of genetic immune response deficiency. In one case, Hartley guinea pigs incapable of responding with production of antibodies or with delayed hypersensitivity to dinitrophenylated (DNP) polylysine were able to produce anti-DNP antibodies when these complexes were combined with a carrier protein such as bovine serum albumin. The other example of genetic immune response deficiency was the response of rabbits to lactate dehydrogenase, which is a tetrameric enzyme composed of two types of subunits, A and B, which can be assembled in all the possible combinations: AAAA, AAAB, AABB, ABBB, and BBBB. In the experiments under discussion, the AAAA,

BBBB, and AABB forms of enzyme composition were used. The principal characteristic of this molecule as antigen is that it permits the arrangement of two antigenic determinants in a single molecule or in different molecules. With these three molecules it was verified that rabbits capable of producing antibodies against only one of two subunits produced antibodies against both subunits when immunized with the hybrid molecules or with molecules composed of two subunits. Thus, a particular animal incapable of producing anti-A when immunized with the AAAA enzyme responded with production of anti-A when immunized with the AABB form of the enzyme and vice versa. In this fashion, one unit served as a type of carrier, permitting an immunologic response to the other. It soon was verified in these experiments that animals tolerant to the carrier unit no longer responded to the hybrid molecules, demonstrating that the recognition of one of the units was indispensable to the immune response.

However, direct evidence of the cooperation of two different cells in the response to the hapten–protein conjugate was not available until the following results were obtained by Mitchison: He took spleen cells from syngeneic mouse donors previously immunized with 4-hydroxy-5-iodo-3-nitrophenylacetyl-ovalbumin (NIP-OVA), injected them into irradiated recipient mice, and obtained a secondary response after a "challenge" with the original immunogen; however with a different protein, 4-hydroxy-5-iodo-3-nitro-phenylacetyl-bovine serum albumin (NIP-BSA), no immune response was obtained.

In other experiments in which recipient mice were injected with spleen cells obtained from donors immunized with NIP-OVA and with spleen cells obtained from animals immunized with BSA, an excellent secondary response was obtained against NIP when the animals were tested with NIP-BSA. This finding demonstrated that the addition of cells specific for carrier protein, in the BSA case, permitted the cells specific for the hapten to exhibit a secondary response against it. This experiment demonstrated further that the humoral response against the hapten requires interaction between carrier-specific and hapten-specific cells in order to stimulate maximally the precursors of those cells that form anti-hapten antibodies. Subsequently, Raff showed that the cells specific for the carrier protein, or "helper" cells, were T cells, whereas the precursors of the antibody-producing cells were B cells. In these experiments, Raff demonstrated that the treatment with anti-Thy-1 serum and complement of spleen cells obtained from donors immunized with BSA, abolished the capacity of such cells to cooperate in the NIP-BSA secondary response with spleen cells obtained from animals immunized with NIP-HGG (NIP-human gamma globulin). However, treatment of the NIP-HGG-sensitized cells with anti-Thy-1 serum plus complement did not affect the capacity of such cells to produce anti-NIP antibodies when the cells were transferred together with cells immunized against BSA and boosted with NIP-BSA.

Raff's experiments were performed using the adoptive transfer technique on spleen cells. With this technique and the related experimental protocols, the following results were obtained:

1. The transfer of spleen cells of animals immunized against BSA permitted a secondary response against NIP when the recipient animals were boosted with NIP-BSA.

2. The transfer of spleen cells primed with NIP-HGG and treated with anti-Thy-1 serum plus complement (C) resulted in the abolition of the secondary response against the hapten when the recipients were boosted with NIP-BSA. This same phenomenon of cooperation can be detected in vivo. For example, guinea pigs immunized with DNP-OVA do not respond to a secondary immunization with a heterologous carrier such as DNP-BGG. However, if the animals immunized with DNP-OVA receive an intermediate injection with BGG, not only do they exhibit a secondary response against DNP but the magnitude of the secondary response can be significantly greater than that produced with a second injection of DNP-OVA immunogen. This phenomenon is not restricted to secondary reactions. When doses of specific size and interval are used, rats, rabbits, and guinea pigs preimmunized with BGG exhibit an enhanced primary response against DNP when tested with DNP-BGG. The mechanism of cellular cooperation is discussed in Chap. 6.

T-Suppressor Cell. Experimental data obtained from diverse sources suggest that T cells have, in addition to a positive regulatory effect (helper cells) upon the activity of B cells (and T effector cells), a negative or suppressor effect upon the latter. For example, in certain situations of T-cell deficiency (thymectomy, injection of antilymphocyte serum), the production of antibodies is enhanced, whereas when an excess of T cells is present, the production of certain antibodies is diminished or halted. The existence of suppressor cells has been elegantly demonstrated by Judith Kapp after it had been postulated by Gershon and his collaborators many years before. There are strains of mice which are phenotypically unable to produce an antibody response to the haptenic terpolymer GAT (glutamine-alanine-tyrosine) coupled to bovine serum albumin (BSA). She immunized one group (1) of mice of this strain with GAT, another group (2) remained untreated. After several days, the spleen cells of mice of these two groups were prepared and half of the cells of each group were mixed and seeded into agar which contained BSA-GAT to induce a response in cells of group 2, and red blood cells coated with GAT as indicator. The remaining half of spleen cells of group 1 mice having received initially GAT was treated with anti-Thy-1 serum to eliminate T cells, and was then mixed with the remaining half of spleen cells of the other group (2) of mice. This mixture was seeded as the first cell mixture in agar containing BSA-GAT and indicator red blood cells. After the secreted antibodies had been allowed to diffuse and to bind to the red blood cell bound GAT, the agar plates were incubated with anti-mouse immunoglobulin antibo-

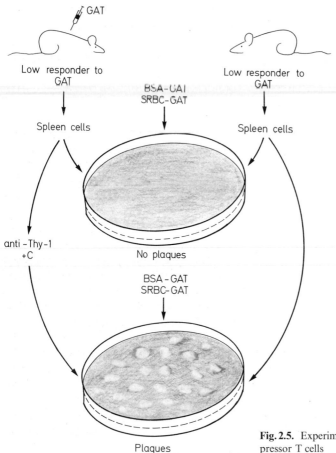

Fig. 2.5. Experiment showing the existence of suppressor T cells

dies and complement. Lysis of red blood cells was observed only in the agar plate of the second, anti-T cell treated mixture, indicating that T cells of GAT primed animals suppressed the normal response (Fig. 2.5).

T suppressor cells probably play an important role in the induction and/or maintenance of tolerance (see Chap. 9 and Chap. 13). The mechanism of the suppressive effect of the T cells is unknown.

Cytotoxic T Lymphocytes. A third subset of T lymphocytes was described at the end of the sixties, capable of specific destruction of allogeneic cells against which the animal had been primed usually by transplanting cells or tissue. They may also be generated in vitro by incubating lymphocytes from a nor-

mal or presensitized individual for a few days with lymphocytes from another individual, differing from the former in its major histocompatibility antigens (see Chap. 6). This type of immunization in vitro by mixed lymphocyte culture (MLC) has made it possible to elucidate the cytolytic T lymphocyte (CTL) system in detail.

In brief, when exposed to foreign antigen on the surface of the stimulator cells, some small lymphocytes of T-lineage will start to differentiate and to proliferate. Initiation of this process may require participation of macrophages and perhaps also some other regulatory T-cells (see below, and Chap. 6). Proliferation leads to the development of highly cytotoxic, medium- to large-sized lymphocytes called early CTL. Upon further maturation, these cells revert to small-sized lymphocytes called memory CTL. When exposed to the same antigen at a later occasion, these memory cells will again transform into larger cytotoxic effector cells now called secondary CTL. These secondary CTL will again proliferate and revert to small memory cells and this cycle may be repeated many times. It is easily seen how these cyclic process will result in an enlargement of the pool of lymphocytes adapted to react with the antigen involved in the initial process of immunization.

The CTL-system has very exquisite specificity requirements. Thus, CTL lyse allogeneic cells carrying H-2 (or HLA, see Chap. 6) antigens different from their own. However, CTL also attack syngeneic cells, i.e., *MHC*-identical cells, but modified in their surface by a virus (see Chap. 6), by tumor transformation, or by introduction of a hapten. CTL recognize target cell antigens by means of specific receptors apparently synthesized by the cells which carry them. Each individual has many different clones of such T cells, each clone with receptors for a given specificity. The CTL-receptors are not conventional antibodies of immunoglobulin-type, and the reaction with the target cells does not require complement but direct contact between the cytolytic T cell and its target. There are some indications that only the contact-reaction is antigen-specific, but the subsequent killing reaction is an independent and nonspecific step. Nothing is known about the mechanism(s) of killing by cytolytic T lymphocytes. These cells possess membrane markers similar to those found on T suppressor cells, Ly-1$^-$, 2$^+$, 3$^+$, but apparently they lack Ly-5 present on the membrane of suppressor cells (see Table 2.1). A more detailed account of the reaction mediated by these cells and their specificity is given in Chaps. 6 and 9.

Killer and Natural Killer Cells. Two additional sets of lymphocytes with the capacity for lytic activity have been described: Killer (K) cells and Natural Killer (NK) cells. The lineage of these cells, whether T or B cells, is not known, and the distinction between these two sets of cells is not sharp.

Killer Cell. The cytotoxic reaction mediated by K-cells is experimentally studied by mixing lymphocytes from normal ("non-immune") donors with target cells in the presence of antibodies against some surface antigens on the latter. This reaction is, therefore, called antibody-dependent cell-mediated cytotoxicity (ADCC) (see Chaps. 6 and 9). The antibody serving as recognition factor for the initiation of cytotoxicity is not made by the K cells themselves. K cells and CTLs are distinct lymphocytes: (1) K cells have receptors for IgG antibodies which mediate the cytotoxic reaction. These Fc-receptors are proteins with low affinity for monomeric IgG, but they have high affinity for aggregated IgG of most subclasses or for IgG which has reacted with antigen, e.g., after having formed immune complexes on the surface of the target cells. (2) K cells are a heterogeneous population in regard to their surface characteristics: about 40% of them possess a T cell specific marker, the receptor for sheep red blood cells in addition to Fc-receptors for IgG; these cells may belong to the subset of peripheral T cells in an immature stage. Another 40% lack this T cell marker as well as surface-bound immunoglobulin M and/or D (S-Ig), a marker of B cells, but they possess receptors for activated complement (C3b, see Chap. 5). The remaining 20% of K cells lacking these markers may include cells of nonlymphocytic lineage.

K cell-mediated target cell lysis is an extremely sensitive reaction; under optimal conditions, a few hundred molecules or less of antibody per target cell are enough to lyse 50% of the target cells in an incubation mixture. The lytic process appears to be identical to that of CTL (see above).

Natural Killer Cell. Natural cell mediated cytotoxicity refers to the lytic activity of lymphocytes from apparently healthy, not deliberately immunized donors against a variety of antigens. Obviously, this definition is ambiguous since it is difficult to know whether or not a "normal" donor has previously in life been immunized, perhaps by exposure to microorganisms carrying antigens which cross-react with antigens on the target cell surface. In most instances these natural cytotoxic reactions are selective, i.e., some target cells are susceptible to the action of lymphocytes from a given donor while others are not. This pattern will often be different when the cytotoxicity of the lymphocytes from different individuals is compared. In other words, the reactions are "specific". However, since we usually do not know the antigens which are involved and since we even do not know whether or not this phenomenon has an immunological basis in a strict sense, the term selective rather than specific is commonly applied in this context. Natural killer cells are the least well defined population of cytotoxic cells, and may resemble in part K cells. The effector cells are lymphocytes of unknown lineage, but believed to be (at least in their majority) pre-T cells originating from preprogrammed precursor cells in the bone marrow; they are found in the blood and the spleen. The generation and activity is thymus-independent, and they are found in high numbers in young individuals. Part of their activity can be inhibited by purified Fab-fragments of rabbit antibodies to immunoglobulin, suggesting that NK cell-mediated cytotoxicity is in part identical to that mediated by K cells. However, the origin of the immunoglobulin involved in the NK-cytotoxicity is not known; it might be produced by contaminating B cells and taken up by the NK cells, or NK cells may have them adsorbed to their surface when removed from the donor. On the other hand, when lymphocytes from healthy donors are added to target cells the surface of which has been modified by an acute or persistent virus infection, natural cytotoxicity is strongly enhanced. This enhancement is a common phenomenon which is obtained with lymphocytes from practically every healthy donor. The phenomenon is distinct from CTL mediated cytotoxicity. It seems to be non-specific and to be unre-

lated to the possible presence of anti-viral antibodies in the lymphocyte donor's serum. It is obtained with a great variety of viruses. The effector cells in this virus dependent "natural" cytotoxicity have Fc-receptors for IgG but no surface-bound immunoglobulin. On the basis of surface marker analysis, 30%–40% may be T cells, distinct from the majority of the human blood T cells. However, this enhanced natural cytotoxicity is not an antibody-dependent reaction since it is not inhibited by anti-immunoglobulin. There is evidence that factors such as interferon (see Chap. 11) or similar substances are involved in the cytotoxic reaction in an unspecific manner.

The NK-system is believed to protect the organism against growth of certain tumors, particularly those of the lymphatic system itself. It may also have a general regulatory role on the normal function of the entire hemopoietic system. Hence, the role of this NK-system would be similar to that of the CTL system. However, while the CTL system requires the presence of a functioning thymus, the NK system does not. Therefore, the two systems seem to complement each other in their biological function.

B Lymphocytes

B lymphocytes are cells that migrate to thymus-independent areas (areas not affected by thymectomy, see Chap. 1) of the secondary lymphoid organs: the follicles and medullae of the lymph nodes, the peripheral regions of the white pulp of the spleen, and follicles of the lymphoid tissue associated with the intestine. The majority of these cells are sedentary: Once they have reached the secondary lymphoid organs, they survive there for about 10 days, not having been stimulated by antigen.

Each of the B lymphocytes expresses on its membrane about one hundred thousand antibody molecules with the same specificity. Two types of antibodies apparently can be concomitantly expressed on the membrane: IgD molecules and monomeric IgM, different from the pentameric form normally encountered in the circulatory system (see Fig. 1.6). These two types of membrane antibodies can execute different functions when they come in contact with the specific antigen. It has been calculated that each organism possesses between 10^6 and 10^7 different types of B lymphocytes in its lymphoid tissue and that any particular antigen is able to bind to 10 million B lymphocytes when injected into the organism. This cell population, which binds antigen, includes cells of many different clones of B lymphocytes, expressing antibodies of different specificities. In some cases, the antibodies bind the antigen with great affinity; in other cases, the linkage may be loose and insufficient to activate the cell. Depending upon the antigen dose, the activated population is either comprised exclusively of more avid cells (low antigen dose) or contains both highly avid and weakly avid cells (high antigen dose).

The activation of the B lymphocytes induces the cell to enlarge and to divide. The transformation (blast transformation) can be measured biochemically by incorporation of DNA precursors such as thymidine, or morphologically. The blasts are large (15–20 µm) cells with abundant basophilic (pyroninophilic) cytoplasm, large nuclei with prominent nucleoli – quite different from lymphocytes in the resting phase. The blasts divide repeatedly and differentiate during each division, each time generating a greater number of small cells more adapted to the synthesis of antibodies. The final cell, known as plasma cell, does not resemble either a blast or a lymphocyte. Plasma cells are small, and have eccentric nuclei, with the chromatin arranged as in a cartwheel and with endoplasmatic reticulum and well-developed Golgi apparatus in the cytoplasm (see p. 11, and Fig. 1.5 D).

The specific B-cell activation requires at least two signals; the binding of the antigenic determinant to the membrane-bound immunoglobulin receptors and another, as yet undefined, signal from T helper cells. Some types of antigens are called thymus-independent because they are capable of stimulating directly the B lymphocyte to differentiate in-

to plasma cells without the interaction of T lymphocytes. This stimulation leads to the differentiation of IgM-synthesizing plasma cells but does not extend to the synthesis of IgG – nor to the formation of memory cells. Thus, there is no secondary response; repeated contact with the antigen, induces a repeated transitory synthesis of IgM antibodies. The thymus-independent antigens are polymeric substances containing large numbers of the same antigenic determinants on the molecule. This characteristic facilitates enormously the linkage of these substances to the antibodies on the B lymphocyte membranes: a strong global interaction results from the simultaneously occurring individual weak interactions. In addition, these substances function as polyclonal mitogens for B lymphocytes; that is, they are capable of inducing the activation of all B and not merely the specific B lymphocytes that possess antibodies capable of combining with the antigenic determinants present on the antigen. Nevertheless, the specific B lymphocytes are much more sensitive to every thymus-independent (T-independent) antigen than to nonspecific antigens, for they concentrate the antigen much more easily through their antibodies. The concentrations of T-independent antigen necessary for polyclonal activation of B lymphocytes are much higher than those necessary for the activation of these cells by the antigen. The T-dependent antigens are neither nonspecific (polyclonal) mitogens for B lymphocytes nor are they necessarily polymeric. It has not been determined whether the simple linking of T-dependent antigens is merely inefficient for activating B lymphocytes or whether there is incomplete activation, which leads only to division and differentiation to IgM-synthesizing cells. Regardless of their form, when B lymphocytes that bind T-dependent antigens are exposed to T lymphocytes also capable of recognizing the antigen, the proliferation of B lymphocytes is greatly amplified, IgM antibodies are formed in greater quantities, and, more characteristically, they differentiate into plasma cells that synthesize IgG, IgA, and

IgE. Furthermore, the level of reactivity to the antigen is augmented, and memory cells appear that permit secondary responses to greatly reduced doses of antigen.

The differentiation signal given by T lymphocytes to B lymphocytes drastically modifies the activation sequence of these cells. During clonal expansion, a portion of the activated cells revert to a B lymphocyte morphology instead of differentiating progressively into plasma cells. However, these are different B lymphocytes. They survive for months and not merely a few days. They are recirculating rather than sedentary cells. In the event of new contacts with the antigen, they are capable of differentiating rapidly for the synthesis of IgG, IgA, and IgE – not being limited to IgM synthesis. It has been suggested that the antibodies expressed on the membranes of these "memory" B cells are different from those expressed by the original B cells. The original B cells express only monomeric IgM on their membranes; the memory B cells have a mixture of monomeric IgM and IgD on their membranes or even have IgG, IgA, or IgE.

Localization of the Immunoglobulin on the B Lymphocyte Membrane. It is calculated that the number of immunoglobulin molecules on the B lymphocyte surface varies from 50,000 to 150,000 and averages 100,000. The immunoglobulin molecules are apparently distributed randomly over the surfaces of the B lymphocytes. Exactly how they are bound to the membrane is not known; presumably, however, the Fab fragments of the molecule are exposed, since the immunoglobulin on the lymphocyte surface can combine with the antigen. Some of the Fc fragments also must be exposed to explain the fact that the antibodies specific for the heavy chains react with the immunoglobulins on the cell surface. The localization of the immunoglobulin molecules on the lymphocyte surfaces has been studied principally with the use of fluorescein or ferritin-conjugated anti-immunoglobulin antibodies.

The first observations with this technique revealed two types of labeling: (1) diffuse distribution of immunoglobulin over the cell surface, which microscopically resembled a ring-like pattern, or (2) a polar position giving the appearance of polar "caps" (see Chap. 6). It was soon verified that this difference in localization was due to a redistribution of the immunoglobulin molecules induced by their interaction with the anti-immunoglobulin. Electron-microscopic observation of the lymphocytes incubated with anti-immunoglobulin conjugated with ferritin showed that lymphocytes treated at 4 °C exhibited diffuse distribution of immunoglobulins, whereas those treated at 20 °C exhibited polar-capping distribution. Under the light microscope, the direct redistribution of the immunoglobulin molecules was observed by permitting the lymphocytes to react with the fluorescent anti-immunoglobulin at 4 °C and then observing the behavior of the cells as the temperature was increased to 37 °C. Within about 2 min after the temperature reached 37 °C, the immunoglobulin molecules assumed a polar distribution. After 5 min at 37 °C, the fluorescent material was localized within the lymphocytes. These lymphocytes no longer reacted with the anti-immunoglobulin, showing that the redistribution of the surface immunoglobulin is followed by pinocytosis and disappearance of the majority of the membrane immunoglobulin molecules. These observations suggest that the redistribution of the molecules of the receptor immunoglobulins may be an important phenomenon in the activation of lymphocytes by the antigen.

When the lymphocytes that had lost their surface immunoglobulin were maintained in culture, there was a gradual reappearance of the surface immunoglobulins, which showed up initially at one pole of the cells and then later diffused over the entire surface. The kinetics of the appearance and disappearance of the lymphocyte surface immunoglobulin molecules is roughly similar to that of the change of immunoglobulin in untreated lymphocytes and to the turnover of cell membrane components in general, suggesting that this phenomenon constitutes a general cellular phenomenon.

Plasma Cells. The plasma cell is the cell responsible for the production of the immunoglobulins. The search for the location of antibody production in the organism led, at an early date, to the lymphoid organs as the structures responsible for the synthesis of these proteins. Pfeiffer and Marx (1898) appear to have been the first to perform the experiments demonstrating that the spleen, the lymph nodes, to a lesser degree the bone marrow, and possibly the lungs were the organs responsible for the production of the major portion of the antibodies. Some years later, McMaster and Hudack (1935) showed that injections of antigen into the footpads of rabbits gave rise to the production of antibodies, first in the peripheral lymph nodes and then in the other lymphoid organs. Furthermore, they showed that if different antigens were injected into each one of the paws, the antibody concentration in the lymph node was much greater for the antigen injected into the region directly drained by that lymph node than in the central lateral nodes. Since a major percentage of the antigens frequently had been found in the macrophages, it was natural at first to suppose that these cells were those responsible for the antibodies produced by these organs. Later, the observation of a considerable increase in the lymphocyte population of the lymph nodes and of the spleen after antigenic stimulus led to affirmation of the fact that the lymphocytes and not the macrophages were the cells directly responsible for the production of antibodies.

Although some turn-of-the-century histologists had implicated a basophilic cell with an eccentric nucleus in the production of antibodies, only much later did convincing data begin to appear pointing to plasma cells as producers of antibodies. One of the first favorable indications in this regard was the observation that patients with hyperglobulinemia possessed an increased concentration of plasma cells in their tissues. Almost simultaneously, Bjorneboe and colleagues in Scandinavia, showed that hyperimmunization of rabbits caused a considerable increase of immunoglobulins in the serum accompanied by an increase in the number of plasma cells in the tissues. In the meantime, Fagraeus studied the correlation between the histologic alterations of the spleen and the production of antibodies and definitely showed the relationship between plasma cells and antibodies. Fagraeus studied the cell types that appeared in the red pulp of the spleen in response to an antigenic stimulus. The first cells to increase in number were large immature cells indistinguishable from similar cells normally existing in this organ. Subsequently, the relative ribonucleic acid (RNA) content of the cytoplasm of these cells increased, as indicated by the increased pyroninophilia, whereas the nucleus simultaneously diminished in size, condensed its chromatin, and became eccentric, thus acquiring the characteristics of the plasmatic series. Furthermore, simultaneous determination of the level of antibodies in the blood showed a clear correlation between antibody levels and the quantity of plasma cells in the spleen.

After the studies of Fagraeus, numerous other techniques were used to study this problem, giving rise to a more direct demonstration of the production of antibodies by plasma cells. One of the first such demonstrations utilized the phenomenon of bacterial adherence: Bacteria incubated with cells obtained from the lymph nodes of animals previously immunized with the same bacteria adhered specifically and exclusively to the plasma cells. Subsequently, Coons, employing the immunofluorescence technique, arrived at the same conclusion. The most commonly used method is the so-called sandwich technique: Histologic cuttings or cell smears obtained from lymphoid organs of an immunized animal are immersed in an antigen solution that combines with the antibody present in the cells. The preparation is then carefully washed to remove all of the uncombined antigen and only then immersed in a fluorescent antibody solution that combines with the antigen fixed by cells that contain antibodies. Under such conditions, practically all the cells that turn fluorescent are plasma cells; a few weakly fluorescent cells are lymphocytes. The same result is obtained when radioactive antigen and autoradiography are employed.

The intense production and secretion of immunoglobulins by plasma cells is in accord with the ultrastructure of these cells, which possess in their cytoplasm the organelles necessary for the synthesis and secretion of proteins, such as endoplasmatic reticulum, ribosomes, and well-developed Golgi complexes (Fig. 2.6). Notably, these same structures are present in other protein-producing cells such as acinar cells of the pancreas. However, the exact mechanism by which the secretion of immunoglobulins proceeds in plasma cells is not known. It may occur by clasmatosis, i.e., the loss of small portions of cytoplasm. Experimental data from different laboratories using different techniques indicate that each plasma cell synthesizes immunoglobulins of a unique class and subclass, as well as a unique type of heavy (H) and light (L) chain. For example, in individuals heterozygous for a specific allotype of immunoglobulin, even though both the allotypes coexist in the serum, the plasma cells show allelic exclusion; that is, each cell produces only one allotype and not both. This finding suggests that during the differentiation of immunocompetent cells a somatic

Fig. 2.6. Monkey *(Callithrix)* plasma cell. Note the abundant granular endoplasmic reticulum. A Golgi zone is seen at the *right* of the nucleus. Courtesy of LC Junqueira, Instituto de Ciências Biomédicas, Universidade de Sao Paulo (× 21,000)

mechanism enters into action in such a way that one of the allotypic genes is suppressed. In short, each plasma cell produces only immunoglobulins of the same class, type, and allotype. In the same manner, numerous experiments show that the plasma cells synthesize antibodies of a single specificity. Thus, in animals immunized simultaneously with various antigens, or as usually happens, with an antigen containing diverse antigenic determinants in the same molecule, each plasma cell forms antibodies specific for just one of these determinants.

A possible exception to the rule that each plasma cell forms immunoglobulins of a unique class comes from the observation that frequently in a primary response, the synthesis of one immunoglobulin class (IgM) is followed shortly by the synthesis of another (IgG). Examination of plasma cells at the point in time where synthesis of IgM is being followed by synthesis of IgG reveals that a significant minority of plasma cells produces both classes of immunoglobulins simultaneously. This elicited the hypothesis that some cells synthesize IgM first and then go on to synthesize IgG. As we shall see later, this "switch" from IgM to IgG is related to the "maturing of the immune response" through the reciprocal action of T-helper cells under whose influence antigen-stimulated B cells differentiate into antibody-secreting plasma cells and memory cells (see Chap. 6).

While the lymph nodes are in a resting state, only a small number of plasmocytic cells are present (about 1%–3%); after an antigenic stimulus, their number increases significantly. The origin of these cells has been studied in two ways. According to one method, tritiated thymidine is given to an unimmunized animal for a short time followed by an antigenic stimulus. After 3–4 days, labeled plasma cells appear. Such results suggest that the plasma cells originate from immature lymphoid cells ready to divide – lymphoblasts – that exist in lymphoid organs and that differentiate into plasma cells when stimulated by the antigen. With the other methods populations of small lymphocytes, obtained by

cannulation of the thoracic duct, exhibited the capability to restore the capacity for production of antibodies in irradiated animals. These results suggest that the small lymphocyte might be able to differentiate into plasma cells after antigenic stimulation.

Other experimental results support the first alternative. For example, the transformation of lymphocytes into large pyroninophilic cells has been observed in cultures. In addition, it has been verified that lymph node specimens obtained from animals previously immunized with antigens A and B lose the capacity to form antibodies in vitro against antigen A when subjected simultaneously to the presence of this antigen and to 5-bromodeoxyuridine (a substance that blocks cellular division if incorporated in sufficient quantity into the DNA); yet the capacity to form anti-B antibodies is retained. Taken together, these observations suggest that the plasma cells may originate from the small lymphocytes that, under antigenic stimulus, revert to the condition of an immature cell, synthesize DNA, enter rapidly into division, and differentiate into plasma cells. In addition, some small lymphocytes do transform into memory cells.

Differences Between B and T Lymphocytes

The scanning electron microscope was used to detect morphologic differences between B and T lymphocytes. B cells are rich in microvilli whereas T cells tend to be smoother, having fewer and shorter villi. However, such differences are relative: Some cells cannot be classified by these criteria. The B lymphocytes can be differentiated from T lymphocytes by a series of membrane markers:

1. The *B lymphocytes* possess a high concentration of *membrane immunoglobulin;* these immunoglobulins are homogeneous in each B cell in terms of their immunologic specificity. The classes expressed are IgM (monomeric), IgD, or both.

Table 2.1. Differential membrane markers of T and B lymphocytes, and macrophages

Marker	T lymphocytes			B lymphocytes	Macrophages
	Helper cells	Suppressor cells	Cytotoxic cells		
Surface Ig[a,b]	−		−	+	−
Receptor for IgG-Fc[a]	−	+(Tγ)	·	+	+
Receptor for monomeric IgM[a]	+(Tμ)	−	·	·	·
C3b-receptor[a,b]	−	−	−	+	+
Ia/DR antigen[a,b]	−	+[b]	−	+	+
Thy-1[b]	+	+	+	−	−
Ly-1[b,c]	+	−	−	−	−
Ly-2, 3[b,c]	−	+	+	−	−
Ly-4[b]	−	−	−	+	−
Ly-5[b]	−	+	−	−	−
Receptor for SRBC[a,d]	+ (spans Helper/Suppressor/Cytotoxic)			−	−
Histocompatibility antigens[a,b]	+	+	+	+	+

− Absent; + present; · not known

[a] In human

[b] In mice

[c] Recently, Nagy and colleagues have provided some indications that the Ly-phenotype may not correlate to the differentiated *function* of lymphocytes (helper, suppressor, cytotoxic cell) but rather to the *restricting structures* (see Chap. 6), i.e., T cells recognizing antigens in association with K molecules assume the Ly-1^{-2+}, those recognizing antigens in association with A molecules are Ly-1^{+}2^{-}, and those recognizing antigens in association with E molecules are Ly–1^{+}2^{+}

[d] Sheep red blood cells; it is not known which subsets of T cells are involved in the rosette formation with sheep red blood cells

2. In addition to expressing on its membrane self-synthesized immunoglobulins, the B lymphocyte also possesses *receptors for the Fc* parts of other immunoglobulins and is capable of fixing those molecules to its membrane. The immunoglobulins bound in this way belong to a specific IgG subclass (in mice, IgG_1) and are not restricted in specificity. The physiologic function of these receptors is not known, but they can function as an accessory process in the concentration of antigens on the B lymphocyte membrane.

3. In addition to immunoglobulin receptors, B lymphocytes express on their membranes *receptors for C3b*, which is the active form of the third component of the complement system. These receptors make possible the concentration on the B lymphocyte membrane of soluble antigen–antibody complexes that have fixed complement.

4. B lymphocytes express on their membranes *alloantigens* not represented in T lymphocytes. Some of these antigens are also expressed on other cell types such as plasma cells and stem cells. They include antigens defined by heterologous antisera (e.g., rabbit antimouse) such as mouse-specific B-lymphocyte antigen (MBLA), as well as others which can be detected by alloantisera (e.g., mouse antimouse) such as Ly-4 and the Ia antigens (cf. Chap. 6).

B and T cells also differ in characteristics that depend upon the structure of the cell membrane.

5. They differ in their *response to lectins*. Lectins are products of plant or bacterial origin that, for unknown reasons, are capable of inducing activation in lymphocytes when exposed to the latter in vitro. B lymphocytes are relatively insensitive to the action of cer-

tain lectins (phytohemagglutinin, concana-valin A) which are highly effective in the activation of T lymphocytes. On the other hand, B lymphocytes can be strongly activated by mitogens such as lipopolysaccharides (endotoxin) of *Escherichia coli* (T-independent antigen) that do not act upon T lymphocytes. Furthermore, B lymphocytes can be activated by anti-immunoglobulin antibodies that link to their membrane immunoglobulins; this does not occur with T lymphocytes.

6. The fractionation of cell suspensions of lymphocytes indicated that B lymphocytes are slightly smaller and less dense than T lymphocytes. Thus, these cells can be separated, according to their sedimentation rate, in gravitational or centrifugal fields. Furthermore, B lymphocytes adhere more strongly to surfaces such as glass or nylon than do T lymphocytes; thus, when lymphoid cell suspensions are passed through columns containing nylon fibers, the population that passes through the column is enriched in T lymphocytes.

The *T lymphocytes* of certain species are capable of fixing heterologous erythrocytes on their surfaces, forming rosettes. Although the mechanism of the phenomenon is unknown, the formation of rosettes with sheep erythrocytes by human T lymphocytes is a routine test for identification of these cells in humans. The differences between T and B lymphocytes are summarized in Table 2.1.

Cooperation Between B and T Lymphocytes

B and T lymphocytes exhibit a collaborative effect in their immune response against T-cell-dependent antigen. For example, the capacity of mice to respond with the production of antibodies to the presence of sheep erythrocytes is not reestablished by the transfer of thymic cells alone or by that of bone marrow cells alone, yet it is easily restored by the transfer of both cell types. In the immunologic response to hapten-carrier antigen (hapten–protein conjugate), it has

been verified that the T lymphocytes respond specifically to the carrier protein, whereas the B lymphocytes react specifically to the hapten. The immune response to almost all antigens requires the cooperation of the two types of lymphocytes. This can be clearly shown in an experiment using bovine serum albumin as antigen. In this experiment, lethally irradiated mice were inoculated with thymus and bone marrow cell mixtures in varying proportions and were inoculated quickly thereafter with the antigen. About 1 month later, the level of antibodies present in the serum was determined, permitting verification that for a constant dose of thymus cells, the antibody level diminished with decreasing doses of marrow cells; for a constant dose of marrow cells, the antibody level diminished with decreasing doses of thymus cells. These results clearly indicate cooperation between the two types of lymphocytes in the immune response. The phenomenon also has been observed in cell culture, where a primary response to erythrocytes only occurs when both types of lymphocytes are present. Thus, although spleen-cell cultures obtained from mice thymectomized shortly after birth (containing only B lymphocytes) or thymus-cell cultures (containing only T lymphocytes) do not produce antibodies against sheep erythrocytes, a culture containing both types of cells produces hemolytic antibodies. It appears that T lymphocytes assume a helper function in the immune responses of the B lymphocytes. In the experiments, shown in Fig. 2.7, irradiated mice were divided into three groups – A, B, and C. In group A, the animals were inoculated with thymus cells; in group B, with thymus cells plus antigen; and in group C, only with the antigen. Six days later, the animals of the three groups were killed and, from each group, suspensions of spleen cells were prepared. Irradiated mice were then inoculated with each of these suspensions added to bone marrow cells and the antigen under study. The immune responses of these animals were then compared. The experiment demonstrated considerable augmentation of the immune

Fig. 2.7. Protocol of experiments showing the conditioning of T lymphocytes by antigen

response in the animals of group E, which had received spleen cells of the mice from group B, which in turn initially had been injected with thymus cells plus the specific antigen. These results show that the T lymphocytes of the group B animals were conditioned by prior contact with the antigen. Because cooperation between these two types of cells is not necessary for all antigens, one differentiates between thymus-dependent antigens and thymus-independent antigens. In certain cases, depending on the dose used, certain antigens may or may not be thymus-dependent. With high antigen doses, the B lymphocytes are directly stimulated to produce antibodies.

Macrophages

The term macrophage is generally applied to phagocytic cells encountered in the connective tissue that are capable of ingesting bacteria, cellular remains, and foreign substances generally present in the tissues. The prefix "macro-"distinguishes these cells from other smaller phagocytic cells existing in the blood and tissues, the polymorphonuclear neutrophils.

In lymphoid tissue, the macrophages may be of the fixed variety, reticuloendothelial cells that border the lymphatic sinuses and sinusoids; or they may be mobile, like the free phagocytes that move actively in the tissues. The form of the macrophage depends upon its functional status and localization. Fixed macrophages are star-shaped or spindle-shaped, possessing nuclei of delicate chromatin with one or two nucleoli and slightly basophilic cytoplasm. The mobile macrophage is usually round or oval, with a kidney-shaped nucleus. Both types of macrophages possess irregular cytoplasmic membranes with numerous prolongations and entry points that are related to the mechanism of phagocytosis.

Macrophages originate from precursor cells in the bone marrow and pass into the blood as monocytes. They remain in the circulation for some hours (6–12 h in the mouse)

after which they migrate into the tissues, and transform to macrophages. They acquire greater phagocytic activity, more cytoplasm and more cytoplasmic organelles such as lysosomes, microtubules, microfilaments, and Golgi membranes. In addition, the nucleus becomes more irregular and acquires one or two nucleoli. Functionally, the monocytes and macrophages make up part of a system of highly phagocytic mononuclear cells, the mononuclear phagocyte system. The dendritic cells of the follicles of the spleen and lymph nodes, although capable of retaining antigens on their surfaces, are not considered as belonging to this system. The macrophages customarily migrate to the peritoneal cavity and to other serous cavities, the red pulp of the spleen and the lymph node medullae. Fixed macrophages such as the Küpffer cells of the liver probably also originate from monocytes. Epithelioid cells and giant multinucleated cells result from the fusion and transformation of the macrophages.

Monocytes and macrophages are characterized by intense phagocytic activity and by the capacity of adherence to certain materials such as glass. Many techniques for isolating these cells take advantage of these properties.

The process of phagocytosis can be divided into two phases: the adherence of the particle to the surface of the cell and the ingestion of the particle.

Monocytes as well as macrophages possess receptors for the Fc pieces of the immunoglobulins and for the complement system (C 3 b). The adherence phase of the particles is mediated by antibodies or by antibodies plus complement. The time during which the particle is coated with IgM plus C 3 corresponds to the first phase, the adherence phase; if IgG is bound to the particle, ingestion of the particle occurs even in the absence of C 3. Adherence also can be facilitated by other serum factors that in some cases have been identified as immunoglobulins. Apparently, some types of particles can adhere to the macrophages without the intervention of the serum factors.

Phagocytosis mediated by immunoglobulin with or without complement is called immune phagocytosis. The monocytes and macrophages that possess receptors for immunoglobulin and for complement on their cell membranes can be considered "professional" phagocytes to distinguish them from "amateur" phagocytes such as fibroblasts, reticular cells, and endothelial cells, which probably do not possess such receptors but rather ingest the particles independently of the antibodies and complement.

Role of Macrophages in Cellular Immunity. Macrophages play an important role in resistance to many infections by intracellular organisms. Antigens coming into contact with macrophages are either phagocytosed or become trapped in the cytoplasmic membranes of these cells. The immunogenicity of soluble antigens appears to be due particularly to molecules of these antigens that, upon contact, are retained by the membrane of the macrophage. After phagocytosis, the destiny of the antigen depends upon its physicochemical properties. Some antigens such as synthetic polypeptides, composed of D-amino acids, and pneumococcal polysaccharides are degraded slowly, whereas others such as human serum albumin and hematocyanins are degraded rapidly to amino acids by proteolytic enzymes. Still others such as red cells are phagocytosed, partially digested, and then the products of their digestion are released into the medium and are to some extent bound to the outer membrane, where they exercise their antigenicity.

It is important to remember that the antigens phagocytosed by the polymorphonuclear neutrophils are totally digested, losing their antigenic capacity (see below). Usually, the particle to be phagocytosed becomes situated between two pseudopodia; through the fusion of the two pseudopodia, the antigen is enveloped, separated from its surroundings, and ingested. The phagocytosed particle is termed the phagosome. All the antigens inoculated into the organism are phagocytosed in varying degrees by the macrophages. Phagocytosis of the soluble antigens, which proceeds by pinocytosis, is in general inferior to that of the particulate antigens, which not only are phagocytosed more efficiently, but also – perhaps for this very reason – are more immunogenic.

Macrophages obtained from recently infected animals phagocytose and destroy the infecting organism much more rapidly and efficiently than do macrophages obtained from uninfected animals. In this case, it is said that the macrophages are activated. Activated macrophages adhere more strongly to glass or plastic surfaces; they exhibit more intense undulatory movements of the cell membrane; there is an increase in the number of cytoplasmic granules with a consequent increase of hydrolytic enzymes; and there are increased amounts of metabolic enzymes and of adenyl cyclase. The bactericidal activity of the activated macrophages is also considerably enhanced. Activation of the macrophage by lymphocytes depends upon the presentation by macrophages of the specific antigen to lymphocytes that leads to the liberation by the lymphocyte of substances that activate the macrophage. Notably, however, once activated, the macrophages act more efficiently not only against the antigen that specifically stimulated the lymphocytes, but also against any other antigen present. For example, immune spleen cells obtained from tuberculous mice, when transferred to normal animals, are capable of defending the latter efficiently against an infection with *Listeria monocytogenes*, provided that simultaneously with the injection of these bacteria, the animals are injected with a small dose of bacille Calmette Guérin (BCG).

This signifies that there is a specific immunologic mechanism for activation of the T cells that results in the creation of a population of activated macrophages that act nonspecifically against any infectious agent, be it a tumor cell, or a cell that is normal but foreign to the organism. This mechanism is important in the phenomenon of cellular hypersensitivity (see Chap. 10). The activation of macrophages is therefore a cellular hypersensitivity phenomenon (see Chap. 10) and results from the interaction of the sensitized lymphocytes with the antigen. The macrophage can be activated in vitro using the macrophage activation factor (see lymphokines, Chap. 6 and 11). Macrophage activation is associated in vivo with a rapid concentration of these cells in the infection focus, affording the infected animal a defense mechanism against infectious agents that are not easily destroyed. In some cases, however, even the activated macrophages are not capable of destroying the invasive elements, even though the migration of the macrophages to the site of infection continues, resulting in the formation of granulomas. For example, the immunologic mechanism gives rise to the formation of granulomas in certain chronic infectious diseases such as leprosy and tuberculosis, whose pathogenic agents can not easily be eliminated. It should be noted that the macrophages also possess nonimmunogenic and nonspecific bactericidal activity.

Role of Macrophages in the Humoral Response. The initial observation that the antigen or part of it was always encountered within the macrophages gave rise to the belief that these cells produced the antibodies. Later, a wealth of evidence indicated that these cells do not produce antibodies. The demonstration that the macrophages definitely do not produce antibodies raised the question of whether phagocytosis of the antigen by these cells does not in some way modify the immune response to it. The immunogenicity of the antigens after their capture by the macrophages has been studied principally by three methods: (a) Macrophages are incubated with the antigen to permit phagocytosis and afterward are subjected to a cellular fractionation or chemical extraction process. These extracts or subcellular fractions are then injected into another animal to evaluate their immunogenicity in comparison to that of the unphagocytosed antigen. (b) Macrophages are placed in the presence of an antigen and, after phagocytosis, inoculated into another animal of the

same strain. A comparison is then made between the immune response of this animal and that of the other animal that received the same free antigen. (c) The antigen is added to a culture of lymphocytes or to a culture of lymphocytes containing macrophages, and the production of antibodies by the two types of cultures is compared. Experiments such as these have led to the conclusion that the antigens that are poorly phagocytosed when injected in a free state become more immunogenic if they are injected after phagocytosis by macrophages.

The phenomenon is much less evident when one uses antigens that are easily phagocytosed. The immunogenic material in the macrophages has been encountered in the lysosomes, in the cell membrane, and in extracts rich in ribonucleic acid. The antigen present in the live macrophages is more immunogenic than the antigen isolated with the subcellular fractions. Certain antigens encountered on the membranes of the macrophages appear important in the immunogenicity of macrophage transfer systems and in lymphocyte cultures. It should be noted that, for the immune response, it is necessary that the animal inoculated with the macrophages containing antigen be immunocompetent. Recipient animals previously irradiated with X-rays or turned tolerant do not respond to the macrophage–antigen association.

These findings once again demonstrate that the macrophages are not capable of producing antibodies and that phagocytosis of the antigen by the macrophage is not sufficient to produce an immune response, but that beyond this it is necessary that the immunologically competent cells be able to recognize the antigen or antigenic particle presented by the macrophage. It is interesting to observe that antigens contained in macrophages obtained from tolerant donors are just as immunogenic as those obtained from normal animals, which indicates that tolerance does not depend upon a functional modification of the macrophage. The most important evidence of the participation of the macrophages in the immune response

56   Ivan Mota

was obtained in experiments with the production of antibodies in vitro. It was verified
that the addition of antigen to a culture of
lymphoid cells obtained from lymph nodes
or to a culture of macrophages did not result
in the production of antibodies. However,
when the two types of cells were allowed to
coexist in the same culture, antibodies were
produced.

Extracts obtained from macrophages previously incubated with the antigen for about

30 min induced the production of antibodies
when added to a culture of lymphocytes.
The nature of the immunogenic material
contained in these extracts is not known.
Their activity possibly depends upon the existence of a complex comprised of an antigen
fragment and RNA, constituting a species of
"superantigen". Actually, the immunogenicity of the material disappears after
treatment with ribonuclease; whether these
complexes have real significance or merely

```
────────────▶   Development, differentiation to
─ ─ ─ ─ ─▶   Stimulation or suppression
─<,▲,△        Antibody, native and processed antigen
                Phagolysosomal content
```

Fig. 2.8. Interaction of mononuclear cells in the response to antigen (▲ △). The antigen is phagocytized and processed by macrophages (mph), and released together with monokines (see p. 307). Passing T lymphocytes (Tprec)
with receptors for the antigen are activated and differentiate to helper T cells (HTC), suppressor T cells (STC) or
cytotoxic T lymphocytes (CTL); the latter react specifically and antibody-independently with antigens on the surface of target cells (TC), causing target cell lysis (⋯▸). B lymphocytes (BC) are stimulated to mature to plasma cells
(PC) secreting antibodies with specificity for the antigen (─<). Antibodies bind the antigen forming Ab-Ag complexes, or antibody-coated target cells (TC), which are lysed by killer cells (KC) after complexing via Fc-or C3b-
receptors (antibody-dependent cell-mediated cytolysis, ADCC). Regulatory interactions (activation, suppression)
occur between HTC, STC, CTL, BC, and antibodies (─▸)

represent an artifact of the extraction process is not known. It has also been suggested that the substance of these extracts might be a messenger RNA. In any case, the greater immunogenicity of the antigen after its processing by the macrophage is an experimentally proven fact.

It should nevertheless be pointed out that in the case of thymus-independent antigens the direct interaction with immunogenically competent cells can produce a primary response without the intervention of macrophages. In this case, it is possible that the phagocytosis of the antigen by the macrophages impedes or diminishes the primary response. For example, it has been verified that hemocyanin is extremely immunogenic when injected into mice in the soluble form, yet that this immunogenicity is greatly reduced after phagocytosis by macrophages. On the other hand, bovine serum albumin is much more immunogenic after phagocytosis by macrophages. This appears to indicate that some antigens need to be processed by the macrophage in order to stimulate efficiently the immunocompetent cells, whereas others can do this directly.

In summary, based upon experimental data obtained in vitro (which does not necessarily represent that which occurs in vivo), it is clear that macrophages play a role in the production of antibodies. In lymphoid cell cultures containing T and B cells, the production of antibodies against certain antigens is enhanced by the presence of macrophages. The role of the macrophages in this situation is further described in Chap. 6.

Dendritic Reticular Cells

These are cells encountered principally in the germinative centers of the lymph nodes. Their profuse cytoplasmic prolongations are so intricate and extensive as to be suggestive of a three-dimensional spider's web. Unlike macrophages, these cells do not phagocytose antigens, but retain them on their surfaces for considerable periods of time. This retention is accentuated particularly in the secondary response and appears to depend upon the presence of antibodies. Some authors consider these cells a special type of reticular cells, whereas others hold them to be a particular type of macrophage, termed dendritic macrophages. The function of these cells in the immune response is discussed in relation to the response of the lymph nodes to antigenic stimulus.

References

Cantor H, Boyse EA (1976) Functional subclasses of T lymphocytes bearing Ly antigens. I. The generation of functionally distinct T-cell subclasses is a differentiative process independent of antigen. J Exp Med 141:1376

Cantor H, Boyse EA (1976) Functional subclasses of T lymphocytes bearing Ly antigens. II. Cooperation between subclasses of Ly^+ cells in the generation of killer activity. J Exp Med 141:1390

Gowans JL (1971) Immunobiology of the small lymphocyte. In: Good RA, Fisher DW (eds) Immunobiology. Sinauer Associates, Stamford/Conn

Greenwalt TJ, Jamieson GA (eds) (1977) The granulocytes: Function and clinical utilization. Liss, New York

Gupta S, Good RA (eds) (1979) Cellular, molecular, and clinical aspects of allergic disorders. Plenum, New York

Kapp JA, Pierce CW, Schlossman S, Benacerraf B (1974) Genetic control of immune responses in vitro. V. Stimulation of suppressor T cells in nonresponder mice by the terpolymer L-glutamic acid^{60}-L-alanine^{30}-L-tyrosine^{10} (GAT). J Exp Med 140:648

Katz DH (1977) Lymphocyte differentiation, recognition, and regulation. Academic, New York

Möller G (ed) (1980) Unresponsiveness to haptenated self molecule. Immunol Rev Vol 50. Munksgaard, Copenhagen

Moretta L, Ferrarini M, Cooper MD (1978) Characterization of human T cell subpopulations as defined by specific receptors of immunoglobulins. Contemp Top Immunobiol 8:19

Nelson DS (ed) (1976) Immunobiology of the macrophage. Academic, New York

Owen JJ (1971) The origin and development of lymphocyte populations. Ontogeny of acquired immunity. Excerpta Medica, Amsterdam

Perlmann P (1979) The cytotoxic effector function of lymphocytes. Behring Inst Res Comm 63:7

Chapter 3   Antigens

IVAN MOTA

Contents

Antigens (from Greek *anti-*, against; and *gen*, of *gignomai*, to generate) are complex molecules recognized as foreign (nonself) by immunologically competent cells. When introduced into the organism, antigens activate two different sectors of the lymphoid system: They stimulate the production of immunoglobulin molecules, i.e., antibodies, and they lead to the sensitization of cells. Both antibodies and sensitized cells can react specifically with the antigen.

For a substance to function as an antigen, two fundamental requirements must be met: (1) The substance must be of a composition foreign to that of the organism, and (2) it must be a complex macromolecule.

The first requirement means that the antigen must possess certain structures that differ from those encountered on the surfaces of immunocompetent cells, thereby enabling the latter to recognize them as nonself.

Although, as a rule, antibodies are formed only against antigens derived from different species, there are examples of iso- or alloimmunization, that is, immunization against antigens of animals of the same species. This occurs, for example, in maternal–fetal incompatibility for antigens of distinct blood groups and in the rejection of allografts (transplantation alloantigens). In exceptional circumstances, the formation of antibodies that are capable of reacting with constituents of their own organism may occur (autoantibodies).

The specificity of the antibody generally is oriented in relation to the animal species from which the antigen originates (antihorse, antisheep, etc, however, organ-specific antibodies are frequently encountered. For example, if we were to immunize a rabbit with bovine lens crystallin, antibodies would be generated that would react not only with it, but also with crystallins of other species (e.g., horse, sheep, guinea pig). Other examples clearly demonstrative of organ-specificity include spermatozoa, cerebrum, and thyroglobulin.

The second requirement relates to the bulk and complexity of the antigenic molecule. Small molecules (mol. wt. $< 5,000$) generally are not immunogenic, except when conjugated to a larger protein molecule. However, certain low-molecular-weight substances such as compounds of arsanilic acid with tyrosine, and DNP-7-lysine, when injected with Freund's adjuvant become strongly immunogenic. These substances do not combine with the proteins of the organism: The manner in which they induce the formation of antibodies is not understood.

To act as an antigen it is not enough that a substance be macromolecular: Synthetic polymers such as nylon, Teflon, polystyrene, polyacrylamide, etc., possess voluminous molecules; nevertheless, they are devoid of antigenic activity. It is necessary that the molecule have a certain internal complexity, such as that exhibited by proteins. Even the polysaccharides, which can have a monotonous structure with numerous repeated units, may be considered complex molecules when compared to the synthetic plastics. Lipids apparently are not immunogenic, yet they may function as haptens when mixed with human or porcine serum. In this manner, antibodies have been obtained against cholesterol, cephalin, and lecithin. The operative mechanism of the serum is unknown, but it is thought to function as a carrier or *Schlepper* protein. An important lipid from the serologic point of view is cardiolipin, used in the serodiagnosis of syphilis.

Two discrete properties are exhibited by antigens: (1) the capacity to induce the formation of antibodies, or *immunogenicity*, and (2) the capacity to react with antibodies, or *antigenicity*. Only the macromolecules possess both properties. Substances exist that are not immunogenic, yet still are antigenic.

These substances, when isolated, are seen to possess structures too simple to be capable of inducing the formation of antibodies; however, as integral parts of larger molecules they become immunogenic, inducing the formation of antibodies with which they are capable of reacting – even when separated from the larger molecules. When these structures are artificially conjugated to a

protein or when they become a natural part of an antigen, they are called antigenic determinants (epitopes). The specificity of the antibodies and sensitized cells is directed against the haptens or antigenic determinants.

Chemical Basis of Antigenicity

Synthetic Antigen Conjugates

Karl Landsteiner performed a series of brilliant investigations with artificial antigen conjugates that led to an understanding of the chemical basis of antigenic specificity. Landsteiner made use of the observation that the antibodies against a conjugated protein (a carrier protein plus a hapten) react and form precipitates with other proteins when conjugated with the same hapten. In experiments with protein conjugates, the antigen used for obtaining the antisera and those used in reactions in vitro, must be prepared through conjugates of the hapten to different proteins (e.g., serum albumin and gamma globulin) in order to eliminate reactions due to the determinants belonging to the carrier proteins. The method used most by Landsteiner to unite haptens to proteins and obtain artificial antigen conjugates was that of diazotization. This method, ap-

Fig. 3.1. Diazotization reaction used by Landsteiner for preparation of hapten–protein conjugates by diazotization with the tyrosyl residues of a natural protein

plicable in cases in which the hapten is an aromatic amine (arylamine), consists of transforming the hapten into the respective diazo salt in order to couple it with a protein (residues of tyrosine, histidine, lysine) via an -N-N- linkage (Fig. 3.1).

The indicated reaction is run for the first time in acid medium at 0 °C, and for the second time in alkaline medium. A typical result of an experiment of this type is exemplified in Table 3.1.

Table 3.1. Precipitation tests with proteins conjugated by diazotization to sulfanilamide and to sulfapyridine

Antigens	Precipitation with Anti-	
	BSA-azosulfanilamide	BSA-azosulfapyridine
BGG-azosulfanilamide	+ +	−
BGG-azosulfapyridine	−	+ +
BSA	+ +	+ +
BGG	−	−

BSA = bovine serum albumin; BGG = bovine gamma globulin

Utilizing the methodology to be described in the following remarks, Landsteiner investigated the importance of different factors in the determination of the specificity of antigen conjugates. DNP conjugates are other frequently used synthetic antigen(s) that can be preserved by nucleophilic substitution through halogen derivatives, e.g., 2,4-dinitrofluorobenzoyl. The coupling can be made over the α- or the ε-NH_2 group, as is illustrated with α,ε-DNP lysin:

Spatial Configuration. The influence of this factor can be illustrated by studying the serologic specificity of the proteins conju-

Table 3.2. Serologic specificities of the tartaric acids

Antigens	Antisera		
	Levo	Dextro	Meso
Levo	+ + +	±	+
Dextro	0	+ + +	+
Meso	±	0	+ + +

gated to isomers of levo-, dextro-, and meso-tartaric acid (Table 3.2).

As indicated in Table 3.2, each antiserum reacts strongly with its homologous antigen without there being appreciable cross-reaction between the levo- and dextrotartaric acids; however, as one could anticipate, the serum against the mesotartaric acid exhibits conspicuous cross-reaction with the levo- and dextro-forms.

Another good example of the influence of isomerism in antigenic specificity is the capacity of antibodies to distinguish specifically between glucose and galactose, which differ only by the inversion of the position between a hydrogen atom and a hydroxyl group linked to the same carbon atom.

Polar Groups. The radicals that exhibit electrostatic charges of contrary signs and that act as dipoles are highly active as determinant groups of antigenic specificity. This can be verified, for example, in the reaction between the antisera produced to meta-aminobenzenic and meta-aminobenzenesulfonic acid, in the presence of the following antigens whose formulas are reproduced, in the order indicated, in the horizontal column of Table 3.3: aniline, para-aminobenzoic acid, meta-aminobenzoic acid, a methylated derivative of the preceding substance, and meta-aminobenzenesulfinic acid.

Specific Determinants of the Natural Antigens

What part of the antigenic molecule participates in immunologic specificity? The classic investigations of Obermayer and Pick (1904) demonstrated that proteins treated with io-

Table 3.3. Importance of the polar groups and of their positions in the specificity of antibodies

Antiserum against	Haptens used in the precipitation reaction				
	NH$_2$ (benzene)	NH$_2$ / COOH	H$_3$C–NH$_2$ / COOH	NH$_2$ / COOH	NH$_2$ / SO$_3$H
NH$_2$ / COOH	0	0	+++	+++	+
NH$_2$ / SO$_3$H	0	0	0	0	+++

In this table the following is clearly verified:
1. The determinant action of the polar groupings COOH and SO$_3$H
2. The influence of the position (meta or para) of the COOH radical
3. The lack of action of the CH$_3$ radical
4. The co-reactivity of the COOH and SO$_3$ groups when they occupy the same position

dine lost their original specificity (species-specificity) but acquired a new specificity (chemical), becoming reactive with the iodo-proteins of other species. The same is true, to a certain extent, with the azoproteins; however, in this case the original species specificity does not disappear.

The secondary and tertiary structures of the protein molecule are also important, i.e., the manner in which the peptide helices are coiled so as to constitute a three-dimensional protein molecule. Depending upon such structure, miniscule reactive areas on the surface of the globular molecule are exposed. The antibodies attach themselves to these areas, which correspond to the determinant groups of antigenic specificity.

The determinant groups are numerous (the number rising as the molecular weight increases), and not all of them are alike: To each determinant of distinct specificity there corresponds a homologous antibody. This fact was demonstrated elegantly by Lapresle (1955) in immunoelectrophoresis experiments with human serum albumin fragmented by means of a cathepsin.

As with a key fitting a lock, immunologic specificity evidently depends upon the perfection with which the determinant matches the cavity of the antibody. If the fit is perfect (homologous reactions), the antigen and the antibody come within sufficient proximity for effectual action of the short-reaching secondary valence forces (Coulomb forces, Van der Waals forces, and hydrogen bonds) and the stabilization of the union. The same does not occur, however, in the case of cross-reactions, in which the fit is imperfect and thus does not foster a firm union of the components involved.

In agreement with the theory of clonal selection, one lymphoid cell, carrying one specific combining site, corresponds to each antigenic determinant. Lymphocytes are able to recognize the substitution of a single amino acid (the minimum size of one determinant has been measured to be about 6 amino acids) in the antigenic determinant, which leads to a shift in the specificity of the respective antibody.

Antigenic Determinants of Polysaccharides

The most simple polysaccharide antigens are represented by homopolymers of glucose, among which the most studied from the immunologic point of view is dextran, which is composed of principal chains of polyglucose

Fig. 3.2. α-1,6 and α-1,3 glucose chains of dextran

in an α-1,6 linkage and secondary chains in an α-1,3 linkage (Fig. 3.2).

As that synthesized by certain microorganisms (e.g., *Leuconostoc mesenteroides*), native dextran has a high molecular weight (10^7–10^8 daltons), whereas clinical dextran, used as a plasma substitute, is partially hydrolyzed so as to reduce its molecular weight to about 75,000 daltons. Even so, clinical dextran still is capable of producing antibodies in man – sometimes in high titers.

A more prolonged hydrolysis of dextran yields oligosaccharides, of which those with two to seven glucose molecules (isomaltose and isomaltose triose, pentose, hexose, and heptose) are of particular interest.

Pioneering studies by Kabat on the quantitative inhibition of the dextran-antidextran reaction by the oligosaccharides permitted measurement of the maximum size of binding site of the antibody. Evidently, this size must correspond to that of the oligosaccharide capable of producing maximum inhibition; this was found to be hexose or heptose. The maximum size of the antibody binding was therefore estimated in terms of the dimensions of the distended isomaltose hexose molecule, i.e., $34 \times 12 \times 7$ Å

Aside from this, the study of various human antidextran antisera has yielded different inhibition curves for the various oligosaccharides, which came to demonstrate the heterogeneity of the antibodies with respect to the size of the combining sites, i.e., from two to six or seven glucose molecules.

Data obtained later with other systems, in particular with synthetic polypeptides, confirmed the maximum size established with the dextran oligosaccharides – five to six amino acid residues.

Antigenic Determinants and Cross-Reactions

When two antigens possess common or structurally similar antigenic determinants, the antibodies obtained to one of these antigens tend to react with the other antigen. These reactions are called cross-reactions. The antigen used as the immunogen is usually termed the homologous antigen, whereas the antigen that cross-reacts is called heterologous. Cross-reactions occur not only between phylogenically related antigens, but also between substances of phylogenically remote origins – or even between substances that bear no known relationship. In the first case, known cross-reactions occur between the ovalbumins of different fowl and between the serum albumins of different species. A typical example of the cross-reaction between phylogenically unrelated antigens is that of the Forssman antigen, which is a substance encountered in many animal species and in diverse bacteria. Rabbits immunized with sheep erythrocytes form two types of hemolytic antibodies: isophilic, which are species-specific (recognizing only the antigenic determinants of the species) and heterophilic, which are specific for the Forssman antigen. The Forssman antigen is but one example; there are many other examples distributed among phylogenically distant species that can cause totally unexpected cross-reactions. Antigens of this type are called heterophilic antigens.

Conformation and Antigenic Specificity

Numerous observations have evidenced the importance of steric conformation in antigenic specificity. In natural protein antigens and in synthetic polypeptides, it is possible to distinguish determinants whose specificity is due to the sequence of amino acids (sequential determinants) and determinants whose specificity depends on the conformation of the molecule (conformational determinants). Antibodies produced against a sequential determinant react with other determinants of a similar sequence, whereas antibodies of a specificity directed against a conformational determinant cannot react with a determinant that exhibits the same sequence of amino acids but does not possess the original steric conformation of the immunogen. For example, it is possible to digest a lysozyme molecule and thus to isolate a polypeptide composed of 20 amino acids that, in the molecule as a whole, form a "loop" united to the former by a disulfide bridge, situated between the cysteines that occupy positions 64 and 80. Antisera prepared in rabbits using as antigen the intact peptide conjugated to lysine are capable of reacting with the isolated "loop" as well as with the entire lysozyme molecule (in this case, evidently, through the loop region), but not with the peptide "loop" opened by the rupture of the disulfide bridge through reduction and alkylation. Similarly, antibodies produced against pancreatic ribonuclease do not react with it after denaturation and rupture of its disulfide bridges.

Myoglobulin is an even better example: Not only is its primary structure known, but its tertiary structure as well – established by Kendrew through crystallographic diffraction studies with x-rays. As with hemoglobin, myoglobin is a heme molecule where the heme is lodged in a "cavity" of the protein molecule, bound to the Fe^{2+} by hydrogen bridges to two histidines that occupy positions 64 and 93. These linkages ensure that the metamyoglobin will have a conformation different from the apomyoglobin.

In inhibition studies of the precipitation of antiapomyoglobin by apo- or metamyoglobin in the presence of six chemotryptic peptides, it was verified that two of them (A 2 and A 4) were producing the same degree of inhibition, even though the A 2 contained 15 amino acids and A 4 contained 19 amino acids. The four additional amino acids in A 4 corresponded, however, to amino acids "buried" in the myoglobin molecule and therefore not participating in the antigenic determinant.

A third peptide (B 1), composed of amino acids 56–69, was capable of inhibiting the reaction with apomyoglobin but not that with metamyoglobin, showing that the union through the heme of the 64 and 93 histidines creates a conformational specificity (Fig. 3.3).

Of the remaining peptides studied, D 1 and D 2 were active and included external amino acids; D 3, being inactive, contained only internal amino acids.

It is possible that the antigenic specificity of the globular proteins and even of some fibrillar proteins such as collagen are principally of the conformational type.

Chemical Basis of Immunogenicity

The chemical basis of immunogenicity is not understood as fully as that of antigenic specificity.

It has been known for a long time that certain proteins are potent antigens whereas others are weak, and that, generally speaking, this difference is related to molecular size. However, other characteristics undoubtedly participate in immunogenic capacity – in particular, the nature of the amino acids that make up the immunogenic

Fig. 3.3. Three-dimensional structure of the myoglobin molecules, determined by crystallographic and amino-acid sequence methods (Reproduced from Kabat, 1976)

pacity – in particular, the nature of the amino acids that make up the immunogenic determinant (but not necessarily that of the specificity) and also the accessibility of this determinant. An example is that of gelatin, a fibrillar protein obtained by boiling collagen in water or in acid; its lack of immunogenicity has been imputed to a deficiency in aromatic amino acids (tryptophan, tyrosine). Although other factors cannot be excluded, there is no doubt that the addition of a small quantity of tyrosine, under certain experimental conditions, can enhance the immunogenicity of gelatin, notwithstanding the nonparticipation of this amino acid in the antigenic specificity. The weak immunogenicity of gelatin, meanwhile, appears to be due to its strong constitutional similarity to collagen in various species; the substitution of only a few amino acids renders it barely distinguishable for various organisms.

An enormous impetus to the study of the chemical determination of immunogenicity was imparted by the investigations under-taken with synthetic polypeptides, in particular by Sela and associates, in Israel. The synthetic polypeptides are polymers of α-amino acids prepared by the polymerization of monomeric amino-acid derivatives, usually carboxyanhydrides, which can be prepared with either ramified or linear chains. Such polymers offer, with respect to the proteins, a great advantage in that at the will of the experimenter the nature and the positions of the amino acids that constitute them can be varied to facilitate their study relative to immunogenic capacity.

Investigations with such polymers permitted a considerable advance in the understanding of immunogenicity. For example, it has been verified that the homopolymers (polymers composed of a single amino acid) such as polylysine (PLL) usually are not immunogenic in rabbits; however, when conjugated to proteins or simply precipitated by oppositely charged proteins, they can induce an immune response. On the other hand, many copolymers (polymers of differing amino acids) of two amino acids are immunogenic principally when they contain a cyclic amino acid. These copolymers frequently are immunogenic only for some individuals or for some isogeneic strains. For example, whereas the polymers of glutamic acid and alanine are not immunogenic for strain 13 guinea pigs, they are immunogenic for strain 2; at the same time, the polymers of glutamic acid and tyrosine, although nonimmunogenic for strain 2, are immunogenic for strain 13. When "outbred" guinea pigs are immunized with these polymers, some react with strain 2, others with strain 13, and others behave as hybrids by responding to both polymers. Copolymers of three or more amino acids are immunogenic for all animal species.

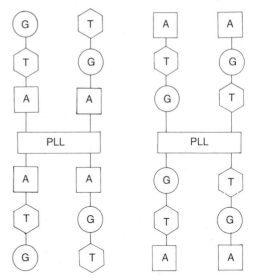

Fig. 3.4. External grouping of the antigen molecule in immunogenicity. *T*, tyrosine; *G*, glutamic acid; and *A*, DL-alanine

Importance of the External Groupings of the Antigen in Immunogenicity

The immunogenicity of the antigen depends upon the groupings present on its surface and not upon those localized in the interior of the molecule. For example, polymers composed of an axial skeleton with internal groupings of DL-alanine (nonimmunogenic) and external groupings of tyrosine-glutamic acid (immunogenic) are in fact immunogenic; however, when the order of the grouping is inverted – by placing the nonimmunogenic DL-alanine grouping on the surface – the polymer becomes nonimmunogenic (Fig. 3.4).

Experiments with polymers of D-amino acids, which are poorly immunogenic, also confirm the importance of the accessibility of the immunogenic groupings: ramified polymers with 95% L-amino acids (which are immunogenic), and 5% D-amino acids (which are nonimmunogenic) on their surfaces are as poorly immunogenic as polymers that contain 100% D-amino acids; on the other hand, polymers with 95% D-amino acids and with 5% L-amino acids on the molecule exterior are as immunogenic as those with 100% L-amino acids.

Adjuvanticity

Substances or treatments that augment the immunogenicity of antigens are termed adjuvants (Latin *adjuvans*, aiding). The observation that certain substances potentiate the production of antibodies when applied simultaneously with the antigen (though not necessarily mixed with it) was made about 45 years ago, some decades after the discovery of antibodies. Ramon was one of the first to note this phenomenon. He observed that the production of antitoxoid antibodies in horses was greatly increased when these substances were injected adsorbed to a particulate substance rather than in their pure state. The adjuvant concept also originated from the use of toxoid-associated vaccines plus bacterial vaccines, e.g., the so-called triple vaccine, in which it was observed that one of the components reinforced the humoral response to the other. Currently, many heterogeneous substances are known to be capable of augmenting immunogenicity: alum, aluminum phosphate, aluminum hydroxide, beryllium sulfate, saponin, alginate of calcium, guanidine silica, mineral oil emulsions, double-helix synthetic nucleic acids such as the complexes of polyadenylic (poly A) and polyuridylic (poly U) acids and of polyinosinic (poly I) and polycytidylic (poly C) acids, and lipopolysaccharides obtained from numerous gram-negative bacteria such as *S. typhi*, *B. pertussis*, and *E. coli*. Although the operative mechanism of the adjuvants is poorly understood, it is accepted that they augment the production of antibodies in three ways: (1) by continuous and gradual liberation of the antigen (depot effect), (b) by stimulation of phagocytosis, and (c) by activation (nonspecific) of the lymphocytes (mitogenicity).

One frequently used adjuvant mixture is Freund's adjuvant. It is composed of a mixture of a mineral oil (Bayol F), an emulsifying agent (Aquafor, Falba, Arlacel), and an aqueous antigen solution. This mixture is prepared to obtain a water–oil emulsion. In this manner, the antigen is dispersed with the finest fat dioplets, from which it is slowly liberated. In the so-called complete Freund's adjuvant, the mixture also contains dead mycobacteria in suspension (*M. tuberculosis* or *M. butyricum*); the adjuvant without mycobacteria is called incomplete adjuvant. The operative mechanism of Freund's adjuvant has three principal effects: (1) a depositing action that retards the systemic absorption of the antigen, (2) local formation of a granuloma rich in macrophages and immunocompetent cells, and (3) farther-reaching action in the lymphoid organs (there is an almost immediate dissemination of the emulsion droplets through the lymphatics to the lymph nodes). With the complete adjuvant, the addition of mycobacteria is indispensable for production of a state of delayed hypersensitivity. Complete adjuvant is therefore essential for the production of the experimental autoallergic diseases such as encephalomyelitis, thyroiditis, arthritis, and others (see Chap. 13).

Cytologic examination of the lymph of the efferent lymphatic vessels of the granuloma produced by the injection of the Freund's adjuvant into the tissues has revealed an intense outpouring of lymphocytes. This fact and the older observations that the injection of antigen into a tuberculous granuloma induces a state of delayed hypersensitivity for the injected antigen, suggests that the encounter of the antigen with the immunocompetent cells within or near the granuloma cells is important for the establishment of a hypersentivity state.

The adjuvant activity of the mycobacteria has been attributed to various substances extracted from them – particularly to wax D (peptidoglycolipid composed of mycolic acid esters with different polysaccharides, united by an amide linkage to a heptapeptide) and also to ribonucleic acid.

The strong adjuvant effect of the gram-negative bacteria appears due in large part to the endotoxin contained in these bacteria. The term endotoxin is applied to complex, high-molecular-weight substances existing in the cell walls of many bacteria; they are extremely toxic, pyrogenic, immunogenic, and produce an adjuvant effect. These complexes are composed of polysaccharides, lipids, and proteins. The biologic activity of the endotoxins is present in a smaller molecule, a lipopolysaccharide (LPS), that is free of proteins. There appears to be a direct relation between the toxic effect of LPS and its adjuvant effect. For example, rabbits that have been made tolerant to LPS simultaneously become refractory to the adjuvant effect of this substance. The lipopolysaccharide, in addition to being a thymus-independent antigen, is also a specific mitogen of the B lymphocytes that stimulates the proliferation of specific cellular clones in the absence of the antigenic stimulus. It is possible that the adjuvant effect of LPS is related to its mitogenic effect upon the B cells.

Certain adjuvants appear to favor specific classes of antibodies to the detriment of others: Guinea pigs immunized with ovalbumin and complete Freund's adjuvant produce preferentially antibodies of the IgG_2 type, whereas under the same conditions, incomplete adjuvant induces a greater production of IgG_1. The adjuvant effect of *B. pertussis* gives rise to the preferential production of IgE-class antibodies in rats, mice, and guinea pigs. In the first two species, the preferential formation of IgE appears to be due to the histamine-sensitizing factor (HSF), whereas in the guinea pig, the adjuvant effect is directly associated with the LPS. It is probable that the adjuvants act particularly at the cellular level and that the type of cell affected determines the class of antibody predominating in the humoral response.

Curiously, many immunosuppressive agents also possess adjuvant activity when applied at the right moment in relation to contact with the antigen. These agents include, among others, X and gamma rays, 6-mercaptopurine, 5-fluorouracil, and 5-fluorodeoxyuridine (see Chap. 14).

References

Borek FF (1972) Immunogenicity. Physico-chemical and biological aspects. North-Holland, Amsterdam

Kabat EA (1976) Structural concepts in immunology and immunochemistry, 2nd edn. Holt, Rinehart & Winston, New York, Chap 2

Landsteiner K (1962) The specificity of serological reactions. Bover, New York

Sela M (1965) Immunological studies with synthetic polypeptides. Adv Immunol 5:29

Sela M (ed) (1973) The antigen, vol I. Academic, New York

Staub AM, Raynaud M (1971) Cours d'Immunologie générale et de Sérologie de l'Institut Pasteur, vol I. C.D.U., Paris

WHO Scientific Group on Immunological Adjuvants (1973) Report Series No 595. World Health Organization, Geneva

Chapter 4   Antibodies

OTTO G. BIER and DIETRICH GÖTZE

Contents

Antibody Formation at the Level of the Organism

Preparation of Immune Sera

A prerequisite to the study of antigens (from Greek *anti* = against, and *gen* = gignomai, to create, see Chap. 3) and antibodies is the production of antisera (immune sera), i.e., of sera that react specifically with antigens. In laboratory experiments, small animals, i.e., the rabbit, are used for the production of antisera. However, when it is necessary to produce therapeutic or diagnostic antisera on a large scale, larger animals are used – primarily the horse.

Antisera produced by injecting animals with antigens obtained from a different species are termed xenoantisera (from Greek *xenos* = foreign), i.e., rabbit anti-chicken ovalbumin serum, or horse anti-diphtheria toxin serum. On the other hand, antisera may be raised to detect lesser antigenic differences, for example, the Rh antigens on human erythrocytes. In this case, it is advisable to utilize an animal of the same species that does not possess the antigen in question. Thus, if a rabbit is immunized with Rh^+ human erythrocytes, antibodies would be produced against other predominant human erythrocytic antigens, thereby masking or impeding the formation of anti-Rh antibodies. If, however, an Rh^- person were immunized with blood from an Rh^+ individual both sharing the same ABO antigens, the species-shared erythrocytic antigens would be ignored and only anti-Rh antibodies would be produced. This intraspecies immunization is termed alloimmunization (from Greek *allos* = the other), and the antiserum obtained is called alloantiserum.

Adjuvants. The techniques for immunization, largely empirical, vary according to the nature of the antigen and the manner of inoculation; yet in the case of soluble antigens they fall into two principal categories: (1) repeated intravenous or intraperitoneal injections of increasing doses of antigen in an aqueous solution, and (2) administration of single or repeated subcutaneous injections of a fixed dose of antigen in an oil emulsion.

An example of the first category is a method seldom used today, the immunization of rabbits to obtain hemolysin or antibacterial antibodies (antipneumococcic or antisalmonella serum). For the production of precipitating antibodies against soluble proteins such as ovalbumin or bovine gamma globulin, method 1 or method 2 can be applied. One effective scheme consists of intraveneous injection into rabbits of an aluminum hydroxide-precipitated protein solution. The use of aluminum hydroxide as an adjuvant diminishes excretion and fosters phagocytosis. Immunization is initiated with 0.5 mg protein, and the dose is increased progressively until it reaches 5 mg; a series of 4–5 injections per week, on consecutive days, follows until a total of 20–30 mg is reached.

At the end of 4–6 weeks, the process of immunization is interrupted and a blood sample is drawn 5–6 days after the last antigen injection. If a sufficient titer of antibody is present, a large blood sample (about 50–60 ml) is drawn by cardiac puncture; if the titer is still not high enough, immunization is continued for another 2–3 weeks. Today, preference is given to the injection of a single dose of antigen emulsified in complete Freund's adjuvant and injected subcutaneously on each side of the nape of the neck at four or five points (0.2 ml in each site). Generally, a single injection is sufficient to yield antisera of satisfactory titers within 4–6 weeks. If an even higher titer is desired, an intravenous or intraperitoneal booster injection of 2–5 mg of aluminum hydroxide-precipitated antigen can be administered.

In the case of cellular antigens, for example for the production of anti-lymphocytic sera, about 2 to 20×10^6 cells are injected with or without Freund's adjuvant subcutaneously; 3–4 weeks later, the same number of cells is injected either subcutaneously, or on three consecutive days intravenously. Six to eight days later, the serum is tested for antibody activity. If the titer is satisfactory, a larger sample of the blood is obtained; if the titer is not sufficiently high, the immunization is continued by injecting the same number of cells every other week. Again, 6–8 days after each antigen injection, the serum is tested for antibody activity.

The antisera obtained in the final bleeding are then separated under aseptic conditions. A bacteriostatic agent is added (Merthiolate at 1:10,000, or sodium azide at 1:1,000) and the sera are then frozen.

Two fundamental rules must be remembered in the preparation of antisera: (1) Before the initiation of immunization, a sample of serum must be collected to verify the possible pre-existence of antibodies reacting with the antigen in question. (2) Because the responses of the individual animals vary, it is advisable to assay the antisera individually. Making mixtures or pools of antisera before assaying them frequently results in the loss of important information available from an individual antiserum.

Dynamics of Antibody Formation

The dynamics of the formation of antibodies in the organism is expressed by the two types of the immune response: primary and secondary. In both cases, the magnitude of the response depends upon the sensitivity of the method used for its detection. Thus, in measuring the titer or the quantity of antibodies, we must be conscious of the fact that we are detecting only the antibodies that react with the antigen utilized under the conditions employed for the measurement.

Primary Response. The name primary response was given to the reaction observed to the first antigen stimulus. This reaction occurs only after a determined latent period (days to weeks), the duration of which varies as a function of the parameters inherent in the animal immunized and in the immunizing antigen.

In rabbits, appreciable titers of antibodies against red blood cells, bacteria, and other particulate antigens can be observed after 5 days, whereas antibodies against diphtheria toxin are first detectable 2–3 weeks after injection of the toxoid. At birth, man is

Fig. 4.1. Time course of specific antibody activity (concentration) after a single injection of antigen: primary response

immunologically much more mature than the mouse; it is estimated that the human embryo of 5–6 months has attained immunologic maturity comparable to that of the newborn mouse. In the mouse, lymphoid tissue attains a degree of development sufficient to assure immunologic maturity only after 1 or 2 months of extrauterine life. In any case, the curve representing the production of antibodies after antigenic stimulation inclines toward a maximum, remains at a plateau for a long period of time, and then declines at varying speeds, depending upon the balance between the metabolism and the biosynthesis of the antibody (Fig. 4.1). Accordingly, the disappearance of the antibodies from the blood requires periods ranging from several weeks to several years, depending upon the antigen involved.

The persistence of the antigenic stimulus and the rate of metabolic destruction are the determining factors in the decline of the antibody titer. Particulate (insoluble) antigens produce a more prolonged stimulus than do soluble antigens, and for this reason give rise to elevated antibody levels that persist over long periods. The same occurs with the polysaccharides, e.g., the pneumococcic polysaccharides, which are poorly attacked by enzymes in the organism. Proteins, on the other hand, are destroyed in vivo with relative rapidity. In many cases, the persistence of the antigenic stimulus and its catabolism are the primary factors responsible for the discontinuity and the duration of antibody formation.

Secondary Response. In an animal previously sensitized by a primary stimulus, a second dose, or booster, produces an accelerated and more elevated response than that associated with the first dose (Fig. 4.2). The secondary response, also called the anamnestic response, is attributed to what has been termed immunologic memory, i.e., part of the cells stimulated by the first antigen stimulation differentiate and proliferate not to become plasma cells but to become "committed lymphocytes" which after restimulation with the same antigen immediately turn into plasma cells.

Adopting the terminology introduced by Sercarz and Coons, using X to indicate the immunocompetent (sensitive to antigen) cell, Y to indicate the primed or memory cell, and Z for the antibody-forming cell, we can schematically follow the primary and secondary response:

$$X \xrightarrow[\substack{\text{Primary} \\ \text{Stimulus}}]{\text{Antigen}} Y \xrightarrow[\substack{\text{Secondary} \\ \text{Stimulus}}]{\text{Antigen}} Z$$

In both the primary and secondary responses, the phase during which the antibodies increase is logarithmic in relation to time; this strongly suggests a multiplication of the cells that form antibodies – more rapid in the case of the secondary response by virtue of the prior accumulation of memory cells.

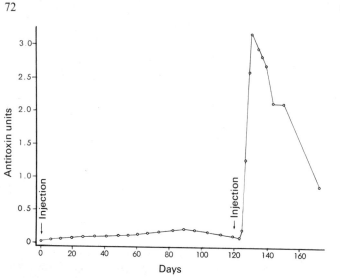

Fig. 4.2. Time course of antibody activity (concentration) specific for diphtheria toxin in the horse after booster injection: secondary response

Antibody Formation at the Cellular Level

For the study of antibody formation at the cellular level and its cytodynamics several methods have been utilized: (1) the Jerne plaque technique, (2) the rosette technique, (3) the microdrop technique, and (4) the hybridization of plasma cells with myeloma cells.

Jerne Plaque Technique

In the Jerne plaque technique, a suspension of lymphoid cells of the immunized animal is mixed homogeneously with an adequate quantity of melted agar, and red cells bearing the same antigen used for immunization are added to the culture medium. Once the mixture is solidified, complement is added. The antibodies diffuse radially from the cells that synthesize them, and produce circular plaques of hemolysis in the layer of agar (Fig. 4.3).
The plaque-forming cells (PFC) are generally plasma cells, and the antibodies revealed by the described technique are of the IgM type (see below). To detect IgG antibodies that do not fix complement, the addition of complement must be preceded by the addition of anti-IgG serum. In this manner, both

IgG and IgM types of antibodies can be detected – the first being distinguishable by noting the difference in relation to the plaque test done without antiglobulin serum.

Rosette Technique

Also called immunocytoadherence, the rosette method was developed by Biozzi and his colleagues. It consists of microscopic verification of the formation of rosettes from erythrocytes (Fig. 4.3) in a suspension of lymphoid cells from immunized animals, and of red cells bearing the antigen used for immunization. For the same suspension of lymphoid cells and the same erythrocytes, the number of plaques is much smaller than the number of rosettes, because the latter technique is capable of revealing much smaller quantities of both classes of antibodies. Almost all cells that form rosettes are lymphocytes, but rosettes may also be encountered around plasma cells, blasts, and even macrophages that have adsorbed cytophilic antibodies.

Microdrop Technique

This method, utilized extensively by Nossal and his colleagues, requires separation of

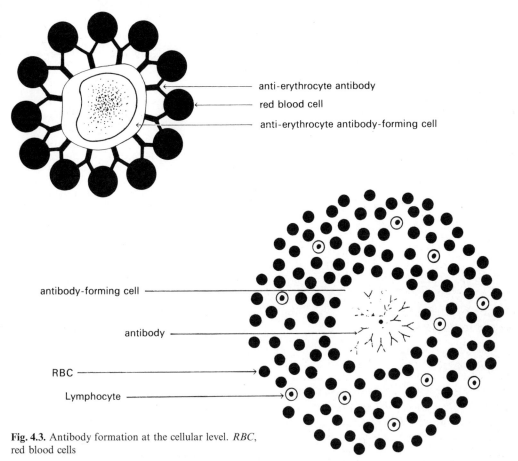

anti-erythrocyte antibody

red blood cell

anti-erythrocyte antibody-forming cell

antibody-forming cell

antibody

RBC

Lymphocyte

Fig. 4.3. Antibody formation at the cellular level. *RBC*, red blood cells

microdrops that contain single lymphocytes, and involves a search in these for bacteria-immobilizing antibodies (by direct microscopic observation) or phage-neutralizing antibodies (by observation of areas of lysis in agar). With the help of these methods it was possible to establish that lymphoid cells are capable of producing immunoglobulins of a single specificity only, and at a given time produce only one class of immunoglobulin. From this, it was concluded that all plasma cells derive from one stem cell, which itself does not form antibodies, but has the capacity to generate as many differentiated plasma cell clones as there are different antibody specificities (Fig. 4.4).

Since antigens in general are complex molecules, they possess several structural "patches" which are recognized by specific receptors on lymphocytes; these patches are called antigenic determinants or *epitopes* (see Chap. 3). From this, it follows that immunization with any antigen, even highly purified, will lead to the stimulation of several clones, each recognizing a different or only partially identical epitope on the same antigen molecule, i.e., immune sera are polyclonal and therefore, heterogeneous in respect to specificity and immunoglobulin class of single antibodies. Attempts to obtain oligoclonal antisera, or monoclonal antibodies of known antigen or epitope specificity have been made. For this, very simple antigens, for example synthetic polypeptides (see Chap. 3, p. 65) or certain bacterial polysaccharides, have been used as antigens,

Stem cell

Differentiation

"Inner" selection

B Cell

Antigen

Plasma cell clone

"Outer" (clonal) selection

Antibody

Fig. 4.4. Differentiation of antibody-forming cells. The undifferentiated stem cell is multipotent. It has the ability to generate approximately 10^6 different, antigen-specific B cells. Each B cell is only "unipotent" (monopotent). After contact with an antigen, the corresponding B cell differentiates to a plasma-cell clone with only one specific antibody

and indeed have produced rather homogeneous antisera.

Hybridomas

A new approach to obtaining specific monoclonal antibodies became possible in 1975 after Köhler and Milstein succeeded in demonstrating that, when fused with plasma cells from immunized donors, plasmocytoma cells growing in vitro secreted the specific antibody of that plasma cell in addition to their own. Such specific antibody-producing hybrid cells derived after fusion of a myeloma cell with a plasma cell are called *hybridomas* (*hybrid* myel*oma*). The procedure for obtaining such hybridoma lines is shown in Fig. 4.5. The myeloma cell lines (derived from BALB/c mouse plasmocytomas) used for the production of monoclonal antibodies were selected for thymidine-kinase (TK) and/or hypoxanthine-guanine-phosphoribosyl-transferase (HGPRT) deficiency. Neither of these enzymes is needed by the cells under normal culture conditions. However, if the main pathway for the synthesis of pyrimidine and purine is blocked by the folic acid antagonist aminopterin (or methotrexate), the cells die. Normal plasma cells that are not TK or HGPRT deficient compensate this deficien-

cy by complementation when fused with the myeloma cell, and the hybrid cell can grow, provided that the culture medium contains *H*ypoxanthine and *T*hymidine in addition to *A*minopterin (HAT-medium) (nonfused normal spleen cells die naturally in culture). The fusion is performed with plasma cells from the spleens of immunized donors 3–4 days after the last intravenous antigen injection, and myeloma cells in a ratio of 2 to 5:10. Polyethylenglycol (PEG, mol. wt. 1,000–4,000) in a concentration of 35%–50% (v/v)

$$HO\!-\!\overset{\displaystyle H}{\underset{\displaystyle H}{C}}\!-\!\overset{\displaystyle H}{\underset{\displaystyle H}{C}}\!-\!O\!-\!\left(\overset{\displaystyle H}{\underset{\displaystyle H}{C}}\!-\!\overset{\displaystyle H}{\underset{\displaystyle H}{C}}\!-\!O\right)_{\!x}\!\!-\!\overset{\displaystyle H}{\underset{\displaystyle H}{C}}\!-\!\overset{\displaystyle H}{\underset{\displaystyle H}{C}}\!-\!OH$$

x = 25 for mw. of 1,000

is used as a fusion reagent. The plasma cell-myeloma cell mixture is incubated for 1–8 min with 0.2–0.5 ml of PEG, the PEG is then diluted out with about 30 ml medium, the cells are washed and placed in wells of microtiter plates, and then incubated in HAT-medium. After 5–7 days, the medium is exchanged, and 5–7 days later the supernatants of growing cultures are tested for antibody activity (binding test, hemag-

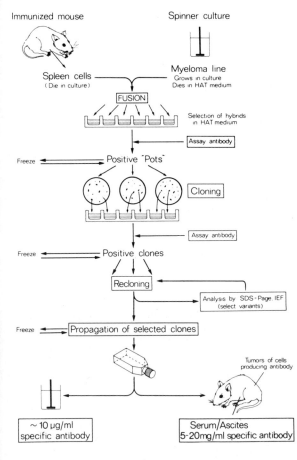

Fig. 4.5. Procedure for the production of monoclonal antibodies by fusion of primed spleen cells with myeloma cells, and selection of specific antibody-producing cell hybrid clones. (With permission reproduced from Milstein and Lennox 1980)

glutination, complement-dependent cytotoxicity, see Chap. 7).

The positive cultures are then cloned by limiting dilution; the cloned cultures are (a) propagated to produce mass cultures, (b) injected into BALB/c mice to obtain ascites, (c) recloned, and (d) frozen for storage in liquid nitrogen. The monoclonality of the produced antibody is proven by isoelectric focussing (IEF). This technique allows production of specific antibodies even when highly complex antigens such as cells are used or whenever the antigen of interest cannot be purified from contaminating substances (Fig. 4.6). Moreover, the production of monoclonal antibodies has proven to be a highly valuable tool for medical applications (diagnostic and therapy) as well as for research purpose, i.e., estimation of the size of specificity repertoire, classification of biological systems, etc.

Antibody Formation at the Protein Level

The production of antibodies at the molecular level has been studied in vitro using experiments with extracts of myelomas capable of producing large quantities of immunoglobulins (up to 40% of the total quantity of protein). Such extracts are much more convenient for studies of this nature than are those obtained from normal lymphoid organs, because they exhibit a high degree of heterogeneity of the synthesized immunoglobulins (see above).

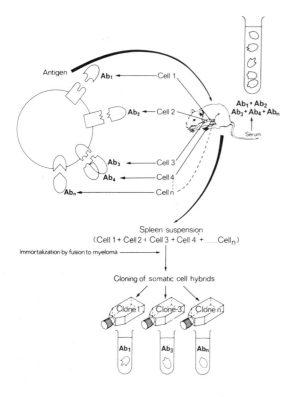

Fig. 4.6. Production of pure antibodies from impure antigens. Different antigenic determinants on a cell surface are recognized by B cells producing different antibodies. Single determinants can be recognized by different antibodies (Ab_3 and Ab_4), and the overlap in the antigenic determinants could be such that *different* antibody molecules recognize exactly the *same* determinant. Each antibody is made by a cell but the products are all mixed in the serum, so that the antiserum of an immune animal is a very heterogeneous mixture of antibody molecules. The hybrid myeloma method permits the separation of each antibody molecule by cloning the antibody-producing cell (with permission reproduced from Milstein and Lennox, 1980)

Myeloma cell extracts were incubated with labeled amino acids (along with those not labeled) to determine the time required for the heavy and light chains (see below, p. 80) to appear in the supernatant and in the sediment after sucrose-gradient centrifugation. The results indicated that the light chains appear in the ribosome fraction which sediments at 190 S after only 30 s, whereas the heavy chains associated with polyribosomes, which are considerably larger (250 S), do so only after 60 s. The times indicated (30 and 60 s) correspond to peaks in the formation of the respective chains. Before and after, the counts of labeled isotope fall considerably, indicating either that the chains were still being synthesized at the level of the polyribosomes, or that they were already being "excreted" in the liquid phase. It is important to mention that the fraction with the sedimentation coefficient of 250 S was found to obtain, in addition to heavy chains, small quantities of light chains, suggesting that the assembly of the immunoglobulin half-molecule takes place at the level of the polyribosome arrays.

Purification of Antibodies

For the determination of antibody structure as well as for medical application in prophylaxis, diagnosis, and therapy, antibodies must be isolated and purified from other contaminating serum proteins. They can be purified by nonspecific or specific methods. The former are based on the physical or physico-chemical characteristics of immunoglobulins, and do not allow separation of the normal gamma globulins from the antibodies. Specific methods, on the other hand, are based on the dissociation or elution of immune complexes, thus permitting the isolation of antibodies to a high degree of purity, free of nonspecific immunoglobulins. Specific methods are used chiefly for experimental studies; they cannot be applied to therapeutic antisera because of the low yield inherent in the purification process.

Without entering into detailed techniques, we might examine some representative examples of the different methods of purification, as outlined below:

1. Nonspecific methods
   (a) Precipitation with neutral salts ("salting out")
   (b) Chromatographic fractionation
   (c) Ethanol fractionation
   (d) Enzymatic digestion

2. Specific methods
   (a) Dissociation with 15% NaCl (antipolysaccharides)
   (b) Dissociation in acid pH (antiproteins)
   (c) Dissociation by means of haptens
   (d) Immunoadsorbents.

Nonspecific Methods. Precipitation with neutral salts (salting out) is a frequently used method employing ammonium sulfate and sodium sulfate as the preferred salts. When the aim is to precipitate the total globulin fraction, ammonium sulfate at a saturation concentration of up to 50% or sodium sulfate in a 22% concentration (at 37 °C) can be added to the serum. Sometimes, however, there is an advantage in separating only the fraction that precipitates between 33% and 50% saturation; this is easily obtained in the following manner: (1) Add to 2 volumes of serum, 1 volume of saturated ammonium sulfate solution (hence 33% saturated). Centrifuge. The precipitate contains the fraction called "euglobulin," insoluble in distilled water and composed predominantly of gamma globulin (IgG). (2) To the supernatant (approximately 3 volumes), add 1 additional volume of saturated ammonium sulfate to produce a 50%-saturated solution. The "33%–50%" precipitate contains significant quantities of gamma globulins plus most of the beta globulins (IgA, IgM).

In the sera of horses hyperimmunized with toxins, the antitoxins are concentrated principally in the "33%–50%" fraction, which can also be obtained by precipitation with semisaturated ammonium sulfate, followed by dialysis of the precipitate against distilled water. Under these conditions, the "euglobulins" precipitate, leaving only the "pseudoglobulins" in solution. Salting out does not permit satisfactory separation of the different globulins identified by electrophoresis. However, although the fractions obtained by salting out may indeed be impure and reveal numerous components upon electrophoresis, there is relative purification, for certain components predominate (Table 4.1).

Greater purification is achieved through chromatography in diethylaminoethyl (DEAE) cellulose. If the serum, or the serum fraction obtained through salting out, is eluted with 0.02 M phosphate buffer, pH 8.0, the IgG can be obtained in a nearly pure form.

In alkaline pH, the ionization of DEAE cellulose decreases and the ionized proteins (Pr-COO$^-$) are eluted in ascending order of

Ammonium sulfate, % saturated	Sodium sulfate, % saturated	Characteristic components	% of total proteins	g/ml plasma
25	10	Fibrinogen	3	0.2
34	15	γ globulins	20	1.4
40	19	γ, β	15	1.0
50	27	α, β, A	14	1.0
70	–	Albumin	46	3.4

Table 4.1. Human serum fractions obtained by "salting out" and their relation to components identified by immunoelectrophoresis

their electrophoretic mobilities (γ, β, α, and albumin).

$$RN^+H(C_2H_5)_2 \cdot Pr-COO^- \xrightarrow{\text{NaOH}}$$
$$(DEAE^+)$$
$$RN(C_2H_5)_2 + Pr-COO^-Na^+$$
$$(DEAE)$$

Among the chromatographic methods, we might also mention gel filtration and affinity chromatography.

In gel filtration, dextran (Sephadex), agarose (Sepharose) or polyacrylamide (Biogel) is used. The Sephadex beads are obtained from fractions of dextran with distinct gradations of cross-linkages, having greater or lesser capacity to swell (take up more or less water), thus permitting the separation of molecules of different sizes. Beads are prepared with varying porosities, from G 10 to G 200. The former have an inhibition capacity of 1 ml/g and permit penetration only by molecules below 700 daltons; the G 200 beads absorb 20 ml/g and permit penetration by molecules up to 800,000 daltons. For column chromatography, the Sephadex grains are first swollen in water and then, under appropriate pressure (without provoking the formation of air bubbles) are poured into the column. The large molecules pass directly into the liquid surrounding the beads (void volume, V_o), whereas the small molecules penetrate through the beads (inner volume V_i). The large molecules must only traverse the distance V_o, whereas the elution volume of the small molecules is equivalent to the sum of $V_o + V_i$. Therefore, the molecules are eluted in the order of their size. However, this observation is true only for gel particles that completely exclude or completely absorb a substance, i.e., when the molecules are dispersed either completely within the beads (dispersion coefficient $K_d = 0$) or outside ($K_d = 1$) them. Because K_d can vary from 0 to 1, the general equation for the elution volume is $V_e = V_o + V_i \times K_a$. A gel with small pores, e. g., G 10 or G 25, is particularly suitable for the exclusion of electrolytes (substituting for dialysis),

whereas G 100 to G 200 permit the separation of macromolecules, e.g., IgG and IgM. Gel filtration and ion-exchange chromatography can be combined, e.g., with DEAE-Sephadex or CM-Sephadex.

Sepharose is used principally for the separation of large molecules such as DNA, RNA, viruses, and polysaccharide polymers, and is also useful as a matrix for the immobilization of ligands through chemical groupings that are coupled on the dextran beads, such as cyanogen bromide, 6-aminohexanoic acid, and others. The preparation called "Sepharose 4 B activated with CNBr" is particularly useful for the direct coupling of proteins or of other molecules that contain amino groups. After the coupling of an antigen, it is possible through affinity chromatography to bind the corresponding antibody and to isolate it by elution, and vice versa.

Fractionation with ethanol, introduced by Cohn and associates (1940) for the separation of the human plasma proteins, is performed through gradual addition of ethyl alcohol in varying concentrations and pH levels, and at a temperature close to that of the freezing point of the mixtures, in order to avoid the denaturation of the proteins (Table 4.2). Cohn's method is commonly used for fractionating proteins on an industrial scale to obtain two fractions of great therapeutic importance: albumin (fraction V) and gamma globulin (fractions II, III). In the latter case, fractionation by ethanol is especially advantageous because it permits elimination or inactivation of hepatitis B virus. Only those donors should be chosen who are proved free from HB antigen.

Table 4.2. Fractionation of the plasma proteins by Cohn's method 6

Ethanol (%)	pH	Fraction	Principal components
8	7.2	I	Fibrinogen
25	6.8	II + III	β and α
40	4.8	V	Albumin

Deutsch described a variant technique for alcohol fractionation on a laboratory scale: The serum, diluted 1–4 in distilled water and then chilled to 0 °C, is combined with a 50% solution of alcohol previously chilled to $-20°$, under slow but continuous agitation, to a concentration of 20%, in order to maintain the mixture at a temperature near the freezing point ($-5°$ to $-6°$). The immunoglobulin precipitate (precipitate A) is resuspended in a buffer of 0.01 ionic strength, pH 5.1; ethanol at a concentration of 15% is then added. The IgA and IgM fractions remain soluble; the IgG fraction is precipitated with a yield of about 65% and at a purity of 90%–98%.

The technique of enzymatic digestion was developed empirically by Parfentjev (1936) and by Pope (1939); today it is utilized only for the purification of the antitoxins destined for therapeutic use. It consists essentially of the partial digestion of plasma with pepsin at pH 3.2, followed by thermocoagulation of the inert proteins (at 56 °C, pH 4.2) and by isolation of the digested antibody through precipitation with ammonium sulfate.

Specific Methods. The fact that the amount of antibody precipitated by pneumococcic polysaccharide of a given quantity was less when the reaction was carried out in 1.8 M NaCl than in 0.15 M NaCl, permitted Heidelberger and Kendall in 1936 successfully to dissociate pneumococcic antibody through the extraction of the specific precipitate with 15% NaCl. Antibody solutions with a purity of 80%–100%, which were homogeneous after electrophoresis and ultracentrifugation, could be obtained by this method – sometimes in relatively high yields (30% for horse antisera). The same method can also be applied to the purification of the anticardiolipin of syphilitic sera. Dissociation in 15% NaCl, however, does not permit the purification of antiprotein antibodies. In this case, other eluents are utilized, particularly acid buffers at pH 3.0.

Special reference must be made to the elution of antibodies by haptens, exemplified by the purification of antidinitrophenyl (DNP) antibodies by means of DNP-OH. In its general outlines, this method of purification, developed by Eisen, consists of the following steps:

1. *Precipitation* of the antibody by the hapten linked to a support protein different from that used to prepare the conjugate utilized in the immunization, e.g., anti-DNP prepared by immunization with DNP-BCG and precipitated with DNP-BSA.

2. *Dissociation* of the anti-DNP/DNP-BSA complex with DNP-OH, pH 5.0, in the presence of streptomycin. The DNP-BSA molecules, dislocated from their combination with anti-DNP by the competitive action of an excess of DNP-OH, because of their negative charge, are precipitated by the basic streptomycin molecule.

3. *Dialysis* to remove the DNP-OH.

4. *Passage* through a column of Dowex 1-RX ion-exchange resin, which permits removal of the remaining DNP-OH or DNP-BSA, leaving the anti-DNP antibody in a free state.

Most recently, immunoadsorbants have been successfully used for the purification of antibodies. This method was first utilized by Campbell in 1951 in the conjugation of diazotized proteins to p-aminobenzylcellulose. The antigen is bound to the insoluble immunoadsorbent-column and later eluted with an acid buffer. Identical results are obtained with protein antigens coupled by diazotization to polyaminostyrene or with insoluble polymers of protein obtained with ethyl chloroformate or glutaraldehyde.

Nature and Heterogeneity of Antibodies

Although it had long been known that the antibodies were contained in the globulin fraction of the serum, it was not until 1939 that Tiselius and Kabat identified them conclusively as gamma globulins:

1. In the *serum of hyperimmunized animals*, the electrophoretic peak corresponding to the gamma globulins exhibits abnormal elevation, being reduced to normal propor-

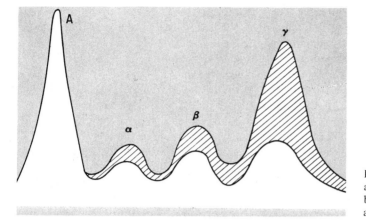

Fig. 4.7. Electrophoretic profile of an anti-ovalbumin rabbit serum before and after absorption of the antibody

tions in the supernatant of the antiserum after precipitation with the specific antigen (Fig. 4.7).

2. *Antibodies purified by specific methods* behave under electrophoresis in a similar fashion to the slow protein of the serum that Tiselius had previously termed gamma globulin.

Two years earlier, Heidelberger and Pedersen had studied the sedimentation rates of antibodies purified by ultracentrifugation and had established that certain antibodies, e.g., the pneumococcal antibodies of horses, cattle, and swine, sedimented rapidly (sedimentation constant 19 S, mol. wt. close to 900,000); others, however, such as human and rabbit pneumococcal antibodies, exhibited a 7 S sedimentation constant with a molecular weight of about 160,000. The former were identified as slow beta globulins (β_2), and the latter were called slow gamma globulins (γ_2).

Twenty years later, with the advent of immunoelectrophoresis, Grabar and associates demonstrated that what until then had been called gamma globulin in reality corresponded to a family of molecules that, although antigenically identical, possessed extremely diverse charges, imparting to them anodic mobility in alkaline pH (8.6), in a broad band that extended from the slow gamma (γ_2) to the slow alpha (α_2) region. They furthermore found that two other globulins, antigenically related but not identical

to the gamma globulins, exhibited antibody activity. These two globulins, which under immunoelectrophoresis appeared as distinct arcs of precipitation, were at first called β_{2A} and β_{2M}, and were later changed to γ_A and γ_M, with the γ_G designation being used for the classic gamma globulin.

Following the suggestion of Heremans, all proteins that exhibit antibody activity or that are antigenically related to the antibody molecules are collectively called immunoglobulins; as proposed by a group of experts of the World Health Organization, they are designated by the Ig abbreviation, e.g., IgG, IgA, IgM, IgD, and IgE.

Immunoglobulin Structure

The 7 S immunoglobulin molecule (mol. wt. 150,000) is composed of four polypeptide chains: two heavy chains (mol. wt. 50,000) and two light chains (mol. wt. 25,000), linked together by disulfide bridges (S-S) (Fig. 4.8). Two lines of research led to this conclusion: (1) separation of the chains by reducing agents; and (2) digestion of the immunoglobulin molecule by enzymes.

Separation of the Chains. In 1950, Porter investigated the number and the identity of the N-terminal amino acids in the 7 S immunoglobulin of the rabbit using the reaction with dinitrofluorobenzene and encountered only one N-terminal residue of alanine per mole-

Fig. 4.8. Structural model of the IgG molecule

cule. Consequently, he concluded that the molecule was composed of a single polypeptide chain. However, when the same technique was applied to the immunoglobulins of other species, different results were obtained (2 N-terminal residues for the human immunoglobulin and 4–5 for the horse immunoglobulin, for example), suggesting that in the rabbit the N-terminal ends of the other chains might have been blocked, perhaps by acetylation.

This caused Edelmen and associates in 1959 to attempt a technique for determining the number of peptide chains of the immunoglobulin molecule based on the reduction of the S-S bridges that covalently united the polypeptide subunits in numerous proteins. Under these circumstances, they showed that the molecular weight of the immuno-

globulin fell from 150,000 to 50,000; furthermore, chromatography of the reduced material revealed another subcomponent of lower molecular weight (25,000). Such a finding strongly suggested that in the rabbit immunoglobulin molecule there were four polypeptide chains: two with a molecular weight of 50,000 each, and two with a molecular weight of 25,000 each.

The experiments of Edelman and his associates were conducted in the presence of urea or guanidine. These substances acted as a denaturant, promoting the uncoiling of the peptide chain and the exposure of the intrachain S-S bridges; as a result, insoluble products that lacked any biologic activity were formed.

This inconvenience was overcome by Fleischman, Pain, and Porter in 1962 by reduction with mercaptoethanol at pH 8.2, followed by alkylation with iodoacetamide in order to avoid the reoxidation of the SH groupings, and by acidification with organic acids (acetic or propionic acid) to prevent the hydrophobic linkages and to confer positive charges upon the chains to impede their reassociation. Under these conditions, filtration in dextran gel (Sephadex G 75) equilibrated with acetic or propionic acid resulted in the distinct separation of two peaks – the former corresponding to the heavy chains and the latter to the light chains.

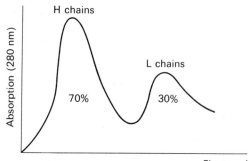

Fig. 4.9. Separation of H and L chains by Sephadex G 75 gel filtration. The gel was equilibrated with 0.1 M propionic acid. The protein was reduced and alkylated before being applied to the column

Separation of the H and L chains of the 7 S rabbit immunoglobulin

IgG (150,000)
↓
Reduction of the S-S bridges between the chains with mercaptoethanol pH 8.2.
↓
Blockage of the S-H groups with iodoacetamide
↓
Dialysis against 1.0 M propionic acid.
↓
Filtration in G 75 Sephadex equilibrated with 1.0 M propionic acid.

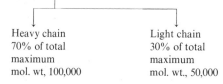

Heavy chain	Light chain
70% of total	30% of total
maximum	maximum
mol. wt, 100,000	mol. wt., 50,000

Under the experimental conditions used by Porter and others, the secondary structure of the chains is preserved because the mild conditions under which the reaction proceeds permit reduction of only four or five of the 20–25 S-S bridges that exist in the immunoglobulin molecule. Thus, only the S-S linkage points between the chains are attacked; points within the chains are not. The diagram at the end of this section shows the general outlines of the fractionation method used by Porter; Fig. 4.9 illustrates the peaks he obtained with gel filtration.

Since there was almost complete recovery of the heavy and light chains, with approximately 70% in the first peak (H chain) and 30% in the second peak (L chain), it was

possible to conclude by simple arithmetic that of the total molecular weight of the immunoglobulin, about 100,000 daltons corresponded to the heavy chain, and 50,000 daltons to the light chain. Moreover, since ultracentrifugation disclosed that the heavy chain had a molecular weight of 50,000 and the light chain a molecular weight of 25,000, it was concluded that the IgG molecule possessed two heavy chains and two light chains.

The manner in which these four chains are associated in the molecule was solved by enzymatic fragmentation experiments.

Enzymatic Fragmentation

In 1959, Porter subjected rabbit IgG to papain digestion in the presence of cysteine and verified that the sedimentation constant of the digested material fell from 7 S to 3.5 S, indicating a cleavage into fragments of about 50,000 daltons. When the digested material was dialyzed against a phosphate buffer at pH 7 and passed through a column of carboxymethylcellulose at pH 5.2, three peaks were separated. In the order of their elution (using a pH 5.2 acetate buffer gradient) they were designated fragments I, II, and III (Fig. 4.10). Fractions I and II possessed the activity of monovalent antibody, for they inhibited precipitation by the com-

Fab

I

II

Fc

III

Eluate, ml

Fig. 4.10. Chromatographic separation in CM-cellulose of papain-digested rabbit IgG. Elution with acetate buffer, pH 5.5, gradient from 0.1 to 0.9 M. The Fc fragments crystallize when dialyzed against a low-ionic strength buffer. Two-thirds of the total IgG correspond to the Fab, and one-third to the Fc

plete antibody; fraction III was biologically inactive. Upon dialysis of the digested product against a buffer of low ionic strength, fragment III crystallized. Fragments I and II were antigenically identical and came from IgG molecules with different mobilities, thus appearing in separate peaks. These are now called Fab (antigen-binding) fragments because of their ability to combine with antigens. Fragment III is designated Fc (crystallizable fraction). The antigenic relationships among fragments I, II, and III are illustrated in Fig. 4.11.

Nisonoff and his associates (1960), by digesting rabbit IgG with pepsin instead of papain, and in the absence of cysteine, showed that the molecular weight of the digested

product dropped to just 100,000 (5S), with the capacity for precipitation being preserved, which is a property of the bivalent antibody. If, in a second phase, cysteine was added, the molecular weight fell to 50,000 and precipitation no longer occurred, only inhibition of precipitation (monovalent fragment).

The monovalent pepsin fragments have a molecular weight slightly greater than that of the Fab fragment and thus were termed Fab′ fragments. Prior to the cysteine reduction, the two Fab′ fragments are united by an S-S bridge, forming a bivalent 5S fragment called the F(ab′)₂ fragment. The Fc fragment is not recovered by pepsin digestion because it is digested into smaller fragments.

Interpretation of the results of digestion by papain and by pepsin leads to the conclusion that the points of attack for the two enzymes are situated, respectively, to the left and to the right of the S-S bridges that unite the heavy chains (Fig. 4.12).

Relation Between Chains and Fragments. The relationship between the fractions obtained via reduction and the enzymatic fragments, which led to the currently accepted molecular model for the 7S immunoglobulins (see Fig. 4.12), was elucidated through gel precipitation experiments between anti-Fab sera or anti-Fc sera and the heavy and

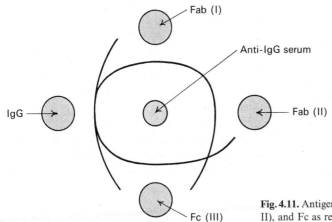

Fab (I)

Anti-IgG serum

IgG

Fab (II)

Fc (III)

Fig. 4.11. Antigenic relationships among IgG, Fab (I or II), and Fc as revealed by gel precipitation

Otto G. Bier and Dietrich Götze

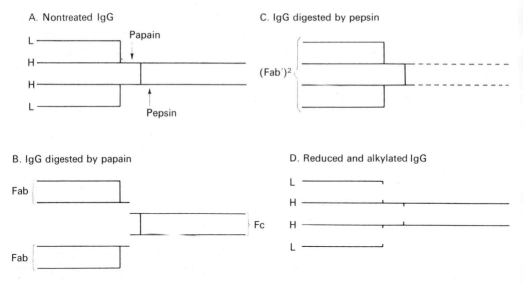

Fig. 4.12. Fragmentation of the immunoglobulin G molecule. IgG (mol. wt. 150,000), when digested by papain, produces three fragments of approximately 50,000 daltons each (2 Fab + 1 Fc). Digestion by pepsin leads to the destruction of Fc, leaving a divalent fragment (mol. wt. close to 100,000) designated (Fab′)$_2$. If the S-S bridges between the chains of IgG are reduced and the SH-groups are stabilized by alkylation, 2 L chains (mol. wt. 25,000) and 2 H chains (mol. wt. 50,000) are separated

light chains of the immunoglobulin (Table 3.3).

The results shown in Table 4.3 clearly demonstrate that the Fab fragment is composed of part of the heavy chain plus the light chain, whereas the Fc fragment is made up of the other part of the heavy chain not included in the Fab, i.e., not associated with the light chain.

Functions of the Fragments. The Fab fragments of the immunoglobulin molecule possess the antigen combining sites that enable the antibody to unite to the antigen in bivalent form; these must necessarily possess a large variety of forms, corresponding to the many antigenic determinants that come into contact with the organism. On contrast the

structure of the Fc fragment remains relatively constant within the same immunoglobulin class.

Among the multiple functions of the Fc fragment, the following merit special mention: the capacity of this fragment to bind complement and to produce cytotoxicity reactions; the capacity to become fixed to the tissues and to provoke anaphylactic reactions; the ability to adhere to macrophages and to make possible phagocytosis, and the ability to cross the placenta; the distribution of the antibody in the organism, in particular in the external secretions; and its catabolism index, which controls the blood level of the immunoglobulins.

Heterogeneity and Structure of the Chains. Simple immunoelectrophoretic analysis demonstrates that the immunoglobulins are composed of heterogeneous populations of molecules with highly different mobilities that, in the case of IgG, extend from the gamma region to that of the alpha-2 globulins (see Fig. 9.8).

This heterogeneity, typically observed with normal immunoglobulins, is much less evi-

Table 4.3. Reaction of anti-Fab and of anti-Fc with H and L chains

Antisera	H chain	L chain
Anti-Fab	+	+
Anti-Fc	+	−

dent in the pathologic proteins that appear in the serum of patients with myeloma–tumors of monoclonal plasma cells that produce immunoglobulins that are relatively homogeneous.

In cases of myeloma, special proteins called Bence-Jones proteins appear in the urine as fragments of the same pathologic proteins encountered in the serum [1]. Since these proteins occur in such large quantities, they are particularly useful for the study of the light chains, because they are composed of dimerized light chains with molecular weights of approximately 45,000.

The Bence-Jones proteins differ from one individual to another, yet when studied immunologically with rabbit antisera they have been found to fall into two groups, originally designated I (or B) and II (or A). Today, they are called "K" and "L," after the initials of the authors who studied them (Korngold and Lipari, respectively). The light chains that correspond to these two classes of proteins are termed κ (kappa) and λ (lambda). In the immunoglobulin molecule, the light chains can be either κ or λ, there being no hybrid molecules. In normal human serum, about two-thirds of the G immunoglobulins carry the κ chains, with the remaining one-third bearing λ chains.

The structure of the immunoglobulin chains can be analyzed by gel electrophoresis with amide or acrylamide gel. Under these conditions, the heavy chains normally produce a single, diffuse, slow band; the light chains are resolved into a number (7–10) of relatively rapid bands. Myeloma and Bence Jones proteins are relatively homogeneous, exhibiting a small number of light-chain bands.

The intrinsic heterogeneity of the normal immunoglobulins renders simple amino acid analysis even in purified preparations impossible. For this reason, the best approach to the solution of this problem is the use of monoclonal myeloma proteins or affinity-chromatographically purified antibodies or their fragments to determine the amino acid sequence. Studies of this sort have been undertaken principally with the Bence-Jones proteins of humans and mice.

Of the 214 amino acids that constitute the light chains, the N-terminal half (from 1 to 107) is variable (V_L), whereas the C-terminal half is constant (C_L), as exemplified in the following words:

$$\begin{array}{cc} V_L & C_L \\ \text{PHYSI} & \text{OLOGY} \\ \text{GYNEC} & \text{OLOGY} \\ \text{IMMUN} & \text{OLOGY} \end{array}$$

In these words, the first five letters represent the V_L region and the last five letters represent the C_L region.

Similarly, in the heavy chains, the first 110 N-terminal amino acid residues are variable (V_H), whereas the rest of the chains (3 or 4×110 residues, see below) are composed of constant segments (domains; C_H1, C_H2, C_H3) as represented in Fig. 4.13. The δ, γ, and α chains are composed of three segments, C_H1, C_H2, and C_H3, and the μ and ε chains, of four segments, C_H1, C_H2, C_H3, and C_H4. Structural studies and comparisons with the immunoglobulins of primitive fish suggest that the "primordial" C chain corresponds to the present-day μ chain with four homologous segments (domains); the shorter γ and α chains arose through the loss of the C_H2 (μ) domain during phylogenic development.

The homologous areas of the L_V and H_V region suggest the doubling of an ancestral gene during evolution, and that subsequent mutations led to the variable regions with antibody function and species-specific residues in the constant regions of the L and H chains.

Domains. Edelman suggested the subdivision of immunoglobulin molecules into domains, on the basis of homologous regions. According to the domain hypothesis, the antibody molecule consits of compact regions (domains) of 102 to 110 amino acids that are stabilized through S-S chemical

---

1 Described in 1847 by Dr. H. Bence-Jones in the urine of a patient with myeloma, these proteins are characterized by the fact that they coagulate at 50°–60 °C at pH 4–pH 6; these proteins dissolve upon further heating, only to precipitate again upon cooling

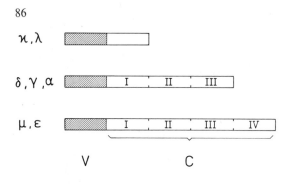

Fig. 4.13. Length of different Ig chains. The variable (V) regions of all types of chains have about 110 amino acids and approximately the same length. The constant region of the L chain consists of 1, the constant regions of the γ, α, and δ heavy chains of 3, and the constant regions of the μ and ε heavy chains of 4 homologous segments (domains), each consisting of about 110 amino acid residues. (Reproduced with permission from Hilschmann et al., 1978)

bond bridges and that engage in one or more functions:

1. *The L_V and H_V areas on the N-terminal of the Fab fragment,* which serve to bind antigens: The specificity of the antibody-combining site probably depends on the specific order of the amino acids in the hypervariable regions of this area, as well as on the variable angles between the V and C regions of the Fab fragments (quaternary structure).
2. *The C_H2 region,* to which complement binds.
3. *The C_H3 region,* which clings to receptors on macrophages or other cells.

These different functions and the corresponding domains for IgG are summarized in Table 4.4. The domain hypothesis offers a theoretical concept on which an understanding of the structural and functional characteristics of immunoglobulin can be based.

Chemical Structure of the Combining Site.
The chemical structure of the combining site of the antibody cannot yet be defined with

precision; it must await crystallographic studies that will establish its spatial structure. However, some facts are already well established:

1. The *maximum size of the combining site* may be inferred from its accommodation of molecules with the dimensions of a hexasaccharide or a hexapeptide; this approximates a molecular size similar to that of the molecule of the lysozyme substrate. In these molecules, 15–20 "contact amino acids" have been identified, and the same presumably holds true for the antibody combining site. If any residue can occupy one of these 15–20 positions, the possible number of variations is extremely large.
2. If the *constant regions of the immunoglobulin chains* of different species are compared, e.g., the λ chains of human and murine Bence-Jones proteins, identical amino acid residues occur in 44 positions. This finding indicates that during the phylogenic evolution, the C_L region remained extremely well preserved.

On the other hand, the amino acid sequences of the V_L regions of the same molecules are extremely similar, there being exactly three hypervariable regions, corresponding to positions 24–34, 50–56, and 89–97 (Fig. 4.14). Homologous hypervariable regions were shown in human H chains (area V_H) in positions 31–35, 50–65, and 95–102. These homologous, complementary areas together form the antigen binding site.

There are also variable residues on C_L. However, whereas in V_L, nonvariable glycine residues are in the majority, these residues in the C_L region consist primarily of hydrophobic amino acids. It appears that, during

Table 4.4. Functions of the domains of the immunoglobulin-G molecule

Domain	Verified or probable function
$V_H + V_L$	Antigen recognition (antigen combining site)
$C_H1 + C_2$	Noncovalent bond between L and H chains; S-S bridges between the distal Fd- and Fc ends
C_H2	Binding of CIg and control of catabolism
C_H3	Cytotropy for macrophages, lymphocytes, and mast cells. Noncovalent bond between the H chains

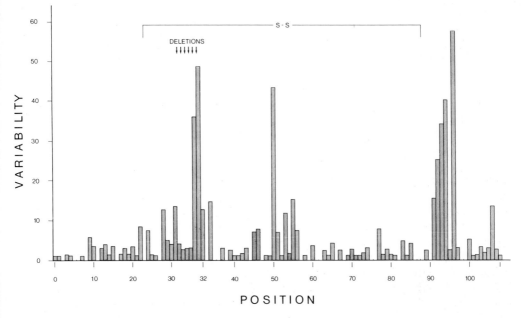

Fig. 4.14. Histogram of the variability of V_L chains. In V_L as well as in V_H chains, three hypervariable sections can be recognized between the positions 28–34, 45–56, and 91–98. (Reproduced with permission from Hilschmann et al., 1978)

evolution, certain regions of the V_L skeleton were unable to break free; consequently, the glycine was kept in a specific position (particularly in positions 99 and 101) in order to guarantee the necessary flexibility for adaptations on the antigenic determinants.

Sequence data also indicate that the three hypervariable complementarity-determining regions (CDR's) of human V_L are inserted between four framework (FR) segments which were remarkably preserved during phylogeny: FR 1, FR 2, FR 3, and FR 4, corresponding to residues 1–23, 35–49, 57–88, and 98–107, respectively. The sequences of each FR are grouped into different sets of 1–18 residues and the same set of FR 1, for example, can be associated with different sets of FR 2, FR 3, and FR 4. This led Kabat to the stimulating hypothesis that the complete framework for the L and H chains V-regions is assembled during ontogeny from sets of minigenes for each FR segment. A considerable degree of diversity is generated by this assembly of FR pieces from different FR segments and if we con-

sider further that the positions corresponding to the hypervariable CDR's may be occupied by any one of 20 possible amino acids, the number of resulting specificities is largely sufficient to cope with the epitopic universe.

Affinity-Labeling Technique. The so-called affinity-labeling technique is particularly suitable for defining the structure of the combining site. With this technique, a labeled, chemically modified hapten, which through an additional reactive group (e.g., diazonium-, bromacetyl-, or arylnitro-bindings) is capable of forming a covalent bond on or near the combining site, is added to the antibody. Then the amount of labeled hapten in the peptides, which is maintained through hydrolysis of the antibody (H and L chains), is determined. Finally, the amino acid sequence of the labeled peptide is determined.

The principle of the method can be shown schematically as follows:

$$B(y) + H^{\star}(x) \rightarrow B.y - x.H^{\star},$$

in which B is the antibody combining site, H*, the labeled hapten, y and x are the structures that lie in or near B or H* and that form a stable B.y − x.H* complex through a covalent bond.

Certain controls must be considered: (1) the absence of labeled haptens in nonspecific immunoglobulins and (2) inhibition of labeling through previous administration of unmarked haptens.

The total results of such experiments with different antibodies and labeling agents support the hypothesis that tyrosine and lysine residues in the hypervariable regions of the V_H and V_L domains play a primary role in the specific binding of the antigen.

Classes and Subclasses of Human Immunoglobulins

The human immunoglobulins are presently divided into five classes, designated IgG, IgA, IgM, IgD, and IgE (Fig. 4.15). They are characterized by specific antigenic determinants in their heavy chains, respectively designated by the Greek letters γ (gamma), α (alpha), μ (mu), δ (delta), and ε (epsilon). The light chains are identical in all classes; κ (kappa) and λ (lambda).

Since the immunoglobulin molecules possess two heavy chains and two light chains, IgG is expressed as $\gamma_2\kappa_2$, or $\gamma_2\lambda_2$, and IgA as $\alpha_2\kappa_2$ or $\alpha_2\lambda_2$, and so on.

To differentiate the classes, rabbit antisera are used that have been absorbed with immunoglobulins of classes different from those used for immunization, e.g. anti-IgG antiserum absorbed with IgM (specific for the γ determinant); or vice versa, anti-IgM absorbed with IgG (specific for the μ determinant).

IgG. Immunoglobulin G, which is quantitatively the major serum immunoglobulin (ca. 1,300 mg-% compared to 160 or 90 mg-% for IgA and IgM, respectively), has four "subdeterminants" on its Fc part (1, 2, 3, and 4) that characterize four subclasses (IgG$_1$, IgG$_2$, IgG$_3$, and IgG$_4$). Rabbit

antiserum used to differentiate these subclasses is produced with a myeloma-G antigen and is absorbed with other IgG myeloma proteins. The chief characteristics of the different classes of human immunoglobulins and the particulars of the IgG subclasses are summarized in Tables 4.5 and 4.6.

IgG (with the exception of IgG$_4$) and IgM, but not the other immunoglobulins, have the ability to fix Clq – a bond that appears to occur on the C_H2 domain. Except for IgG$_2$, IgG can also bind to heterologous skin, thereby inducing the anaphylactic reaction. Only IgG can pass through the placenta and bind to macrophages. This bond occurs in the middle of the C_H3 domain and, in contrast to the binding of opsonizing IgG and IgM antibodies, it is independent of any previous antigen binding.

IgM. IgM (M stands for macroglobulin) consists of a pentamer whose 7S units are held together by a peptide of about 25,000 daltons, called the "J" (junction) chain. This peptide consists of a single amino-acid chain with a high content of cysteine (12 residues) and asparagine, and is also involved in the formation of IgA polymers by an as yet unknown mechanism.

Immunoglobulin M has a molecular weight of about 900,000 and a somewhat greater electrophoretic mobility than IgA, IgD, and IgE. The heavy chain is composed of four homologous segments (domains): $C_\mu3$ has a cysteine in position 102 that mediates the binding of the IgM subunits to pentamers (Fig. 4.16). IgM is much more active than IgG in the Clq binding; a single molecule suffices for the sensitization of an erythrocyte.

Theoretically, IgM should have a valence of 10. However, this occurs only with small hapten molecules such as DNP. In most cases, for stereochemical reasons, only five antigen molecules can be bound (steric hindrance).

IgA. Immunoglobulin A usually circulates in monomeric (7S) and dimeric (9S) forms,

CLASSES   CHAIN -TYPES

IgG1		γ_1	$\varkappa,\lambda$
IgG2		γ_2	$\varkappa,\lambda$
IgG3		γ_3	$\varkappa,\lambda$
IgG4		γ_4	$\varkappa,\lambda$
IgA1	$[\quad]_n$	α_1	$\varkappa,\lambda$
IgA2	$[\quad]_n$	α_2	$\varkappa,\lambda$
IgD		δ	$\varkappa<\lambda$
IgE		ε	$\varkappa,\lambda$
IgM	$[\quad]_5$	μ	$\varkappa,\lambda$
		H	L

Fig. 4.15. Immunoglobulin classes and subclasses. The class or subclass of an antibody molecule is determined by the nature of the H chain. The different H chain types are distinguishable by their amino acid sequences and by the number of their interpeptidal disulfide bridges (vertical lines). L chains can be of λ- or κ-type. The complete structure of IgG, IgM, IgA$_1$, and IgE is known. The other molecules represent tentative structures which are sometimes only based on the analyses of disulfide-containing peptides. In one allotype of the IgA$_2$ subclass, the L chains are not covalently linked to the H chains but are linked to each other. The specificity is determined by the V parts (----). (Reproduced with permission from Hilschmann et al., 1978)

Table 4.5. Physicochemical and biologic properties of the different classes of human immunoglobulins

Properties	IgG	IgA	IgM	IgD	IgE
Average concentration in serum mg/ml[a]	13.1	1.6	0.9	0.12	0.33×10^{-3}
Sedimentation coefficient (S)	7	7	19	7	8
Mol. wt. 10^3	160	170[b]	900	185	185
Carbohydrate (%)	2.9	7.5	11.8	13	12
J chain	−	+	+	−	−
Lability at 56 °C	−	−	−	−	+
Mercaptoethanol resistance	+ +	±	−	+ +	−
Isotypic determinants	$\gamma1, \gamma2,$ $\gamma3, \gamma4$	$\alpha1, \alpha2$	μ	δ	ε
Allotypic determinants					
Gm (H chains)	+	−	−		
Inv (L chains)	+	+	+		
Synthesis (mg/kg/day)	28	8–10	5–8	0.4	
Catabolism (%/day)	3	12	14		2.5
Half-life (days)	23	5.8	5.1	2.8	2.5
Agglutinating activity	1	−	100		
Fixation of complement	+	−	+	−	−
Transplacental passage	+	−	−	−	−
Binding to macrophages	+	−	−	−	−
Binding to mast cells[c]	−	−	−	−	+
Reaction with staphylococcus A protein	+	−	−	−	−
Reaction with rheumatoid factor	+	−	−	−	−

[a] According to Johansson, 1967
[b] Secretory IgA is a dimer and is associated with a secretory piece. Secretory IgA has a molecular weight of ca. 390,000, that is, the sum $(2 \times 170,000) + 58,000$ (secretory piece)
[c] IgG$_1$, IgG$_3$, and IgG$_4$ bind to xenogeneic skin (see Table 6.6)

Table 4.6. Principal properties of human IgG subclasses

Property	IgG$_1$	IgG$_2$	IgG$_3$	IgG$_4$
% Total IgG	67	24	6	3
% in IgG myeloma	77	14	6	3
Half-life (days)	23	23	8	23
Fixation of complement	+ +	+	+ + +	0
Placental passage	+	+	+	+
Hetero-PKA (gumea pigs)	+	0	+	+
Homo PKA				
Macrophage cytophilia	+	0	+	0
S-S bridge between H chains	2	4	5	2
Reactivity with staphylococcus A protein	+	+	0	+
Gm allotypes	Many	Many	1 (No. 23)	0

but also occurs as 11 S and 13 S polymers. The units of this chain are connected by the J chain. Like the other immunoglobulins, IgA also has a carbohydrate part that is about three to four times larger than that on the IgG.

IgG and IgM are found in small quantities in secretions, e.g., saliva, tears, intestinal secretions, and colostrum; however, IgA, particularly IgA$_1$, is the predominant immunoglobulin in these secretions. Secretion IgA has a molecular weight of approximately 390,000 daltons. In 1963, Tomasi showed that two 7 S units are held together by an additional glycoprotein, mol. wt. 58,000, the "secretion piece" or "transport piece." This component is excreted from epithelial cells of the mucosa or from exocrine glands. Apparently, it confers a protection against proteolytic enzymes and assures the passage of secretory IgA synthesized in subepithelial regions to the surface of the mucous membranes (Fig. 4.17).

Although IgA does not bind complement and has no bactericidal effect, it is thought to play an important role in the localization

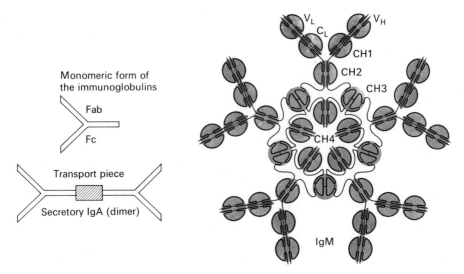

Fig. 4.16. Structural forms of immunoglobulins: IgG is monomeric; IgA exists in mono-, di-, tri-, and tetrameric forms; and IgM is pentameric. (IgM is reproduced from Hilschmann et al., 1978)

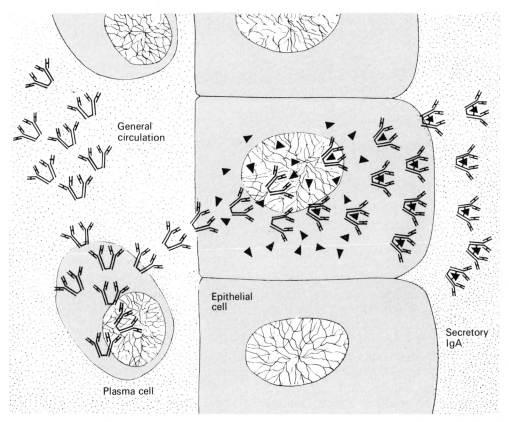

Fig. 4.17. Synthesis and transport of secretory IgA (Adapted from Tomasi, 1970)

of certain infectious agents (e.g., influenza and polio viruses on the mucous membranes of the intestine or the nose) and in the neutralization of some bacteria toxins.

IgD. This immunoglobulin was discovered in 1965 in the serum of a myeloma patient; because of the low serum concentration, it had remained undiscovered. The discovery of IgD-myelomas made possible the isolation of a large enough quantity of the immunoglobulin to make a physico-chemical characterization. It is a 7S immunoglobulin with a high carbohydrate portion, whose H chain has a molecular weight of about 70,000 daltons and is bound by a single disulfide bridge. No antibody activity can be assigned to this immunoglobulin. New findings concerning IgD specificities against specific antigens (nucleoproteins, insulin) are questionable. It should be emphasized that

IgM as well as IgD is found on the surface of lymphocytes, particularly in cases of lymphatic leukemia (see p. 11).

IgE. IgE corresponds to the reaginic antibody responsible for the PK test. It was identified as a distinct immunoglobulin in ingenious studies performed by Ishizaka and associates (1966): Rabbits were immunized with the serum of a patient sensitive to ragweed pollen. The antisera obtained were absorbed with immunoglobulins G, A, M, and D. The "empty" antiserum could contain only antibodies against immunoglobulins not belonging to these four classes, presumably against the immunoglobulins associated with the reaginic activity (later called IgE).

When the "empty" antiserum was mixed with a reaginic-rich serum (R), the supernatant lost the capacity to give a positive

Fig. 4.18. Demonstration of the reaginic (IgE) antibody by gel precipitation and autoradiography

PK test – which had been strongly positive with the untreated R serum.

Furthermore, if a mixture of "empty" (anti-IgE) antisera plus labeled antigen (^{131}I) was located in the central well of an Ouchterlony plate, and IgG, IgA, IgM, IgD, and R were placed in the peripheral wells, a line of precipitation developed only between the anti-IgE and the R wells (Fig. 4.18). After careful washing of the plate and subjecting it to autoradiographic examination, the radioactivity was located about the line of precipitation.

The three facts just mentioned (specific immunoprecipitation, inactivation of PK activity in the supernatant after precipitation,

and localization of radioactivity in the precipitation line) led Ishizaka and his associates to postulate that the reaginic antibodies were identical to a new immunoglobulin class (IgE) and not with IgA, as previously thought.

The later discovery of an atypical IgE-producing myeloma permitted the physicochemical study of the immunoglobulin and the elucidation of its structural characteristics (Fig. 4.19): (1) a molecular weight of approximately 200,000 daltons, arising from the fact that their heavy chains weigh 75,000 daltons and not 50,000 daltons as with IgG, because, like the Hμ chain, they have four C domains; (2) a sedimentation

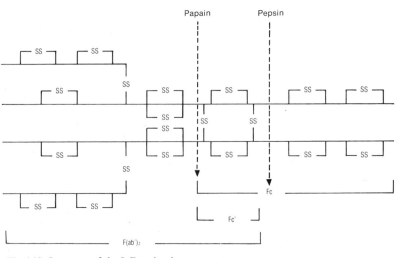

Fig. 4.19. Structure of the IgE molecule

constant of 8 S; (3) an abundance of carbo-hydrate (11%), methionine, and SH groups; and (4) thermolability at 56 °C after 4 h, probably due to destruction of a structure contained in the Fc part, which ensures fixation of the immunoglobulin into the masto-cyte surfaces (C_H4 domain). Its serum level is low (like that of IgD) and its activity is revealed by the PK test. Because its serum concentration in most cases lies in the range of picograms to nanograms, it can be proved by precipitation only in exceptional cases. To determine its presence, the PK test or special methods are used.

former migrating more rapidly in immunoelectrophoresis. These two fractions are designated as IgG_1 and IgG_2 in the guinea pig, and as IgG_1 and IgG_{2a} in the mouse. They differ in biological properties in regard to complement fixation ($\gamma_1 -, \gamma_2 +$) and to passive sensitization of homologous skin ($\gamma_1 +, \gamma_2 -$) (cf. Chap. 10). Studies on the mouse immunoglobulins have been greatly facilitated by the availability of myeloma proteins produced by the intra-peritonial injection of mineral oil in BALB-c animals. With the exception of IgI (γ_3), myeloma proteins and antibodies of all classes have been found (Table 4.7).

Classes and Subclasses of Animal Immunoglobulins

Horse. In the sera of horses immunized with bacterial exotoxins (diphteria, tetanus) or snake venoms *(Crotalus, Bothrops)*, two major types of antibodies have been identi-fied: the usual IgG of a slow β_2 mobility and an antibody of faster mobility (α_2 or β_1), termed the T component or IgG(T) (cf. p. 201). The main antibody in horse anti-pneumococcal sera is of the IgM type, but on continued immunization IgA and IgG(T), as well as slow IgG are also found. Equine anti-LAC(lactosyl) antibodies could be separated chromatographically on DEAE-cellulose into two slow β_2 fractions (IgGa, -b) and IgGc, of a faster mobility starting in the α_1 region, like IgA.

Rodents. Benacerraf et al. have identified in guinea pig and mouse antibodies to DNP-proteins two fractions termed γ_1 and γ_2, the

Genetic Markers of the Immunoglobulins: Allotypes and Idiotypes

It was long believed that the immunoglobulins possessed only isotopic antigenic specificities, i.e., specificities common to their own species.

In 1956, however, Oudin showed that specificities, termed allotypes, could be identified with the help of alloantisera produced by immunization of one rabbit with immunocomplexes or immunoglobulins of another rabbit. These allotypic determinants from protein molecules (not necessarily immunoglobulins) were inherited according to simple Mendelian rules[2]. With minor differences, they correlate in the amino acid sequences.

---

2 Todd's surprising observation that allotypic specificities of the system occur on the H chain of IgG as well as on those from IgM and IgE, necessitated the assumption that there the gene for isotypic and allotypic specificities is translocated

---

Table 4.7 Nomenclature of animal immunoglobulins

Species	Classes or subclasses of immunoglobulin						
Horse	IgM	IgA	IgG a	IgG b	IgG c	IgG (T)	
Mouse	IgM	IgA	IgF (IgG_1)	IgG (IgG_{2a})	IgH (IgG_{2b})	IgI (IgG_3)	IgE
Guinea pig	IgM	IgA	IgG_1	IgG_2			IgE
Rat	IgM	IgA	IgG_1	IgG_2			IgE
Rabbit	IgM	IgA	IgG	IgG_2			IgE

In the rabbit at least five systems of allotypic markers are recognized – a (H chain, variable region), b (κ chain, variable region), c (λ chain, variable region), d (γ chain, C_H2 domain), and e (γ chain, hinge):

V_H	a_1	a_2	a_3
V_κ	b_4	b_5	b_6	b_9
V_λ	c_7	c_{21}	
C_γ	d_{11}	d_{12}	e_{14}	e_{15}.

Each system is determined through multiple alleles of different loci, e.g., a^1, a^2, b^4, b^5, and each animal shows a minimum of two, and a maximum of four, allotypic specificities. At the molecular level, however, only two alleles are expressed, so that both H and L chains always carry the same allotype (allotypic restriction). If the animal is a homozygote, e.g., $a^1a^1b^4b^4$, only molecules of allotypes a^1b^4 are synthesized. However, if it is a heterozygote, molecules of different allotypes can be synthesized, e.g., for the genotype $a^1a^2b^4b^5$, the allotypes a^1b^4, a^1b^5, a^2b^4, and a^2b^5, so that four allotypic specificities can be found in the serum.

Thus far, numerous allotypic variations have been described in man, in the heavy chains (Gm factors) as well as in the light chains (Inv factors). The Gm (gamma globulin) factors, described by Grubb, number 23 and are located in the Fc or Fd fragments of the IgG molecule, most often in specific subclasses. Thus, Gm groups 1, 2, 3, 4, 17, and 22 are located in the IgG_1 subclass; group 23 exclusively in IgG_2; and groups 5, 6, 10, 11, 14, and 21 in IgG_3. Subclass IgG_4 does not possess any known Gm determinant.

There are three Inv factors (In from "inhibitor" and v from the patient's initial), and they occur in the kappa chains of all of the immunoglobulin classes. The specificity of the Inv determinants depends upon the substitution of a unique amino acid in position 191 of the kappa chains – leucine for Inv 1 and valine for Inv 3 [3].

In addition to the Gm and Inv systems, there is the ISF (San Francisco) system, of which a single determinant is known, localized in the Fc fragment of IgG_1.

The Gm groups are identified by the inhibition reaction in a system composed of Rh(D)-positive erythrocytes, incomplete anti-Rh(D) serum, sera from rheumatoid arthritis patients containing antigamma globulin (rheumatoid factor, RF), and the immunoglobulin whose Gm allotype is sought to be determined. If the allotype of the immunoglobulin under examination is identical to that of the anti-D immunoglobulin, RF agglutination is inhibited (Fig. 4.20).

3 In the chains that have no Inv specificity, the amino acid 191 is serine, and amino acid 153, alanine. In λ chains, position 191 contains either lysine (O^+) or arginine (O^-) and position 154, serine (Kern$^-$) or glycine (Kern$^+$)

Fig. 4.20. Method for detecting human IgG allotypes

Obviously, it is not possible to use any anti-D and any anti-RF, but only the combinations that correspond to the same specificity.

In addition to the allotypes, Oudin demonstrated that specific individual determinants, or idiotypic determinants, exist in rabbits. Although allotypic specificities are encountered in normal immunoglobulins and in certain groups of individuals, the specificities termed idiotypic can be demonstrated only in the antibodies of certain individuals. Such specificities persist even after repeated absorption with the antibodies of the same subclass and allotype, appearing thus to be related not only to the sequence of amino acids in the variable regions of the heavy and light chains, but also to the quaternary structure of the combining site.

Electron-Microscopic Studies of the Antibody

Valentine and Green verified that the soluble complexes formed by rabbit IgG from antidinitrophenyl (DNP) with di-DNP-octamethylendiamine [DNP-NH-$(CH_2)_8$-NH-DNP], when examined under the electron microscope, exhibit predominantly triangular or rhomboidal designs with lateral extensions at their corners (see Fig. 4.21).

The length of the sides of these geometric figures is about 120 Å i.e., twice the length of the Fab fragment (the antigen is disregarded because of its extremely small size and its position within a cavity of the antibody). The lateral extensions are interpreted as Fc fragments: They do not appear in antigen-antibody complexes digested by pepsin. The flexibility provided by the hinge region permits considerable variation in the angle between the two Fab fragments connected to the same Fc fragment, permitting the formation of trimers, tetramers, and pentamers.

IgM antibodies, because of their relatively large dimensions, can be observed directly with the electron microscope in purified and concentrated preparations. They appear in the form of stars with a central "wheel" of 100 Å and five lateral "arms" of 125 Å Af-ter reduction and alkylation, the star-shaped structure disappears. Excellent electron photomicrographs have been obtained of IgM antibodies attached to viral particles (phages, polio viruses) or to the surfaces of erythrocytes.

Antibody Formation at the Gene Level

Antibodies are proteins with specific binding sites for any antigens, be they cells, bacteria, viruses, proteins, carbohydrates, in fact, almost all natural substances, provided they are macromolecules (see Chap. 3), and they are foreign or "non self" to the organism (see Chap. 6, 9 and 13).

Where does the information for the millions of antibodies which one individual can synthesize come from? This question has been fundamental since the foundation of modern immunology. The first theory proposed for the formation of antibodies was the "side-chain" theory (1900) by Paul Ehrlich. He developed the idea that antibodies are preformed constituents of the cell surface which multiply under the influence of the antigen and are finally secreted into the blood plasma. This predetermination hypothesis was practically the only theory of antibody formation until the 1930s. Under the influence of the work of Landsteiner, who demonstrated that antibodies can arise even against antigens which normally do not exist in nature, an "instructive theory" became more and more accepted; according to this theory, the antigens act as a mold, or template, at some stage of the antibody formation. This theory reigned for about 25 years until Burnet, inspired by the ideas of Jerne (1955), formulated a new selection theory – the "clonal selection" theory – the essentials of which can be summarized thus: (1) mesenchymal cells, precursors of the cells that form antibodies, are made up of innumerable clones; (2) the clones capable of reacting with "self" components are eliminated (or suppressed) in the prenatal period; (3) the not-eliminated (or suppressed) clones specific for foreign substances react with the

Fig. 4.21. Formation of active immunoglobulin genes from germline DNA by somatic recombination and deletion

antigen fitting to the receptor, which leads to the proliferation of that clone (Fig. 4.4).

According to the theory of clonal selection, the sequence of the amino acids in antibodies of different specificities would be determined by the sequence of the nucleotides in the messenger RNA of the respective clone, which accordingly could form antibodies of a single specificity only. Experiments with isolated cells from animals immunized against three or four antigens have effectively shown that, indeed, single cells were capable of producing antibodies of only a single specificity (see above, p. 73).

The greatest problem for proponents of the clonal selection theory (as for any other previously formulated theory about antibody formation) was how to explain the extreme diversity of immunologically competent cells (generation of diversity = GOD). Thanks to the work of Susuma Tonegawa and his group in particular, this problem is almost solved today.

Organization of Immunoglobulin Genes and Their Expression

The capacity of the organism to form antibodies with a practically unlimited number of specificities presupposes the existence of a similarly unrestricted mechanism for the recognition of the respective immunogen. The differentiation of the lymphoid cells that leads to immunologic competence must at the same time generate a mechanism through which each immunologically competent cell becomes capable, when stimulated by the antigen, of forming immunoglobulins of the corresponding specificity.

There is evidence that this mechanism of diversification – which operates not only in relation to immunoglobulin class but also in relation to specificity of the combining site of the antibody – is genetically controlled; at least two pairs of cistrons[4] are responsible for the synthesis of each of the heavy and light chains. The cistrons for the heavy (H) and light (L) chains of the five classes of human immunoglobulins IgG, IgM, IgD, IgA, and IgE are indicated by $C_\gamma V_H$, $C_\mu V_H$, $C_\delta V_H$, $C_\alpha V_H$, and $C_\varepsilon V_H$; the cistrons for the kappa and lambda chains are termed $C_\kappa V_\kappa$ or $C_\lambda V_\lambda$, respectively.

There is experimental evidence from amino-acid-sequence analysis of myeloma proteins for the hypothesis that the DNA segments responsible for the coding of the constant and variable regions unite at specific areas in order to build a cistron, so that a single mRNA is produced that codes for the amino-acid-sequence of the entire chain. These genetic regions which are not linked to each other and which can even be on separate chromosomes, are called "translocon" regions. At least three translocon areas, termed κ, λ, and H, which form the cistrons for the κ, λ, and H chains have been postulated. The V and C segments are supposed to arise from different gene structures, corresponding to the L and H subgroup chains that differ in the composition of the first 23 amino acids. The V and C regions involved in the coding of human immunoglobulins are summarized in Table 4.8.

DNA cloning and sequence studies have now confirmed this hypothesis which was formulated on the basis of amino-acid-sequence data from many myeloma proteins in the mouse, and from the inheritance and

Table 4.8. System for genes important in coding for human immunoglobulin

Translocon	V subgroup gene	C gene
$\varkappa$	$V_\varkappa I$–III	$C_\varkappa$
λ	$V_\lambda I$–V	C_λ Kern $-O_2+$
		C_λ Kern $+O_2-$
		C_λ Kern $-O_2-$
H	$V_H I$–IV	C_γ 1–4
		C_α 1, 2
		C_μ
		C_δ
		C_ε

occurrence of Ig-allotypes in man. There are three gene families (translocons), one for the λ light chain, another for the κ light chain, and a third for the heavy chains (μ, δ, γ_1, γ_{2b}, γ_{2a}, γ_3, ε, and α in the mouse). The three translocons are unlinked; the κ and H chain loci of the mouse have been found to reside on chromosomes 6 and 12, respectively (Fig. 4.21).

Lambda Chain Translocon. In contrast to the more complex kappa and heavy chain systems (see below), the mouse lambda translocon contains only one or very few germline V_λ genes separated from the C gene by a rather large DNA segment of about 4.5 kilobase (kb) pairs, and preceded a few base pairs apart by a leader (L) sequence. The V genes code only the 95 N-terminal amino acids; the remaining 13 amino acids (positions 96–108) of the light chain are encoded by a separate region, called the joining (J) region, about 1.2 kb pairs "upstream" from the C region. In the mouse, there is a second, very rare λ chain designated λ_{II}. $V_{\lambda I}$ and $V_{\lambda II}$ are closely related, while $C_{\lambda I}$ and $C_{\lambda II}$ are very different. Since there is no λ chain known of the composition $V_{\lambda I}C_{\lambda II}$ or $V_{\lambda II}C_{\lambda I}$, it is likely that λ_I and λ_{II} form two distinct loci. It is reasonable to suppose that the scarcity of λ chains in mouse immunoglobulin molecules ($\sim 5\%$) is related to the very small number of V_λ genes.

---

4 "Cistron" is defined as functional unit made from different structural genes, which codes for the entire amino-acid sequence of a polypeptide chain.

Kappa Chain Translocon. There is strong evidence from V_κ hybridization experiments and cloning of V_κ genes that there are up to 600 (or more) V_κ genes. It appears that there are several distinct subsets of V_κ, with V_κ genes more similar within subsets than between them; whether or not the gene subsets correspond to the subgroups defined from N-terminal amino acid sequences of polypeptides remains to be seen.

The available data indicate that each V_κ gene is separated from the next by an intervening noncoding DNA sequence (exons) of about 14 kb pairs. Each V_κ gene is also preceded by a leader sequence.

Cloning and subsequent sequencing of segments of embryonic DNA which included the kappa C gene and 4.5 kb pairs upstream from the C gene revealed five J segments. The J segments are in a cluster, separated from each other by about 300 base pairs; the nearest to the C gene is about 2.5 kb from it. Of the five J segments, examples of four can be found in known kappa protein sequences; the J_3 sequence is not found in any known protein.

V-C Joining. During lymphocyte maturation, DNA undergoes somatic rearrangment (translocation) which brings the V gene into precise alignment with the J gene but leaves the J-C intervening sequence intact (Fig. 4.21). Findings on nuclear precursor RNA suggest that the entire V-J-C genomic sequence is transcribed and the intervening sequences excised and deleted from the nuclear precursor RNA by RNA splicing, leaving a messenger RNA (mRNA) in which V, J, and C are contiguous. The intervening sequence within the leader peptide sequence preceding the V region is also removed by splicing. The exact mechanism of VJ recombination is not yet clear. However, DNA sequence analysis revealed that it involves deletion of the exons, and that two short conserved sequences 5' to each germline J_κ gene are inverse complements of sequences 3' to germline V_κ genes close to the point of recombination. These structures are thought to be recognized by joining enzymes.

Apparently, in the case of the kappa genes, any V_κ can reassort with any of the J segments (except maybe J_3); this increases the variability of the variable region at least fourfold since the J segment encodes part of the third hypervariable region of the light chain (see p. 87, Fig. 4.14). Furthermore, additional variation is introduced into the first J_κ codon (amino-acid residue 96): by adjusting the point of recombination within the three nucleotides which follow the V coding sequence and the three nucleotides of residue 96 in the five J segments, one can generate all residue 96 amino acids known in mouse myeloma kappa proteins. This is exemplified by the myeloma MOPC-41 V segment and J_1:

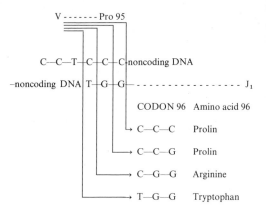

Since amino acid residue 96 is near or even at the antigen combining site, it is safe to assume that, in some cases at least, diversity generated by V-J joining can alter the antigen binding properties of immunoglobulins.

H Chain Translocon. The translocon for the H chains harbors the V_H as well as the C_H genes of all immunoglobulin classes and subclasses, although the localization of C_ε relative to the other C genes is not known. Here too, cloning of V_H genes lends strong support to the idea that there are at least 400 V_H genes arranged in tandem arrays, and again grouped into subsets; the V_H are separated by noncoding sequences of at least 14 kb, and preceded by a leader sequence. Comparison between the DNA sequence of a germline V_H gene and the corresponding rearranged sequence expressed in a myeloma has shown that the germline V_H segment ends at the sequence coding for the third hypervariable region before the end of the expressed V_H sequence. This suggested that the missing sequence should be found in J segments near the C_μ gene, which is first expressed during B-cell ontogeny. Indeed, the J segments were found about 8 kb upstream from C_μ, although they did not account for all of the third hypervariable region. This suggested that the missing residues are separately encoded in yet another set of genes termed D segments (for diversity). How many D segments exist is not known, but there are at least three. At least four J_H segments have been identified. Whether or not heavy chain diversity is fully accounted for by random combination of V, D, and J segments and codon variation at the joins of these segments ($> 400\ V_H \times 3\ D \times 4\ J_H = >4{,}800$) is controversial. Further diversity may arise from point mutations at the other two hypervariable regions during the differentiation of B lymphocytes, although one might also expect separate sets of sequences for these two regions.

The heavy chain constant region genes are aligned in the order μ (C_1, hinge, C_2, C_3, C_4), δ, γ_3, γ_1, γ_{2b}, γ_{2a}, ε, and α – for C_ε, see above –, C_μ being the first about 8.3 kb downstream from J_4. Each C_1 gene is preceded by a small sequence (S) involved in the switching mechanism (see below), and each gene for the terminal C domain is followed by two sequences separated by about 1.6 kb, the one coding for a piece of polypeptide typical of secreted proteins, and the other typical of membrane immunoglobulins.

Heavy Chain Switches. Unlike the light chains, for which there is only one C-region gene for each set of V regions, each heavy-chain V gene (V_H gene) may be expressed with any of eight different heavy-chain constant genes which define the different classes of immunoglobulin molecules. All V_H regions are first expressed with C_μ, but upon differentiation of lymphocytes into plasma cells the same V_H region may associate with any of the other C genes (heavy-chain class switch). Several hypotheses have been proposed to explain the mechanism of this switch, but the deletion model of Honjo and Kataoka now seems to be the most likely explanation, as evidenced by hybridization kinetics and gene counting with cloned probes. These investigations suggest that V-D-J first aligns with S-C_μ and then the intervening sequence is deleted; recombination between a switch site within the J-S element and one within the 5′ flanking sequence of another C_H gene relocates the active V-D-J gene, together with much of the J-S element, to a site near the C_H gene to be expressed next. It is not known whether a clone can switch more than once. The deletion mechanism for V/J joining and C_H switching has strong implications for immunoglobulin expression as it is an irreversible process. Therefore, the order of C_H gene expression becomes tied to the linear gene order.

In general, there is no simultaneous expression of two types of immunoglobulins, with the exception of IgM and IgD. In order to explain this in accordance with the deletion mechanism, one may expect to find that C_μ and C_δ are jointly transcribed and spliced in two different ways to generate μ and δ mRNAs with the same V_H region. The problem of allelic exclusion, i.e., that only the genes of one chromosome are expressed, cannot be explained yet.

The question of the generation of membrane-bound and secreted immunoglobulins which differ in the end portion of their terminal C domain has been resolved recently by showing that two chemically and functionally distinct mRNAs can be derived from a single C gene, apparently by alternative modes of RNA splicing.

How much diversity can be generated with all the enumerated gene elements? There are at least $>600\ V_\kappa \times 4\ J_\kappa = >2{,}400\ V_\kappa$ combinations which can be associated with any of $>4{,}800\ V_H$ combinations; therefore, one arrives at a number of $>1.15 \times 10^7$ different combining sites. Variations occurring at joining or switching segments are not counted.

In conclusion, the information for the antibody specificity is genetically determined and encoded in several hundreds of V genes which are linked to but separated from single C genes in the germline and stem cells. When multipotent stem cells possessing *all* genetic information for the synthesis of *all* specific antibodies divide and differentiate, translocation and fusion of V and C genes occurs. Probably, all V genes have an equal chance of fusing with their corresponding C gene. This differentiation process is antigen-independent and irreversible, an "inner" selection process which results in a differentiated and committed "virgin" B cell with a newly recombined DNA and the synthesis of *one* type of antibody with *one* specificity which is incorporated as receptor into the cell membrane (see Fig. 4.4; p. 74). There are as many different "virgin" B cell clones as there are antibody structures.

From the enormous number of different possibilities, the antigen selects that particular B cell which carries the corresponding receptor ("outer", clonal selection). The contact of the antigen with the receptor stimulates this cell; proliferation then leads to the formation of a clone of cells bearing the same determinant (clonal expansion). Finally, part of the B cells are transformed into plasma cells, which no longer have receptors but secrete antibodies. Some of the B cells undergo persistent multiplication and develop to "memory cells" which, at a second contact with the antigen, give rise to a stronger and faster immune reaction.

Regulation of Antibody Formation

The production of antibodies is modulated and regulated by the interaction of a series of factors associated with the immunizing antigen, the immunized organism, and the immune system itself.

Factors Relating to the Antigen

The nature of the antigen, its dosage, and the manner of administration, have a definite influence on the formation of antibodies, not only in connection with the quantity and type of the immunoglobulin produced, but also in respect to its affinity for the binding.

Influence of the Antigen on the Magnitude of the Immune Response. Under standardized experimental conditions, it is possible to determine the relative immunologic potency of different antigens. If one uses as a reference antigen a single 100 µg dose of bovine serum albumin (BSA) that produces a threshold immunogenic effect and compares it to the minimum doses necessary to achieve the same effect with other antigens, one sees that 10 µg bovine gamma globulin, 10^{-2} µg polymerized flagellin, and 10^{-9} µg *Salmonella* "O" antigen, respectively, have immunogenic potencies that are 10, 10^4, and 10^{11} times greater than that of BSA.

The principal parameters to which one might attribute these differences are molecular size, host capacity of the lymphoid system, and phylogenetic distance between the origin of the antigenic material and the reacting organism.

Molecular Size. Molecules below 10,000 daltons, such as glucagon (mol. wt. 2,500), insulin (mol. wt. 5,700), and protamines and histones (mol. wt. 6,000) are weakly immunogenic. The smallest known immunogen is hepta-L-lysine coupled by its α-amino group to a dinitrophenyl (DNP) group. Similar compounds with fewer than seven lysine residues are not immunogenic. At above 10,000 daltons, the protein molecules begin to exhibit distinct immunogenic activity that increases with the rise in molecular weight (Table 4.9).

Polysaccharides are less potent immunogens than are proteins unless polymerized to higher molecular weights. A typical example is dextran: In its native polydispersed form,

Table 4.9. Approximate molecular weight of protein antigens

Protein	Molecular weight
Ribonuclease	14,000
Myoglobin	17,000
TMV peptide[a]	17,000
Crotoxin[b]	30,000
Flagellin[c]	40,000
Ovalbumin	45,000
Diphtheria toxin	62,000
Serum albumin	69,000
γ-Globulin (IgG)	160,000
Octopus hemocyanin	2,800,000

[a] Tobacco mosaic virus protein
[b] Primary component of the Brasilian rattlesnake poison
[c] Monomeric form

with a molecular weight of tens of thousands of daltons, dextran possesses immunogenic power about 3.5 times greater than that of clinical dextran (mol. wt. $75,000 \pm 25,000$ daltons). Preparations degraded by mild acid hydrolysis that contain molecules from 35,000 to 50,000 daltons were only weakly immunogenic. When the molecular weight fell below 10,000 daltons, the immunogenic capacity was totally abolished.

Similarly, the meningococcic A and C polysaccharides used in prophylaxis of meningococcic meningitis only exhibit immunogenic activity when polymerized to a molecular weight of 150,000 daltons or more.

Ability to Lodge in the Lymphoid Organs. The capacity to localize in strategic regions of the lymphoid organs where they could be recognized by the immunocompetent lymphocytes, also constitutes an important characteristic of antigens. Factors favoring this localization are, for example, the particulate nature of the antigen (erythrocytes, bacteria, viruses, grains of pollen, etc.), and the existence in the organism of antibodies arising from previous immunization with the same antigen or with cross-reacting antigens.

Phylogenic Distance. Finally, the phylogenic distance between the antigen and the constituents of the immunized organism – or the degree of foreignness – is a characteristic with direct bearing on the antigen's immunogenicity. An organism is immunologically tolerant to its own constituents and, by extension, to those that are similar to them. For this reason, antigenic variants of the constituents of the organism that are present in different individuals of the same species (isoantigenic variations) are recognized as "self" and usually exercise only weak antigenic activity. An exception should be made only for certain antigens that control the transplantation of tissues (transplantation antigens) such as those determined by the H-2 locus in mice, or by the HLA region in man (cf. Chap. 6).

Influence of the Antigen on the Type of Immune Response. Aside from influencing the magnitude of the immune response, the antigen also determines the type of the response (cellular or humoral), and the type of immunoglobulin produced. Although the majority of antigens possess determinants capable of interacting with both T and B lymphocytes, certain antigens activate almost exclusively one or the other of these types of cells. Accordingly, pneumococcic polysaccharides stimulate only B lymphocytes, and consequently induce the formation of antibodies and the development of anaphylactic reaction of the immediate type, but not delayed-type hypersensitivity reactions. Conversely, oxasolone stimulates only T lymphocytes, inducing delayed hypersensitivity but not the formation of antibodies.

When referring to the preferential production of immunoglobulins, a discussion of the problem of successive synthesis of the immunoglobulins IgM and IgG is pertinent. Although the simultaneous presence of IgM and IgG in the same plasma cell is possible and can be shown by immunofluorescense, plasma cells usually do not synthesize the two concomitantly. From all indications, during immunization, a signal derived from

T helper cells diverts the process of synthesis from the production of IgM to that of IgG. The particulate antigens, such as erythrocytes, trypanosomes (not *Trypanosoma cruzi*), or the plasmodia of malaria, induce preferentially the synthesis of IgM, resulting in prolonged 19-S-antibody production. The antigens from helminths or from pollens, on the other hand, selectively stimulate the production of IgE. In respiratory virus infections, IgA antibodies are produced that appear in appreciable concentrations in the mucus in which they are secreted, but not in the blood.

Other examples suggestive of the influences of the antigen in relation to the type of immunoglobulin produced are the following: (1) The guinea pig, when immunized with the majority of antigens, produces varying quantities of IgG_1 and IgG_2, depending upon the adjuvant utilized and the manner of immunization. However, when immunized with the lipopolysaccharide of *Escherichia coli*, it produces only IgG_2. (2) Also in the guinea pig, the anti-DNP antibodies, which appear late in the course of immunization, carry only $\varkappa$ chains. (3) In guinea pigs, the antibodies against dextran and against teichoic acid belong predominantly to the IgG_2 subclass.

The interpretation of these facts remains problematic; yet the evidence suggests that certain antigens might selectively stimulate different subpopulations of lymphocytes involved in the syntheses of the different types of chains, from which the molecules of the different classes and subclasses of immunoglobulins are integrated.

Influence of the Antigen Dose on the Specificity and Affinity of Antibodies. Antisera produced after long periods of immunization contain a heterogeneous population of antibodies having specificities directed towards different antigenic determinants, and also having different affinities. These facts can be interpreted as a consequence of the simultaneous stimulation of distinct lymphocyte clones that correspond to different antigenic determinants — the latter possessing varying degrees of affinity.

This problem can be analyzed with greater clarity by considering the production of antibodies against a small dose of one monovalent immunogen, e.g., a hapten conjugate: Such an experiment shows that the antibodies formed constitute a relatively homogeneous population of immunoglobulins of high affinity ("perfect fit"), even though the quantity of antibody produced may be small. However, if we were to inject repeated doses of the same antigen over a long period of immunization, the affinity mediated by the antibodies, measured in terms of the occupation of 50% of the combining sites, would decline considerably. In complex antigens, e.g., large molecules carrying many antigenic determinants, the phenomenon is masked by the multiple uniting bridges provided by the antibodies directed against each determinant, which results in the formation of antigen–antibody (Ag-Ab) complexes that dissociate only with difficulty.

A mechanism of regulation exists, however, that permits the formation of antibodies of high affinity even after repeated antigenic stimulation. As immunization runs its course, the antigen, in addition to suffering excretion and metabolic degradation, undergoes a process of metabolic elimination; this occurs as the same antibodies formed in response to the antigen compete with the antigen in relation to the lymphocyte receptors. Because the quantity of antigen diminishes considerably; there is a concomitant increase in the availability of lymphocytes with high-affinity receptors – thus reestablishing conditions conducive to the formation of antibodies of heightened affinity. This mechanism is sometimes referred to as "the maturation of the immune response".

Factors Relating to the Organism

Of special note are age, nutritional state, and genetic factors.

Age. Generally speaking, young animals immunize poorly. This may be attributed to the immunologic incompetence of the lymphoid tissues not yet sufficiently differentiated, or it might be attributed to a deficiency in those mechanisms for capture and processing of antigens at the level of the dendritic and macrophage cells of the secondary lymphoid organs – particularly of the spleen and the lymph nodes (cf. Chap. 2 and 11).

Highly elucidating results in relation to the ontogeny of immunologically competent cells were obtained in sheep fetuses that had been immunized in utero. In this animal species, whose gestation period is 150 days, immunization of the fetus at 40 days only elicited production of antibodies against phages (detectable in minimum quantities). At 80 days, the animals began to demonstrate the capacity for rejecting allografts; and at 120 days, there was formation of antibodies against ovalbumin. For certain antigens, however, such as the flagellar antigen *Salmonella typhi*, antibodies were formed only when the immunization was performed after birth (cf. Chap. 1 and Fig. 1.18).

Similar observations were made in human-newborns, including premature individuals, in whom immunization even during the first day of extrauterine life provoked the formation of antibodies against the flagellar antigen *S. typhi*, but not against the flagellar antigens *S. paratyphi A* and *B*. The antibody produced was of the 19-S type, so as to exclude passive maternal transmission, which is found only with 7-S antibodies. Prophylactic immunization of infants is common within the first trimester of life (see Chap. 11).

Nutritional State. Clinical and experimental observations indicate that even in cases of grave nutritional deficiency, the production of immunoglobulins does not diminish. This has been verified, for example, in Kwashiokor, a syndrome observed in children with deficiencies in protein and certain amino acids, particularly methionine. Such children can have extremely low levels of albumin in their serum yet have normal or even augmented levels of immunoglobulins. From all indications, the diminished resistance to infections associated with nutritional deficiencies depends upon biochemical processes that affect nonspecific defense mechanism, but not the specific mechanisms involved in the synthesis of immunoglobulins.

Genetic Factors. Hereditary characteristics can significantly affect the production of antibodies, as demonstrated experimentally in many animals, and as observed naturally in man (see Chap. 6 and 13). In man, the influence of heredity can be exemplified by a condition known as atopy – by the incidence of certain allergic ailments due to a state of immediate hypersensitivity to inhalable antigens, foods, etc., associated with a particular class of immunoglobulins (see Chap. 10).

Experimental evidence accumulated over the last two decades clearly demonstrates that the production of antibodies (but also the generation of specific effector cells), or in other words, the recognition of antigens, depends upon genetic factors (see Chap. 6). The first evidence derived from experiments by Benacerraf in guinea pigs with polylysine as antigen (*PLL* gene); his observations were extended by McDevitt using another synthetic polypeptide as antigen in the mouse (*Ir*-gene). This genetic control of antigen recognition is regulated by the genes and their products of the *major histocompatibility complex (MHC)*, and will be described in detail in Chap. 6.

Factors Inherent to the Immune System

Immunologic Memory. Previous immunologic stimulation is without doubt among the most relevant factors in determining the magnitude and speed of the immune response. As a consequence of previous immunization, the number of cells in the lymphoid system capable of being stimulated by the antigen (memory cells) increases. Thus the secondary response sets in with greater rapidity and intensity, even in response to weaker concentrations of antigen. This phenomenon constitutes the basis for the "booster" immunization utilized routinely in immunoprophylaxis of toxic-infectious illnesses (cf. Tables 11.18–11.20).

Because memory cells include lymphocytes with considerable longevity (more than 1 year in the rat and more than 10 years in man), immunologic memory is frequently demonstrated after long periods of time. With regard to specificity, immunologic memory can manifest itself among macromolecules that are carriers of common antigenic determinants or among immunogens of similar configurations. In the first case, antibodies are produced only in relation to the common determinants, and, consequently, intensity of production varies according to the number of these determinants; the secondary response elicited by the determinants of similar configuration can result in the formation of antibodies against the original antigenic stimulus that is more intense than that against the antigen used in the second immunization.

In antigen conjugates (see Chap. 3), immunologic memory manifests itself not merely against the hapten, but also against certain carrier-protein determinants that otherwise are not necessarily contiguous with the implantation point of the hapten.

Feedback Control of Antibody Synthesis. As in numerous other biochemical processes, the synthesis of antibodies is inhibited by the products of its own reaction – the antibodies themselves. This phenomenon, called "feedback inhibition," is absolutely specific and can be reproduced easily by passive immunization with the homologous antibody or its $F(ab)_2$ fragment (or Fab). Evidently, there is competition for the antigen between the combining site of the antibody and the specific receptor on the lymphocyte surface. The covering of the antigenic determinants by the homologous antibody prevents further recognition of the antibody as "non-

self," a condition essential to the formation of antibodies.

IgM antibodies are capable only of inhibiting the synthesis of IgM, whereas IgG antibodies suppress the production of IgM as well as that of IgG. Antibodies of low affinity are incapable of inhibiting the synthesis of antibodies of high affinity because they do not compete efficiently with the lymphocyte receptors.

Theobald Smith demonstrated in 1909 in studies of the immunization of guinea pigs with mixtures of diphtheria toxin and antitoxin that antigen–antibody complexes with an excess of antibody have an inhibitory action; however, when there is an excess of antigen the immune response can even be enhanced by the adjuvant effect (phagocytosis of the complex and processing of the antigen). We shall see later that inhibition by feedback is utilized with success in the immunoprophylaxis of erythroblastosis fetalis (see Chap. II).

Idiotypic Network Interaction. Feedback inhibition as just described is a major expression of a sophisticated active regulatory system of homeostasis involving many more elements. We are still at the beginning in our understanding of this regulatory system. Before we briefly outline the essentials of the current concepts of immune regulation, we shall introduce the necessary terminology and the already known elements.

An antigenic determinant is called *epitope;* this is a certain structural patch on an antigen molecule that can be recognized with various degree of precision by complementary patterns of antibody combining sites *(paratopes)*. Antibody molecules themselves present epitopes to complementary paratopes. Epitopes of antibodies located at the constant parts of framework are called allotypes, those formed by the variable part are called idiotypes (see p. 93). Each single idiotypic epitope is called an *idiotope*. An idiotype then denotes a certain set of idiotopes (note that there is no principal difference between epitope and idiotope; the term idiotope only draws attention to the peculiar

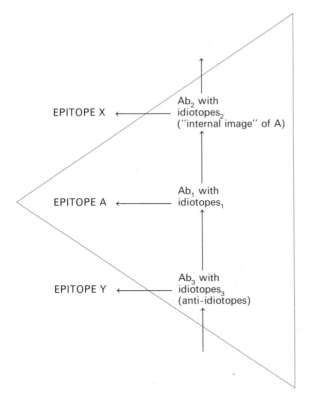

EPITOPE X ←——————— Ab$_2$ with
idiotopes$_2$
("internal image" of A)

EPITOPE A ←——————— Ab$_1$ with
idiotopes$_1$

EPITOPE Y ←——————— Ab$_3$ with
idiotopes$_3$
(anti-idiotopes)

Fig. 4.22. Triad of epitopic and idiotopic antibodies forming an idiotopic network according to Jerne's theory. Ab$_1$ recognizes A, but also idiotopes on paratopes of a set of antibodies Ab$_2$ ("internal image" to A), which by themselves recognize epitope X, and idiotopes on still another set of antibodies. Idiotopes present in paratopes of the Ab$_1$ set are recognized, in turn, by paratopes of a set of antibodies Ab$_3$ (anti-idiotopic antibodies), themselves specific for epitopes Y unrelated to A. Again, idiotopes present in paratopes of these antibodies will serve as "internal image" for still other sets of antibodies, and so on. The triangle contains the elements of the basic triad

location of an epitope, namely at the antigen-binding site of an antibody).

The demonstration that animals can be stimulated to make antibodies to the idiotopes of antibody molecules produced by other animals of the same species or strain indicates that a given animal possesses available paratopes that can recognize any idiotope occurring in the species, i.e., within the immune system of any given individual, any idiotope can be recognized by a set of paratopes, and any paratope can recognize a set of idiotopes.

Thus, the immune system is an enormous and complex network of paratopes and idiotopes, and since antibody molecules occur both free and as receptor molecules on B and T (here, at least the important variable, idiotypic structure, see Chap. 6) lymphocytes, this network intertwines cells and molecules.

An important property of antigen-sensitive lymphocytes is their ability to respond either positively or negatively to a recognition signal, i.e., in this network, there are provisions for on/off switches; the suppression of an immune response by anti-idiotype antibodies has first been shown by Köhler and Cosenza, and Nisonoff.

Antibody Idiotopic Network. With these elements in hand, in 1974 K.N. Jerne proposed a network theory for the regulation of the immune response (Fig. 4.22). In this, a set of antibodies (Ab$_1$)[5] recognizes an epitope A of an antigen. The same set of antibodies Ab$_1$ will also recognize idiotopes present in paratopes of many antibodies Ab$_2$ within the immune system (internal image of epitope A). On the other hand, the paratopes of the antibodies Ab$_1$ consist of sets of idiotopes recognized by other sets of antibodies,

5 Paratopes of antibodies recognizing a particular epitope must not be identical; also, idiotopes recognized by certain paratopes may belong to different paratopes

Ab_3 (anti-idiotope antibodies). Since, for the sets of antibodies Ab_2 and Ab_3, and for all others, the same interconnections exist, this is an open-ended (infinite) network; however, as the effects of distal regulatory interactions will have to be transmitted along a chain, losses of definition can be expected at each step, resulting in a finite network. It is obvious that Ab_3 has suppressive, and that A and Ab_2 have stimulatory, properties with respect to Ab_1.

On the basis of these idiotopic interactions several properties of the immune response can be accounted for: Activation of specific antibody responses and their regulation: The elimination by the antigen of antibodies of set Ab_1 removes their inhibitory effect on the "internal image" (Ab_2) as well as their stimulatory effect on the anti-idiotypic set (Ab_3). Both effects favor an escape from suppression of cells of set Ab_1. On the other hand, the enhancement of set Ab_1 will tend to reverse these effects. The network attempts to restore its equilibrium.

Feedback inhibition of passively administered 7S antibodies as described above removes the stimulatory effect of antigen A before antigen epitope A can activate the Ab_1 set, but beyond that may also suppress the set of internal-image antibodies, Ab_2, which diminishes the stimulatory effect for the Ab_1 set.

Low-zone tolerance (see Chap. 9) might be induced by an imbalance of activation: Low amounts of epitope A stimulate few Ab_1 producing cells; after proliferation the stimulation of the anti-idiotypic antibody set Ab_3 becomes dominant. In addition, unsaturated Ab–Ag complexes may provide a stronger stimulus to the Ab_3 set.

By now, the idiotypic network theory is widely accepted in its basic form. When Jerne proposed his theory, antibody molecules had been the best known part of the immune system; it laid, therefore, the groundwork for the theory. The firm existence and importance of various other parameters in this regulatory system such as helper and suppressor T cells have become clear only since then.

Control of Antibody Formation by Regulatory Cell Circuits. The development of T and B lymphocytes from precursors to effector cells follows similar differentiation patterns. Initially, virgin precursor cells already committed with respect to effector function (see Chap. 2) and antigenic specificity (see p. 74) arise in the absence of antigen. Antigenic exposure triggers virgin precursors to differentiate to memory and effector cells. These antigen-dependent differentiation steps require help from (and are therefore regulated by) specific populations of T helper cells (THC_1). The recruitment of THC_1, in turn, is regulated by T suppressor cell populations (TSC_1) capable of specifically depleting individual THC_1. Recently, Cantor, Gershon and their colleagues demonstrated that the differentiation of TSC_1 from precursors to functionally active cells also requires help from T cells (THC_2), and these helper cells are distinct from the THC_1 which help precursor B cells to differentiate to antibody forming cells (feedback inhibition). It is not unreasonable to expect that the supply of the second population of THC_2 is specifically controlled by another suppressor cell population (TSC_2), and so on.

The regulation of these regulatory cells is thought to be realized via idiotope recognition whereby THC_1 possess paratopes (id^-) [6] complementary to the B cell receptor (id^+) and the TSC_2 paratopes (id^+); TSC_2 paratopes are, in turn, complementary to idiotopes of the THC_2 paratopes (id^-); the latter are again complementary to TSC_1 paratopic idiotopes (id^+); the paratopes of TSC_1 are complementary to idiotopes of THC_1. Each paratope consists of sets of idiotopes. The activation of these cells requires antigen as well (which, however, does not necessarily imply that a given T cell

---

6 Complementary *idiotypes* are referred to as id^+ and id^-; id should not be read as implying a single variable region structure but rather as a collective group of id^- structures complementary to several id^+ V_H. The id structure produced by the B cell is assigned as id^+, the anti-id V_H structure of THC that helps the B cell is assigned id^-

possesses two *different* paratopes, see Chap. 6), whereby T and B cells recognize different epitopes.

On the basis of these data and other considerations, Herzenberg and colleagues extended Jerne's hypothesis and proposed a network of closed circles of regulatory interactions among cells and cell products which they termed circuits (in analogy to closed electronic circuits), capable of being switched between responsive (help), and nonresponsive (suppression) states. The basic or *Core Regulatory Circuits* (CRCs) are constructed by sets of overlapping TSC–THC triads in which TSC is flanked by two different THCs, one which helps the TSC and the other which is its target; THCs will be similarly flanked by two different TSCs, one which is helped by the THC and the other which depletes it (for a given TSC, recognition restriction exists that prevents the depletion of its own THCs; a paratope X possessing an idiotope x recognized by a paratope Y_x needs not be complementary to any of the idiotopes y of paratope Y_x):

pand. On the other hand, if the THC(2) becomes activated first, the circuit will drive itself into the suppression configuration and lock there. The configuration of the CRC depends, therefore, ultimately on the regulatory interactions that control THC(1) or THC(2) stimulation. Such regulatory interactions can be constructed as *Auxiliary Regulatory Circuits* (ARCs) by inclusion of antibodies and antigens in the circuit.

However, before we go on, three points should be emphasized and kept in mind: (1) None of the different lymphocytes (B, T helper, T suppressor lymphocytes) are stimulated without the help of macrophages which have to present the epitope to lymphocytes with appropriate receptors; when macrophages, epitope, id^+Ig, and lymphocytes form a complex (bridge), macrophages release a stimulatory factor for the bridged lymphocyte. (2) The same receptor on lymphocytes recognizing id also recognizes an epitope on the antigen, and since $THCid^-$ and Bid^+ as well as $TSCid^+$ have different receptors (although complementary), they

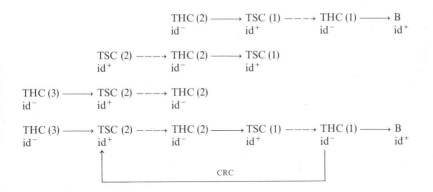

A solid arrow in this diagram indicates help, a broken arrow suppression. This circuit configuration assumes that a THC that helps an id^+ B cell can also help an id^- TSC. Depending upon which THC population is stimulated initially, the CRC tends to lock into either suppression or help configuration: if the THC(1) becomes activated first, it stimulates the TSC(2), which, in turn, suppresses the THC(2); therefore, the TSC(1) remains unactivated and the THC(1) can ex-

probably recognize different antigenic epitopes; the epitope recognized by T cells is called "carrier", the epitope recognized by B cells is called hapten. And (3), for one epitope there is not only one but many CRCs; and further, for each antigen with numerous different epitopes, there will be even more CRCs involved in the overall reaction to them. In some of the CRCs, THC(1) will have an id^- fitting better to that id^+ which has high affinity for the epitope than that of THC(2); in others, THC(2) will have the better fitting id⁻.

Under these provisions, ARCs may look as follows: At the beginning of an immune response, macrophages presenting the antigen-epitopes bound to any badly or well-fitting id⁺Ig to THCs (and B cells) will stimulate those THCs (and B cells) that are bridged. Different B cells will secrete id⁺Ig with different affinity; soon, the poorly-fitting id⁺Ig will occur freely displaced from the epitope by the better-fitting id⁺Ig. The free id⁺Ig will bind to "its" THCid⁻ and will prevent its further stimulation, i.e., will cause suppression of this THC. Those id⁺Ig fitting best an epitope will prevail and continue via macrophages to stimulate "their" THC; this process will go on, and more and more specific antibodies (with high affinity) will be stimulated until all the antigen is eliminated. Then, even the best-fitting id⁺Ig will occur freely, and stimulation of THCs (and B cells) possessing complementary (best-fitting) id⁻ will cease. Of the many CRCs involved in the response to one particular antigen, only a few may have the constellation THC(1)id⁻high fit-THC(2)id⁻low fit, but these will secure a positive immune response overall. In cases where antigens with few repetitive epitopes are used, such constellations may not arise, and the result might be one of no response. There are known parameters, influencing the availability of certain CRC combinations in respect to certain antigen-epitopes, which will be discussed in Chap. 6. There, we shall also discuss how the immune system may distinguish those epitopes against which a positive reaction is desired from those against which, if possible, no reaction should arise, namely the constituents of the individual's own organism.

References

Avremeas S, Terninck T (1969) The cross linking of proteins with glutaraldehyde and its use for the preparation of immunoadsorbents. Immunochemistry 6:53

Benacerraf B (1969) The mechanism of immunization. In: Miescher PA, Müller-Eberhard HJ (eds) Textbook of Immunopathology. Grune and Stratton, New York

Breinl F, Haurowitz F (1930) Chemische Untersuchungen des Präzipitats aus Hämoglobin und Anti-Hämoglobin-Serum und Bemerkungen über die Natur der Antikörper. Hoppe-Seyler's Z Physiol Chem 192:45

Burnet FM (1959) The clonal selection theory of acquired immunity. Cambridge University Press, Cambridge, England

Cantor H, Hungenberger, J, McVay-Boudreau L, Eardley D, Kemp J, Shen FW, Gershon RK (1978) Immunoregulatory circuits among T cell sets. Identification of a subpopulation of T helper cells that induces feedback inhibition. J Exp Med 148:871

Capra JD, Kehoe JM (1975) Hypervariable regions, idiotypy, and the antibody combining site. Adv Immunol 20:1

Cazenave PA (1974) Similar idiotypes in antibody-forming cells synthesizing immunoglobulins without detectable functions. Proc Natl Acad Sci (USA) 71:4500

Dunnick W, Rabbits TH, Milstein C (1980) An immunoglobulin deletion mutant with implications for the heavy chain switch and RNA splicing. Nature 286:669

Edelman GM (1970) The structure and function of antibodies. Sci Am 123:3

Givol D (1974) Affinity labelling and topology of the antibody combining site. Essays Biochem 10:1

Green NM (1969) Electronmicroscopy of the immunoglobulins. Adv Immunol 11:1

Grubb R (1970) The genetic markers of human immunoglobulins. Springer, Berlin Heidelberg New York

Heremans JF (1968) Immunoglobulin formation and functions in different tissues. Curr Topics Microbiol Immunol 45:131

Herzenberg LA, Black SJ, Herzenberg LA (1980) Regulatory circuits and antibody responses. Eur J Immunol 10:1

Hilschmann N, Barnikol HU, Kratzin H, Altevogt P, Engelhard M, Barnikol-Watanabe S (1978) Genetic determination of antibody specificity. Naturwissenschaften 65:616

Honjo T, Kataoka T (1978) Organization of immunoglobulin heavy chain genes and allelic deletion model. Proc Natl Acad Sci (USA) 75:2140

Ishizaka K (1970) The identification and significance of gamma-E. In: Good RA, Fisher DW (eds) Immunobiology. Sinauer, Stanford, Conn.

Jerne KN (1974) Toward a network theory of the immune system. Ann Immunol (Institut Pasteur) 125C:373

Kabat EA (1978) Variable region genes for the immunoglobulin framework are assembled from small segments of DNA. A hypothesis. Proc Natl Acad Sci (USA) 75:2429

Köhler G, Milstein C (1975) Continuous cultures of fused cells secreting antibody of predefined specificity. Nature 256:495

Koshland ME (1975) Structure and function of the J chain. Adv Immunol 20:41

Low TLK (1975) Structure, function, and evolutionary relationship of Fc domains of human immunoglobulins A, G, M, and E. Science 191:390

Maki R, Trauenecker A, Sakano H, Roeder W, Tonegawa S (1980) Exon shuffling generates an immunoglobulin heavy chain gene. Proc Natl Acad Sci (USA) 77:2138

Melchers F, Potter M, Warner NL (eds) (1978) Lymphocyte Hybridomas. Curr Topics Microbiol Immunol 81

Metzger H (1970) Structure and functions of IgM immunoglobulins. Adv Immunol 12:57

Milstein C, Lennox ES (1980) The use of monoclonal antibody technique in the study of developing cell surfaces. Curr Top Dev Biol 14:1

Molgaard HV (1980) Assembly of immunoglobulin heavy chain genes. Nature 286:657

Nisonoff A (1973) The antibody molecule. Academic, New York

Oudin J (1977)L'allotypie. Congress francophone int. Immunol INSERM, Paris

Richards FF, Konigsberg WH (1973) Speculations how specific are antibodies? Immunochem 10:545

Sakano H, Maki R, Kurosawa Y, Roeder W, Tonegawa S (1980) Two types of somatic recombination are necessary for the generation of complete immunoglobulin heavy chain genes. Nature 286:676

Shur PH (1972) Human gamma-G subclasses. Prog Clin Immunol 1:71

Singer PA, Singer HH, Williamson AR (1980) Different species of messenger RNA encode receptor and secretory IgM u chains differing at their carboxy termini. Nature 285:294

Tomasi TB Jr. (1970) The gamma-A globulins: First line of defense. In: Good RA, Fisher DW (eds) Immunobiology. Sinauer, Stamford, Conn.

Voisin GA (1980) Role of antibody classes in the regulatory facilitation reaction. Immunol Rev 49:3

Woodland R, Cantor H (1978) Idiotypic specific T helper cells are required to induce idiotype-positive B memory cells to secrete antibody. Eur J Immunol 8:600

Chapter 5 Complement

WILMAR DIAS DA SILVA

Contents

Complement

Pfeiffer and Issaeff observed in 1894 that cholera vibrios disintegrated when injected into the peritoneal cavities of previously immunized guinea pigs. Bordet demonstrated that the microorganisms also were lysed within minutes when placed in vitro in the presence of serum obtained from immunized animals; however, if the serum was heated to 56 °C for 30 min, or simply allowed to age for a few days, it lost its lytic activity even though the antibodies were preserved. The addition of fresh serum obtained from nonimmune animals restored the lytic activity of serum. This experiment demonstrated that the bacteriolytic action of serum of immunized animals depended upon two factors, one (the antibody) specific and thermostabile, and another that was thermolabile and nonspecific, existing in immune serum as well as in normal serum. The latter, initially termed alexin, is now called complement (C). Any immunologic reaction, as in the example cited above (Pfeiffer's phenomenon), is initiated by a specific combination of antigens and antibodies. From this point, a series of reactions is unleashed, humoral or cellular in nature, whose final expression is the production of tissue injury.

The union of the antigen and antibody in itself is an innocuous event, and antigen–antibody complexes resulting from this union are capable of producing cellular lesions only in collaboration with accessory systems. Complement is the effector system in reactions between antigens and humoral antibodies. This system may be defined as a group of factors (primarily enzymes) present in normal serum that do not increase with the immunization process and that are capable of interacting with different antigen–antibody complexes. If the antigens make up part of the structure of the cellular membrane, the participation of complement in the antigen–antibody reaction that occurs there causes an irreversible cellular lesion, terminating in lysis of that particular cell. As a result of the cytotoxic effects produced by complement during its activation, various orders of consequences can occur: lysis of bacteria (bacteriolysis); phagocytosis of certain particulate antigens that have been coated by antibodies (opsonization); alterations in the cellular membrane that lead to the lysis of erythrocytes (immune hemolysis) or of nucleated cells (cytolysis); production of substances capable of liberating histamine from mast cells or from smooth muscle cells (anaphylatoxins); formation of substances that attract leukocytes (chemotactic factors), etc. Finally, by the activation of the complement system, factors are formed that are necessary for the initiation of the inflammatory reaction that occurs in certain forms of immunologic tissue injury. Of the models of direct tissue injury mediated by complement, immune hemolysis has been investigated most thoroughly. The advantage of this model, which employs sheep erythrocytes sensitized with rabbit antibodies, and fresh guinea pig or human serum as a source of complement, lies in the precision of the information obtained.

Total Titration of Hemolytic Complement

Immune hemolysis was described by Bordet in 1909, but adequate methods for the rigorous quantitative determination of the hemolytic titer of complement in the serum have only been available since 1945, when advantage was taken of the role of the divalent cations Ca^{2+} and Mg^{2+} in the unleashing of the reaction. Much appreciation is owed to Manfred Mayer for the clarification of many aspects of the kinetics of immune hemolysis. Its general reaction can be represented as follows:

$$E + A \rightarrow EA; \quad EA + C \rightarrow Stroma + Hemoglobin$$

where E represents sheep erythrocytes, A, antisheep erythrocyte antibodies produced in rabbits, EA, sensitized erythrocytes; and C, complement.

For the titration of C, a standardized quantity of EA (5×10^8) is incubated with varying quantities of C, in a constant volume (usually 7.5 ml), with the pH of the medium maintained at 7.4–7.5 by an adequate isotonic buffer (saline veronal or triethanolamine buffer) containing Ca^{2+} ($1.5 \times 10^{-4}\ M$). Incubation is performed for 90 min at 37 °C when guinea pig serum is used, or at 32 °C in the case of human serum. The degree of hemolysis is determined by measuring the quantity of hemoglobin liberated in each mixture. The mixtures are centrifuged, and the supernatants are examined spectrophotometrically at 540 μm. When the percentage of hemolyzed red cells is plotted against the quantity of C added, a sigmoidal dose-response curve is obtained (Fig. 5.1).

The graph shown in Fig. 5.1 verifies that the curve becomes asymptotic at the point where the hemolysis value approaches 100%. For this reason, it is best to titrate the complement at the linear part of the curve, with the unit of complement (CH_{50}) defined as the quantity that produces 50% hemolysis under the standardized conditions described previously. The relation between the percentage of hemolysis, y, and the quantity of complement, x, is given by the equation:

$$y = \frac{x^n}{x^n + K^n}$$

from which is derived the van Krogh equation:

$$x = K \left(\frac{y}{1-y}\right) 1/n,$$

in which x is the quantity of complement; y, the percentage of hemolysis; n, a constant whose reciprocal defines the inclination of the curve; and K, a constant expressing the 50% unit of complement. When there is 50% hemolysis , $y/(1-y) = 1$ and $\times$ becomes equal to K (CH_{50} dose).

Fig. 5.1. Dose-response curve in the assay of complement (arithmetic scale)

The curve described by van Krogh's equation is sigmoidal when $1/n > 1$ and, under normal conditions, the value of $1/n$ should vary around 0.2 ($\pm 10\%$).

When a determination is made of the CH_{50} units in a serum, it is convenient to prepare a graph (Fig. 5.2) plotting $\log x$ along the ordinate against $\log [y/(1-y)]$ along the abscissa. With this formula, a straight line is obtained whose equation is

$$\log x = \log K + \frac{1}{n} \log \left(\frac{y}{1-y} \right).$$

The intersection of this line with the ordinate axis ($x = 0$) gives a quantity of serum that corresponds to one CH_{50} unit, for $\log (y/1-y) = 0$, $y + 0.5$. Guinea pig serum contains 200–300 Ch_{50}/ml and human serum, 40–60 CH_{50}/ml.

Complement as a Multifactorial System

The liberation of hemoglobin in immune hemolysis, or the liberation of other cellular constituents in other forms of cellular injury mediated by complement, represents the final event in a sequential reaction. The multiplicity of components taking part in this reaction was verified in 1912, when Ferrata demonstrated that the serum fractions corresponding to the euglobulins and to the

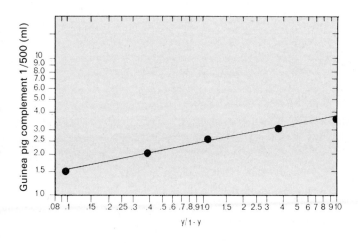

Fig. 5.2. Dose-response curve in determining the concentration of complement: $\log x$ versus $\log (y/1-y)$

pseudoglobulins, obtained by dialysis of fresh guinea pig serum against water, were hemolytically inactive by themselves, but regained their original hemolytic activity upon reassociation. Experiments in which first one fraction was added to the erythrocytes and then, after washing the cells, the other was added, revealed that the euglobulin fraction was fixed first, followed by the pseudoglobulin fraction. The former was thus termed the midpiece, or C 1, and the second was called the end piece, or C 2. Later, two other components were recognized – both thermostable – through the treatment of human serum with cobra venom or zymosan (C 3) and with ammonia or hydrazine (C 4).

The designations R 1, R 2, R 3, and R 4 are given to selectively deficient serums (called R-reactives), which serve, respectively, for the demonstration of C 1, C 2, C 3, and C 4 (Table 5.1).

The availability of the R-reactives also permits the titration of each of the components. For example, the titer of a serum in C 1 is indicated by the greatest dilution that produces 50% hemolysis of EA in the presence of a standardized concentration of R 1.

Until 1958 only four complement components were known. The component that formerly was termed C 3 ("classic" C 3) is today recognized as a mixture of at least six distinct proteins, with individual structures and functions, now called C 3, C 5, C 6, C 7, C 8, and C 9. Moreover, C 1 can be divided into three subcomponents designated C 1 q, C 1 r, and C 1 s. These 11 proteins react sequentially in the fashion of a cascade. Some important properties of the components of complement are reproduced in Table 5.2.

Nomenclature

In accord with the nomenclature recommended by a group of experts convened by the World Health Organization, complement is designated by the symbol C, and the components are expressed by that symbol

Table 5.1. Separation of the classic components of complement

Treatment of the serum	R-Reactive	Components Present
Dialysis against		
pH 5.5 buffer, $\mu = 0.02$		
Supernatant	R1	C2, C3, C4
Precipitate	R2	C1, C3, C4
Zymosan (2–3 mg/ml), 1 h at 37 °C	R3	C1, C2, C4
Hydrazine 0.02–0.03 M		
1 h at 37 °C	R4	C1, C2, C4
30 min at 56 °C	Inactivated serum	C3, C4

Table 5.2. Properties of the components of human complement

Components	C1q	C1r	C1s	C4	C2	C3	C5	C6	C7	C8	C9
Synonyms	–	–	C1–esterase	$\beta_1 E$	–	$\beta_1 C$	$\beta_1 F$	–	–	–	–
Approx. mol. wt. ($\times 10^3$)	388	168	79	230	117	185	185	125	120	150	79
Sedimentation constant	11 S	7 S	4 S	10 S	6 S	9.5 S	8.7 S	6 S	7 S	8 S	4 S
Electrophoretic mobility	$\gamma 2$	β	$\alpha 2$	$\beta 1$	$\beta 2$	$\beta 1$	$\beta 1$	$\beta 2$	$\beta 2$	$\gamma 1$	$\alpha 2$
Concentration in serum (µg/ml)	20–30	–	120	430	30	300	75	60	60	Trace	Trace
Congenital deficiency				Guinea pig	Man	Guinea pig	Mouse	Rabbit			
Thermolability at 56 °C, 30 min	+	+ +	+	–	+	–	+	–	+	+	+

followed by a corresponding number (C 1, C 4, etc.).

The activated components are designated by a horizontal bar over the numeral of the respective symbol, e.g., $C\bar{1}$ = activated C 1. The small letter "i" at the end of the symbol indicates a component that has lost its activity, e.g., C 4 i = inactivated C 4. The products resulting from the cleavage of peptide linkages are represented by the general formulas Cna and Cnb, e.g., C 3 a and C 3 b or C 5 a and C 5 b.

Sequential Reaction of Components in Immune Hemolysis

Figure 5.3 shows the reaction sequence of the complement components as established for immune hemolysis. This sequence is also valid for the lysis of other animal cells and for bacteria, and it is the same in cell-free systems with soluble preformed antigen–antibody complexes. The hemolysis of sheep erythrocytes (E) produced by rabbit anti-

sheep red cell antibodies (A) and human or guinea pig complement, proceeds in eight steps:

(1) $E + A \longrightarrow EA$

(2) $EA + C1 \xrightarrow{Ca^{2+}} EA\overline{C1}$

(3) $EA\overline{C1} + C4 \longrightarrow EA\overline{C1, 4b}$

(4) $EA\overline{C1, 4b}, + C2 \xrightarrow{Mg^{2+}} EA\overline{C1, 4b, 2a}$

(5) $EA\overline{C1, 4b, 2a}, + C3 \longrightarrow EA\overline{C1, 4b, 2a, 3b}$

(6) $EA\overline{C1, 4b, 2a, 3b}, + C5 + C6 + C7 \longrightarrow$
$EA\overline{C1, 4b, 2a, 3b, 5b, 6, 7}$

(7) $EA\overline{C1, 4b, 2a, 3b, 5b, 6, 7} + C8 + C9 \longrightarrow E^*$

(8) $E^* \longrightarrow Stroma + Hemoglobin$

First Step

$E + A \rightarrow EA$.

In the first step, there is a specific union between antibodies (A) and antigens (E) localized on the surfaces of erythrocytes. There is indirect evidence that a single molecule of IgM or two molecules of IgG localized near

Fig. 5.3. Cascade reaction of the complement components in specific cytolysis

one another on the cell surface are sufficient to sensitize it, making it capable of initiating the activation of complement. This idea agrees with the finding that, if an excess quantity of cells is mixed with a given quantity of IgM, the number of sensitized cells remains constant, whereas the same would not occur if IgG were used in place of IgM. Thus, antibodies of the IgM class tend to be much more efficient than those of the IgG class.

The necessity of having a pairing of the IgG molecules is implied in the fact that the corresponding groups with which they combine must be extremely close on the surface of the erythrocyte. Because the antigens of the Rh system, and some other isoantigens, are widely dispersed over the erythrocyte membrane, the foregoing considerations explain the inefficiency of antibodies for such antigens in sensitizing erythrocytes for immune hemolysis.

The antigenic determinants involved in immune hemolysis do not necessarily need to be natural constituents of the cellular membrane. Antigenic groups can be artificially linked to the membrane, and one can achieve hemolysis by the binding of antibodies specific for this group and the addition of complement. Immune complexes prepared in the zone of equivalence, or in slight antigen excess, activate complement more efficiently than do those found in regions with extreme antigen excess, where lattice-type structures do not form. Moreover, hybrid antibodies artificially prepared (antibodies synthesized from two half-molecules – one heavy and one light chain – from two antibodies with different specificities), having only one combining site, do not form lattices, nor do they activate complement.

The initial activation appears to depend at least upon a pair of heavy chains properly arranged and spaced with respect to one another for exposure of the Fc fragment sites responsible for aggregation with C1q. F(ab')$_2$ fragments, obtained by the cleavage of IgG with pepsin, form complexes with corresponding antigens that do not activate C. This last appears decisive for the localization of C1q combining sites in the parts of the heavy chains that form the Fc fragment.

Not all antibodies that form complexes are capable of fixing guinea pig complement, which is usually used in routine tests. For example, the antibodies of birds do not activate mammalian complement. Moreover, in species whose antibodies are capable of fixing complement, only antibodies belonging to specific classes of immunoglobulins are really efficient. Thus, IgM and some subtypes of human IgG can fix complement, whereas IgA and IgE cannot.

Nonspecific aggregates of IgG, formed by warming at 63 °C for 10 min or by chemical aggregation with BDB (bis-diazobenzidine) also activate complement efficiently.

Second Step

$$EA + C1 \xrightarrow{Ca^{2+}} EA C\overline{1}.$$

The reaction between complement and red blood cells requires Ca^{2+} and Mg^{2+} ions, and the velocity of the reaction is greater at 37 °C than at 0 °C. These observations suggest that at least some of the complement components are enzymes that under normal conditions are encountered in serum in the form of proenzymes.

C1 forms a macromolecular complex composed of three subunits, designated C1q, C1r, and C1s, joined together by Ca^{2+} ions. Breaking this down with chelating agents such as EDTA (ethylenediaminetetraacetic acid), the complex dissociates into its subunits, which themselves can be separated by DEAE-cellulose (diethylaminoethyl-cellulose) column chromatography. In its macromolecular form, C1 combines, through receptors localized in C1q, with special sites positioned on the Fc portion of the antibody molecule, which become accessible when the antibody molecules combine with the antigen. C1q appears to be formed of five or six subunits. Four or five of these subunits have a molecular weight of 70,000 daltons, with one or two weighing 52,000 daltons. Ultrastructural analysis sug-

Fig. 5.4. Esterolytic activities of activated C 1

gests that C 1 q can assume two molecular forms: One consists of five units arranged symmetrically around a central unit, the whole measuring approximately 200 Å The other takes on a more-or-less cylindrical shape, measuring about 400 Å apparently possessing the same number of subunits. Because C 1 q possesses five or six valences per antibody molecule, each valence therefore could localize in the peripheral subunits. C 1 q also is capable of interacting with IgG molecules and of precipitating preformed antigen–antibody complexes. Analysis through ultracentrifugation of the complexes formed by IgG and C 1 q molecules indicates that they have a 15 S sedimentation coefficient; apparently they are composed of six IgG molecules per single C 1 q molecule. Complexes of IgM and C 1 q are formed in an analogous manner.

Study of this stage of immune hemolysis has revealed that (1) after attachment to the EA membrane, C 1 takes on the activated C$\overline{1}$ form, capable of hydrolyzing certain synthetic amino acid esters such as ATEE (N-acetyl-L-tyrosine-ethyl ester); and (2) the hemolytic activity as well as the esterolytic activity of C 1 is blocked by DFP (diisopropyl fluorophosphate) and other inhibitors of esterase activity.

If EA or an adequate antigen-antibody complex interacts with C 1, two esterase activities, distinct in terms of specificity, (Fig. 5.4) occur. The first, associated with

C 1 r, hydrolyzes AAME (N-acetyl-arginine-methyl ester), whereas the other, associated with C 1 s, hydrolyzes ATEE (N-acetyl-L-tyrosine-ethyl ester) or TAME (N-p-toluenesulfonyl-methyl ester). The latter is commonly called C 1-esterase and represents the hemolytically active form of C 1. The component C 1 treated with EDTA loses its macromolecular form by virtue of the removal of the Ca^{2+} ions. DEAE-cellulose column chromatography of C 1 thus treated permits its resolution into three subcomponents C 1 q, C 1 r, and C 1 s (Fig. 5.5). Activation of C 1 s only occurs, however, when the three subcomponents reassociate following the addition of Ca^{2+} ions. In these, the

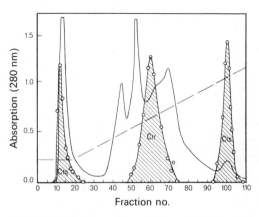

Fig. 5.5. Chromatographic resolution of C 1 treated with EDTA. [Lepow IH, et al., (1962) J Exp Med 117:983]

Ca^{2+} ions would be integrally part of the macromolecular C 1 complex.

The normal serum of diverse species, including human and guinea pig, contains an inhibitor of C 1-esterase. The inhibitor is an acid-labile α_2 globulin with a 3 S sedimentation constant and a molecular weight of 90,000. It is destroyed by heating to 63 °C and by treatment with ether. Highly purified preparations of this inhibitor impede the activity of C 1-esterase in the proportion of one unit of inhibitor for ten units of enzyme.

Third Step

$$EAC\overline{1} + C4 \rightarrow EAC\overline{1, 5b}.$$

After the formation of $EAC\overline{1}$, the ensuing stage of immune hemolysis involves reaction with C4 to form the intermediate complex $EAC\overline{1,4}$ (see Fig. 5.3). The formation of this complex occurs efficiently only when C 1 is present in its enzymatically active form on the surface of the sensitized erythrocyte. The inhibition of C 1 with DFP, with anti-C 1-es-

terase antibodies, or with purified preparations of C 1-esterase inhibitor impedes the formation of the $EAC\overline{1,4}$ complex. Once this complex is formed, C 1 can be inactivated by EDTA without affecting the activity of C4. This indicates that C4 is not itself linked to C 1, but rather to receptors located on the membrane of the red blood cell or on the antibody molecule, probably through covalent bonds.

Human C4 has been obtained in a highly purified form. It is a protein with a sedimentation constant of 10 S, that migrates under electrophoresis with the β proteins, and is designated $\beta_1 E$. Antibodies prepared against this protein block the hemolytic activity of C 4. When these antibodies are labeled with fluorochromes such as fluorescein isothiocyanate, they can be used to detect the presence of C 4 in antigen-antibody complexes existing in tissues.

The treatment of a purified preparation of C 4 with C 1-esterase results in modifications of its electrophoretic mobility and in a small but detectable reduction in its sedimentation constant to 9.5 S (Fig. 5.6). These modifi-

Fig. 5.6. The effect of purified C 1-esterase on purified C 4, demonstrable by **a** immunoelectrophoresis, **b** electrophoresis, and **c** through ultracentrifugation. [Müller-Eberhard JM, Lepow IH (1965) J Exp Med 121:819]

cations result from the cleavage of the $C4$ molecule into a small fragment ($C4a$) with a molecular weight of approximately 15,000, and into a larger fragment that combines with the membranes of red blood cells ($C\overline{4b}$), having a molecular weight of 230,000. This larger fragment also contains the acceptor sites for $C2$ molecules. The availability of purified preparations of $C4$ has permitted a series of studies regarding the biochemistry of this stage of immune hemolysis. It has been ascertained, for example, that $C1$-esterase probably acts upon the $C4$ molecules in two ways: first, in creating the conditions necessary for the linking of $C4$ molecules to the cellular membrane or to antigen–antibody complexes; later, in preparing them for combination with the $C2$ molecules (see Fig. 5.3). The sites of the $C4$ molecule responsible for its combination with $C2$ molecules are different from the sites responsible for its fixation to the cellular membrane. These last sites are unstable, and easily inactivated if the $C\overline{4b}$ molecules do not encounter their receptors on the cellular membrane. However, the sites for the fixation of $C2$ molecules are more stable, remaining active long after activation by $C1$-esterase.

Fourth Step

$$EAC\overline{1,4b} + C2 \xrightarrow{\text{Mg}^{2+}} EAC\overline{1,4b,2a}$$

$C2$ is a β_2-globulin with a molecular weight of approximately 117,000 daltons. Treatment of $C2$ with iodoacetic acid or with p-chloromercuribenzoate destroys its hemolytic activity, whereas treatment with iodine increases this activity. This suggests that $C2$ molecules possess sulfhydryl groups essential for their activity. The reaction proceeds in two stages. In the first, in a reaction that requires Mg^{2+} ions, $C2$ molecules are linked, reversibly, to the EA $C\overline{1,4b}$ complex; in the second stage, depending upon temperature, $C1$ cleaves the $C2$ molecules that have just joined, producing two fragments: one active ($C\overline{2a}$) that binds firmly, but not irre-

versibly to $C4$, the other inactive ($C2b$ – mol. wt. 34,000 daltons), which dissociates in the liquid phase (see Fig. 5.3). The $C\overline{2a}$ fragment has a molecular weight of 83,000 daltons and contains the active sites for the $C\overline{4b}$–$C\overline{2a}$ complex, an enzyme provisionally termed $C3$-convertase because of its action in "converting" $C3$, in terms of electrophoretic mobility, from a protein that migrates to the β region into one that migrates to the α-protein region.

The complex $EAC\overline{1,4b,2a}$ is unstable, with a half-life of approximately 12 min at 32 °C. If $C2$ loses its activity, it is liberated in the aqueous phase, the complex thus reverting to the $EAC\overline{1,4b}$ stage. This last phenomenon is usually referred to as "decay".

The $C\overline{4b}$–$C\overline{2a}$ ($C3$-convertase) complex has a molecular weight of 305,000 daltons, which corresponds approximately to the sum of the values for $C\overline{4b}$ and $C\overline{2a}$. Its formation thus involves four distinct steps: (1) reversible interaction between the $C4$ and $C1$ molecules; (2) cleavage of $C4$ by $C1$-esterase into $C\overline{4a}$ and $C\overline{4b}$, whereby the latter carries acceptor sites for activated $C\overline{2}$; (3) by action of $C1$-esterase, $C2$ is split into $C\overline{2a}$ and $C\overline{2b}$; (4) finally $C\overline{2a}$ binds tightly to $C\overline{4b}$. Although Mg^{2+} is necessary for this reaction, EDTA causes neither dissociation nor inhibition of activity once the complex is formed. $C3$-convertase, formed from $C2$ oxidized with iodine ($C2^{\text{oxi}}$), is a considerably more active and more stable enzyme than that formed with native $C2$. This finding suggests that the transformation of S–H groups in S–S bridges is important for the enzymatic activity as well as for the stability of the bimolecular complex. It can also be assumed that the S–S bridges on the $C2$ molecule are close neighbors of the $C4b$ combining region.

Fifth Step

$$EAC\overline{1,4b,2a} + C3 \rightarrow EAC\overline{1,4b,2a,3b}.$$

$C3$ is a β-protein with a 9.5 S sedimentation constant and a molecular weight of approximately 185,000 daltons. It consists of two polypeptide chains (α and β) with molecular weights of 120,000 and 75,000 daltons, respectively, linked by disulfide bridges. Upon activation, the C3 molecules are split, giving rise to a large fragment, $C\overline{3b}$, which is responsible for the hemolytic activity of C3, and a small fragment, $C\overline{3a}$, with an approximate molecular weight of 9,000 daltons, which is liberated in the liquid phase and possesses pharmacologically important properties (see Fig. 5.3). This fragment ($C\overline{3a}$) can be liberated by treatment of highly purified preparations of C3 with the $C\overline{4b,2a}$ (C3-convertase) complex, as well as by the action of trypsin or cobra venom. During activation, $C\overline{3a}$ is separated from the N-terminal end of the C3 α chain. The remaining part of the C3 molecule ($C\overline{3b}$) is immediately bound to the membrane and forms an intermediate complex $EAC\overline{1,4b}$, $\overline{2a, 3d}$ (C5-convertase). C1 does not take part in this reaction, because the reaction also occurs when C1-free $EAC\overline{4b,2a}$ complex is used. If the $C\overline{3b}$ molecule does not attach quickly enough to the cell membrane, it loses its activity and is converted into the hemolytically inactive form, C3bi.

The influence of the $C\overline{3b}$ inactivator (conglutinin activating factor) or of trypsin on the bound $C\overline{3b}$ causes its decay into a large fragment, $C\overline{3a}$ (mol. wt. ca. 25,000), which remains in the membrane, a small piece that represents the C3 α chain, and the remaining part of the α chain with the entire β chain, which passes into the liquid phase. The binding of $C\overline{3b}$ apparently occurs via the C3d fragment. All available findings indicate that all physiologically active fragments of C3 are derived from cleavage of the α chain: $C\overline{3a}$, $C\overline{3b}$, $C\overline{3c}$, and $C\overline{3d}$.

Sixth Step

$EAC\overline{1, 4b, 2a, 3b} + C5 + C6 + C7 \rightarrow EAC\overline{1,}$
$\overline{4b, 2a, 3b, 5b, 6, 7}$.

Little is known about the mechanisms involved in the reaction of C5, C6, and C7.

Analysis of the interactions of C6 and C7 with C5 through ultracentrifugation indicates that each of these can interact independently of the other; however, it is not clear whether the two components compete for the same site on the C5 molecule. It appears that the peptidase activity encountered in $C\overline{3b}$ is essential for the cleavage of the C5 molecules. This was suggested by the observation that peptides containing residues of aromatic amino acids – e.g., glycyl-L-tyrosine – that are hydrolyzed by the intermediate complex $EAC\overline{1,4b,2a,3b}$, inhibit the conversion of this complex to the succeeding stage $EAC\overline{1,4b,2a,3b,5b,6,7}$. The first phase of this reaction would therefore be the cleavage of the C5 molecule into $C\overline{5a}$ and $C\overline{5b}$, followed by the aggregation of $C\overline{5b}$ with $C\overline{6}$ and $C\overline{7}$, to form the trimolecular complex $C\overline{5b,C6,C7}$. This aggregate attaches immediately to the cellular membrane, though there is some evidence that activated $C\overline{7}$ acts upon the membrane without linking to it permanently. Treatment of the $EAC\overline{1,4b,2a,3b,5b,6,7}$ complex with anti-C5 antibodies inhibits the combination of C8 with the cell membrane, suggesting that C6 and C7 are components responsible for the activation of C8 (see Fig. 5.3).

Seventh Step

$EAC\overline{1, 4b, 2a, 3b, 6, 7} + C8 + C9 \rightarrow E^\star \rightarrow$ Hemolysis.

Müller-Eberhard and co-workers suggested that the production of lesions by complement on the cell membrane was provoked by a decamolecular complex involving components C5–C9. After the cleavage of C5 into $C\overline{5a}$ and $C\overline{5b}$ by the $C\overline{4b,2a,3b}$ (C5-convertase) enzyme, C5b, C6, and C7 could link to the membrane in the form of a complex. The geometric form of this suggested complex is triangular, each component contributing a molecule in order to form a triangle. Because the molecular weight of C5b is 165,000 daltons and the molecular weights of C6 and C7 are 100,000 daltons each, the complex has a total weight of 365,000 daltons. The central region of the triangle accommodates a C8 molecule that is linked by simple adsorption to each of the components of the trimolecular complex. The complex, now tetramolecular, assumes the form of a tetrahedron. The connected C8 molecule is also capable of fixing, by simple adsorption, six C9 molecules. Because the molecular weight of C8 is 150,000 and that of C9 is 79,000, the decamolecular complex $C5b_1–C6_1–C7_1–C8_1–C9_6$ has a molecular weight of 995,000.

This molecular arrangement of the six last components was proposed based upon the following information: (1) $C\overline{5b}$, C6, and C7 are tied to the membrane of the target cell in intimate proximity with one another; (2) the $C\overline{5b,C6,C7}$ complex consitutes the combining site for C8; and (3) C8 possesses many combining sites for C9. This model is in accord with the possible allosteric effector functions of C9, suggested by earlier observations, in which C9 can be substituted by chelating compounds such as 1–10–phenanthrolene and 2,2′-bipyridine.

The mechanism by which this decamolecular complex injures the cellular membrane is unclear. The initial suggestion as to the activation of phospholipases was not confirmed in experiments using artificial membranes

Fig. 5.7. Production of holes in the cell membrane (sheep and human erythrocytes) during cytolysis by complement

containing labeled phospholipids as substrates for the terminal components of complement. These experiments suggested that the lesion could occur by hydrophobic interactions between complement and the lipids of the cellular membrane.

The morphologic characteristics of the lesions on the surface of the cellular membrane (Fig. 5.7) become apparent immediately after fixation of C5. These "ultrastructural" lesions occur by the detergent action of $C\overline{5b}$ after cleavage from C5, which becomes strongly hydrophobic for the other phospholipids of the membrane. The subsequent interaction of the other two components only enhances the detergent action of $C\overline{5b}$, transforming the "ultrastructural lesions" into "functional lesions."

Quantitative Determination of Components

A method for the quantitative determination of the individual components of complement based upon hemolytic activity was introduced by Meyer in 1961, following the formulation of his "one-hit theory" for immune hemolysis. This theory takes the position that a single molecule of any of the components of complement, at some stage in the sequence of reactions, is sufficient to produce a lesion on the surface of the erythrocyte that in turn is sufficient for lysis. The number of hemolytically active sites of each component could then be represented by $[Z = -\ln(1-y)]$, the negative natural logarithm of the number of cells not lysed. For 63% hemolysis, $Z = 1$, which corresponds to one hemolytically active site per cell. Because this method does not compute the unsuccessful reactions, the results represent the estimated minimum and thus are expressed in terms of "effective molecules." From an operational point of view, the method consists of making a graph in which the arithmetic values of Z are plotted against the dilutions of serum. To obtain the number of effective molecules of a specific complement component, it suffices to multiply the graphically obtained value corresponding to $Z = 1$ by the reciprocal of the dilution and by the number of erythrocytes in the mixture, and then to convert for 1 ml of serum.

Morphologic Consequences of the Immunocytotoxic Reactions

Lesions produced in the cellular membrane by the action of antibody and complement have been visualized with the electron microscope using negative staining techniques. The lesions produced in the membranes of erythrocytes and in bacterial membranes are exhibited as relatively circular holes 80 Å–100 Å in diameter (Fig. 5.7). These lesions are called type I, whereas the membrane lesions induced by the properdin system, which have a larger diameter (150 Å) and which are surrounded by a light halo about 80 Å wide, are called type II.

Studies of the effect of complement upon the lipopolysaccharide *Veillonella alcalesens* suggest that the lesions produced in the membrane are not actual orifices, but only the accumulation of micelles in the lipoprotein layer of the erythrocyte surface.

Nucleated cells, such as those of Kreb's ascites tumor, after interacting with antibodies reveal invaginations and interdigitations of the cellular membrane. The addition of complement to these cells produces swelling of the mitochondria and of the membranes of the endoplasmic reticulum; larger perinuclear pores are also noted. Disturbances in control of cellular permeability are manifested initially by the loss of K^+, amino acids, and riboneucleotides. The cell swells and, as a consequence of osmotic lysis, macromolecules such as proteins and nucleic acids are liberated.

Immunobiologic Activities of Complement

During the sequential reaction of the complement system, various biologic activities emerge, associated alternatively with activated components or with products of cleav-

Table 5.3. Biologic activities associated with products resulting from the sequential reaction of complement

Biologic activity	Components involved in the process of production									Originating component (s)
	C1	C2	C4	C3	C5	C6	C7	C8	C9	
Hemolysis	+	+	+	+	+	+	+	+	+	C8
Bacteriolysis	+	+	+	+	+	+	+	+	+	C8
Anaphylatoxins	+	+	+	+	+	−	−	−	−	C3 and C5
Chemotaxis	+	+	+	+	+	+	+	−	−	C3, C5, C5–C6, C7
Opsonization	+	+	+	+	+	−	−	−	−	C3
Immunoadherence	+	+	+	+	−	−	−	−	−	C3
Conglutination	+	+	+	+	−	−	−	−	−	C3
Immunoconglutination	+	+	+	+	−	−	−	−	−	C3
Activation of kinin	−	+	+?	−	−	−	−	−	−	C2? C4?
Enzymes	+	+	+	+	−	−	−	−	−	C1 r, C1 s, C4–C2, C3
Liberation of histamine	+	+	+	+	+?	+?	−	−	−	C5 ? C6 ?
Production of glomerulonephritis	+	+	+	+	?	?	?	?	?	?
Production of pulmonary edema	+	+	+	+	?	?	?	?		?

age. Table 5.3 shows these different activities and the component or components that participate in their production.

Hemolysis

Immune hemolysis utilizes the 11 complement components for its realization. Due to its great reproducibility and its considerable ease of execution, this reaction has been frequently used in studies of the biochemistry of the activation of complement.

Bacteriolysis

Gram-negative bacteria are susceptible to the action of antibody and complement; all 11 components, apparently, are also necessary. The final lesion involves the cell wall, leading to the formation of spheroplasts (cf. Chap. 7, Immunocytolysis).

Anaphylatoxins

The term "anaphylatoxin" was employed by Friedburger in 1910 to describe the property of inducing a syndrome similar to anaphylactic shock that some sera acquire when treated with preformed antigen–antibody aggregates. It was later verified that sera treated with polysaccharide complexes such as agar, zymosan, dextrans, etc, also acquire

this property. Subsequent investigations demonstrated that the sera containing anaphylatoxin exhibited the following pharmacologic properties: (1) production of spasmodic contractions in smooth muscle (guinea pig ileum), followed by tachyphylaxis after administration of another dose; (2) capacity to liberate histamines from mastocytes and to produce degranulation (in guinea pigs) or extrusion (in rats and mice) of the metachromatic granulations encountered in the cytoplasm of these cells; (3) inability to contract the smooth musculature of the uterus of the rat in estrus; and (4) capacity to produce an increase in vascular permeability.

Based on the fact that sera previously heated to 56 °C did not form anaphylatoxin, Friedburger suggested in 1911 that complement could be involved in its formation. For nearly 50 years, this hypothesis remained unexplored, probably because of lack of greater knowledge of the biochemical events related to the activation of the complement system. This hypothesis was tested only after it became possible to obtain components of complement in a highly purified form. These investigations demonstrated that during the sequential reaction of complement, two products of cleavage were formed, one derived from C3 and the other from C5, both biologically similar to anaphylatoxin.

Anaphylatoxin Derived from C3. The biologically active fragment $C\overline{3a}$ originates from the cleavage of C3 by C3-convertase, according to the following reaction:

$$C3 \xrightarrow{\overline{C4b-2a}} C\overline{3a} + C\overline{3b}$$

The fragment $C\overline{3a}$ represents approximately 4% of the original C3 molecule, has a molecular weight of around 7,200, and migrates during electrophoresis at pH 9 toward the cathode. The basic character of this fragment was confirmed by amino-acid analysis, which revealed a ratio of 1.65 between the basic and the acid residues. The $C\overline{3a}$ fragment is composed of a small carbohydrate portion bound to the peptide portion, which contains four residues of cysteine, serine as the N-terminal residue, and leucine as the C-terminal residue. This residue of leucine links $C\overline{3a}$ to the remaining portion of the original C3 molecule.

Aside from C3-convertase, other enzymes such as trypsin, plasmin, thrombin, and the complex resulting from the combination between the 7S factor present in cobra venom (CVF) and a 5S serum protein (C3PA) also break down C3 molecules, forming fragments analogous to $C\overline{3a}$. The fragment resulting from the action of trypsin possesses arginine as a residual C-terminal, which sug-

gests that the region of the C3 molecule susceptible to enzymatic attack is formed by more than one peptide linkage.

Anaphylatoxin Derived from C5. The biologically active fragment $C\overline{5a}$ originates from the cleavage of C5 by the activating enzyme $C\overline{4b,2a,3b}$ according to the reaction:

$$C5 \xrightarrow{\overline{C4b, 2a, 3b}} C\overline{5a} + C\overline{5b}$$

This $C\overline{5a}$ fragment has a molecular weight of 10,000–15,000. It can also be formed by treating purified preparations of C5 with trypsin. Data are not yet available concerning either its chemical composition or the mechanism of its formation.

The two fragments $C\overline{3a}$ and $C\overline{5a}$ possess all the properties attributed to anaphylatoxin. Table 5.4 shows the similarities as well as the differences in the pharmacologic behavior of these two products.

As Table 5.4 indicates, the anaphylatoxin derived from C3 ($C\overline{3a}$) degranulates and liberates histamine from mastocytes in rats and guinea pigs, whereas the anaphylatoxin derived from C5 ($C\overline{5a}$) is active only for guinea pig mastocytes. These differences in biologic specificity suggest that the two anaphylatoxins act upon chemically distinct re-

Table 5.4. Biologic properties of the fragments $C\overline{3a}$ and $C\overline{5a}$ obtained by cleavage of components C3 and C5, respectively

Fragment	Enzymes responsible for cleavage	Contraction of guinea pig ileum	Morphologic alterations of mastocytes		Liberation of histamine by the tissues	
			Rat	Guinea pig	Rat	Guinea pig
C3a	C4b–2a	+	+	+	+	+
C3a	Trypsin	+	+	+	+	+
C3a	Plasmin	+	+	+	+	+
C3a	9S Complex (CVF+C3PA)	+	+	+	+	+
C5a	C4b–2a–3b	+	−	+	−	+
C5a	Trypsin	+	−	+	−	+
Anaphylatoxin generated in guinea pig serum	Agar	+	−	+	−	+

ceptors. In these terms, guinea pig mastocytes would have receptors for both anaphylatoxins, whereas rat mastocytes would only have receptors for $C\overline{3}a$. It has been determined that preparations of guinea pig ileum desensitized to one of the anaphylatoxins, for example, by successive additions of $C\overline{3}a$, respond fully to the addition of the same dose of $C\overline{5}a$. These results also suggest that the two anaphylatoxins act upon different receptors.

In normal human serum there is an anaphylatoxin inhibitor. It is a β-globulin, thermolabile at 56 °C, which inactivates $C\overline{3}a$ as well as $C\overline{5}a$. It has a molecular weight of 300,000 and the activity of carboxypeptidase B, and probably is identical to carboxypeptidase N. The presence of this inhibitor in the serum could explain the absence of anaphylatoxic activity in samples of human serum treated with antigen–antibody complexes, agar, C 1-esterase, or anaphylatoxin-forming agents.

Chemotactic Factors

Also called chemotaxins, these are substances that promote the migration of leukocytes from an area of lesser to an area of greater density in a concentration gradient of the chemotactic substance. Studies of chemotaxis originally were performed in vivo by local injections of the chemotactic factor, in order to follow histologically the movement of leukocytes to the injected locale. Experiments of this type are now carried out in vitro, using appropriate chambers formed into two equal compartments of nonoxidizing metal separated by a microporous disk. The pores of this disk measure 650 mµ and permit penetration of cells from the compartments. The chemotactic substance to be tested is placed in one compartment and the leukocytes in the other. Leukocytes migrating to the compartment that contains the chemotactic substance penetrate, by ameboid movements, into the membrane and are retained there (Fig. 5.8). Development of this in vitro method permitted the study of various chemotactic ac-

tivities formed during the activation of the complement system. Chemotactic activity was shown by fragments of $C\overline{3}a$ and $C\overline{5}a$, by a fragment of C 3 after cleavage by plasmin, by proteolytic enzymes obtained from β-hemolytic streptococci of group A, and in the macromolecular complex formed by C 5-C 6-C 7.

The chemotaxis induced by any of these factors is related to the activation of an esterase linked to the leukocytes, from which the increased directional motility of these cells results. In human serum, there are at least two inactivators of the chemotactic effect (CFI-A and CFI-B) of $C\overline{3}a$ or $C\overline{5}a$.

Opsonization

Opsonins are substances that modify particles that are to be phagocytosed so as to cause them to be more easily ingested by phagocytic cells. Experiments designed to verify that complement components sensitize particulate substances by direct opsonization were conducted by inducing the adhesion of these substances to the surfaces of red blood cells. The results of these studies indicated that erythrophagocytosis could occur only after fixation by C 3 and was not augmented by the addition of the other complement components.

Complement-Dependent Liberation of Histamine

Whenrat mastocytes isolated from the peritoneal cavity are incubated at 37 °C with antimastocytic sera or with antigamma globulin inactivated at 50 °C, liberation of histamine occurs only with the addition of fresh serum. To verify that complement components were necessary, experiments were performed with purified preparations of complement. It was thereby possible to demonstrate that the liberation of histamine occurred only in the presence of C 1, C 4, C 2, C 3, and C 5, with the necessity for C 6 remaining in doubt. With the use of inhibitors whose spectrum of inhibition is well defined, the activation of an esterolytic en-

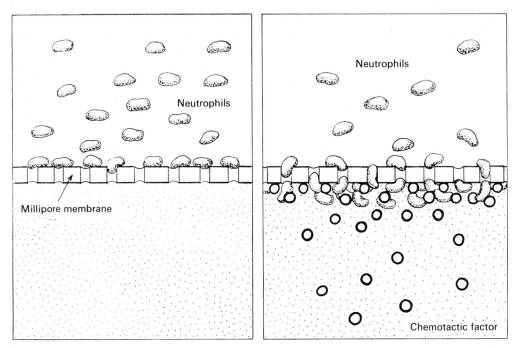

Fig. 5.8. Schema of the technique for demonstrating chemotactic factor

zyme in mastocytes was shown; it appears to be related to the process of liberation of histamine in anaphylaxis. The demonstration that C 5 initiates the lesion in the erythrocyte membranes suggests that the factor responsible for the liberation of histamines is related to this component.

A similar phenomenon was observed when mastocytes isolated from the peritoneum of mice were treated in vitro with 19 S fractions of rabbit anti-Forssman serum. The presence of heterophilic antigens on the surfaces of mastocytes was thus demonstrated.

Formation of Kinins

Numerous attempts to demonstrate the formation of kinins during the activation of complement have furnished inconclusive results. The first indirect evidence that this could occur was encountered in sera of patients with hereditary angioneurotic edema. In such sera, in addition to an accentuated increase of C 1-esterase and a depression of the titers of C 4 and C 2, a pep-

tide has been found that increases the vascular permeability of the rat uterus, but that differs, in certain respects, from bradykinin and from lysobradykinin. Subsequent experiments have shown that treatment of purified preparations of C 4 and C 2 with C 1-esterase induces an activity similar to that of kinins, but in the conditions under which the experiments were performed, it was not possible to determine the nature of its relationship to C 4 or to C 2.

Activation of Enzymes

During the sequential activation of complement, four enzymes were activated, each with an already well-characterized spectrum of activity. These enzymatic activities are the esterases associated with C 1 r and C 1 s, the proteolytic activity associated with the bimolecular C 4–C 2 complex, and the dipeptidase associated with C $\overline{3b}$. Although the natural substances of these enzymes are encountered in the complement system itself, the possibility cannot be excluded that structural substrates also appear to be localized in plasma components not related to complement or making up a part of the composition of cellular membranes.

Immunologic Glomerulonephritis

Glomerulonephritis produced by nephrotoxic sera or by deposit of preformed antigen–antibody complexes involves the participation of complement.

The Properdin System or Alternative Pathway

A second pathway of complement activation has been described that bypasses C 1, C 4, and C 2, called the alternative pathway or properdin–complement activation. Nomenclature for the components of this pathway was suggested by the First International Congress of Immunology (Washington, 1972). The alternative or properdin-complement-activating system consists of seven components: properdin (P), the third complement component C 3 (factor A), the proactivator (factor B), the proactivator-convertase (factor D), the initiation factor (IF), the C 3 b-inactivator (KAF), and the activator of the C $\overline{3b}$ inactivator (C $\overline{3b}$-INA). In the following sections, the biologic, chemical, and physicochemical properties of these components are described (Table 5.5).

Properdin (P) is a euglobulin that occurs in the serum of various species of animals and in man. Usually P is isolated from the serum in the form $\overline{P}$. The protein has a molecular weight of 220,000 daltons and binds directly to surface-bound C $\overline{3b}$; C $\overline{3b}$, together with the factors B, D, and Mg^{2+}, forms the P-C 3-convertase. In serum, P occurs in its precursor form, which does not bind directly with C $\overline{3b}$ and does not form a soluble enzyme complex. P is bound to and activated by a complex of particle-bound properdin receptors and activated factor B (S-C $\overline{3b}$-B, whereby S represents the surface binding site). The binding and activation of P is a nonenzymatic process in which approximately one P molecule is bound per 50 C 3 b molecules. The P → $\overline{P}$ conversion is accompanied by a conformational change in the properdin molecule.

C 3 or Factor A is a protein whose properties were discussed in the description of the fifth step of the classic activation of complement.

Proactivator or Factor B is a thermolabile (52 °C) β-protein with a molecular weight of 80,000 daltons. If the serum is treated with substances that activate the properdin system (complex polysaccharides such as zymosan, inulin, agar-agar; preformed immune aggregates of IgA, IgE, or IgG, etc.), factor B is cleaved into at least two fragments. The large fragment (factor $\overline{B}$; mol. wt. 60,000) exhibits the electrophoretic

Table 5.5. Physico-chemical properties of components of the properdin system

Component (synonym)	Mol. ($\times 10^3$ dalton)	Sedimentation coefficient (S)	Serum concentration (mg/100 ml)	Electrophoretic mobility	Thermo-lability (56 °C, 30 min)
IF	160	7	Traces	β/γ_1	–
Properdin (P)	220	5.2–5.4	1.0–2.5	γ_2	
Factor B (C3-proactivator)	94	5–6	20.0–25.0	β_2	+
Factor D (C3-proactivator-convertase)	25	2–3	Traces	α	
C3b-Inactivator (KAF)	100	5.5–6.0	2.5	β_1/β_2	+

mobility of a gamma globulin; the small fragment (mol. wt. 20,000) is an acidic peptide. Factor $\bar{\text{B}}$ can react with the S-C$\overline{3b}$, P-complex and forms the C3 and C5-convertases of the properdin system. Factor B is identical with the glycine-rich β-glycoprotein (GBG), and shares properties with the glycine-glycoprotein (GGG), the 4.2S fragment that stems from GBG.

The toxin of the Indian cobra *Naja naja* contains a glycoprotein with a molecular weight of 144,000 daltons and the electrophoretic mobility of a β-protein at pH 8.6. This protein, termed cobra factor (CoF), converts and inactivates C3 when it is added to the serum. The reaction leads to a labile complex with factor B, B-CoF, which is stabilized through factor D. Antiserum against CoF cross-reacts with human C3 and with a cobra-serum protein, probably cobra C3. CoF apparently is similar to C3b, and its strong anticomplement activity can be explained in terms of its insensitivity to the human C3b inactivator.

Factor D is a protein, traces of which are found in serum (2 mg/100 ml), that stabilizes the B-CoF complex in minimal amounts and enhances its C3-cleaving activity. After conversion from D to $\bar{\text{D}}$, it exhibits serum-esterase activity that can be inhibited through DFP.

C$\overline{3b}$-inactivator (KAF) is a serum protein with a molecular weight of 100,000 daltons. It cleaves C$\overline{3b}$ into two fragments – C3c and C3d. Under the influence of the C$\overline{3b}$ inactivator, C$\overline{3b}$ reacts with bovine conglutinin, from which comes the term conglutinin activating factor (KAF)[1]. Particle-bound C$\overline{3b}$ reacts under the influence of KAF with conglutinin and loses its hemolytic and its immune-adherence activity.

C$\overline{3b}$-INA is a euglobulin with a molecular weight of 150,000 daltons. It consists of a single polypeptide chain with a high percent-

age of carbohydrates. This protein appears to enhance the inactivation of C$\overline{3b}$ through the C$\overline{3b}$ inactivator,and to decrease the activation of C5 through C3b of the classic complement reaction chain and of factor B of the properdin system. It also lessens the activity of the properdin system convertases C$\overline{3b}$,B and C$\overline{3b}$,B,P in that it accelerates their decay.

Initiating Factor (IF) is a 7S-pseudoglobulin that acts like a β-globulin, is stable at 56 °C, and is apparently different from immunoglobulin. This factor was first identified in its active form, $\overline{\text{IF}}$, or NeF, in serum from patients with hypocomplementary chronic glomerulonephritis. In this form, $\overline{\text{IF}}$ acts as a non-7S-gamma globulin that activates exclusively the properdin system. IF is thought to consist of two identical chains, each with a molecular weight of 85,000 daltons, that are linked by disulfide bridges. It is not yet known whether this factor consists of a series of proteins that recognize the surface structures on complement-activating structures resembling benzyl-β-D-fructopyranoside, or of sequential 1–3 and branched 1–6 bonds that are not found on immunoglobulins.

Activation of the Properdin System

On the basis of extensive experimental findings, two activation pathways of the properdin system can be differentiated.

Activation by Solid Particles

This mechanism consists of two steps:

1. *The formation of P-independent C3 convertase*

$$\text{IF} + \text{C3} + \text{B} + \text{D} \xrightarrow[\text{Mg}_{2+}]{\text{Activator}} \overline{\text{S} - \text{IF, B, C3b}}$$

The first event occurs on the surface of the activating particle through reaction of its active area (S) with the I factor. The bound IF reacts with the factors B, D, and native C3,

---

1 In the abbreviation K is used to avoid confusion with complement

which together represent the P-receptor-forming enzyme S-IF, B, C3b, which is the initiating C3-convertase. The effect of the enzyme is limited by its spontaneous decay, whereby B and S-C3b fall apart. It is not known whether factor D represents an integral subunit of this complex.

2. *Formation of the P-dependent C3-convertase*

$$S - C\overline{3b} + B, D \xrightarrow[\mathrm{Mg^{2+}}]{} S - \overline{C3b, B} +$$
$$P \longrightarrow S - \overline{C3b, P, B}$$

The binding of the newly activated $\overline{B}$ on the P receptor, which binds at least two $C\overline{3b}$ in specific alignment, produces the P-activating principle, $C\overline{3b\text{-}B}$. The complex is labile; if it comes in contact with native P, the latter is converted to the bound form $\overline{P}$. $\overline{P}$ gives the complex S-C$\overline{3b, P, B}$ stability. IF apparently is the recognition factor, whereas P has only a reciprocal action with the $C\overline{3b, B}$ complex and stabilizes it.

IF reacts with B, and P reacts with C3 or $C\overline{3b}$; in the complex S-IF, $C\overline{3b, P, B}$ factor B exercises a catalytic activity as C3- and C4-convertase, thereby activating the properdin reaction chain. The complex S-IF, $C\overline{3b, P, B}$ cleaves C3 into $C\overline{3a}$ and C3b, whereby the latter represents new receptors for P. It is probable that the addition of two $C\overline{3b}$ molecules to the S-IF, $C\overline{3b, P, B}$ complex leads to a new complex S-IF, $C\overline{3b_2, P, B}$, which, like the enzyme that catalyses the formation of the cytolytic complex C5b-9, exhibits C5 convertase activity.

Activation by Cobra Venom Factor

Addition of cobra venom factor (CoF) to serum leads to the formation of a CoF-B complex that enzymatically cleaves C3 into $C\overline{3a}$ and $C\overline{3b}$, thereby giving rise to the formation of the cytolytic complex C$\overline{5b\text{-}9}$. Factors B and D and Mg^{2+} are necessary for the formation of this complex. Because CoF appears to be similar to C3b, but insensitive to the effect of human KAF, CoF-B may be similar to $C\overline{3b\text{-}B}$.

The activation of the properdin chain can be regulated in three ways: (1) through spontaneous decay of S-IF, $C\overline{3b}, \overline{B}$ or S-IF, $C\overline{3b_2}, P, \overline{B}$-convertase (these enzymes have a half-life of approximately 2 and 15 min, respectively); (2) through dissociation of the components of the enzyme with a surplus of $C\overline{3b}$ and liberation of inactivated factor B; and (3) through cleavage of the bound $C\overline{3b}$ by KAF into fragments $C\overline{3c}$ and $C\overline{3d}$.

Effect of Complement on the Solubilization of Immune Complexes

Studies show that immunocomplexes in the aqueous phase or bound to the cell membrane can be made soluble through the addition of complement. This reaction appears to be more effective when complement is activated via the properdin system.

Defects in the homeostatic mechanism of circulating immunocomplexes through increased use, or because of a state of genetic deficiency of specific components of the complement or properdin system, are probably the basis for aggregation of immunocomplexes in tissue, leading to subsequent tissue damage.

Biosynthesis of Complement Components and Certain Hereditary Deficiencies

It is not known for all complement components which cell or tissue produces them. Recent studies suggest that C1 is synthesized in epithelial cells of the intestine and genitourinary tract (but not in the kidney); C2, C3, C4, and C5 are most probably synthesized in macrophages; C3, in addition, in parenchymal liver cells, as probably also C6, C9, and C1-inhibitor (Table 5.6).

The complement component C3 exists in different allotypic forms distinguishable by their electrophoretic mobility. C3 polymorphism has been verified in patients subjected to liver transplantation; after engraftment, the C3-allotype of the donor could be dem-

Table 5.6. Cell and tissue synthesizing complement components

Component	Species	Organ	Cell
C1	Human, guinea pig	Intestine, GU[a]	Epithelial
C1q	Human	Intestine, GU	Epithelial
C1r	—	?	?
C1s	Human	Intestine, GU	Epithelial
C2	Human, guinea pig	Wide distribution	Macrophage
C3	Human	Liver	Parenchymal cell
C4	Human	Wide distribution	Macrophage
C5	Human, mouse	Wide distribution	Macrophage
C6	Rabbit	Liver	?
C7	—	?	?
C8	Pig	Wide distribution	?
C9	Rat	Liver	Parenchymal cell
C1-inhibitor	Human	Liver	Parenchymal

[a] GU, genitourinary tract, excluding kidney. (According to Lachman, 1979)

onstrated. C4 also displays a polymorphism detected by electrophoretic mobility and serological markers, known in man as Chido and Rodgers.

The structural genes for the components C2, C4, and factor B are linked to the major histocompatibility complex.

Hereditary deficiencies of each complement component of the classical pathway have been studied in man; they are described in more detail in Chap. 12. Among inbred strains of laboratory animals, several deficiencies have been found: C5 in mice, C6 in rabbits, and C4 in guinea pig.

References

Alper CH, Rosen FS (1971) Genetic aspects of the complement system. Adv Immunol 14:252

Gewurz H (1971) The immunologic role of complement. In: Good RA, Fisher DW (eds) Immunobiology. Sinauer, Stamford

Humphrey JH, Dourmashkin RR (1969) The lesions in cell membranes caused by complement. Adv Immunol 11:75

Lachman PL (1979) Complement. In: Sela E (ed) The Antigen. Academic, New York

Lepow IH (1965) Serum complement and properdin. In: Santer M (ed) Immunological diseases. Little, Brown, Boston

Lepow IH et al. (1968) Nature and biological properties of human anaphylatoxin. In: Austen KF, Becker EL (eds) Biochemistry of acute allergic reactions. Blackwell, Oxford

Mayer MM (1961) Complement and complement fixation. In: Kabat EA, Mayer MM (eds) Experimental immunochemistry. Thomas, Springfield

Mayer MM (1973) The complement system. Sci Am 229:54

Medicus RG, Schreiber RD, Götze OJ, Müller-Eberhard HJ (1976) A molecular concept of the properdin pathway. Proc Natl Acad Sci 73:612

Müller-Eberhard H (1966) A molecular concept of immune cytolysis. Arch Path 82:205

Müller-Eberhard HJ, Schreiber RD (1980) Molecular biology and chemistry of the alternate pathway of complement. Adv Immunol 29:2

Müller-Eberhard H (1969) Complement. Ann Rev Biochem 38:389

Müller-Eberhard H (1975) Complement. Ann Rev Biochem 44:697

Spitzer RE (1977) The complement system. Pediatric Clinics of North America 24:341

Ward PA (1971) The role of complement in inflammation and hypersensitivity. In: Movat HZ (ed= Inflammation and hypersensitivity. Harper and Row, New York

Chapter 6　The Major Histocompatibility Complex

DIETRICH GÖTZE

Contents

Histocompatibility Genes

At the beginning of this century, Tyzzer and Loeb showed that tumors of a strain of mice *(A/A)* grow normally if they are transplanted into mice of the same inbred strain (syngeneic, see Table 6.1); however, they are rejected by mice of another inbred strain (allogeneic, e.g., *B/B*). Mating experiments showed that susceptibility for tumor growth is genetically controlled: all F_1 animals of the cross $A/A \times B/B$ accepted tumors from both parental lines. Based on the percentage of accepted parental tumors in the F_2 generation, Little and Tyzzer calculated that in the mouse at least fifteen genes were responsible for the resistance to the parental tumor, because tumors grew in only 1.6% of the F_2 animals. According to the preceding example, if susceptibility were controlled by one gene, 75% of the F_2 animals would have been susceptible to the parental tumor tissue (50% A/B, 25% A/A, 25% B/B); if susceptibility were controlled by two genes, the number of susceptible animals would be reduced to 56% (9/16). In general, the percentage of F_2 animals in which a parental tumor grows is $(3/4)^n$, where n represents the number of different genes of both parental strains that control susceptibility. From these findings it was determined that susceptibility was controlled by several dominant genes.

In 1933, Haldane postulated that resistance (or susceptibility) is dependent on structures of the surface of the cell membrane which are different for each inbred strain and against which the recipient would react when its own differ from that of the donor. A few years later, Gorer (1936) demonstrated that there were indeed structures on the membranes of cells from inbred strains that could be revealed with antisera, and that were antigenically different for each inbred strain (alloantigen). He also showed that animals of an inbred strain that rejected a tumor from another inbred strain had antibodies in their serum reacting with cells of the inbred strain from which the tumor originated. Thus, Gorer demonstrated that genes responsible for susceptibility to tumor transplantation were identical to those that

Genetic relationship between donor and recipient	Noun (former term)	Adjective (former term)	**Table 6.1.** Terminology of histo-genetic relationships
Different species	Xenotransplant (heterotransplant)	Xenogenic (heterologous)	
Same species, genetically different	Allotransplant (homotransplant)	Allogenic (homologous)	
Same species, genetically identical (identical twins, animals of an inbred strain)	Isotransplant (isotransplant)	Syngenic, isogenic (isologous)	
Donor = recipient	Autotransplant (autotransplant)	Autogenic (autologous)	

coded for alloantigenic structures, and that resistance to tumor transplantation was an immunologic phenomenon.

Shortly thereafter, Medawar showed that these observations were true not only for transplanted tumors but also for normal tissue grafts (e.g., skin); the rejection of normal tissue grafts was an immunological phenomenon. Structures on the cell surface, alloantigens, induced in a genetically different individual an immune reaction against the graft. Snell (1948) termed the antigens responsible for tissue compatibility *histocompatibility antigens* (H antigens) and the genes that control their expression, *histocompatibility genes* (H genes).

To study the effect and function of *H* genes and their products individually, Snell developed the concept of producing mouse strains that differ in only one *H* gene, the so-called congenic mouse strains. By developing such strains, the mouse became the experimental model par excellence in immunobiology.

In experiments with congenic mouse strains, Snell observed that not all the differences among *H* genes were equally strong in causing rejection: in some combinations transplanted tissue (e.g., skin) was rejected more quickly than in others. One gene in particular appeared to be responsible for acute rejection; this gene controlled the alloantigen designated by Gorer as antigen II, and that therefore was named the *H-2* gene. Allelic differences in this gene between recipient and donor of tissue grafts usually cause rejection within two weeks after engraftment,

whereas differences for other *H* genes led to delayed or chronic rejection. Tumor transplants were always rejected in cases of allelic differences at the *H-2* locus; however, this was not always true when there were differences in the alleles of other *H* genes. Thus, it appeared reasonable to distinguish two types of *H* genes: those that induce strong (major *H* gene), and those that induce weak (minor *H* genes) immune reaction. The major *H* gene was termed *major histocompatibility complex, MHC*. The minor *H* genes were summarized in general with a negative term, *non-MHC* genes. In the mouse, more than thirty *non-H-2* genes have been detected (*H-1, H-3, H-4, ...,* etc.). In most other species, including man, one may assume the existence of *non-MHC* genes, but they have not as yet been characterized.

Since the first description in the mouse, a major histocompatibility complex has been described for all better studied mammals, birds, and several lower vertebrates. Thus, the mouse *H-2* complex corresponds to the human *HLA* complex, to the *RhLA* complex in rhesus monkey, to the *DLA* complex in dog, to the *GPLA* complex in guinea pig, to the *RTl* complex in rat, and to the *B* complex in chicken. The genetic organization of these complexes appears to be extremely similar in all species thus far examined (with the possible exception of the mouse).

The elucidation of the *MHC* in terms of its phenotypic expression as well as function is based on the serological recognition and analysis of the cell surface molecules controlled by *MHC* genes. This serological and genetic analysis is performed in different ways depending upon the availability of inbred animals (for example, the mouse), or accessibility to outbred populations only (for example, man). The two different approaches will be discussed separately using the mouse as an example in which the analysis is based on inbred strains, and man in which the analysis is based upon population and family studies.

The Major Histocompatibility Complex (H-2) of the Mouse

Congenic Strains

Before we describe the mouse *MHC*, *H-2*, in terms of its serological properties, a brief summary on the laboratory mouse as used in these studies will follow.

Inbred strains are maintained by continuous brother–sister matings; after about twenty generations complete homozygosity for almost all alleles of the genome is achieved. In-

dividuals of an inbred strain are comparable to monozygous twins. An inbred strain differs in many alleles from other inbred strains or wild animals. If one of these alleles is a histocompatibility gene, one can determine the allogeneic difference by analysis of tumor or skin graft rejection and serological typing. If an allele donor strain (wild or inbred strain) A *(a/a)* is crossed with a background inbred strain B *(b/b)*, both genomes, *a* and *b*, will be "diluted" by half in the F_1 generation. Repeated crossing of the heterozygote *(a/b)* with the background strain B *(b/b)* and simultaneous selection for the allele H^a brings about in every subsequent generation a dilution of the A genome by half. In this way, after about 12 generations one has a mouse strain that has up to 99.999% the genome of the background strain B together with the H^a allele of the donor strain A (Fig. 6.1). Such a new inbred strain is now designated with the name of the background strain from which the genome originated (e.g., B 10) together with the symbol of the selected allele $(H-2^a)$:

Production of H-2 complex congenic lines

Breeding system		Generation	Selection	% Genome of the background strain
Marker Donor (A)	Background Donor (B)			
a a	b b			
a/b a/b	b b	N 1		50
b/b a/b	b b	N 2	Acceptance of A-(a/a) skin; positive reaction with anti-A	75
b/b a/b	b b	N 3	''	87.5
b/b a/b	a/b	N 12	''	99.999...
b/b a/b a/a a/a		N 12FI	Rejection of B-(b/b) skin; negative reaction with anti-B	

Fig. 6.1. Backcross system (NX) for the production of congenic strains of mice. Gen., backcross generation (N); A, donor strain; B, "background strain" (inbred); $a = H\text{-}2^a$; $b = H\text{-}2^b$, $H\text{-}2^a/H\text{-}2^b$ heterozygotes are selected through serotyping. [Modified from Klein J (1975) The biology of the mouse histocompatibility-2 complex. Springer, Berlin Heidelberg New York]

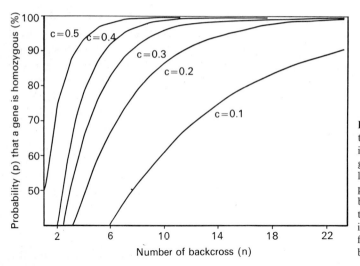

Fig. 6.2. Probability p (in percent) that any gene is homozygous if it is segregated from the selected gene ($c = 0.5$) or is linked to the selected gene ($c = 0.4$ to $c = 0.1$), depending upon the number of backcrosses. Calculated according to the equation $p_n = 1 - (1 - c)^{n-1}$, in which c is the recombination frequency and n, the number of backcrosses

B 10. H-2^a. This strain is H-2 congenic to B 10 (B 10. H-2^b); in a simpler form, only the allele symbol is written: B 10. A.

The degree of congeneity, i.e., the probability (p) that a desired gene will achieve homozygosity, can be calculated according to the equation,

$$p_n = 1 - (1 - c)^{n-1}, \tag{1}$$

where c is the recombination frequency between the H gene and any other gene and n, the number of backcrosses. To achieve homozygosity for all possible unlinked genes, 12 backcrosses are sufficient (Fig. 6.2.). However, to obtain homozygosity for all possible linked genes up to a distance of 10 recombination units, about 48 backcrosses are necessary (Fig. 6.2, curve $c = 0.1$).

The most frequently used congenic inbred strains, together with their H-2 allele, donor strain, background strain, and inbred strains with the same H-2 type, are shown in Table 6.2.

Table 6.2. Congenic inbred strains: H-2 haplotype, H-2 donor strain, background strain, and inbred strains with the same H-2 haplotype

Strain	H-2 type	H-2 donor	Background strain	Inbred strains with the same H-2 type
C57BL/10(B10)	b	C57BL/10(B10)	C57BL/10(B10)	129, C57BL/6 (B6), LP, A.BY, C3H.SW
B10.D2	d	DBA/2	B10	DBA/2, BALB/c
B10.A	a	A/WySn	B10	A/J
B10.M	f	Not inbred	B10	A.CA
B10.BR	k	C57BR	B10	C3H, CBA, AKR
B10.Q	q	DBA/1	B10	DBA/1, SWR
B10.RIII(71NS)	r	RIII	B10	RIII, LP.RIII
B10.S	s	A.SW	B10	A.SW, SJL
B10.PL	u	PL	B10	
A/WySn(A)	a	A/WySn	A/WySn(A)	A/J
A.BY	b	B10	A	C57BL/10, B6, 129, LP, C3H.SW
A.CA	f	Caracul	A	B10.M
A.SW	s	Swiss	A	B10.S, SJL

Serology

In the mouse, serology deals with planned immunizations using genetically uniform strains. The antisera obtained in such a reproducible way are then analyzed for their activity in such detail as to define as many antibodies as possible present in a given serum, and to establish all the determinants recognized by them. This is usually accomplished by testing the sera directly (hemagglutination, complement-dependent cytotoxicity test (see Chap. 7), after which absorption analysis with cells of all cross-reacting strains is performed. This analysis is then followed by specifically designed mating experiments to establish linkage and, if possible allelism, of the genes coding for the detected determinants by segregation analysis.

Thus, let us consider an antiserum produced by immunization of a congenic strain B.B with tissue of another strain congenic to B (e.g., B.A). The B anti-A serum, which contains antibodies against alloantigens that are controlled by *H-2* genes, agglutinates or lyses (in the presence of complement) all cells that carry H-2^a molecules. Using a large number of allogeneic strains, e.g., A, B, C, D, ..., etc., one will find that anti-A also reacts with cells from C, D, ..., etc. (cross-reaction with determinants shared by molecules of different alleles). Selective absorption permits the detection of a complete spectrum of alloantigenic specificities (determinants) for the strains examined. For example, if the B anti-A serum reacts with cells of strains A, C, and D, one can assume the presence of at least one alloantigen, though more probably two or three. If after absorption with cells of C, the serum still reacts with A and D, it indicates that A and D cells possess a common alloantigen 1 which the cells of B animals (in which the serum was produced) and of C animals lack. If the serum still reacts with A and C after absorption with D cells, there is a second alloantigen 2 which is common to A and C cells but which the B and D cells lack; finally, if the reactivity against A cells remains after the antiserum has been absorbed with C and D cells, it means that A cells have an alloantigen 3 that neither B, C, nor D cells carry. In the hypothetical example, B has none of the alloantigens, A has all three (1, 2, and 3), whereas C (antigen 2) and D (antigen 1) each have a different antigen in common with A (Table 6.3).

Table 6.3. Determination of antigenic determinants by cross-absorption

Reacting test cells	Reactivity of B anti-A serum after absorption with cells of				
	A	B	C	D	C+D
A (1, 2, 3)	−	+	+	+	+
B (0)	−	+	−	−	−
C (2)	−	+	−	+	−
D (1)	−	+	+	−	−

Using this scheme, one can choose all possible combinations to produce antisera and to analyze the sera by cross-absorption. Antigenic specificities (determinants) which can be detected on cells of the donor strain (against which the antiserum was produced) after the serum has been absorbed with cells of all cross-reacting strains, are called "private" antigens. These are characteristic for a specific *MHC (H-2)* allele when produced, analyzed, and applied within a limited test panel (here, A, B, C, and D). In our example, the private antigen for strain A is 3. Antigenic determinants found on cells of genetically different strains, i.e., cross-reacting antigens, are called "public" antigens (in our example, these are the antigens 1 and 2). The distinction between private and public determinants is only operational; in sufficiently large test panels, there is no difference in principle between these two types of determinants except that private determinants appear to occur less frequently than public determinants. In wild populations, private determinants are not characteristic of a specific allele; only sets of determinants define alleles.

H-2 K,D Genes: Class I Genes. An accidental observation by Snell (1953) indicated that the *H-2* locus consisted not only of one gene. He observed that offspring of crosses between two strains of mice k/k and d/d accepted tumor grafts of a third inbred strain a/a, but that the parents of the k/d-F$_1$ hybrids did not. He explained this unexpected result with the hypothesis that the *H-2* locus consisted of two genes (*K* and *D*), and that the mice of strain a/a possessed one gene (*K*) from the k/k and the other (*D*) from the d/d parent, the combination being derived by recombination of the two chromosomes:

Mouse strain		
Phenotype	Genotype	
k/k	*kk/kk*	} Parents
d/d	*dd/dd*	
k/d	*kk/dd*	F$_1$ hybrid
a/a	*kd/kd*	recombinant

Since then, numerous additional recombinants for the *H-2* complex have been described. For historical reasons, one gene has kept the symbol *K*, and the other *D*. Different alleles are characterized by a small letter suffix with signifies the origin of the allele, e.g., the *K* allele of a b/b mouse is written *K^b*, the *D* allele *D^b*. The combination *K-D* is called a haplotype. Different haplotypes are indicated with small letters (e.g., *H-2^b* represents the haplotype of a B10 mouse, *H-2^a* the haplotype of an A or B10.A mouse, see Table 6.2. If such recombinant mouse strains are used to produce antisera, it can be shown that both genes control different alloantigens (K and D molecules, class I molecules, see p. 155), although both genes express a large number of shared determinants, e.g., each of the two genes controls one antigenic determinant that is typical for the specific *K* or *D* allele (private antigen), and several antigenic specificities that are shared by different *K* and/or *D* alleles (public specificities). The antigenic specificities are designated numerically in order of their detection, preceded by the designation of the encoding locus, for example K 33, D 2 (Table 6.4). Since the first description more

Table 6.4. Antigen specificities of K and D molecules in inbred strains

Allele	Private	Public specificities																	
		3	5	8	11	25	34	35	36	37	38	39	42	45	46	47	52	53	54
H-2. K molecules																			
b	33	—	5	—	—	—	—	35	36	—	—	39	—	—	46	—	—	53	54
d	31	3	—	8	—	—	34	—	—	—	—	—	—	—	46	47	—	—	—
f	26	—	—	8	—	—	—	—	—	37	—	39	—	—	46	—	—	53	—
j	15	—	—	—	—	—	—	—	—	—	38	—	—	45	46	47	—	—	—
k	23	3	5	8	11	25	—	—	—	—	—	—	—	45	—	47	52	—	—
p	16	—	5	8	—	—	34	—	—	37	38	—	—	—	46	—	—	—	—
q	17	3	5	—	11	—	34	—	—	—	—	—	—	45	—	—	52	—	54
r	?	3	5	8	11	25	—	—	—	—	—	—	—	45	—	47	52	—	54
s	19	—	5	—	—	—	—	—	—	—	—	—	42	45	—	—	—	—	—
u	20	—	5	8	—	—	—	35	36	—	—	—	—	45	—	—	52	53	—
v	21	3	5	—	—	—	—	—	—	—	—	—	—	45	—	—	—	—	—

Allele	Private	Public specificities													
		3	6	13	35	36	41	42	43	44	49	50	51	55	56
H-2. D molecules															
b (j)	2	—	6	—	—	—	—	—	—	—	—	—	—	—	56
d (u)	4	3	6	13	35	36	41	42	43	44	49	50	—	—	—
f	9	—	6	—	—	—	—	—	—	—	—	—	—	—	56
k	32	3	—	—	—	—	—	—	—	—	49	—	—	—	—
p	22	3	6	—	35	—	41	—	—	—	49	—	—	—	—
q (v)	30	3	6	13	—	—	—	—	—	—	49	—	—	55	56
r	18	—	6	—	—	—	—	—	—	—	49	—	51	—	—
s	12	3	6	—	—	36	—	42	—	—	49	—	—	—	—

than 11 private K and 12 private D antigens have been found in standard inbred strains. When wild mice are typed with these reagents produced in inbred strain combinations, two remarkable results are obtained: first, the frequency of alleles encoding the different molecules is extremely low for all of them, in general below 2%; and second, the number of alleles which cannot be defined so far is extremely high, i.e., more than 60% of the naturally occurring alleles are undetected by the available reagents. The number of alleles may turn out to be several hundred; we must keep in mind (see above) that the employed reagents do not truly characterize alleles. Thus, a molecule reacting with, say, anti-K 23, may not react with anti-K 25, a combination which defines the H-$2 K^k$ allele of the inbred strain against which the antisera had been produced. These numbers indicate a serological and molecular complexity and a genetic polymorphism unknown in any other genetic system (except antibody binding sites, see p. 100).

Immune Response Region Genes: *Class II* Genes. Specifically designed mating experiments between recombinants and inbred strains yielded new recombinants in which the new cross-over occurred between the K and D genes either extremely close to the K or near the D gene:

Mouse A.AL *(H-2ᵃˡ)* × Mouse A.SW *(H-2ˢ)*

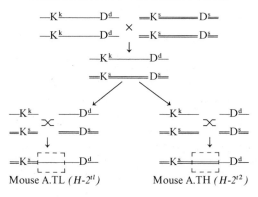

Mouse A.TL *(H-2ᵗˡ)*   Mouse A.TH *(H-2ᵗ²)*

When such recombinants having identical K and D alleles were reciprocally immunized,

it was found, surprisingly, that the chromosomal section between the K and D genes also controlled alloantigens on the surface of cell membranes. Because genes of this region of the chromosome had already been characterized functionally, namely as genes that control the humoral immune response (*Im-mune response genes, Ir* genes), these genes were called I genes and the molecules that they control I region *associated* (Ia) molecules (class II molecules, see p. 155). Thus far, two loci have been identified with serological methods: I-A which maps near the K locus, and I-E which is located to the right of I-A. Both loci are polymorphic with numerous antigen specificities designated by continuous numbers in order of their detection, preceded by the designation Ia (Table 6.5). Recent findings indicate that the I-E locus (and by analogy, the I-A locus) actually consists of two genes, E_α and E_β (and A_α and A_β), each encoding a polypeptide chain, which together form the membrane Ia molecule (see also p. 153). The E_α gene exists in two allelic forms, one expressing the E_α-polypeptide chain with the marker antigen Ia.7 (E_α^7), the other expressing no chain in the membrane (E_α^0). The E_β gene is highly polymorphic but is expressed only if combined with the E_α^7 allele, either in cis-position (linked on the same chromosome, recombinants) or in trans-position (located on the other chromosome, F_1 hybrids) (Table 6.6).

Ia molecules are characterized by two peculiarities that distinguish them both genetically and serologically from the K and D molecules: Ia molecules are found primarily on B lymphocytes and macrophages as well as stimulated T lymphocytes, but not in any other tissue.

The general terminology for the I region alleles corresponds to that of the K or D alleles, i.e., the I region of haplotype H-$2ᵃ$ is called $Iᵃ$, that of the haplotype H-$2ᵇ$, $Iᵇ$. In recombinant haplotypes, the individual MHC loci are identified by the haplotype symbol of the parent strain from which they originate; e.g., for the previously described recombinant A.TL: $Kˢ$-$Iᵏ$-$Dᵈ$ or $s\,k\,d = H$-

Table 6.5. Antigen chart of some specificities encoded at the $I-A$ locus (inbred strains)

$H\text{-}2$ Haplotype	Ia Antigens of the $I-A$ locus																						
	1	2	3	4	5	6	8	9	10	11	12	13	14	15	16	17	18	19	20	24	25	26	27
b	–	–	3	–	–	–	8	9	–	–	–	–	–	15	–	–	–	–	20	–	–	–	–
d	–	–	–	–	–	6	8	–	–	11	–	–	–	15	16	–	–	–	–	–	–	–	–
f	1	–	–	–	5	–	–	–	–	–	–	–	14	–	–	17	18	–	–	–	25	26	27
j	–	–	.	–	5	.	–	.	10	–	–	–	–	15	.	–	.	–	–	–	.	.	.
k	1	2	3	–	–	–	–	–	–	–	–	–	–	15	–	17	18	19	–	–	25	26	–
p	–	–	–	–	5	6	–	–	–	–	–	13	–	–	–	–	–	–	–	–	.	.	.
q	–	–	3	–	5	–	–	9	10	–	–	13	–	–	16	–	–	–	–	–	–	–	–
r	1	–	3	–	5	–	–	–	–	–	12	–	–	–	–	17	–	19	–	24	25	26	–
s	–	–	–	4	5	–	–	9	–	–	12	–	–	–	–	17	18	–	–	24	–	–	27
u	1	–	.	–	5	.	–	.	–	–	–	–	–	–	.	17	.	–	–	24	.	.	.
v	–	–	.	–	5	.	8	.	–	–	–	–	–	15	.	–	.	–	–	–	–	.	.

Table 6.6. Ia determinants controlled by E_β and E_α loci

$H\text{-}2$ haplotype	E_β determinants[a]						E_α det.
	21	22	23	32	41	42	7
b	(–	22	–	32	.[b]	·)	0
d	–	–	23	–	–	–	7
j	.	.	.	32	–	–	7
k	–	22	–	32	–	42	7
p	21	–	–	32	–	–	7
q	(·	·	·	·	·	·)	0
r	–	–	–	32	–	–	7
s	(–	22	–	·	·	·)	0
u	.	.	.	32	–	–	7
v	.	.	.	32	41	42	7

[a] Determinations in parentheses are expressed on the cell surface only when the controlling E_β allele occurs in combination with the E_α^7 allele.
[b] Dot indicates unknown

2^{t1}, and A.TH: $K^s\text{-}I^s\text{-}D^d$ or $s\ s\ d=H\text{-}s2^{t2}$. The most common $H\text{-}2$ recombinants, their origins, and the composition of their haplotypes are depicted in Table 6.7. The same numerical designation of alloantigens controlled by K and D genes indicates identical serological antigenic specificities; identical numerical designations for Ia antigens, however, characterize antigenic specificities that differ from those of the K and D antigens.

Linkage Analysis of the Mouse $H\text{-}2$ Complex. On the basis of serologically determined phenotypes and corresponding breeding experiments, at least four genetic regions in the MHC of the mouse can be differentiated, linked in the following order: $K\text{-}I\text{-}S\text{-}D$. The D region consists of at least two loci, D and L, the order of which is unknown. The L gene product has been defined by capping (see p. 150) and a mutant $H\text{-}2^d$ allele.

The S region also consists of at least two loci, the Ss (serum substance) gene, and the Slp (sex-limited protein) gene; the latter is expressed only in males within inbred strains

Table 6.7. H-2 recombinant strains and their origin

F$_1$-hybrid origin	H-2 type	H-2 complex alleles K A$_\beta$ A$_\alpha$ E$_\beta$ J E$_\alpha$ S D	New H-2 haplotype K A$_\beta$ A$_\alpha$ E$_\beta$ J E$_\alpha$ S D	Strain	H-2 type
X[a]	k	k k k k k 7 k k			
Y	d	d d d d d 7 d d	k k k k k│[b] 7 d d	B10.A	a
B10.A	a	k k k k│k 7 d d			
B10	b	b b b b│b 0 b b	b b b b│k 7 d d	B10.A(5R)	i5
B10.A	a	k k k│k k 7 d d			
B10	b	b b b│b b 0 b b	k k k│b b 0 b b	B10.A(4R)	h4
B10.A	a	k k k k k 7 d│d			
B10	b	b b b b b 0 b│b	k k k k k 7 d│b	B10.A(2R)	h2
B10.A	a	k│k k k k 7 d d			
T138	q	q│q q q q 0 q q	q│k k k k 7 d d	B10.AQR	y1
DBA/2	d	d d d d d 7 d│d			
C3H	k	k k k k k 7 k│k	k k k k k 7 k│d	A.AL	a1
A.AL	a1	k│k k k k 7 k d			
A.SW	s	s│s s s s 0 s s	s│k k k k 7 k d	A.TL	t1
A.AL	a1	k k k k k 7 k│d			
A.SW	s	s s s s s 0 s│s	s s s s s 0 s│d	A.TH	t2
A.TL	t1	s k k k k│7 k d			
B10.S	s	s s s s s│0 s s	s s s s s│7 k d	B10.HTT	t3
B10.A	a	k k k k k 7 d│d			
B10.S	s	s s s s s 0 s│s	s s s s s 0 s│d	B10.S(7R)	t2
A.TL	t1	s k k k k 7 k│k			
A.CA	f	f f f f f 0 f│f	s k k k k 7 k│f	A.TE	an1
B10.AKR	k	k k k k k 7 k│k			
M	q	q q q q q 0 q│q	k k k k k 7 k│q	B10.AKM	m
DBA/2	d	d d d d d 7 d│d			
C3H	k	k k k k k 7 k│k	d d d d d 7 d│k	C3H.OH	02
DBA/2	d	d d d d d 7│d d			
C3H	k	k k k k k 7│k k	d d d d d 7│k k	C3H.OL	01

[a] The H-2 haplotype of B10.A was already existent before inbreeding; the parental strains of the F$_1$-hybrid are not known

[b] Bar designates position of cross-over

– however, in wild mice it also occurs in females. The products of both genes are detectable in the serum and (passively?) attached to the membrane of erythrocytes. The Ss gene product has been shown to be the fourth complement component; the Slp substance has similar physicochemical properties, however, it is functionally not active as a complement component.

Within the I region, several loci can be identified: the A locus (most probably two genes, A$_\alpha$ and A$_\beta$), the E$_\beta$ locus, the I-J locus, and the E$_\alpha$ locus. A product of the I-J locus has not yet been detected, its proposed existence is based on functional tests; it is supposed to control the suppression of an immune response, and is expressed on a subset of T cells only.

Closely linked to the H-2 complex are several genes which also control the expression of membrane components: the Qa loci and the Tla locus to the right of the D region. The

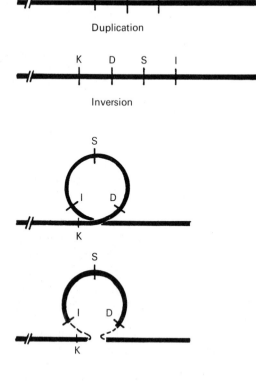

H-2 COMPLEX

Fig. 6.3. Genetic map of the *H-2* complex and its vicinity. *T*, *T/t* complex (brachyury or short tail); *tf*, tufted; *Glo*, glyoxalase; *H-2*, major histocompatibility complex; *Ce-2*, kidney catalase; *C3*, complement component 3; *Ea-2*, erythrocyte antigen 2; *Ir-5*, immune response-5. The order of $A_\beta A_\alpha E_\beta$ and of *D, L* loci is not known. Also linked are: *Pgk-2*, phosphoglycerate kinase-2; *Apl*, acid phosphatase-liver; *Pg-5*, pepsinogen-5; *C3b*-receptor; *H-31; H-32; H-33;* and *H-39*

former express molecules on subsets of B and T lymphocytes, the latter controls differentiation antigens on thymus cells. The relationship of these loci to the *H-2* complex proper is unclear.

To the left of the *K* locus is linked the *T/t*-complex, the genes of which control early ontogenic differentiation.

Several other genes syntenic to the *H-2* complex are also found in linkage with the *MHC* in other species: *Glo* (glyoxalase), *Pgk* (phosphoglycerate kinase), *C3* (third complement component), *Pg-5* (urinary pepsinogen-5).

Cytogenetic studies of translocation indicated that the mouse *MHC* is localized on the seventeenth chromosome, and that the *K* locus lies nearer to the centromere than the *D* locus does (all chromosomes of the mouse inbred strains are acrocentric).

Figure 6.3 is a genetic map of the *H-2* complex. As will be evident, the gene structure of the *MHC* of the mouse differs from that of

Fig. 6.4. Hypothetic scheme of the origin of the *MHC*-(*H-2*) gene sequence in the mouse

other species, including that of human: In the mouse, the *I* region is located between the two *H* loci, *K* and *D*; in all other species thus far examined, the genes that correspond to those included in the *I* region are found outside the *K* and *D* analogues. It is thought that the *K* and *D* genes originated by duplication of an ancestral gene during evolution and came to their present-day position by inversion; thus, the *I* and *S* regions were confined between the *K* and *D* loci (Fig. 6.4).

Fig. 6.5. Histogram of anti-4^a and anti-4^b reactions with leukocytes of a test panel (Van Rood)

The Major Histocompatibility Complex of Man (HLA)

Serology

Leukocyte antigens, later defined as gene products of the human MHC, were first described by Dausset in 1956. Sera of patients who have had multiple transfusions and of multiparous women contain antibodies that agglutinate leukocytes and have specificity other than that exhibited by erythrocyte-agglutinating antibodies. It took almost ten years to discover that the leukocyte antigens were components of one exceedingly complex genetic system: the human major histocompatibility complex, HLA.

Serological analysis of MHC molecules of a species consisting of outbred individuals only has to be performed differently from that of a species in which inbred strains are available, e.g., the mouse. In the outbred human population, no two unrelated individuals are genetically identical. Since the genetic differences are also reflected in antigenic differences, antisera generated by immunization of an individual A by cells of an individual B will be unique. Although different antisera may contain antibodies to the same determinant(s), they will also contain antibodies to other determinants; and those other antibodies tend to obscure the determination of specificities. To analyze such

antisera, it is necessary to apply a different approach from that used for the analysis described above of antisera produced in inbred mouse strains. Here, a large number of antisera has to be tested against a large panel of cells in order to find identical or antithetic reactivity patterns. The reactivity of each antiserum with each single cell of a large panel has to be compared with the reactivity of all other antisera individually. In order to find significant positive (identical reactivity) or negative (antithetical reactivity) associations of reactivity patterns, statistical methods are applied by first constructing a 2×2 contingency table, and then to determine the significance of the associations in this table by either the χ^2-test or the correlation coefficient test.

An example of such an analysis is given in Fig. 6.5. Here, van Rood and his colleagues analyzed the reactivity of 63 antisera with a panel of 40 individuals. The positive and negative reactions with each cell were compared with those of all others, i.e., that of lymphocyte 1 was compared with that of 39 others, that of lymphocyte 2 with the remaining 38, etc. In this way, 820 (20 × 41) independent comparisons had to be performed. Only for one pair were all reactions identical, and only four pairs showed 95% identical reactions.

Applying this approach and analyzing sera from multiparous women which contain antibodies against leukocyte antigens of the paternal haplotype transmitted to the children, it was possible to describe groups of antigens that acted as though they were controlled by alleles of the same gene (i.e., they never appeared together), and others that occurred together indicating that the products of at least two closely linked genes could be demonstrated. Family studies confirmed this contention of at least two genes: *HLA-A* and *HLA-B*. Studies in the past few years have shown that a third gene is located between *HLA-A* and *HLA-B* which controls membrane antigens, but which appears to be less polymorphic than the two others: *HLA-C*. Most recently, as a result of the search for antigenic determinants that are similar to the Ia antigens in the mouse, antibodies were discovered in anti-HLA sera that reacted with antigens found primarily on B lymphocytes. The gene(s) controlling these antigens are linked to the *HLA* complex and appear to map outside but close to the *HLA-B* locus, actually between the *HLA-B* and *HLA-D* (see below) locus. Molecules expressed by these genes are called DR (*D* region related) antigens.

To date, more than 40 HLA antigens have been identified on leukocytes; they represent the alleles of at least four closely linked loci: *HLA-A* (formerly *first* or *LA* locus), *HLA-B* (formerly *second* or *FOUR* locus), *HLA-C* (formerly *third* or *Aj* locus), and loci controlling DR antigens. Of the 58 serologically detectable antigens thus far described, 16 antigens are controlled by alleles of the *A* locus, 26 antigens by alleles of the *B* locus, 6 antigens by alleles of the *C* locus, and 7 antigens controlled by *DR* loci (Table 6.8).

A part of the population that is not homozygous (which can be determined by family studies) cannot be characterized completely ("full house") for all alleles; this indicates that in addition to those already described, there are other alleles not yet identified by any antiserum ("blanks"). Furthermore, the more refined the serological analysis becomes, the more specificities are recognized as a group of specificities giving evidence for two or more antigens detected by a standard reagent (splitting). Thus, in the future, many more specificities will be added to the present chart.

Lymphocyte-Activating Determinants (LAD)

If lymphocytes of two unrelated individuals are cultivated together in vitro (mixed lymphocyte culture, MLC), after a few days (3–5) the culture contains lymphoblasts that are not observed when the cells of each person are cultivated individually for the same period of time. This transformation, from small lymphocytes to lymphoblasts, is called blast transformation. If ^{3}H-thymidine is added to the MLC after 3–4 days, it can be shown after an additional 16 h incubation that the label has been incorporated into the DNA. These findings indicate not only that the lymphocytes are transformed but also that they synthesize new DNA, i.e., they proliferate. This entire process, transformation and proliferation, is called mixed lymphocyte reaction, MLR, and is, in the preceding example, a two-way reaction, because the lymphocytes of both individuals react.

This reaction occurs between lymphocytes only if they originate from histogenetically different individuals. It was thought originally that this reaction was caused by HLA-A and B antigens since there was a correlation of MLC reactivity and identity or disparity for HLA antigens in families. However, it was soon learned that A, B-identical lymphocytes of unrelated persons also exhibited strong MLC reactivity, i.e., they stimulated each other to transform and pro-

Table 6.8. Antigens of the *HLA-A, -B, -C, -D,* and *DR* loci and their average gene frequency in the North American population, Bodmer et al. 1977

HLA-A		HLA-C		HLA-B		HLA-D		HLA-DR	
Antigen	Gene Fre-quency	Antigen	Gene Fre-quency	Antigen	Gene Fre-quency	Antigen	Gene Fre-quency	Antigen	Gene Fre-quency
A1	0.12	Cw1[a]	0.03	B5	0.06	Dw1	0.07	DRw1	0.06
A2	0.23	Cw2	0.07	B7	0.11	Dw2	0.12	DRw2	0.14
A3	0.17	Cw3	0.10	B8	0.09	Dw3	0.09	DRw3	0.12
A11	0.04	Cw4	0.11	B12	0.12	Dw4	0.05	DRw4	0.12
A19	0.11	Cw5	0.04	B13	0.02	Dw5	0.06	DRw5	0.12
A23	0.06	Cw6	0.06	B14	0.05	Dw6	0.09	DRw6	0.15
A24	0.06			B15	0.05	Dw7	0.10	DRw7	0.12
Aw25	0.01			Bw16	0.05	Dw8	0.02		
Aw26	0.02			B17	0.08				
A28	0.05			B18	0.03				
A29	0.02			B21	0.04				
Aw30	0.08			Bw22	0.04				
Aw31	0.04			B27	0.03				
Aw32	0.03			Bw35	0.10				
Aw33	0.03			B37	0.05				
Aw43	>0.00			Bw38	0.02				
				Bw39	0.01				
				Bw40	0.05				
				Bw41	0.02				
				Bw42	0.00				
				Bw44	>0.00				
				Bw45	0.01				
				Bw47	0.05				
				Bw51	0.02				
				Bw52	>0.00				
				Bw53	0.01				
Blank[b]	0		0.60		0.06		0.41		0.14

[a] w in front of the antigen notation indicates that the antigen was tested in a histocompatibility workshop but has not yet been recognized by the nomenclature committee of the World Health Organization (WHO)
[b] Blank gives the percentage of alleles not yet defined

liferate. Eventually, a family was found in which the lymphocytes of HLA-A and B-identical siblings exhibited MLC reactivity, indicating that the genes coding for HLA-A and -B molecules are different from those coding for lymphocyte-activating determinants (LAD) termed *HLA-D* gene(s).

If one of the reacting cell samples in the mixed lymphocyte culture is treated with mitomycin C or is irradiated with 2,500 R, these cells are no longer able to proliferate, but they are able to stimulate the untreated lymphocyte population to transform and proliferate. This set-up is called a "one-way reaction," and its use permits one to distinguish which of the two lymphocyte populations stimulates which. Applying this test, individual determinants can be defined.

Like the HLA-A, B, and C antigens, the membrane determinants responsible for the MLR are expressed codominantly, i.e., each individual has a maximum of two (if heterozygous) determinants on its lymphocytes. The testing of unrelated donors showed that

Fig. 6.6. Determination of HLA-D phenotype(s) with homozygous typing cells (HTC); a, b, and c represent *HLA-D* alleles

there must be more than 20 allelic forms of this gene. Investigating selected families, one can in rare cases find persons who have inherited the same allele from both parents and are, therefore, *HLA-D* homozygous. Cells from this individual will stimulate all other cells that do not possess this allele; however, they will not stimulate those that carry the same allele in heterozygous or homozygous form (one-way stimulation) (Fig. 6.6). Using such homozygous typing cells (HTC), it is possible to characterize other, unknown lymphocytes in terms of

their HLA-D determinants by testing their ability to be stimulated by reference cells (Fig. 6.7). In this way, eight homozygous reference cells with determinants HLA-D 1 through D 8 have been defined (Table 4.6; the small w (= workshop) indicates that this term is used only temporarily until the nomenclature commission of the WHO officially accepts this designation). Lymphocyte-activating determinants defined by HTCs are probably identical with or includ DR antigens with the same specificities (numbers, see Table 6.8).

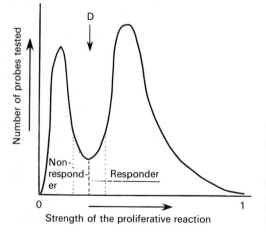

Fig. 6.7. MLR typing with homozygous reference cells as stimulator cells. D, discrimination value. Responder cells that exhibit a reaction < D are *nonresponders*, i.e., they have the *HLA-D* determinants of the reference cells; responder cells that exhibit a reaction > D are *responders*, i.e., they have *HLA-D* determinants that differ from those of the reference cells. D must be tested for each reference cell

Genetics

The genetic analysis of the HLA system is based on two factors: population and family studies.

In the genetic sense, a population is not only a group of individuals, but also a self-reproducing group whose gene constitution is described in terms of gene frequency. This frequency can be calculated from the corresponding phenotype frequency by direct counting of individuals that have a specific phenotype and division of the sum by the number of individuals in the population (in case of dominant genes). The frequency is expressed as a percentage. For example, we have two alleles, A and B, which present three phenotypes (genotypes): AA, AB, and BB (2%, 19%, and 79%, respectively). Because each individual has two genes, the percentages for A and B are: $2+9.5=11.5$ or $9.5+79=88.5$, i.e., the frequency of $A(p)$ and $B(q)$ is $p+q=0.115+0.885=1$.

In an ideal, large, panmictic population, in which the factors of migration, mutation, and selection play no role, there is a state of genetic equilibrium; i.e., genotype, as well as gene frequency, is constant from one generation to another. This characteristic is described by the Hardy-Weinberg theorem, expressed in the equation

$$(p+q)^2 = p^2 + 2\,pq + q^2 , \qquad (2)$$

in which p and q are the gene frequencies of A and B. The gene frequency (p_A) can be calculated from the frequency of the phenotype frequency (f_A) with the help of equation (2), if $q=(1-p)$ is substituted (because $p+q=1$, see above):

$$f_A = p_A^2 + 2\,p_A(1-p_A) = 2\,p_A - p_A^2$$
$$1 - f_A = 1 - 2\,p_A + p_A^2 = (1-p_A)^2 \qquad (3)$$
$$p_A = 1 - \sqrt{1-f_A}.$$

Antigen-phenotype frequencies and the gene frequencies calculated from them are summarized in Table 6.8 for the alleles of the four HLA loci.

Linkage Equilibrium.

According to the Hardy-Weinberg theorem, two conclusions can be drawn: (1) after one generation, the genotype of a gene with two alleles (A and B) will be present with a frequency of $p^2\,AA$: $2\,pq\,AB$: $q^2\,BB$, and (2) the frequency distribution will not change during the next generations, i.e., the population remains in equilibrium.

These conclusions apply to all autosomal gene loci, as long as they are considered individually. If two or more gene loci are considered at the same time, a state of equilibrium is not achieved after one generation. For example, in a population with the same number of $A_1A_1B_1B_1$ and $A_2A_2B_2B_2$ individuals (A and B are two loci each with alleles A_1 and A_2 or B_1 and B_2), the gene frequency for the two loci is then one-half, and from the nine possible genotypes, only one will appear after the first generation ($A_1A_2B_1B_2$). The others will appear in the subsequent generations, however, not exactly in equilibrium frequency. If one represents the frequency of each gene A_1, A_2, and B_1, B_2 with r, s, t, and u ($r+s+t+u=1$) and the frequency of the four gamete combinations: A_1B_1, A_1B_2, A_2B_1, and A_2B_2 with x_1, x_2, x_3, and x_4, whereby $x_1+x_2+x_3+x_4=1$ and $r=x_1+x_2$, $s=x_3+x_4$, $t=x_1+x_3$, and $u=x_2+x_4$, then the population reaches equilibrium when $x_1x_4=x_2x_3$. The difference, Δ,

$$\Delta = x_1x_4 - x_2x_3 \qquad (4)$$

describes the magnitude of the deviation from equilibrium, i.e., the magnitude of a linkage disequilibrium or a gametic association. The time necessary to achieve equilibrium is dependent upon the linkage relationship between the two genes and the initial value of Δ; if the two genes are not linked, Δ is halved with each generation. If both genes are linked, the value of Δ likewise decreases, but is dependent on the recombination frequency between A and B, according to the equation

$$\Delta_n = \Delta_0 (1 - rf)^n \rightarrow 0, \text{ if } n \rightarrow \infty , \qquad (5)$$

where Δ_o is the initial value, Δ_n the Δ value after the nth generation, n the number of generations, and rf the recombination frequency in a generation. The smaller rf is, the longer it will take until an equilibrium ($\Delta = 0$) is reached.

Linkage disequilibrium can occur in various ways: (1) migration, i.e., two populations with different gene frequencies, each of which is in equilibrium, mix; (2) selection, i.e., specific haplotypes (or alleles) have above all an advantage (disadvantage) for the survival of a population; and (3) gene drift, i.e., chance fluctuations of gene frequencies from one generation to another.

Haplotypes. If there is equilibrium, linked genes exhibit a basic difference in their behavior in families and populations. In a family, linked genes (haplotypes) show a "linkage association," whereas in the population no association is observed. If there is disequilibrium (which, with only a few exceptions, is the case in the human population), one can discover favored associations in population studies that would not be observed from family studies. Haplotype frequencies can be calculated using Δ according to the equation

$$x_{ij} = p_i P_j + D_{ij}, \qquad (6)$$

where p_i is the frequency of the allele i of the A locus, P_j the frequency of the allele j of the B locus, and D_{ij} the linkage association (see eq. 4 and Table 6.9) between the alleles. As

Table 6.9. Significant associations of *HLA-A* and *-B* alleles in the North American population. Bodmer et al. 1977

Haplotype	Frequency	Δ value
A1 − B8	67.9	59.2
A3 − B7	38.0	27.6
A25 − B18	8.3	7.5
A26 − Bw38	10.0	9.2
A26 − Bw21[a]	11.4	10.3
A28 − B14	13.3	12.7
Aw30 − B18	7.2	7.2
Aw32 − Bw35[a]	13.5	13.0

[a] Significant among North American Blacks

shown in Tables 6.9 and 6.10, there are several haplotypes in the North American population that do not occur in proportion to the frequency of the alleles of both genes, but rather more frequently. Of these, the *HLA-A1-B8* haplotype occurs most frequently and is the characteristic haplotype for a Caucasian population.

Closely linked genes (with an rf between the loci of 0.001) are generally observed inherited as "one" gene in family studies, and different phenotypic characteristics of both genes can therefore be viewed incorrectly as being controlled by the same gene. Genetic studies of populations can uncover the difference between the gene and its linkage. Thus, family studies of the genetics of reactivity in a mixed lymphocyte culture clearly show that the genes responsible for the mixed lymphocyte culture are apparently identical to those that control the ex-

Table 6.10. Significant associations of *HLA-B* and *-D* as well as *HLA-B* and *-DR* alleles in the North American population (Bodmer et al., 1977)

HLA-B and *-D* associations			*HLA-B* and *-DR* associations		
Haplotype	Frequency	Δ value	Haplotype	Frequency	Δ value
B5 − Dw5	12.6	9.7			
B7 − Dw2	41.0	31.0	B7 − DRw2	48.9	37.2
B8 − Dw3	57.6	56.9	B8 − DRw3	63.6	54.2
B12 − Dw2	41.1	30.0	B13 − DRw7	15.4	12.7
B14 − Dw5	16.5	15.3	B17 − DRw7	22.4	17.4
Bw44 − Dw4	24.4	19.4	Bw38 − DRw4	15.6	11.3
Bw51 − Dw5	12.9	10.6	Bw52 − DRw2	22.0	18.0

pression of the HLA-A and HLA-B antigens, because both characteristics are transfered together. Population studies, i.e., studies of the reactivity of lymphocytes of unrelated donors who were HLA-A and HLB-B identical, disclosed that *HLA-D* represents a different gene, which then could be proved by the finding of recombinant haplotypes in family studies. Particularly frequent associations between *HLA-B* and *HLA-D* are presented in Table 6.10.

Linkage Analysis of the HLA Complex

Until recently, linkage analyses in man were difficult, and with the exception of the sex chromosome-linked genes, few linkage groups were known. In the last few years, it has been possible, due to progress in somatic genetics and cell hybridization[1], to analyze linkage groups on autosomal chromosomes. The *HLA* complex forms a linkage group with phosphoglucomutase-3 (PGM-3), glyoxalase (GLO), and urine-pepsinogen-5 (Pg-5) on the short arm of the sixth chromosome. Complement components C 2 and C 4, with the allotypes Chido and Rodgers for C 4, belong to the same linkage group. Analysis of recombinant haplotypes in families has shown that the loci of the *HLA* complex are linked in the order *HLA-D-- -----B--C----A---*. The genes controlling the expression of DR antigens are found in the segment between *HLA-D* and *HLA-B*; the gene that controls the expression of the C 3-proactivator (C 3 PA, factor B or BF, or GBG – glycine-rich β-globulin) also maps within the same chromosomal stretch. Family studies also revealed that the loci controlling susceptibility for specific diseases are located between the *HLA-B* and *HLA-D* locus: *DS* genes (Disease Susceptibility) for the diseases mul-

Fig. 6.8. Gene (chromosome) map of human chromosome no. 6. *HLA*, human leukocyte antigen locus (human MHC); *PGM-3*, isoenzyme of phosphoglucomutase (in leukocytes); *GLO*, glyoxalase; *PG-5*, urine-pepsinogen-5; *BF*, C3 proactivator; *DS*, disease susceptibility; *MS*, multiple sclerosis; *AS*, ankylosis spondylitis (Bechterew's disease); *CD*, celiac disease

tiple sclerosis (MS), Bechterew's disease (ankylosis spondylitis, AS), and coeliac disease (CD), as well as others (see below, pp. 164–167). Another gene closely linked to *HLA* is that which regulates the immune response to pollen grain antigen (antigen E), and which is responsible for several asthmatic reactions. The data are summarized in Fig. 6.8.

Gene Structure of MHC in Other Species

The gene structure of MHC is similar for all species of animals examined thus far (Table 6.11). In addition to the two species already discussed at length, man and mouse, the following species have been studied in some detail: primates, particularly rhesus monkey and chimpanzee, cattle, pig, dog, guinea pig, rabbit, rat, and among the birds, the chicken. Analysis of *MHC* in primates, dogs, and cattle were carried out by family and population studies, those in the other mentioned animals with the help of inbred strains. In primates and dogs, two loci could be distinguished which control cell surface antigens like *HLA-A* and *B* or *H-2 K* and *D*,

---

1 By this method, cells of different species are fused; after passage of such hybrid cells, chromosomes from one parent are usually lost. Parallel to the loss of certain chromosomes, certain phenotypic markers disappear. It is, therefore, possible to assign the genes of these markers to specific chromosomes which are, in turn, identified by banding patterns

Table 6.11. Genetic organization of major histocompatibility systems

Species	Designation	Genetic organization	Linkage	Remarks
Man	HLA	- - - - - - - -D-Bf,C4,DR - B- - - C- - - - -A- - - - (>8)[a] (>8)(>28)(>6) (>17)	Chromosome 6, Ir, C2, GLO, Pg-5 Chido, Rodgers	Disease association (ass.)
Chimpanzee	ChLA	- - - - - - - -D- - - - - - -B- - - - - - - - - - - -A- - - - (>1) (>7) (>4)		Gene order arbitrary
Rhesus monkey	RhLA	- - - - - - -D, Bf- - - - B- - - - - - - - - - - -A- - - - (>10) (>13) (>13)	Ir, Ia	
Cattle	BoLA	- - - - - - -D_1,D_2- - - - - - - - - - - - - -A- - - - (>6) (>6)		
Pig	SLA	- - - - - - - -D- - - - - - - - - - - - - - - - - -A- - - - (>4) (>4)	Ir	
Dog	DLA	- - - - - - -D- - - - - -B- - -C- - - - - - - -A- - - - (>9) (>5)(>3) (>6)	Ir	Gene order arbitrary
Rabbit	RLA	- - - - - - -D- - - - - -B- - - - - - - - - - - -A- - - - (>5) (>1) (>13)	LG VII, He	Gene order arbitrary
Guinea pig	GPLA	- - - - - - -I- - - - - - -B- - - - - - - - - - - - - - (>4) (>3)	C4, Ir, Ia, Bf	Autoimmune disease ass.
Rat	RT1	- - - - - - -B- - - - - - - - - - - - - - - - - -A- - - - (>9) (>15)	C, D, E, Ir	Autoimmune disease ass.
Mouse	H-2	- -K- - - - I- - - - S- - -D- - - -L- - - - - - - - - - - (>50)(>20) (>50)(>2)	Chromosome 17 C4 (=S), Ir, Is GLO, Pg-5, C3	Autoimmune disease ass.
Chicken	B	- - - - - - -B- F- - - - - - - - - - - - - - - B-G (>1) (>10)	Chromosome 21, Ir	Ass. with Marek's disease

[a] Number of known alleles in parentheses; in addition, *MHC*'s are known in horses, hamsters, and some amphibian species

and one locus that controls reactivity in mixed lymphocyte culture like *HLA-D*. In the cattle, pig, and chicken, only two loci have thus far been found with certainty, one that controls reactivity in MLC, and one that codes for serologically detectable cell surface antigens like *HLA-A, B* or *H-2 K, D*. In the guinea pig and rat, it could be shown by biochemical methods that also here there are at least two genes controlling the expression of antigens analogous to the mouse K and D molecules. Furthermore, in the rat, two loci have been identified by their products which are analogous to the mouse *I-A* and *I-E* locus, respectively.

In most of these species, genes were demonstrated which appear to be closely linked to the *MHC* and control the immune response (*Ir* genes) against certain antigens; in most cases in which a linkage order could be established, these genes are closely linked to or are identical to those controlling the mixed lymphocyte reactivity.

In the rhesus monkey and dog, the gene controlling the expression of the C 3 proactivator (factor B) has been also shown to be linked to the *MHC*; the same has been found to be true for the gene controlling the expression of C 4 in guinea pigs.

Tissue Distribution of MHC Molecules

Molecules whose phenotypic expression is controlled by MHC genes are demonstrable in different concentrations on different tis-

	H-2				HLA-			
	K	I	S	D	A	C	B	D
B lymphocytes	+	+	−	+	+	+	+	+
T lymphocytes	+	(+)ᵃ	−	+	+	+	+	(+)
Thymus cells	+	(+)ᵃ	−	+	+	+	+	·
Macrophages	+	+	+	+	+	·	+	+
Granulocytes	·	·	·	·	+	·	+	−
Reticulocytes	+	·	·	+	+	·	+	·
Erythrocytes	+	−	−	+	+	·	+	−
Thrombocytes	+	−	·	+	+	+	+	−
Fibroblasts	+	−	+	+	+	+	+	−
Endothelial cells	+	·	·	+	+	·	+	+
Epidermal cells	+	+	−	+	+	·	+	+
Liver	+	−	·	+	+	·	+	−
Kidney	+	−	·	+	+	·	+	−
Cardiac muscle	+	−	·	+	+	·	+	−
Skeletal muscle	+	−	·	+	+	·	+	−
Brain	+	−	·	+	(−)	·	(+)	·
Placenta	+	·	·	+	+	·	+	·
Spermatozoa	+	+	−	+	+	·	+	+
Ova	(+)	·	−	(+)	·	·	·	·
Trophoblasts	−	·	·	−	(+)	·	(+)	·
Blastocysts	+	·	·	+	·	·	·	·
Embryo	+	·	·	+	+	·	+	·

Table 6.12. Tissue distribution of antigens whose phenotypic expression is controlled by genes of the *H-2* or *HLA* complex

+ = present; − = absent; · = not tested; ( ) = demonstrable in extremely small amounts or only by absorption or conflicting results
ᵃ Clearly demonstrable on conA-stimulated (and allogen-stimulated) T (thymus) cells

sue cells. Detailed studies on this topic were carried out in the mouse. It is generally accepted that *K* and *D* molecules are present on all tissue cells with the exception of trophoblasts and the chorionic membrane. H-2 antigens were shown on embryos after the fourth day (late blastocyst); and HLA antigens were found also on human fetal tissue. The tissue distribution of MHC antigens is summarized in Table 4.12.

However, the concentration of MHC antigens varies noticeably for individual tissues: Liver cells exhibited only ca. 20%, kidney tissue ca. 5%, skeletal muscle tissue 0.5%, and brain cells only ca. 0.1% of the amount found on lymphatic cells. Erythrocytes also possess only a small amount of H antigen; mouse erythrocytes have about 10% in comparison to lymphatic cells, and human erythrocytes have considerably less.

I gene products (Ia antigen) exhibit restricted tissue distribution. They can best be demonstrated on lymphocytes, particularly on B lymphocytes; they are, however, also demonstrable on T lymphocytes (particularly on stimulated T lymphocytes), macrophages (and their tissue specific forms such as monocytes, Langerhans cells in the epidermis, Kupffer cells in the liver), and spermatozoa. They have not been found on thymus cells (provided they are unstimulated), nor on any other tissue studied thus far.

The antigens are distributed evenly over the cell surface. By "capping" experiments (see below), it was shown that K, D, and Ia antigens are present on the membrane independently of each other (Fig. 6.9). In these experiments, the cells were first incubated with an antiserum that reacted specifically with the antigen of a locus, e.g., with the K antigen. After incubation at room temperature for 30 min, the serum was rinsed off and the cells were incubated with an antimouse Ig -

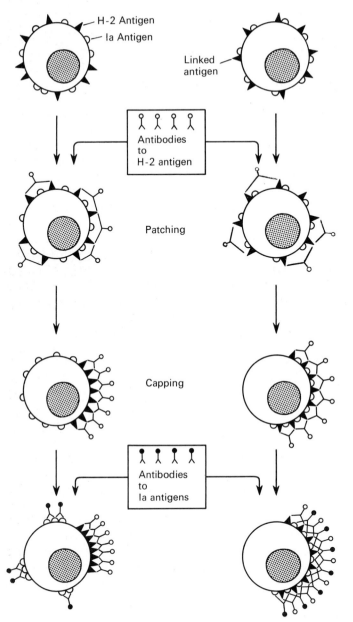

Fig. 6.9. Schematic representation of capping

serum to completely "cap" the K antigen. After an additional 30 min incubation (room temperature) the cells were washed and divided into several aliquots. The following steps were carried out at 0 °C: One aliquot was reincubated with the previously used antiserum; the other aliquots were incubated with an anti-H-2 D and an anti-Ia serum respectively. Finally, after washing

out the second antiserum, the cells were once again incubated with fluorescein-labeled antimouse-Ig (from goat or rabbit). After washing, the labeled cells were examined under a fluorescence microscope. Cells that were incubated twice with the same antiserum (anti-K) showed no label, whereas cells that in the second step were incubated with anti-H-2D or anti-Ia serum exhibited fluorescence, i.e., antigens that had bound antibodies of the first serum and were complexed by the anti-Ig serum on the membrane were pinocytosed and had not reappeared on the cell surface. On the other hand, antigens that were structurally independent of the K antigen were still demonstrable on the cell membrane. By the same method, public and private antigenic determinants have been shown to be on the same molecule.

Biochemistry of MHC Molecules

Elucidation of the biochemical structure of molecules controlled by genes of the *MHC* was considerably impeded because they are integrated into the cell membrane and as such are not soluble in aqueous solutions. Cell membranes consist of a double layer of fatty acids and phospholipids whose polar groups are directed toward the inner and outer surfaces and whose nonpolar groups are pointed toward the interior of the membrane. The arrangement of the proteins on or in this layer can be imagined according to the model developed by Singer and Nicholson in 1972, in which the globular proteins "swim" in the double layer and have contact either with one surface or with both (Fig. 6.10); they are kept stabilized in the membrane by hydrophobic sections in their structure immersed in the lipid phase. The pioneering work on MHC biochemistry was done in the late 1960s by R.A. Reisfeld

and his colleagues as well as S. Nathenson and his collaborators. Nathenson is credited with two methods that are in general use today: 1. Solubilization of membrane proteins by careful digestion of the cell membrane with papain, a proteolytic enzyme; and 2. Solubilization of membrane components, previously labeled with radioactive markers (either by external iodination with lactoperoxidase, or by internal labeling with ^{3}H- or ^{14}C-labeled amino acids) using a nonionic detergent, NP 40.

The detergent solubilized material is then ultracentrifuged. The MHC molecules are enriched by passing the preparation through a column of Sepharose B4 to which lentil lectin (a plant protein that binds sugars like glucose and mannose) is coupled. Since MHC molecules are glycoproteins they are retained on the lectin; after all not-bound proteins have been washed out, the MHC molecules are eluted with α-methyl mannoside. The MHC molecules in the partially purified fraction are then reacted with specific alloantisera. The complexes of MHC molecules with antibodies are precipitated with either a second antiserum (from rabbits or goats) specifically reacting with mouse immunoglobulins, or staphylococcus aureus–protein A which binds to the Fc portion of most mammalian IgG. The precipitate is then isolated by centrifugation, and the MHC molecules are released from the complex by boiling in sodium dodecylsulfate (SDS) in the absence (non-reducing condition) or the presence (reducing condi-

Fig. 6.10. "Fluid mosaic" membrane model according to Singer and Nicolson. Proteins swim like icebergs in the lipid-cholesterol double layer. [Singer SJ (1973) Architecture and topography of biological membranes. Hosp Prac 8:31–90]

tion) of 2-mercaptoethanol. The MHC molecules are separated from the immuno-globulins by SDS-polyacrylamide electro-phoresis.

H-2 K, D, L and HLA-A, B, C Molecules: Class I Molecules

With these two methods, the following re-sults were obtained for the molecules K, D, and L, and HLA-A and B: After digestion with papain, a soluble component with a molecular weight of about 45,000 daltons or two components with molecular weights of about 34,000 and 12,000 daltons were ob-tained. If the purified molecules are dis-solved in urea and analyzed either in this form or after reduction and alkylation by SDS-polyacrylamide electrophoresis, one finds two forms: a fraction with a molecular weight of 34,000 daltons and another with a molecular weight of 11,500 daltons. This finding leads to the conclusion that these molecules consist of two polypeptide chains held together by non-covalent bonds.

If H-molecules are isolated with detergent NP 40, different relationships are found. Analysis of H antigen isolated and purified by gel filtration yields a fraction with a mo-lecular weight of ca. 140,000 daltons. Under mild denaturing conditions, these fractions split into two or three components with mo-lecular weights of ca. 90,000, 45,000, and 11,500 daltons, respectively. After being dis-solved in urea, one finds, after SDS electro-phoresis, two fractions with molecular weights of 45,000 and 11,500 daltons. If the larger protein is digested with papain, one obtains one piece of 34,000 daltons and one of ca. 12,000. These findings yield the fol-lowing picture of the structure of H mole-cules (Fig. 6.11): They are transmembrane glycoproteins with a molecular weight of 45,000 daltons (heavy chain), non-covalent-ly associated with a large polypeptide (Fs = soluble fragment) of about 11,500 daltons (light chain). A polypeptide fragment of about 12,000 daltons can be cleaved from the heavy chain by papain. This fragment (Fm = membrane fragment) appears to re-main in the membrane after isolation of the H molecule by papain digestion. The larger polypeptide, ca. 34,000 daltons, (F$_H$ = heavy fragment) consists of a 30,000-dalton protein portion to which sugar is bound. Ac-cording to Strominger, the polypeptide con-tains four half-cystines that form two intra-molecular loops via S–S bridges. The light, 11,500-dalton chain can be characterized serologically as a protein that is also present

Fig. 6.11. Molecular structure of class I molecules (K,D or HLA-A,B): Solubilization with detergent (NP 40) yields a dimer composed of two heavy chains (H) and two light (β$_2$-microglobulin) chains. Solubilization through papain digestion yields a monomer (*Fs*, soluble fragment) of a shortened heavy chain and the light β$_2$-microglobulin chain (together their mol. wt. is 46,000 daltons). A polypeptide fragment of mol. wt. 10,000–12,000 daltons (*Fm*, mem-brane fragment) remains in the membrane

in serum: β_2-microglobulin (β_2-MG). β_2^--microglobulin has no H-antigen specificity; however, it appears to be important for the occurrence of the H molecule on the cell surface. In fact, it was discovered that transformed cells that grow in suspension culture and exhibit no H molecule on their cell surface (Daudi cells) also have no β_2-MG. If such cells are hybridized with other cells that normally have β_2-MG on their membranes, Daudi's own H-antigens whose specificity is known from the donor of the Daudi cells are expressed on the hybrids.

A particularly exciting finding was the realization that β_2-MG had an unexpected high homology to certain C domains (see Chap. 4) of immunoglobulins; this homology concerns not only the amino-acid sequence, but also the number and position of two half-cysteines, both of which correspond exactly to the immunoglobulin domains.

MHC molecules are cleaved with bromcyan or trypsin and the peptide mixture thus obtained is separated into two dimensions by thin-layer chromatography, the peptide divides in a characteristic manner. A comparison of MHC molecules of different serologic specificities indicates that they differ in up to 50% of their peptides.

Using refined methods, primary structure (amino-acid sequence) analysis can be carried out on MHC molecules isolated by immunoprecipitation. In one of these methods, instead of iodinating the cells with lactoperoxidase, the cells are incubated with radiolabeled amino acids (e.g., ^{14}C amino acid or ^{3}H amino acid) so that they incorporate these in newly synthesized proteins, including H antigen. The cells are then lysed according to method (2) and the antigen is precipitated. After electrophoretic separation, the radioactive gel slices are dissolved and the radiolabeled protein is analyzed in an automatic sequencer. After every step, the cleaved amino acids are tested for radioactivity; thus, it can be determined where the amino acids that were added to the culture for incorporation are located in the primary structure.

Thus far, partial sequences have been obtained from several H molecules; the sequence of the first 25 amino acids is shown in Table 6.13 together with the amino acid sequence of human HLA antigen, determined by Strominger and colleagues using conventional methods. It is evident from a comparison of the sequences of different K and D alleles of mouse-H, and human-H antigens, that there is considerable concordance in the primary structure; H-2K and H-2D molecules differ in approximately 35% to 45% of their amino acid residues, whereby neither K nor D molecules exhibit a typical sequence; HLA molecules (A, B) differ in still fewer amino-acid residues: 5–10%. Even in a comparison of HLA-A, B and H-2K, D molecules, about 40% of the amino-acid residues are identical; three positions appear particularly conservative. These findings clearly indicate a close relationship of the MHC products. Complete sequence data are only available for a few alleles of the H-2K and HLA-A and -B molecules. However, they indicate that there are three stretches of the primary structure that differ in 60% or more of their amino acids in different alleles, whereas the remainder part of the polypeptide chain shows only 10% or less variation. The highly variable areas are between the positions 65 and 80, and between 105 and 115. These areas are considered to be exposed to the outside and to represent the sites which are recognized by immune cells. On the other hand, the sequences within the disulfide loop including the residues 181–271 are totally conserved; this part of the sequence is homologous to Ig constant domains and β_2-MG.

HLA-C molecules are also studied using immunoprecipitation and they do not appear to differ from HLA-A, B molecules in their physico-chemical characteristics. Structural studies have not yet been carried out.

Ia and HLA-DR Molecules: Class II Molecules

Human DR molecules and mouse Ia molecules (controlled by the *A* and *E* locus) are

Table 6.13. N-terminal amino-acid sequence from mouse H-2 and human HLA molecules

Antigen	1	2	3	4	5	6	7	8	9	10	11	12	13	14	15	16	17	18	19	20	21	22	23	24	25
H-2K^k	Met	Pro	His	·	Leu	Arg	**Tyr**	Phe	His	·	Ala	**Val**	·	Ile	**Pro**	·	Leu	·	Lys	Pro	Phe	Ala	·	·	·
H-2K^b		Pro	His	·	Leu	Arg	**Tyr**	Phe	Val	·	Ala	**Val**	·	Arg	**Pro**	·	Leu	·			Arg	Tyr	·	·	·
H-2K^b	–	Pro	His		Leu	Arg	**Tyr**	Phe	Val	·	Ala	**Val**	·	Arg	**Pro**	·	Leu	·	–	–	Arg	Tyr	·		
H-2D^b	–	Pro	–		–	Arg	**Tyr**	·	–	·	Ala	**Val**	·	Arg	**Pro**	·	Leu	·	–	Pro	Arg	Tyr			
H-2D^b		Pro	His		Leu	Arg	**Tyr**	·		·	Ala	**Val**	·	Arg	**Pro**	·	Leu	·	–	Pro	Arg	Tyr			
H-2D^d	Met	Pro	His	·	–	Arg	**Tür**	–	Val	·	Ala	**Val**	·	Arg	**Pro**	·	–	·	–	Pro	Arg	Tyr			
HLA-A2	Gly	Ser	·	Ser	Met	Arg	**Tyr**	Phe	Phe	Thr	Ser	**Val**	Ser	·	·	Gly	·	Gly	Glu	·	·	Phe	Ile	·	Val
HLA-B7	Gly	Ser	·	Ser	Met	Arg	**Tyr**	Phe	Tyr	Thr	Ser	**Val**	Ser	Arg	**Pro**	Gly	·	Gly	Glu	·	·	Phe	Ile	·	Val
HLA-B12	Gly	Ser	·	Ser	Met	Val	**Tyr**	Phe	Tyr	Thr	Ala	**Val**	Ser	Arg	**Pro**	Gly	·	Gly	Glu	·	·	Phe	Ile	·	Val

Boxes indicate different amino acids and bold types indicate constant amino acids

The *dotted lines* indicate the absence of amino acids that are found in this position in other alleles. *Dots* indicate that the amino acids in this position have not yet been characterized

Summarized from Ewenstein B M, Freed J H, Mole L E, Nathenson S G. (1976) Studies on the location of papain cleavage site of H-2 glycoproteins. Proc Natl Acad Sci (USA) 73:915; Henning R, Milner R, Reske K, Cunningham B, Edelman G (1976) Subunit structure, cell surface orientation and partial amino acid sequences of murine histocompatibility antigens. Proc Natl Acad Sci (USA) 73:118; Silver J, Hood L (1976) Structure and evolution of transplantation antigens: Partial amino-acid sequences of H-2K and H-2D alloantigens. Proc Natl Acad Sci (USA) 73:599; Terhorst C, Parham P, Mann D, Strominger J (1976) Structure of HLA antigens: Amino acid and carbohydrate compositions and N-terminal sequences of four antigen preparations. Proc Natl Acad Sci (USA) 73:910; Vitetta E S, Capra J D, Klapper D G, Klein J, Uhr J W (1976) The partial amino acid sequence of an H-2K molecule. Proc Natl Acad Sci (USA) 73:905

also glycoproteins and are composed of two polypeptide chains with molecular weights of about 32,000 and 28,000 daltons, termed α and β (i.e. $A_\alpha A_\beta$ and $E_\alpha E_\beta$ in mice, and $DR_\alpha DR_\beta$ in man). The molecules are not associated with β_2-microglobulin. Peptide mapping and N-terminal amino acid sequencing have provided the following information: The four murine chains A_α, A_β, E_α, and E_β are not homologous to one another or to H molecules. Murine A_α and A_β are not homologous to any known human DR molecules; however, murine E_α and E_β are homologous to human DR_α, DR_β (and rat Ia_α and Ia_β). The human and rat equivalent of the mouse A locus has not yet been detected. The A and E α-chains of different alleles appear to differ only in a few amino acids or about 10% of their peptides. The A as well as E β-chains, however, show between 10% and 45% allelic variations.

S Protein: Class III Molecule

The Ss protein has also been characterized: It represents the complement component C 4, and is a protein with a molecular weight of about 200,000 daltons, composed of three polypeptide chains with molecular weights of about 95,000, 70,000, and 33,000 daltons, respectively (see also Chap. 5).

Function of MHC Genes

Control of Antigen Recognition by T Cells

Transplantation and transplantation reactions obviously are unnatural situations and under the best of circumstances reveal only a special facet of the function of the *MHC* genes that is inherent in its cooperation in a specific immune response. The most attractive theory of the physiologic function of *MHC* genes has been presented by Burnet: *MHC* gene products signify SELF, i.e., indicate what the immune system should not react against unless this self is altered, for example by the occurrence of new antigenic determinants. Burnet's theory has become more plausible, particularly since the discovery that the MHC controls not only the humoral immune response but also the cellular immune response.

On the basis of serological, biochemical, and functional data the *MHC* genes can be divided in three classes (Table 6.14): *Class I* consists of genes that control the expression of the classical transplantation antigens on

Table 6.14. Synopsis of *MHC* gene classes

Characteristics	Class I	Class II	Class III
Designation	H molecules	Ia molecules	C3 activators
Loci(mouse/man)	K,D,L/A,B,C	A, E/D, Dr	S($=$C4)/C4, C2, BF
No. of alleles	>100	>20	≥ 2
No. of specificities	>100	>50	≥ 2
Tissue distribution	All cells	Lymphocytes, macrophages	Serum
Biochemistry: chains	2	2	3
mo. wt.	45,000 D 11,5000 D(β_2-MG)	α: 32,000 D β: 28,000 D	α: 95,000 D β: 78,000 D γ: 33,000 D
Physiology	Target antigen for allo-antibodies and cyto-toxic T cells (effector cells), self for cyto-toxic T cells	Stimulation antigen for allogeneic immune reaction (MLR), self for helper/suppressor T cells (T-T, T-macro-phage, T-B cell interaction)	Activation of lytic enzymes; opsonization; generation of anaphyla-toxin, chemo-(leuko)-tactic substances

all cells of an individual; these substances have a molecular weight of 45,000 daltons and are associated with β_2-microglobulin. In the mouse, these are the *H-2K* and *H-2D* (and *L*) genes, in man, *HLA-A*, *B*, and *C*. *Class II* consists of genes that control the expression of surface structures (Ia antigens) on lymphocytes and macrophages; these molecules consist of two polypeptide chains with a molecular weight of about 33,000 daltons (α-chain) and 28,000 daltons (β-chain); they are not associated with β_2-microglobulin. These molecules are probably identical with lymphocyte-activating determinants and the components that control the humoral immune response. In the mouse, these are the *I-A*, *I-J*, and *I-E* genes. In man, these genes are localized in the *HLA-D* region.

Finally, *class III* genes are those that control a series of serum proteins which are part of the complement system: C4, C2, and factor B in man, and C4 (Ss) in the mouse.

The involvement of *class I* genes in the regulation of the immune response was first discovered 1974 by Doherty and Zinkernagel. They apparently play a significant role in the

production of cytotoxic effector (T) cells against *self* in association with virus antigens. *Class II* genes are involved in the activation of another set of T cells, which exercise a regulatory effect on B lymphocytes in the production of IgG antibodies as well as on effector T lymphocytes in the generation of killer cells. They were first described in 1965 by Benacerraf, and independently at the same time by McDevitt.

Genes belonging to *class III* control complement components involved in the activation of C3. C3 is the key component of both complement activation systems, the classical and the properdin system (see Chap. 5). Activated C3 can bind to macrophages and B lymphocytes which leads to opsonization, it liberates anaphylatoxin, it causes the formation of chemo(leuko)tactic factors, and it activates the lytic chain of complement enzymes $C5 \rightarrow C9$.

Control of the Cellular Immune Response by *Class I* Genes

If mice are infected with lymphochoriomeningitis (LCM), vaccinia, Sendai, influenza, or other viruses and if lymphocytes are subsequently removed and incubated in vitro with ^{51}Cr-labeled peritoneal cells or tissue culture cells previously infected with the same virus, free ^{51}Cr can be detected in the supernatant after 8–16 h, indicating that the labeled cells have been lysed. This lysis is observed only if the labeled target cells were obtained from the same mouse strain from which the lymphocytes (effectors) originated (syngeneic target cells). If target cells are used from mouse strains that have *class I* alleles different from those of the effector cells, the target cells are not lysed. Also, the target cells and the effector cells must have been infected with the same virus. That is, the effector cells are only activated to lyse target cells when they recognize their own class I molecules in association with virus-antigen (Table 6.15). If virus-infected cells from *MHC* recombinant strains are used as target cells that share either the *K*, *I*, or *D* allele with the effector cells, only those target

Table 6.15. Specificity and H-2K, D restriction of virus-specific cytotoxid T effector cells

Target cell lysis		Effector cells stimulated with virus1	
		A(K^kD^k)	B(K^dD^d)
A	(K^kD^k)	−	−
A_{v1}	(K^kD^k)	+	−
A_{v2}	(K^kD^k)	−	−
B	(K^dD^d)	−	−
B_{v1}	(K^dD^d)	−	+
B_{v2}	(K^dD^d)	−	−
C	(K^kD^b)	−	−
C_{v1}	(K^kD^b)	+	−
D	(K^bD^k)	−	−
D_{v1}	(K^bD^k)	+	−
E	(K^dD^b)	−	−
E_{v1}	(K^dD^b)	−	+
F	(K^bD^d)	−	−
F_{v1}	(K^bD^d)	−	+

V1 = infected with virus 1
V2 = infected with virus 2

cells are destroyed that share the K or D allele with the effector cells. Target cells that are identical with the effector cells only for the I allele but that differ in their K and D alleles from the effector cells, are not (in general) destroyed. Such effector cells are also unable to lyse self, noninfected cells, or cells infected with a virus other than that used to sensitize the effector cells. The specificity of the effector cell is *restricted* to the sensitizing virus (non-self) in association with its own class I molecules (K or D) (self).

This phenomenon can be observed not only with virus-infected cells but also with syngeneic cells, the outer membranes of which are modified in some other way, for example by coating syngeneic cells with TNP (trinitrophenol), or by sensitizing with cells which are identical in their class I molecules with the effector cells, but differ for their non-MHC genes.

The formation of specific effector cells against virus-associated K or D molecules underlies the control of K or D alleles. Thus, when in association with vaccinia or Sendai virus, the D^k allele is a low-responder allele, i.e., animals that possess the D^k allele and are infected with vaccinia or Sendai virus are unable to produce cytotoxic effector cells against D^k-vaccinia or D^k-Sendai (but they do generate cytotoxic effector cells against K-vaccinia or K-Sendai). The same animals are, however, capable of producing T cells that react specifically with D^k in association with LCM virus, i.e., D^k is a low responder allele only for vaccinia and Sendai virus but not for LCM virus.

A similar situation exists for the D^b allele. In this case, however, the formation of effector cells is regulated by the linked K allele: If the D^b allele is linked to a K^k or K^d allele, no cytotoxic effector cells are generated that react specifically with D^b-vaccinia or D^b-Sendai antigens. However, if the D^b allele is linked to K^b or K^q, effector cells are formed that react specifically with D^b-vaccinia or D^b-Sendai antigens (Table 6.16).

Little is known about the mechanism of the reaction against self-modified cells. The virus antigen that is recognized by the effec-

Table 6.16. Control by H-2K and H-2D genes of cellular immune response against virus-infected, syngenic cells

Antigen (H-2 virus)	Responser H-2 Allele	
	High	Low
D^k-Vaccinia		D^k
D^k-Sendai		D^k
D^k-LCM	D^k	
D^b-Vaccinia	K^q, K^b	K^k, K^d
D^b-Sendai	K^q, K^b	K^k, K^d
K^b-Influenza		K^b

tor cells is an early antigen, i.e., an antigen that appears on the cell membrane soon after infection and before the virus proliferates. Soluble antibodies play no role in the reaction. The reaction proceeds via direct cell contact between the target cell and the effector cell. The effector cell is a $Ly-2^+3^+$ positive T lymphocyte. Since the T cells that recognize the virus together with the D molecule differ from those that recognize the virus in association with the K molecule, it is thought that different T-cell clones exist. The nature of the receptor itself remains unclear; there are reports suggesting that T-cell receptors carry a variable region similar or identical to that of variable regions of immunoglobulin heavy chains (V_H). The molecule carrying this variable region (antigen binding site) appears to exist in the T-cell membrane as a monomer or dimer with a molecular weight of 65,000 or 130,000 dalton. This molecule is for its "constant part" antigenically different from known immunoglobulin proteins since it does not react with antisera specific for μ, δ, γ, or α heavy chains. With the help of anti-idiotypic antisera, it could be shown that the binding site of the T-cell receptor has specificity for MHC determinants. An analogue to the antibody light chain has not been identified so far.

Many hypotheses have been proposed to explain the K (D) restricted antigen specificity of these cells. To these concepts we will turn after the following section.

Control of the Immune Response
by *Class II* Genes (Ir Genes)

In the 1960s, the work of McDevitt in particular indicated that the antibody response to certain synthetic polypeptides is genetically controlled. Different mouse strains produce a large number of antibodies (high responder, HR) or only a small number (low responder, LR) of antibodies against specific antigens. Experiments with congenic strains showed that the ability to form antibodies was associated with the *MHC* genotype. Studies with mouse *MHC* recombinant strains resulted in the identification of the gene(s) responsible for the immune-response control; it could be demonstrated that it is located within the *MHC*, between the *K* and *S* locus: the *immune response-1 (Ir-1 A)* locus. Since then, two more genes have been detected in the *MHC* which also specifically control the immune response: *Ir-1 C* (Tables 6.17 and 6.18) and *Is-J*; the latter locus functions as suppressor (immune suppression, Is) of a specific immune response. Two of these loci are probably identical to the loci *I-A (Ir-1 A)* and *I-E (Ir-1 C)* which control the expression of serologically demonstrable class II molecules (Ia antigens).

Indirect evidence favors this suggestion: 1) Antisera against class II molecules (anti-Ia sera) suppress the formation of IgG against T cell-dependent antigens in the Jerne plaque assay but not the IgM response (see below); 2) the presence of certain Ia antigens on lymphocyte membranes from inbred strains is apparently identical with high response to certain antigens; 3) anti-Ia sera specifically inhibit the immune response to antigens against which the immune response is controlled by *Ir* genes. Cells from F_1 hybrids between low and high responders are inhibited on the *Ir* gene-controlled immune response by antisera that are specific for the high responder haplotype but not by antisera that are specific for the low responder haplotype – although the F_1 cells react with both sera; 4) Lonai and McDevitt demonstrated that high-responder cells could be stimulated to proliferate in vitro by antigens against which the immune response is *Ir*-gene controlled, but that the low-responder cells could not; 5) *Ir* genes, class II molecules, and LAD controlling genes cannot yet

Strain	H-2 complex loci								Response
	K	A_β	A_α	E_β	J	E_α	S	D	
1. *Ir-1A (I-A)* locus controlled response to (H, G)-A-L[a]									
B10	b	**b**	**b**	b	b	0	b	b	Low
B10.D2	d	**d**	**d**	d	d	7	d	d	Low
B10.BR	k	**k**	**k**	k	k	7	k	k	High
B10.S	s	**s**	**s**	s	s	0	s	s	Low
B10.A(4R)	k	**k**	**k**	b	b	0	b	b	High
A.TL	s	**k**	**k**	k	k	7	k	d	High
B10.A(5R)	b	**b**	**b**	b	k	7	d	d	Low
2. *Ir-1C (I-E)* locus controlled response to GLT[b]									
B10	b	b	b	**b**	b	**0**	b	b	Low
B10.D2	d	d	d	**d**	d	7	d	d	High
D2.GD	d	d	d	**b**	b	**0**	b	b	Low
HTG	d	d	d	**d**	d	7	b	b	High
B10.A(5R)[c]	b	b	b	**b**	k	7	d	d	High

Table 6.17. Mapping of *Ir-1A (I-A)* and *Ir-1C (I-C)* loci in the *H-2* complex

[a] (H, G)–A-L: synthetic polymer of alanin (A) and lysine (L) with histidin (H) and glutamine (G) as end groups
[b] GLT: linear terpolymer of $(Glu^{57}-Lys^{38}-Tyr^5)$
[c] E^b is a high-responder allele; it is, however, not expressed in B10 *(H-2^b)* mice because of the E_α^o allele (see p. 137)

Table 6.18. Immune response to GL$\varnothing^a$ by the *I-E* genes

Strains	H-2 complex loci								Response
	K	A_β	A_α	E_β	J	E_α	S	D	
B10	b	b	b	**b**	b	**0**	b	b	Low
B10.D2	d	d	d	**d**	d	7	d	d	High
B10.BR	k	k	k	**k**	k	7	k	k	Low
B10.S	s	s	s	**s**	s	**0**	s	s	Low
B10.A(5R)	b	b	b	**b**	k	7	d	d	High
B10.S(9R)	s	s	s	**s**	k	7	d	d	High
B10.S(7R)	s	s	s	**s**	s	**0**	s	d	Low
B10.A(2R)	k	k	k	**k**	k	7	d	b	Low
B10.A(4R)	k	k	k	**b**	b	**0**	b	b	Low
B10.HTT	s	s	s	**s**	s	7	k	d	High
D2.GD	d	d	d	**b**	b	**0**	b	b	Low

^{a} GL$\varnothing$: polymer of glutamin, lysine, and phenylalanin

Whenever the high-responder alleles E_β^b, E_β^d, E_β^s are expressed, i.e., linked to the E_α^7, the high-response phenotype appears; E_β^k is a low responder allele

be separated genetically, either in inbred strains or in wild populations.

An additional immune response locus, *Ir-1 B* (formerly *Ir-IgG*) located between *I-A* and *I-J* has been proposed to explain the response pattern to an immunoglobulin allotype (IgG), lactate dehydrogenase-B (LDH$_B$), and ribonuclease (RNase). Extensive serological, biochemical, and cellular (MLC, CML) analysis did not suggest the existence of a product of such a proposed gene. Furthermore, the response to RNase can easily be explained as a result of control by the *I-E* genes after it has been found that the E$_\beta$-chain is not expressed in the sole presence of the E_α^0 allele (see p. 137). Therefore, it appears likely that the control of the immune response against IgG and LDH$_B$ is controlled by both the *A* and the *E* genes, and in order to obtain high response both genes must be present as high-responder alleles. Actually, the response to LDH$_B$ was thought to be controlled by two genes, the proposed *Ir-1 B* and E_α.

Regulation of the immune response by MHC-linked *Ir* genes occurs at the level of T-B cell and macrophage-T cell interaction; thymectomized mice that are high responders to a certain antigen form only minimal amounts of antibodies (IgM) comparable to that of low-responder animals. However, if mice that are low responders for a certain antigen are immunized with this antigen after it has been coupled to a carrier (e.g. BSA), these mice are capable of forming antibodies against the antigen (Fig. 6.12).

(In addition to *Ir* genes mentioned so far, there are other genes influencing antibody formation. Some of these are closely linked to genes that control antibody allotypes, and it is thought that the failure to form antibodies in this case is due to the lack of a gene coding for the antigen-specific variable region (antigen binding site) of the immunoglobulin. Here, antibody formation cannot be restored by coupling the antigen on a carrier.)

Detailed studies have shown that B and T cells from low and high responders bind the antigen to the same degree (this is true of T cells only if the antigen is presented to them by macrophages or B cells). Only high-responder T and B cells are stimulated to proliferate and differentiate by the presented antigen. The *Ir*-gene control occurs on the level of macrophage-T cell, T-T cell, and T-B cell cooperation. The *Ir* gene regulation may act either as augmentation or suppression of the immune response, in the latter case suppression is dominant over non-suppression.

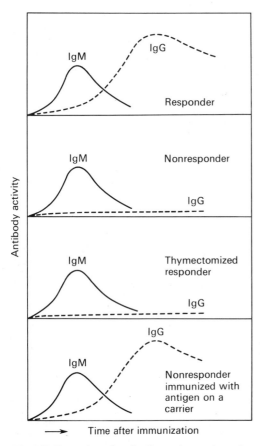

Fig. 6.12. Formation of antibodies against antigens for which the immune response is *Ir-1* controlled. Responders exhibit normal IgM and IgG responses, whereas nonresponders show only an IgM response. If the responder is thymectomized, it behaves like a nonresponder; on the other hand, if nonresponders are injected with antigen after it is linked to a carrier, normal IgM and IgG responses can also be shown

Originally, it was thought that *Ir* genes in the *MHC* control the antigen binding site of the T-cell receptor. However, the finding that the antigen binding site of T-cell receptors (but not the remainder of the receptor structure!) are controlled by genes that also control the antigen binding site for immunoglobulins, which are not linked to *MHC* genes, rendered this hypothesis untenable.

Reconstitution and transfer experiments designed and performed in several laboratories (Kindred, Katz, Sprent) provided a clue to the role of *Ir* genes or their products (class II

molecules, Ia antigens) in immune-response regulation. Their results indicated that T cells must cooperate with macrophages and B lymphocytes in order to become activated to react with an antigen; and this cooperation can only take place when the *Ir* gene alleles of the cooperating cells are identical. In other words, the T-cell activation is *restricted* to the recognition of non-self (antigen) in the context of self (class II molecules). The antigen has to be presented together with self class II molecules – this parallels the activation of cytotoxic T cells which have to recognize cell-bound antigens (non-self) in association with class I molecules (see above). T cells restricted in their specificity to the recognition of class I molecules + antigen bear the characteristic Ly-2$^+$ 3$^+$ markers and function as killer cells. T cells restricted in their specificity to the recognition of class II molecules + antigen bear a characteristic Ly-1$^+$ marker and function as regulator cells (augmentation or suppression) in the immune response, either by turning on B cells to mature and differentiate into plasma cells (IgG secreting) and memory cells, or by augmenting the recruitment of T effector cells. The interaction of the different kinds of cells involved in the immune response is accompanied by the secretion and action of various factors which are not antigen or *MHC* specific.

Two such factors have been characterized to some extent (Table 6.19). Ly-1$^+$ T lymphocytes (helper cells) are triggered to respond antigen-specifically by two signals: 1) the antigen–self complex presented by macrophages and recognized via antigen–self receptors that are antigen-specific and MHC-restricted; and 2) a factor produced by macrophages, interleukin-1. In turn, stimulated T helper cells release another factor, interleukin-2, which together with the antigen–self complex (restricting signal 1) activates cytotoxic T cells and B lymphocytes.

There are at least three hypotheses to explain the restricted activation of T lymphocytes: Cytotoxic T cells recognize their own class I or class II molecules and the virus antigen with a receptor that recognizes a

Table 6.19. Properties of interleukin-1 (IL-1) and interleukin-2 (IL-2)

Chemical and biological properties	Interleukin-1		Interleukin-2	
	Murine	Human	Murine	Human
Produced by	Macrophages		Ly-1$^+$ T cells	Lymphocytes
Size (gel filtration)	16,000		30,000	15,000
Elution from DEAE ion exchange resin pH 7.5	0.05–0.1 M NaCl		0.15 M NaCl	0.05 M NaCl
Isoelectric points	5.0–5.5	6.5–7.5	4.3, 4.9	6.0–6.5
Stable in pH range	2.0–9.0		2.0–9.0	
Absorbed on activated murine T cells	unknown		Yes	Yes
Stimulate growth of murine T-cell lines	No	No	Yes	Yes
Stimulate proliferation of murine thymocytes in presence of ConA or PHA under culture conditions where these mitogens alone are limiting	No	No	Yes	Yes
Generate CTL in murine thymocyte cultures and nude spleen cultures	No	No	Yes	Yes
Stimulate antibody response to heterologous erythrocyte antigens in nude spleen cultures	Yes	Yes	Yes	Yes
Activity MHC restricted	No	No	No	No
Activity antigen-specific	No	No	No	No

neoantigen formed by association of class I or II molecules and virus or macrophage-bound antigen (interaction antigen). Another theory postulates that T cells possess two receptor units, one specific for class I (self) determinants and the other specific for the non-self antigen (dual recognition). A third hypothesis is that T cells, like B cells, do express only *one* V$_H$ *gene, however, restricted to paratopes complementary to histocompatibility epitopes carried by the organism.* As we have seen at the beginning of this chapter, the number of epitopes each individual can express is extremely high. These receptors might possess a broader range of recognition, i.e., they might be less specific, and might be, in general, less fitting to epitopes than B-cell receptors or antibodies, since they apparently consist only of the V$_H$ variable region but do not express V$_L$ variable regions. As a consequence, they have lower affinity and broader "cross-reactivity"[2].

The antigen-presenting cell is the active cell, i.e., whenever one H-molecule epitope and one receptor molecule are complexed, this cell releases an antigen-unspecific factor conveying an activation signal to the next cell to be activated. Thus, whenever the antigen is presented by macrophages, T cells with those receptors for Ia epitopes which happen to bind also to an epitope of the antigen will interact with the macrophages causing then to release IL-I, which activates the T cell to a helper cell (Fig. 6.13). The activated T helper cell will now be able to interact with B cells that have bound the antigen, or with T cells.

---

2 Richards and Konigsberg (1973) summarized evidence favoring the view that one antibody may recognize several structurally different epitopes; in the present context, this might be expected since only half of a binding site (V$_H$) appears to be expressed. With this in mind, the concept of dual recognition (one T cell recognizing a foreign epitope in association with an epitope expressed by the individual's own MHC) is not so far from the concept outlined above, except that it postulates two receptors for what can be accomplished by one

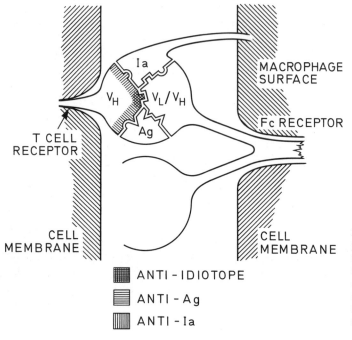

Fig. 6.13. Interaction of macrophage-bound antigen-receptor (antibody), Ia molecule, antigen and T-cell receptor. V_H, heavy chain variable region; V_L, light chain variable region; Ia, I region associated antigen; Ag, antigen

In the former case, the activated T helper cell binds to the epitope of the antigen bound to the membrane immunoglobulin of the B cell and to an identical Ia epitope expressed by this B cell. The activated T helper cell then releases IL-II which stimulates the B cell to proliferate and differentiate to Ig- producing cells and memory cells.

In the latter case, the activated T helper cell interacts with T cells endowed with receptors specific for epitopes present on the antigen as well as the individual's own K, D, or J molecules. Upon interaction, the released IL-II factor activates these T cells to proliferate and differentiate to T killer cells (those with receptors for K, D epitopes) or suppressor cells (those with receptors for J epitopes).

Those T cells expressing receptors for Ia (class II) molecules are predetermined to become helper cells; those expressing receptors for K, D (class I) molecules differentiate to killer cells; and those expressing receptors for J molecules develop into suppressor cells. Suppressor cells may also occur when

there is a paratope (receptor) on T cells containing an idiotope to which a paratope exists, i.e., in cases in which MHC alleles of an individual express complementary epitopes.

The type of receptor (anti-K, D, Ia, J) to be expressed is random but clonal, and is an internal differentiation process induced in the thymus. Which of the many mature but virgin T cells are to be activated, is an external process initiated by the antigen.

In this concept, low responsiveness is simply explained by lack of certain epitopes (no single MHC allele expresses all epitopes!) and, therefore, lack of T cells endowed with receptors for this epitope (no response, recessive), or it happens that the individual possesses a MHC allele which expresses complementary epitopes. In this case, T cells would develop with complementary receptors (anti-idiotype), suppressing the proliferation of each other (suppressed response, dominant).

This concept is in line with the concept of idiotype network regulation for antibody formation (see Chap. 4, p. 104), and also with experimental findings. In addition, with this concept, the high number of alloreactive cells and their apparent lack of restriction (see Chap. 9) is easily understood in view of the large number of shared epitopes of MHC molecules within a species. And, probably even more important, it may explain the association of MHC alleles with certain diseases found in man (see this Chap., last section).

Function of Class III Genes in the Immune Response

A number of genes in this class that together control the expression or regulation of the level of serum proteins have recently been recognized as parts of the complement system. In man, these are the components C2 and C4 of the classical complement pathway, and factor B of the properdin pathway. In mice, the only class III gene that has been identified so far, controls the expression of the complement component C4 (Ss protein).
The complement components C4 and C2 make up the C3-convertase of the classical pathway. This enzyme cleaves C3 to C3b, the active form of C3. Factor B represents the C3-convertase of the properdin pathway, also turning C3 into its active form C3b (Fig. 6.14).
The C2,4 complex (C3-convertase) is formed when Ag–Ab complexes are present; particularly active Ab–Ag complexes are those formed with IgM as antibody, i.e., the kind of antibody that is already present in the serum and exhibits a high cross-reactivity (so-called preformed or natural antibodies), and is generated very early in the immune response, right after the first encounter of B cells with the antigen (and without the activating help of T cells). On the other hand, factor B is activated without antibodies, but when it is bound to certain structures like zymosan present on or in bacterial cell walls. In both instances, be it through the activated C2,4 enzyme or the activated factor B, the complement component C3 is converted into its active form C3b, which in turn facilitates opsonization by macrophages through binding the antigen via C3b receptors. Possibly through activation of B lymphocytes, it effects liberation of chemo(leuko)tactic substances, and activates C5 to C5b, the active component turning on the late complement chain enzymes, resulting in the lytic complex C$\overline{5,6,7,8,9}$ (see Chap. 5).

Classic complement activation ←———————— Ag-Ig complexes

Factor B–bacterium complex ————————→ Properdin system

C3

C4b2a ————————————→ $\perp$ ←———————— Factor B'
(C3-convertase)   (C3-convertase)

C3b

C3b:
Receptor on
Macrophages → opsonization, phagocytosis

Convertase for
C5 → C5a,b → Anaphylatoxin, activator of lytic complement components C6 → C9

Underlined components are controlled genetically by MHC

Fig. 6.14. *MHC*-linked complement components that exhibit C3-convertase activity

The products of the class III genes fulfill a significant helper and enhancer function for the specific immune response, in particular for the digestion and elimination of infectious material such as bacteria, parasites, and particular antigens. The fact that the MHC has a significant regulative influence on an organism's defense against infections, and that certain alleles of the *MHC* cause a low responder status in relation to certain infections, may explain the extreme polymorphism and genetic complexity of this genetic system. Homozygosity for a low-responder allele is considerably reduced by multiplication of a gene to several loci with similar functions, and the formation of multiple alleles for each of these loci. Furthermore, the observation that in populations certain alleles occur in association or linkage disequilibrium might be explained as minimizing unresponsiveness.

In summarizing the functions of the *MHC* (Table 6.20) one has the impression that it plays a significant role in the final differentiation of immunocompetent cells, particularly for the development of specificity of maturing T lymphocytes that come in contact with a substrate foreign to the organism (antigen), and a deciding role in the differentiation between *self* and *non-self* when the organism is infected by viruses, bacteria, parasites, or soluble antigens.

In this context – discrimination between *self* and *non-self* – can also be seen the phenomenon of linkage of specific *MHC* alleles with susceptibility to specific diseases, as is observed in the mouse and in man, particularly because most of these diseases involve a combination of infection and autoimmunity.

MHC–Disease Association in Man

The finding that inbred strains of mice exhibited different susceptibility to a tumor-inducing (oncogenic) virus (Gross virus), initiated the search for genes that play a specific role in viral oncogenesis. It was found that viral leukemogenesis is influenced by genes of the *H-2* complex. A similar relationship between susceptibility and the *H-2* haplotype could be determined for many other viruses: Tennant virus (RNA virus, lymphocytic leukemia); Friend virus (RNA, erythremia); Bittner virus (RNA, mammary carcinoma); lymphochoriomeningitis virus (RNA); vaccinia virus (DNA); and radiation-induced leukemia virus (RNA). In none of these cases, however, are genes of the *H-2* complex the only factors that control susceptibility.

These findings, and the fact that the immune response is controlled by genes of the *MHC*,

Table 6.20. Control of the immune system by the *H-2* complex

System	Expression	Effector	Interaction	Controlling H-2 locus
Humoral immunity	Antibody formation	B-plasma cells	T-helper cells, macrophages	A, E
Cellular immunity	Cell-mediated cytotoxicity, graft rejection	T-killer cells	T-helper cells macrophages	K, D
	Immunosuppression	T-suppressor cells	T-helper, killer cells	J
Auxiliary system	Phagocytosis, opsonization, chemotaxis	Complement factor B, C2, C4	Macrophages, monocytes, Ag-Ab complexes, B'-bacterium complex	S

Chromosome No. 17   C ————— K-A-J-E-S-D —————

H-2 complex

Table 6.21. Examples of HLA-disease associations

Disease	Associated antigen	Relative risk	Disease	Associated antigen	Relative risk
Rheumatology:			Endocrinology:		
Ankylosing			Juvenile onset insulin		
spondylitis (AS)	HLA-B27	90.09	dependent diabetes	HLA-B8	2.42
AS among japanese	HLA-B27	324.49	(JOD)	HLA-Cw3	2.0
Reiter's disease	HLA-B27	35.89		HLA-DRw3,Dw3	3.8
Yersinia arthritis	HLA-B27	17.59		HLA-DRw4,Dw4	3.5
Psoriatic arthritis	HLA-B27	8.58	Subacute thyreoiditis	HLA-Bw35	16.81
	HLA-B13	4.79	Idiopathic addison dis.	HLA-Dw3	8.8
	HLA-Bw38	9.09	Adrenocortical		
Acute anterior uveitis	HLA-B27	9.43	hyperfunction[a]	HLA-Bw47	15.4
Rheumatoid arthritis (RA)	HLA-Dw4	3.9	Gastroenterology:		
RA among females	HLA-DRw4	5.20	Coeliac disease	HLA-B8	8.62
Neurology:				HLA-Dw3	73.0
Multiple sclerosis	HLA-Dw2	4.3	Ulcerative colitis	HLA-B5	3.8
	HLA-DRw2	4.2	Atrophic gastritis	HLA-B7	2.55
Myasthenia gravis	HLA-B8	4.4	Autoimmune chronic		
	HLA-Dw3	2.3	active hepatitis	HLA-Dw3	6.8
	HLA-DRw3	2.1	Healthy HBsAg Carriers	HLA-Bw41	11.16
Paralytic poliomyelitis	HLA-Bw16	4.28	Idiopathic hemo-	HLA-A3	8.34
Harada's disease	'LD-Wa'	10.5	chromatosis	HLA-B14	9.23
Dermatology:			Allergology:		
Psoriasis vulgaris (PS)	HLA-B13	4.67	Dust allergy	HLA-Aw33	11.68
	HLA-B17	4.69	Immunopathology:		
	HLA-B37	6.35	Systemic lupus		
PS among japanese	HLA-A1	10.50	erythematodes	HLA-B8	2.11
	HLA-B37	19.67	Sicca syndrome	HLA-Dw3	19.0
Dermatitis herpetiformis	HLA-Dw3	13.5	Other diseases:		
	HLA-B8	8.74	Congenital heart		
Behcet's disease	HLA-B5	7.43	malformation	HLA-A2	4.92
Recurrent herpes labialis	HLA-A1	3.72	Cryptogenic fibrosing		
Alopecia areata	HLA-B12	3.60	alveolitis	HLA-B12	9.39

[a] 21-hydroxylase deficiency (21-OH-def); controlling locus is closely linked to *HLA-B* and *HLA-D*

induced investigators to search for associations between diseases and specific HLA antigens or haplotypes. An association of *HLA* alleles and tumor disease has not yet been convincingly presented, although in some neoplastic diseases certain HLA antigens are increased in long-term survivors, which probably indicates an association between HLA and resistance. A number of diseases do exhibit a distinct association with certain *HLA* alleles or *HLA* haplotypes. Primarily these are autoimmune diseases, infectious diseases, and the se-

quelae (which may themselves be autoimmune diseases) of certain infectious diseases. A summary of the associations is given in Table 6.21.

The most significant association found is that between Bechterew's disease (ankylosing spondylitis) and HLA-B 27: 85% of patients with the disease are HLA-B 27-positive. The association is one-sided only: the presence of the antigen does not indicate that the person is susceptible to the disease. Terasaki extensively examined association phenomena. His analysis showed that HLA-

Table 6.22. Association of diseases with different *HLA-B27* haplotypes. Summarized form Terasaki PI, Mickey MR (1975) *HL-A* haplotypes of 32 diseases. In: Möller G (ed) Transplant. Review 22: 105–124, Munksgaard, Copenhagen

HLA haplotype (A-B)	Bechterew's disease	Reiter's syndrome	Juvenile rheumatoid arthritis
1–27	– [a]	–	–
2–27	+ [b]	+	+
3–27	–	+	–
9–27	+	+	–
11–27	–	+	–
30–27	+	–	–
32–27	–	–	+

[a] –, Frequency the same or lower than average in the normal population
[b] +, Frequency significantly higher than average

B 27 occurs with increased frequency in patients with Bechterew's disease, Reiter's syndrome, and juvenile rheumatoid arthritis, *and* the frequency of HLA-B 27-carrying haplotypes is different for each of the diseases (Table 6.22). In Bechterew's disease the frequency of haplotypes *HLA-A 1-B 27*, *HLA-A 3-B 27*, *HLA-A 11-B 27*, and *HLA-A 32-B 27* is normal, but that of haplotypes *HLA-A 2-B 27*, *HLA-A 9-B 27*, and *HLA-A 30-B 27* is higher than average. In juvenile rheumatoid arthritis the frequency of haplotypes *HLA-A 32-B 27* and *HLA-A 2-B 27* is higher than average. In Reiter's syndrome haplotypes *HLA-A 3-B 27* and *HLA-A 11-B 27* occur with highest frequency (in addition to *HLA-A 2-B 27*).

Reiter's syndrome and juvenile rheumatoid arthritis thus clearly differ from Bechterew's disease and from each other. Haplotype *HLA-A 30-B 27* is characteristic for Bechterew's disease, haplotypes *HLA-A 3-B 27* and *HLA-A 11-B 27* for Reiter's syndrome, and haplotype *HLA-A 32-B 27* for juvenile rheumatoid arthritis.

Two conclusions can be drawn: 1) that the *HLA-A* or *HLA-B* genes themselves are probably not responsible for susceptibility, but are closely linked to the genes that are responsible; and 2) that the linkage is stronger with HLA-B than with HLA-A, because most of the associations with B antigens are stronger than with A antigens.

Studies of the association of HLA and multiple sclerosis showed that susceptibility is controlled by genes found between *HLA-B* and *HLA-D*; this locus is named *DS-MS* (disease susceptibility gene for multiple sclerosis).

Family studies showed that in some cases a specific *HLA* haplotype is inherited together with susceptibility for a specific disease; however, in other cases *HLA* and susceptibility for this disease segregate independently of each other. This may depend on the fact that different syndromes consist of a series of different diseases (e.g., psoriasis manifests itself in many clinical forms, but only a few forms such as acute exanthematic psoriasis show a strong association with Bw 17, and other forms exhibit no association), that there is multigene control of susceptibility, or that, in addition to the genetic disposition, other (environmental) factors (i.e., infection with specific bacteria or hormonal factors) play a role.

At present, there are only hypotheses concerning the underlying mechanisms of the association of *HLA* and disease. Several possibilities are discussed: Since the *MHC* is the major system regulating immune reactions (see p. 155), it is conceivable that under certain circumstances the normal immune response deviates, i.e., becomes suppressed or enhanced. That might be the case if the immunodominant epitope of a pathogen happens to be identical to an epitope of an *MHC* allele to which a complementary epitope (leading to anti-idiotypic reactions, see p. 162) is controlled by the same or the other allele class present in that individual. Indeed, in certain cases an association of susceptibility with *HLA* alleles was only apparent when certain *HLA* alleles occurred together in heterozygotes.

It has been shown that certain microorganisms possess epitopes similar or identical to epitopes of certain *MHC* alleles (i.e., streptococcal protein M and HLA); in these cases, an individual possessing such HLA alleles might be tolerant to those microorganisms (molecular mimicry).

On the other hand, genes that control the expression of complement components may explain the association if some alleles of this gene code for defective products. As discussed previously, the complement system plays a significant role in initiation or enhancement of the immune response. Preferential linkage of such alleles with certain *HLA* alleles could give the impression of an association with *HLA*. A linkage disequilibrium between HLA-B 8 and one of the two *Bf* alleles has been demonstrated (HLA-B 8 is the most frequently occurring antigen associated with a disease; see Table 6.21). Clinically, complement-deficiencies can cause autoimmune disease-like syndromes (see Chap. 12).

Though there is as yet no explanation for the association, the clinical significance of these findings is obvious. HLA typing can be extremely important for diagnosis, particularly in the early phase of a disease. Furthermore, a known association can acquire prognostic and/or therapeutic value when more is known about the course of the disease in patients who either possess or do not possess the specific *HLA* allele. Thus, there is a correlation between the presence of HLA-D 2 allele and the progression of multiple sclerosis. On the other hand, HLA-A 9 and/or HLA-A 2 positive patients with acute lymphatic leukemia appear to have a better prognosis for survival than those who do not have these alleles.

It also appears possible to determine the risk for family members of persons who suffer from an *HLA*-associated disease, and on occasion to take prophylactic measures (e.g., vaccination for an infectious disease). Also, *HLA*-disease associations should also be considered in genetic family counseling.

An association of MHC alleles with specific diseases in which not all diseased persons demonstrate such an association could lead to a new subdivision of certain diseases that today are viewed as units; without doubt, this would have repercussions on therapy and prognosis, and even on prevention.

Finally, an association between *HLA* and a specific disease also provides information about the etiology and pathogenesis of the disease, particularly concerning an infectious or immunologic (autoimmune) mechanism.

References

Albert E, Götze D (1977) The major histocompatibility system in man. In: Götze D (ed) The organisation of the major histocompatibility system in man and animals. Springer, Berlin Heidelber New York, p 7

Binz H, Wigzell W (1975) Shared idiotypic determinants on B and T lymphocytes reactive against the same antigenic determinants. I. Demonstration of similar or identical idiotypes on IgG molecules and T cell receptors with specificity for the same alloantigens. J Exp Med 142:197

Bodmer WF, Batchelor JR, Bodmer JG, Festenstein H, Morris PJ (eds) (1978) Joint Report 1977. In: Histocompatibility testing 1977. Munksgaard, Copenhagen

Burnet FM (1970) Immunological surveillance. Pergamon, Sidney

Cantor H, Boyse EA (1975) Functional subclasses of T lymphocytes bearing different Ly antigens. I. The generation of functionally distinct T cell subclasses is a differentiative process independent of antigens. J Exp Med 141:1376

Cantor H, Boyse EA (1975) Functional subclasses of T lymphocytes bearing different Ly antigens. II. Co-operation between subclasses of Ly$^+$ cells in the generation of killer cell activity. J Exp Med 141:1390

Counce S, Smith P, Barth R, Snell GD (1956) Strong and weak histocompatibility gene differences in mice and their role in the rejection of homografts of tumors and skin. Ann Surg 144:198

Debré P, Kapp JA, Dorf ME, Benacerraf B (1975) Genetic control of specific immune suppression. II. H-2 linked dominant genetic control of immune suppression by the random copolymer L-glutamic acid^{50}-L-tyrosine^{50} (GT). J Exp Med 142:1447

Doherty P, Götze D, Trinchieri G, Zinkernagel RM (1976) Models for recognition of virally-modified cells by immune thymus-derived lymphocytes. Immunogenetics 3:517

Edidin M (1972) The tissue distribution and cellular localisation of transplantation antigens. In: Kahan BD, Reisfeld RA (eds) Transplantation antigens, markers of biological individuality. Academic, New York, p 125

Falconer DS (1960) Introduction to quantitative genetics. Ronald, New York

Fu SM, Kunkel HG, Brusman HP, Allen FH Jr., Fotino M (1974) Evidence for linkage between HL-A histocompatibility genes and those involved in the synthesis of the second component of complement. J Exp Med 140:1108

Götze D, Reisfeld RA, Klein J (1973) Serologic evidence for antigens controlled by the Ir region in mice. J Exp Med 138:1003

Götze D (1976) Serologic characterization of Ia antigens and their relation to Ir genes. Immunogenetics 3:139

Götze D (ed) (1977) The major histocompatibility system in man and animals. Springer, Berlin Heidelberg New York

Götze D, Hofmann L, Huang CM, Vollmers HP (1980) Antigenic complexity of H-2 molecules. In: Protides of the biological fluids, Peeters H (ed), Vol. 28, p. 579. Pergamon Press, London

Götze D, Nadeau J, Wakeland EK, Berry RJ, Bonhomme F, Egorov IK, Hjorth JP, Hoogstraal H, Vives J, Winking H, Klein J (1980) Frequencies of H-2 and Ia antigens in wild mice from Europe and Africa. J Immunol 124:2675

Hämmerling G, Mauve G, Goldberg E, McDevitt HO (1975) Tissue distribution of Ia antigens. Ia on spermatozoa, macrophages and epidermal cells. Immunogenetics 1:428

Jerne NK (1971) The somatic generation of immune recognition. Eur J Immunol 1:1

Jerne NK (1974) Toward a network theroy of the immune system. Ann Immunol (Inst Pasteur) 125 C:373

Klein J (1975) The biology of the mouse histocompatibility-2 complex. Springer, Berlin Heidelberg New York

Klein J, Juretić A, Nagy Z (1980) The *I* region of the mouse *H-2* complex: A reinterpretation. Nature (in press)

Krangel MS, Orr HT, Strominger JL (1980) Structure, function and biosynthesis of the major histocompatibility antigens (HLA-A and HLA-B). Scand J Immunol 11:561

McDevitt HO, Benacerraf B (1969) Genetic control of the specific immune response. Adv Immunol 11:31

McDevitt HO, Bodmer WF (1974) HL-A, immune response genes, and disease. Lancet 1:1269

McDevitt HO, Deak BD, Shreffler DC, Klein J, Stimpfling JH, Snell GD (1972) Genetic control of the immune response. Mapping of the Ir-1 locus. J Exp Med 135:1259

McDevitt HO, Tyan ML (1968) Genetic control of the antibody response in inbred mice. Transfer of the response by spleen cells and linkage to the major histocompatibility (H-2) locus. J Exp Med 128:1

Medicus RG, Schreiber RD, Götze D, Müller-Eberhard HJ (1976) A molecular concept of the properdin pathway. Proc Natl Acad Sci (Wash.) 73:612

Meo T, Krasteff T, Shreffler DC (1975) Immunochemical characterization of murine H-2 controlled Ss (serum substance) protein through identification of its human homologue as the fourth component of complement. Proc Natl Acad Sci (Wash.) 72:4536

Möller G (ed) (1980) T cell stimulating growth factors. Immunol Rev 51

Revised nomenclature for antigen-nonspecific T cell proliferation and helper factors. J Immunol 128:2928 (1979)

Rood J van, Leeuwen A van, Termijtelen A, Keuning JJ (1976) B cell antibodies, Ia-like determinants, and their relation to MLC determinants in man. Transplant Rev 30:122

Selwood N, Hedges A (1978) Transplantation antigens: A study in serological data analysis. Wiley, Chichester

Shreffler DC, David CS (1975) The H-2 major histocompatibility complex and the I immune response region: Genetic variation, function, and organization. Adv Immunol 20:125

Snell GD, Dausset J, Nathenson S (1976) Histocompatibility. Academic, New York

Someren H van, Westerveld A, Hagemeijer A, Mees JR, Meera Khan P, Zaalberg OB (1974) Human antigen and enzyme markers in man/Chinese hamster somatic cell hybrids. Evidence for synteny between the HLA, PGM-3, ME_1, and IPO-B loci. Proc Natl Acad Sci (Wash.) 71:962

Svejgaard A, Platz P, Ryder LP, Staub-Nielsen L, Thomsen M (1975) HL-A and disease association – A survey. Transplant Rev 22:3

Terasaki PI, Mickey MR (1975) HL-A haplotypes of 32 diseases. Transplant Rev 22:105

Thorsby E, Piazza A (1975) Joint report from the VI International Histocompatibility Workshop. II. Typing for HLA-D (LD-1 or MLC) determinants. In: Kissmeyer-Nielsen F (ed) Histocompatibility testing 1975. Munksgaard, Copenhagen, p 414

Chapter 7   Antigen–Antibody Interaction

OTTO G. BIER

Contents

Serologic Reactions for Detection of Antibodies

The union of antibody and antigen gives rise to a series of reactions, the qualitative or semiquantitative study of which is the domain of serology.

The type of reaction observed depends upon the physical state of the antigen (soluble or particulate) and the experimental conditions of the test involved. If the antigen is a soluble protein, the reaction between the macromolecules of the antigen and the antibody, in the proper proportions, results in the formation of an insoluble complex (precipitate). When the antigen is found on the surfaces of particles (such as bacteria or erythrocytes), the molecules of the divalent antibody form bridges with the particles and cause their agglutination (Fig. 7.1). In reactions with erythrocytes, when complement as well as antibody is present, lesion sites form on the erythrocyte membrane through which hemoglobin is liberated. This is the phenomenon of specific hemolysis.

The intensity of a serologic reaction is generally expressed in terms of "titer" – the dilution of serum (or of antigen) in which a specific effect is observed under certain experimental conditions. Thus, for example, if a given serum prepared for experimentation in serial dilutions (1:10, 1:20, 1:40, etc.) produces agglutination at the 1:640 dilution, but does not produce agglutination at 1:1280, it is said to have a titer of 1:640 or to contain 640 agglutinating units per unit of volume. In this type of test, the precision of the reading is obviously subjective and can vary by a factor of $\pm \log 2$ in repeated tests, so that only differences in the titers of two or more tubes of the reaction series are considered significant. In the case of specific hemolysis, however, one can, by using successive dilutions that vary by a factor of less than 2 and through spectrophotometric determination of the quantity of liberated hemoglobin, achieve a precision of $\pm 2\%$.

Although the verification of the intensity of serologic reactions is of inestimable practical value in the diagnosis of infections, it is important to bear in mind that serologic titer does not represent a measure of the

Reaction of the antibody with the antigen in solution

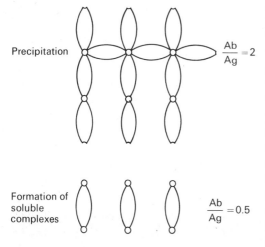

Precipitation $\dfrac{Ab}{Ag} = 2$

Formation of soluble complexes $\dfrac{Ab}{Ag} = 0.5$

Reaction of the antibody with the particulate antigen

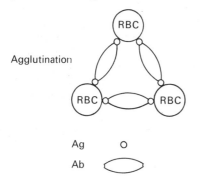

Agglutination

Ag   ○

Ab   ⬭

Fig. 7.1. Mechanisms of specific precipitation and agglutination

quantity of antibody, since it depends also upon the quality of the antibody (as in nonagglutinating or noncomplement-fixing antibody) not to mention variations in function from antigen peculiarities and from conditions inherent in the particular test.

In any case, when comparing the titers of various antisera, one should use the same dosage technique, including, whenever possible, previously standardized reference reagents (sera and antigens).

In Vitro Serologic Reactions

Precipitation

The easiest way of testing the reaction between an antibody and the corresponding antigen in solution consists of layering the two reagents and then observing, at the interface, the appearance of a disk or ring of precipitation (ring test). This reaction, called specific precipitation, occurs whenever the antigenic macromolecule possesses two or three or more combining sites for each of the two combining sites of the bivalent antibody molecule. If the antigen is univalent (hapten) or just bivalent, soluble complexes are formed and a precipitate is not observed (Fig. 7.1). The same occurs when there is an excess of antibody. There is no precipitation when the multivalent antigen reacts with univalent antibody fragments or with antibodies with weak affinity. In the latter case, special methods must be used to detect the presence of the antibody.

The quantitative reactions between antigen and antibody in specific precipitates proceed in variable proportions and are reversible. Accordingly, the antibody (Ab)/antigen (Ag) ratio in the precipitate decreases in proportion to the increase in the quantity of antigen, until a molecular composition of Ag_2Ab is attained, in which soluble complexes are formed:

$$Ag + Ab \longrightarrow AgAb + Ag\ Excess \longrightarrow Ag_2Ab$$
$$\qquad\qquad\quad (Precipitate)\qquad\qquad (Soluble\ complex)$$

$$AgAb + H\ excess \longrightarrow H_2Ab + Ag + H$$
$$\qquad\qquad (Hapten)\qquad (Soluble\ complex).$$

The latter reaction is the basis of the process for purification of antibodies through the elution of specific precipitates by the corresponding haptens.

Precipitation in Liquid Media. If, instead of layering the antigen and the antibody as in the ring test, aqueous solutions of the two reagents are mixed, initially the mixture is perfectly clear; after a while, there is a progressively developing turbidity, or opalescence. After a certain period of time, a flocculate, or precipitate, forms that finally collects in the bottom of the tube. The quantity of precipitate is a function of the quantity of antibody present in the antiserum, as well as of the quantity of antigen added. Under these circumstances, if increasing quantities of antigen are added to a series of tubes containing a fixed quantity of antiserum (e.g., 1 ml), an increasing quantity of precipitate is formed, up to a maximum level. Beyond this level, the amount of precipitate diminishes because of the formation of soluble complexes by the antigen excess. By subtracting the quantity of antigen added from the quantity of precipitate formed at the level of maximum precipitation, one obtains the quantity of antibody present in the antiserum.

One can also measure the antibody (or the antigen) in precipitation reactions through determination of the time of the most rapid precipitation, which corresponds to the optimum proportion in which the two reagents combine (optimal proportions method). In the so-called alpha method (Dean and Webb), the concentration of the antiserum is maintained constant whereas that of the antigen is varied; in the beta method (Ramon), varying quantities of antiserum are added to a fixed quantity of antigen. In both methods, the optimum proportion corresponds to that in the tube in which precipitation first appears.

Titration of antibodies by this method is useful in the measurement of antitoxins produced in the horse (Ramon flocculation), whereby determination of the optimum relation is particularly clear because of the presence of precipitation inhibition (formation of soluble complexes) with excess antigen as well as with excess antibody.

Expressed as Lf, the dose of toxin that produces optimum flocculation in the presence of one unit of antitoxin (abbreviated AU) can easily be measured for an antitoxin (A),

and a toxin (T), as a function of the relation expressed by the equation

$$ml\ A \times AU/ml = ml\ T \times Lf/ml \ .$$

Thus, for example, if 5 ml of a known toxin (30 Lf/ml) produces optimum flocculation in the presence of 0.1 ml of unknown serum, it can be concluded that such serum possesses 1,500 antitoxin units per milliliter, since

$$AU/ml = \frac{ml\ T \times Lf/ml}{ml\ A} = \frac{5 \times 30}{0.1} = 1\,500.$$

Vice versa, the potency of an unknown toxin that flocculates optimally in a 5-ml dose in the presence of 0.1 ml of a serum titrated at 1 500 AU/ml, can be calculated at 30 Lf/ml as follows:

$$Lf/ml = \frac{ml\ A \times AU/ml}{ml\ T} = \frac{0.1 \times 1\,500}{5} = 30,$$

Gel Precipitation. When an antigen mixture reacts with its antibodies (total antiserum) in a gel medium (agar, Agarose), multiple lines of precipitation are formed that correspond to the specific reactions of each component. It is thus possible by means of gel precipitation to analyse, using various techniques, the components of the antigen mixture (Fig. 7.2).

Simple Immunodiffusion. In this method, introduced by Oudin, the antigen, in aqueous solution, is layered in narrow-bore tubes above a column of 0.6% agar in which the antiserum has first been incorporated. As the solution diffuses through the gel, the antigenic components react with the antibodies to which they correspond. They thus form, in an excellent gradient, rings of precipitation. The position of these rings depends upon the concentration of the antigen and the time of diffusion. The greater the antigen concentration, the farther removed from the surface of the gel is the ring of precipitation. For a known concentration of antigen, the distance "h" from the ring to

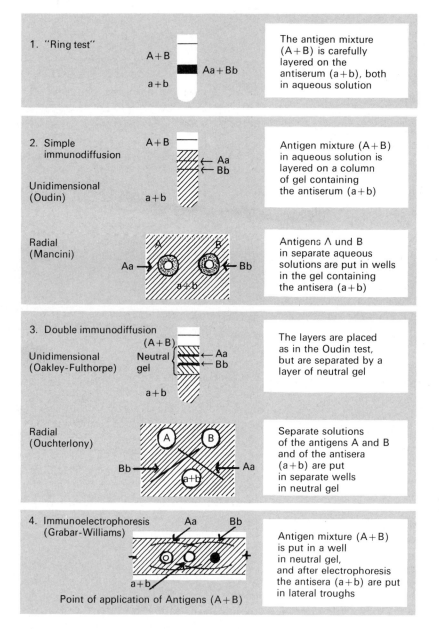

Fig. 7.2. Methods of immunochemical analysis by gel precipitation

the gel–antigen interface is proportional to the square root of the diffusion time, according to Fick's law ($h = k\sqrt{t}$). The distance, therefore, increases after 1, 4, 9, and 16 days by a factor of 1, 2, 3, and 4 respectively; for example, if $k = 2$, the distance would be 2, 4, 6, and 8 mm after 1, 4, 9, and 16 days.

The specificity of the rings formed with the antigen mixture can be demonstrated clearly with absorption experiments, as exemplified in Fig. 7.3. With Oudin's test, the diffusion in the tube operates in only a single dimension. For the titration of immunoglobulins, however, Mancini introduced simple radial

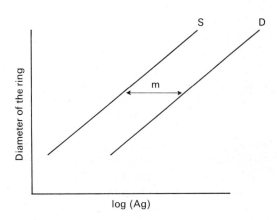

Fig. 7.3. Proof of specificities of the precipitation rings in Oudin's technique through absorption

diffusion [1], in which different dilutions of a standard antigen and of an unknown preparation are placed in separate wells made in a plate of gel in which specific antibody has been incorporated (immunoplate). The antigen diffuses radially, forming rings of precipitation whose diameters are proportional to the logarithm of the antigen concentration. The horizontal distance, m, between the parallel lines obtained with the standard dilution (S) and unknown dilution (D) enables calculation of the relative potency of the latter (Fig. 7.4).

Double Immunodiffusion. Oakley and Fulthrope modified Oudin's technique, interposing a neutral layer of agar between the gel containing the antibody, located in the bottom of the tube, and the aqueous antigen solution, located on the surface. Under these conditions, the antigen diffuses from the bottom upward and the antibody diffuses from the top downward, forming a ring of precipitation in the neutral layer of gel. A variant of this technique (Preer) consists of placing a drop of antiserum in the bottom of

the tube, covering it with a layer of neutral gel, and after solidification, adding the antigen solution.

In Oakley's technique, because the diffusion is double, it proceeds in a single dimension. However, in double radial diffusion, introduced by Ouchterlony, the antigen and the antibody – both in aqueous solutions – diffuse into one another from proximate wells cut in a layer of neutral gel. Figure 7.5 illustrates the formation of the precipitin line in the Ouchterlony plate.

With the latter technique, numerous arrangements can be used, depending upon

Fig. 7.4. Graph of relative antibody concentration in the Mancini test

----

1 This is not to be confused with radioimmunodiffusion or radioimmunoelectrophoresis, in which radioactive antigens are used and the precipitation lines are revealed by autoradiography

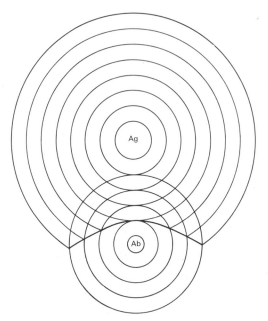

Fig. 7.5. Formation of precipitin line in the Ouchterlony plate

Fig. 7.6. Identical (complete or partial) and nonidentical reactions in double immunodiffusion

the experimental objectives. One of the most commonly used is that shown in Fig. 7.6. If the front wells contain the same (A 2) antigen, a continuous line of precipitation (identity reaction) is formed. In the case of different antigens (A 1 and A 2) the lines intersect; when there is partial identity (e.g., A 2 and A 1, 2), a spur is formed in the direction of the monospecific antigen (here, A 2).

The use of immunodiffusion methods has permitted detailed analysis of the antigenic components of organic materials. For example, simple diffusion has shown that donkey's milk produces, with a homologous immune serum, five rings of precipitation, three of which disappear when the immune serum is absorbed with horse milk. As many as ten antigenic components have been found in eggwhite, and even after three recrystallizations, chicken ovalbumin disclosed three antigenic impurities. Figure 7.7 illustrates, in diagrammatic form, some examples of antigen analysis with the Ouchterlony test.

Immunoelectrophoresis. Grabar and Williams combined electrophoresis with immunodiffusion and obtained a better separation of the lines of precipitation. In immunoelectrophoresis, an antigenic mixture is placed in a well in a plate of gel; after electrophoretic separation of the components, the antiserum (total) is added in a longitudinal trough (see Fig. 7.2, 4) along the path of electrophoretic migration.

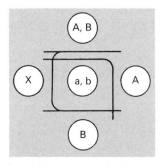

A and B are unrelated antigens;
X is partially identical to B,
but is not related to A

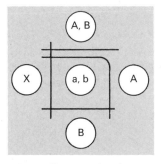

A, B, and X are unrelated

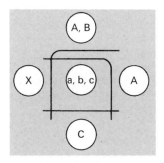

A, B, and C are unrelated
antigens; X is identical to B

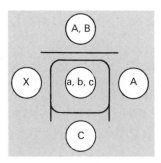

A and B are unrelated antigens;
A and C exhibit partial identity;
X is identical to A

Fig. 7.7. Example of antigenic
analysis in Ouchterlony plate

In alkaline pH, the proteins, negatively charged, migrate toward the anode[2], and the components, separated along the axis of electrophoretic migration, diffuse radially to form a series of precipitation arcs with the specific antibodies diffusing from the lateral troughs in the gel.

Immunoelectrophoresis has a considerably greater power of resolution than that of immunodiffusion, making possible the separation of antigenically distinct components that have differing electrophoretic mobilities. For example, in normal human serum, immunoelectrophoretic analysis permits characterization of up to 30 components, instead of five (albumin, α_1, α_2, β, γ) as disclosed by simple paper electrophoresis or agar-gel electrophoresis. In ascending order of their electrophoretic mobilities, the components are differentiated as: γ and β_2 globulins (IgG, IgA, IgM); β_1 (siderophilin or transferrin); hemopexin (β_1B); β_1C–β_1A, β_1E, and β_F, corresponding to C3, C4, and C5; α_2 (haptoglobin, ceruloplasmin, α_2 macroglobulin), α_{1a} (antitrypsin), and albumin (Fig. 7.8).

Two-Dimensional Immunoelectrophoresis. Laurell has developed a new immunoelectrophoretic technique which, besides giving a marked increase in resolution, is especially

2 The electrophoretic mobilities are not determined from the point of application of the sample, but at a point situated to the left, in the direction of the cathode. This is because a current establishes itself in a direction opposite to that of electrophoretic migration. This current, called endosmosis, results from the fact that agar is not completely neutral and possesses an electronegative charge in relation to the buffer in which it is embedded. Under these conditions, since the support-gel is fixed, it is the buffer that moves in the direction of the cathode

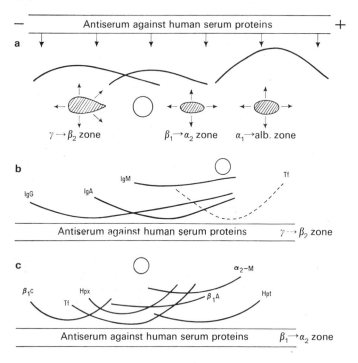

Fig. 7.8. Immunoelectrophoretic separation of the principal protein components of normal human serum

valuable for quantitation. Electrophoresis of the antigen is carried out in one dimension, the gel is cut, unused gel is discarded and warm gel containing the antibody is poured onto the plate. A second electrophoresis is then carried out at a right angle to the initial direction of travel. After diffusion, distinct peaks are obtained whose areas are directly proportional to the concentration of antigen. In the Laurell technique, electrophoretic separation is achieved with a voltage of 10 V/m for at least 60 min (and not at 3–6 V/m as in the technique of Grabar and Williams), so that a cooling device is required.

For the titration of purified antigen the first electrophoretic separation is not necessary. Successive dilutions of the purified antigen are added to contiguous wells of the antibody containing gel, and electrophoresis is carried out at a right angle. As a consequence of the migration of antigen molecules precipitation cones are formed (rather like interplanetary rockets) and the procedure is therefore designated "rocket immunoelectrophoresis".

Counterimmunoelectrophoresis. Another important technique is usually called "counter-immunoelectrophoresis" (a better designation is "immuno-osmophoresis") and consists of cutting wells about 8–10 mm apart in a gel plate. Antigen is added to one well, and antibody to the other. The antigen must migrate more quickly than the antibody at the pH used. After passage of the current, antigen migrates to the anode and antibody, because of endosmotic flow, travels in the opposite direction: $+\overrightarrow{Ab}\ \overleftarrow{Ag}-$. Consequently, the appearance of the precipitation line may occur within 20–30 min, instead of the 24–48 h required in the conventional Ouchterlony technique.

Counter-immunoelectrophoresis has proved to be extremely useful as a routine procedure to detect hepatitis HBs antigen (Australia antigen), in the rapid diagnosis of meningococcal meningitis, etc.

Agglutination

When a suspension of particles that bear antigenic determinants on their surfaces is mixed with the specific antiserum, large granules are formed that quickly sediment. This is the phenomenon of agglutination, described by Gruber and Durham at the beginning of the century.

The phenomenon may be observed with microbes or cells (erythrocytes, leukocytes, or other cells), in the activity of determinants naturally existing on the surface (direct agglutination), with cells (generally erythrocytes), or inert particles (latex, bentonite, etc.) artifically coated with a soluble antigen (indirect or passive agglutination). In any case, the mechanism of agglutination is fundamentally the same as that of specific precipitation, that is, the formation of bivalent antibody bridges that connect the antigenic determinants of adjacent particles (see Fig. 7.1).

As Bordet demonstrated, the presence of electrolytes constitutes a critical factor in agglutination: In the absence of salts, the particles fix the antibody, but are incapable of agglutinating. This fact caused the authors to espouse a two-stage theory, according to which the union of the antigen and the antibody (first stage) constituted the specific immunologic phenomenon, whereas agglutination represented only a secondary, nonspecific phenomenon (second stage) comparable to the flocculation of hydrophobic colloids by electrolytes. If this concept were accurate, mixing a suspension containing particles of two types, A and B, with an antiserum containing anti-A and anti-B antibodies would result in mixed granules of the two particles. However, in experiments with particles easily differentiated via microscopic examination, such as sheep or chicken erythrocytes, granules were observed containing only one or the other of the particles.

According to the currently accepted explanation, the relevance of salinity in its neutralization of the net negative charge that the particles exhibit in neutral pH, nullifies the repulsion between them and fosters a sufficient degree of attraction. In this way short-range noncovalent forces that assure the binding of the antigen by the antibody are able to determine the formation of bridges between adjacent particles.

Titration of Agglutinating Sera. The agglutinin titer of an antiserum is determined in a semiquantitative test in which decreasing quantities of serum (for example, 0.5-ml dilutions 1:10, 1:20, 1:40, etc) are reacted with a constant quantity of antigen (for example, 0.5 ml of a bacterial suspension containing $0.5–1.0 \times 10^9$ organisms per milliliter). After a period of incubation at the proper temperature, readings of the results are taken, noting the degree of agglutination $(++, +, -)$ by the nated eye, or with the aid of a magnifying lens. The agglutination titer is expressed in terms of the greatest dilution that gives rise to complete $(+++)$ or partial $(+)$ agglutination. As pointed out previously, the precision of this type of test is only $\pm 50\%$.

Various factors play an important role in the determination of agglutination titer:

1. The *presence of electrolytes* is essential to the phenomenon, and the pH of the diluent must not be excessively acidic or alkaline in order to avoid nonspecific results. Saline solution is generally utilized as diluent (1.9% NaCl solution), buffered to a pH of 7.2.

2. The *concentration of the antigenic suspension* also constitutes an important factor, for the greater the concentration of particles, the more rapid the agglutination. On the other hand, concentrated antigenic suspensions cause greater consumption of antibody and, consequently, lower agglutination titers.

3. The *temperature* at which the reaction occurs is important. The best temperature for the agglutination of microbes is 37 °C. In hemagglutination, e.g., in the study of the ABO or Rh blood groups, it is convenient to discriminate between the immune antibodies, which react better at 37 °C (warm agglutinins) [3] and the natural antibodies, which agglutinate better at 20 °C; there are also hemagglutinins, such as cryoagglutinins

---

3 Agglutinin is the term used for agglutinating antibodies

of atypical primary pneumonia or the anti-I agglutinins of acquired hemolytic anemias that react intensely only at 4 °C (cold agglutinins).

4. The *duration of incubation* is also important. One usually takes a first reading of the agglutination test after incubation for 1–2 h at 37 °C and then again after 24-h incubation at room temperature or under refrigeration at 4 °C. Agitation hastens considerably the results in tests performed on plates or on slides with concentrated antigenic suspensions (rapid agglutination). When the test is performed in tubes with diluted antigenic suspensions (slow agglutination), the results can be hastened through moderate centrifugation, followed by gradual resuspension of the sediment.

5. Certain antibodies called *incomplete antibodies* are incapable of agglutinating and, when coexisting with agglutinating antibodies, can block the fixation of the latter and produce a "prozone" of inhibition:

Dilution of the serum	1:10	1:20	1:40	1:80	1:160	1:320	1:640
	−	−	+	+	+	+	−
Agglutination	(Prozone)					(Titer)	

Prozones are observed not uncommonly in certain antibacterial sera such as anti-*Brucella* sera. With anti-Rh antibodies, it is common to observe the exclusive occurrence of nonagglutinating antibodies, which may be disclosed for example through the utilization of diluents with high levels of albumin, the trypsinization of red blood cells, or the antiglobulin test.

It was thought at first that the incomplete antibodies were incapable of agglutinating because they were univalent. Today, however, we know that the lack of agglutination of these antibodies is due to an inaccessible location of the antigenic determinants to which they correspond (Fig. 7.9), or to their weak avidity (low association constant).

It is obvious that an agglutination titer, even when determined under standardized conditions, does not denote the total level of antibodies in the serum, but only that of the predominant antibodies. Thus, for example, if A, B, and C antigens exist on the surface of a particle, the agglutination of these particles in the presence of a whole antiserum (antibodies a, b, and c) will be assured, in

Fig. 7.9. Schematic representation of the absence of hemagglutination observed in certain systems, e.g., in the Rh system. According to interpretation I, the antibody, because it has combining sites that are too close together, cannot unite with two antigenic sites; whereas, according to interpretation II, the antibody is incapable of establishing linking bridges because of the deeply recessed location of the antigenic sites in crypts in the surface of the erythrocyte. In either case, the union can be assured by means of an antiglobulin serum (Coombs' test)

weak dilutions of antiserum, for any of the antibodies –

B-b-B-b-B-b-B
A-a-A-a-A-a-A
C-c-C-c-C-c-C

However, in an end-point dilution (titer), only the molecules of the antibody present in greatest quantity enter into play, e.g., for antibody a –

B   B   B   B
A-a-A-a-A-a-A
C   C   C   C

Somatic and Flagellar Agglutination. In motile bacteria such as *Salmonella*, agglutination can be of two types (Fig. 7.10):

1) *Flagellar* (H) *agglutination* occurs when microorganisms unite through their flagella, forming loose floccules that dissociate easily under agitation. This type of agglutination develops rapidly, enabling a reading of the H titer to be taken after 1–2 h of incubation[4].

2) *Somatic* (O) *agglutination* occurs when the union proceeds by way of antibody bridges uniting the bacterial bodies so as to form compact granules, not easily dissociable. This type of agglutination develops slowly, in 24–48 h.

The agglutinogens (antigens that can be detected using agglutinating antibodies) responsible for these two types of reaction can be easily discriminated by heating the bacterial suspension at 100 °C: Such treatment

---

4 The designations H and O are derived from German and were used primarily for the motile and nonmotile strains of *Proteus*: the former an invasive veil on the surface of the agar, which was compared to breath (Ger. *Hauch*) on a window pane; the other variant, O, grows in isolated colonies, without the invasive veil (Ger. *Ohne Hauch*)

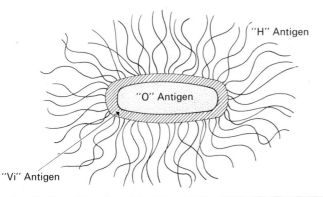

"H" Antigen

"O" Antigen

"Vi" Antigen

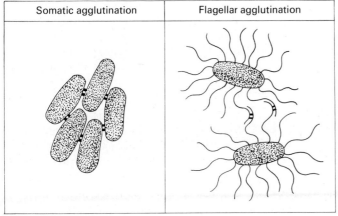

Somatic agglutination	Flagellar agglutination

Fig. 7.10. Somatic and flagellar agglutination

destroys the H antigen without appreciably injuring the O antigen. On the other hand, the agglutinability of the O type is impeded in the presence of 0.5% formalin, which does not act upon H agglutination.

In *Salmonella*, the O antigen is represented by a polysaccharide composed of repeated units (galactose-mannose-ramnose) that – depending upon the mode of linkage among the sugars and/or upon the existence of lateral chains on the basic trisaccharide – exhibit differing specificities (antigenic determinants). As for the flagellar antigens, we know that they are proteins, yet we know nothing about the chemical nature of their determinants.

Cross-Reactions in Microbial Agglutination. When two microbial species exhibit common antigens on their surfaces in addition to their specific antigens, or related antigens, cross-reactions occur among them; that is, the antiserum prepared with the homologous species is capable of agglutinating the heterologous species or vice versa.

We shall not occupy ourselves in this chapter with reactions due to related antigens, which can only be studied properly with the help of precipitation curves. Rather, we shall examine how cross-reactions due to group antigens can be distinguished utilizing the agglutinin absorption test.

Common antigens (group specific) and homologous antigens (type specific) can be represented by distinct molecules or by different regions of the same agglutinogen. In exemplifying this fact, the four species of *Salmonella* represented by the following abbreviated antigenic formulas are considered:

Salmonella paratyphi-B	4/b
Salmonella typhimurium	4/i
Salmonella anatum	3,10/e,h
Salmonella newington	3,15/e,h.

The first two are identical in respect of their somatic antigen (4) but differ in the flagellar antigens (b,i), whereas the last two possess identical flagellar antigens (e, h) but differ in

one of the specificities of the O antigen (10 and 15).

If a rabbit is immunized with *S. paratyphi-B*, the total antiserum contains anti-4 + anti-b and, as such, agglutinates *S. paratyphi-B* (4/b) as well as *S. typhimurium* (4/i). The same occurs with the anti-*typhimurium* (anti-4 + anti-i). However, by treating the anti-*paratyphi-B* serum with a thick suspension of *S. typhimurium*, we cause the absorption of the anti-4 agglutinin and thereby produce a monospecific anti-b antiserum.

Vice versa, the absorption of anti-*typhimurium* serum with *S. paratyphi-B* removes anti-4, leaving just anti-i. In this example, the common antigen and the specific antigens correspond to distinct molecules of the two agglutinogens.

The identical result is obtained, however, with the species *S. anatum* and *S. newington*, whose O specificities correspond to distinct regions of the respective agglutinogens:

$$\underset{10}{\overset{3}{(\text{Gal-}\alpha\ \text{Man-Ra})_n}} \qquad S.\ anatum$$

$$\underset{15}{\overset{3}{(\text{Gal-}\beta\ \text{Man-Ra})_n}} \qquad S.\ newington.$$

The 3,10 serum absorbed with 3,15 becomes monospecific anti-10 and, reciprocally, the anti-3,15 serum, absorbed with 3,10, becomes monospecific for 15.

The agglutinin absorption test has been widely utilized by bacteriologists for the differentiation of serologic types – in the enterobacteria group, for example. Utilizing monospecific sera obtained by absorption, more than 1,000 serotypes in the *Salmonella* genus can be distinguished (White-Kaufman table).

The determination of the agglutination titer of sera is important for the diagnosis of infections, as first demonstrated in typhoid fever (Widal's test). The agglutination absorption test permits differentiation of results due to a group reaction or to a mixed infection (Castellani's test). We might illustrate this by a case clinically characterized as ty-

Table 7.1. Model of Castellani's saturation of agglutinins test for the differentiation between group agglutination and mixed infection

Serum of the Patient	0 Agglutination with			
	T	B	T	B
Nonabsorbed	+	+	+	+
Absorbed with T	–	–	–	+
Absorbed with B	+	–	+	+
Interpretation:	Group agglutination		Mixed infection	

phoid fever, in which the serum of the patient exhibited an O agglutination titer of 1:640 for *S. typhosa* (9, 12) and of 1:80 for *S. paratyphi-B* (4, 12). Castellani's test (Table 7.1) may distinguish the group agglutination in a case of *S. typhosa* infection from that of a mixed infection of *S. typhosa* (T) and *S. paratyphi-B*.

Passive Hemagglutination. It is possible to fix antigens to the surfaces of erythrocytes or inert particles (colloid, latex, bentonite, etc.), making them agglutinable by the respective antibodies. With red blood cells (RBCs), this gives rise to passive or indirect hemagglutination, as opposed to natural or direct hemagglutination, which results from the interaction of antibodies with natural agglutinogens of the RBCs. Various antigens can be fixed simultaneously to the same RBC, which then becomes agglutinable by various antibodies. The same occurs in direct hemagglutination: the anti-RBC serum of sheep, for example, contains a mixture of antibodies with specificities directed against the various natural antigenic determinants of sheep RBCs.

Examples of natural hemagglutination include the agglutination of human erythrocytes by the serum of individuals with different blood groups; the agglutination of sheep erythrocytes by the serum of patients with infectious mononucleosis (Paul-Bunnell reaction); the cryohemagglutination of human O erythrocytes by the serum of patients with primary atypical pneumonia. Examples of passive agglutination include the agglutination of polystyrene (latex) or bentonite particles by the so-called rheumatoid factor; the agglutination of cholesterol crystals coated with cardiolipin by the serum of syphilis patients (Kline and VDRL tests); the passive hemagglutination tests with erythrocytes coated with specific agglutinogens, is utilized in the serodiagnosis of various infections because of their high sensitivity (detection of antibody quantities of the order of 0.003 µg).

Generally speaking, the polysaccharide antigens, when not highly purified [5], can attach directly to erythrocytes. Proteins, however, require prior treatment of the red blood cell with tannic acid (tanning – Boyden's technique), which makes it possible to obtain RBC suspensions specifically agglutinable in the presence of the respective antisera. It is not known for certain how tanning functions; it appears, however, that it not only causes a loose adsorption of the proteins to the red blood cell surfaces, but it also becomes easily agglutinable in the presence of small quantities of antibody. Occasionally, it causes nonspecific agglutination in the control tubes containing no antibody. This last inconvenience generally can be counterbalanced by the use of special diluents (e.g., saline solution with 1% normal rabbit serum).

In addition to tanning, other methods are also available for conjugating proteins to the red cell:

1) *Covalent bonding.* Covalent linkages are achieved by bifunctional molecules such as bidiazotized benzine (BDB), carbodiimide (CDI), glutaraldehyde (GA), and others.

2) *Metallic bridge.* Certain multivalent cations, Cr^+ in particular, modify the red

---

5 Fixation of polysaccharides to red blood cells appears to depend upon the presence of ionized sugars (amino sugars, uronic acids). Thus, for example, the O polysaccharides of *Salmonella* obtained by alkaline hydrolysis, which possess the characteristics described previously, attach more easily to erythrocytes than do highly purified polysaccharides obtained through acid hydrolysis

blood cell surface, making it capable of adsorbing proteins.

3. *Immunologic bridge.* To avoid autoagglutinating suspensions because of the conjugation of erythrocytic proteins, one may resort to an interesting method that consists of the following steps: (1) the protein antigen is conjugated by means of BDB with nonagglutinating anti-Rh antibodies; (2) the conjugate is then fixed to Rh-positive red cells (immunologic bridge).

Regardless of the method employed, the specificity of each amount of erythrocyte suspension must be controlled, for small variations in technique can noticeably affect the degree of autoagglutinability. Today there is a tendency to fix the erythrocytes before or after the fixation of the antigen to obtain suspensions that remain unchanged for months when maintained at 4 °C.

The erythrocytes most commonly used are human erythrocytes or sheep erythrocytes; in certain cases, however, there is an advantage in using erythrocytes from other species.

The quantity of antigen fixed to the erythrocytes is of major importance. It is advisable to determine the optimum quantity in preliminary experiments; that is, the quantity that produces the highest titer in comparison to a reference antiserum. The minimum number of molecules capable of "sensitizing" the erythrocytes can be determined by using antigens labeled with isotopes. The minimum number of molecules of O polysaccharide of *Salmonella* is of the order of 2,000 molecules per erythrocyte.

The hemagglutination reaction itself can be performed in tubes or, more conveniently, on plastic plates with wells in which different dilutions of serum to be tested are distributed along with a constant dose of the erythrocyte suspension. This latter technique is practical because it utilizes only 25 µl of serum. This assemblage, shown in Fig. 7.11, consists of a plastic plate with 75-µl wells and a metal loop titrator with a 25-µl capacity (Takatsy microtitrator). Into each well, 25 µl of diluent is pipetted; then 25 µl

of the antiserum under study is deposited in the first well. The microtitrator is then dipped into the first well, and the solution is mixed well by rotating the stem of the microtitrator between the fingers. Then 25 µl of successive dilutions of serum at 1:2, 1:4, 1:8, etc. are passed successively from one well to another. Subsequently, 25 µl of 1% erythrocyte suspension is added, agitating carefully to mix the reagents. The plate is covered or placed in a humid chamber to prevent evaporation and incubated at the desired temperature. Results are generally read after 2 h at room temperature and after 12–24 h when refrigerated at 4 °C. In the tubes as well as in the plates, the results are interpreted in conjunction with the pattern of the sediment, which exhibits the form of a button in negative reactions ($-$), that of a round plate with irregular borders in strongly positive reactions ($4+$), and with intermediate patterns in the $+$, $2+$, and $3+$ reactions (see Fig. 7.11, bottom). In case of doubt, the reading can be confirmed by gently resuspending the sediment and then observing with a lens the presence and size of the granules.

Immunofluorescence

It is possible to make the antigen–antibody reaction visible by labeling one of the reagents with substances called fluorochromes, which have the capacity to absorb luminous energy, to store it for short periods (10^{-9}–10^{-1} s), and then to emit it in the form of radiation of a greater wavelength. This mechanism of fluorescence is due essentially to the absorption of the energy of photons by electrons of peripheral orbits that move to occupy orbits more distant from the nucleus, inducing a state of excitability in the molecule. Such a state is, however, of extremely short duration, because the electrons quickly return to their former orbits, i.e., to a state of repose, due to the emission of luminous radiation. Because part of it is degraded into thermal or mechanical energy, the quanta of light emitted (fluorescence) have less energy, or greater

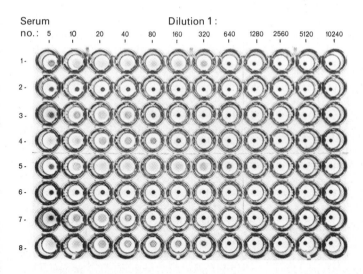

Serum   Dilution 1:
no.: 5   10   20   40   80   160   320   640   1280 2560 5120 10240

Fig. 7.11. Hemagglutination in the microtiter plate (Takatsy's microtitrator)

wavelength, than that of the exciting radiation (Stokes law).

For this reason, anti-DNA antibodies labeled with fluorescein have an absorption maximum at approximately 490 nm [1 nm (nanometer) or millimicron (mμ) is equal to 10^{-9} m, or 10^{-6} mm], whereas its emission maximum takes place at around 530 nm. If a section or cellular smear is treated with labeled antibody, the cytoplasm appears blue, whereas the nucleus exhibits green-yellow fluorescence.

In addition to fluorescein, rhodamine B, which emits an orange-red fluorescence, is also frequently used. Both fluorochromes are used in the isothiocyanate form, which

conjugates easily to proteins in alkaline pH
(>9):

$$\text{Fluorescein—N} = \text{C} = \text{S}$$
$$+ \text{Protein—NH}_2 \longrightarrow \text{Fl—N – C—N—Pr}$$

(Isothiocyanate of fluorescein)

For microscopic observation of fluorescence, the following accessories are necessary: (1) a source of excitatory light; (2) a thermal filter; (3) an excitatory filter; (4) a dark-field (cardioid) condenser; and (5) a "barrier" or protector filter. The source of excitatory light is generally in the form of a quartz bulb with mercury vapor (Osram HB 200 lamp), which emits visible and ultraviolet radiation (below 400 nm).

The light proceeding from the excitatory source passes successively through the thermal filter and the excitatory filter – the latter permeable only to radiation of a wavelength around 435 nm, which is still situated in the band of absorption of the fluorescein. Next, the excitatory light is directed at the cardioid condenser, which projects it along the microscope's optical axis on to the preparation. The light transmitted by the preparation includes not only radiation of the same wavelength, but also radiation having a wavelength longer than that of the excitatory light (fluorescent). The barrier filter interposed between the preparation and the eyepiece protects the eye of the observer from short wavelength radiation that passes through the objective (Fig. 7.12).

In principle, two techniques are utilized for the study of immunofluorescence (Fig. 7.13)

1) *Direct immunofluorescence.* This involves direct coloration of the antigen with labeled antibody. It is commonly used to identify microorganisms by immunofluorescence, e.g., *E. coli* (enteropathogenic serotypes), *Klebsiella* (serotypes), *Streptococcus* (Lancefield groups), *Gonococcus*, *B. pertussis*, *C. diphtheriae*, *Leptospira* (serotypes), and *Candida albicans.*

2. *Indirect immunofluorescence.* The specimen with attached antigen is treated with an

Fig. 7.12. The optical system in fluorescence microscopy

- Eyepiece
- Barrier filter
- Objective
- Preparation
- Condenser
- Exciter filter
- Thermal filter
- Exciter lamp

unlabeled specific antibody and then, after washing, incubated with conjugated anti-gamma globulin produced against the immunoglobulin of the species from which the specific antibody originates.

The double-layer immunofluorescence just described is frequently utilized to demonstrate antimicrobial antibodies (serodiagnosis of syphilis, toxoplasmosis, leptospirosis, schistosomes, Chagas' disease, etc.), as well as to detect autoantibodies, e.g., antinuclear antibodies in lupus erythematosus or intercellular antibodies in pemphigus. There can also be formation of triple layers, as in the so-called sandwich technique. The first layer is an antigen–antibody complex, a second layer, unlabeled antibody against antibodies of the first layer, and the third, labeled antibody with a specificity directed against the second layer. This technique is used to demonstrate antibody on the surfaces of plasma cells, as performed by Coons and his associates.

The immunofluorescence reactions for the demonstration of complement fixation are

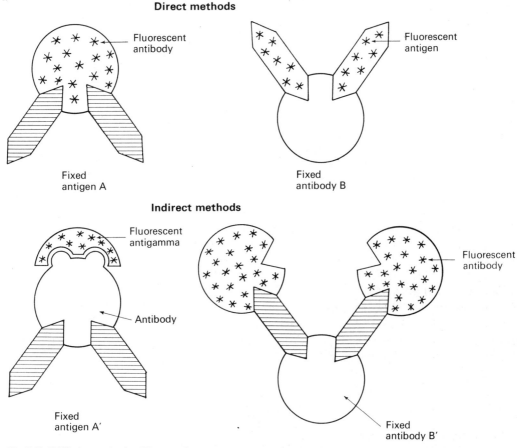

Fig. 7.13. Different methods of immunofluorescence

similar to the sandwich technique. A first layer is composed of an antigen–antibody complex; a layer of complement is adsorbed to it; then a third level of labeled anticomplement is added. [Anticomplement is obtained by immunization with antigen-antibody complex or with zymosan-C3 (production of anti-β^1C serum).] The demonstration of complement fixation in vivo by immunofluorescence suggests that the lesions such as those that occur in the Arthus reaction (vasculitis), in certain forms of glomerulonephritis by the deposition of antigen–antibody complex or by cytotoxic antibodies, are produced by antigen–antibody complexes.

In any case, one must utilize reagents previously characterized as to their activity (titra-tion of the conjugate to determine the optimum dose) and their specificity (absence of nonspecific fluorescence), which generally can be achieved by using conjugates obtained from potent antisera and with discrete labeling (low fluorochrome/protein ratio).

Complement Fixation

In combining with the antigen, certain antibodies affiliated with the IgG and IgM immunoglobulins form complexes capable of fixing complement. The phenomenon was discovered at the beginning of the century by Bordet and Gengou and quickly aroused great interest because of its application in the serodiagnosis of syphilis (Wassermann reaction). Today, numerous other infections are diagnosed by the complement fixation reaction (CF), e.g., Chagas' disease, South American blastomycosis, toxoplasmosis, echinococcosis, gonococcic infections, rickettsiosis, and numerous virus infections (psittacosis, lymphogranuloma, poliomyelitis, arbovirus infections, epidemic parotitis, influenza). Moreover, the CF test is also utilized, through the use of known antisera, to characterize the types and subtype of numerous viruses, such as the aftosa viruses, the arboviruses, and the echoviruses.

The Qualitative Test. The complement fixation test can be summarized in the following manner:

I. Specific antigen (Ag)+C   Free C
 II. Anti-Ag antibody+C   Free C
  III. Anti-Ag+Ag+C   Fixed C.

If EA (e.g., sheep erythrocytes sensitized by rabbit antisheep erythrocytes) is added to mixtures I and II, hemolysis occurs:

EA + free C = Hemolysis .

The addition of EA to mixture III, however, produces little or no hemolysis, for part or all of the complement mixed with the Ag-anti-Ag complex will have been consumed:

EA + fixed C → Absence of hemolysis .

The qualitative test can be limited to the three tubes mentioned previously – I and II being antigen and serum controls, respectively, and III being the reaction tube. The mechanism of the test, in its two stages, is represented schematically in Fig. 7.14.

In the early days of serology, when the Wassermann reaction was introduced, the degree of fixation was evaluated by the percentage of hemolysis observed, expressing the results as + + + + (absence of hemolysis), + + + (25% lysis), + + (50% lysis), and + (75% lysis). Today, however, to evaluate

Positive reaction

Negative reaction

No hemolysis   Hemolysis

Wassermann antibody

Wassermann antigen (cardiolipid)

Complement

Antisheep erythrocyte antibody

Sheep erythrocytes (E)

Antigenic determinants of E

Fig. 7.14. Mechanism of the Wassermann reaction for complement fixation the fixative potency of a serum, increasing dilutions of antiserum are mixed with adequate fixed amounts of antigen and complement, proceeding to a reading of the results in terms of the quantity of hemoglobin liberated in the supernatants, as previously described for the spectrophotometric measurement of complement-mediated hemoglobin release.

Quantitative Testing Methods. Two methods for quantitative testing should be mentioned here:

1) In the *macromethod of Mayer and associates*, dilutions of serum (or of antigen) are incubated for 20 h at 2°–4 °C with an optimum dose of antigen (or of serum) and an excess of complement, e.g., 100 CH_{50} units. Controls containing just serum $+C$ or antigen $+C$ are also included in the test, in order to detect any anticomplement activity in the reagents. After incubation the mixtures are diluted to measure the quantity of unfixed C and to determine the number of fixed CH_{50} units.
2) In *serodiagnostic tests* in which small quantities of complement (2–5 CH_{50} units) are used in such a way that the residual quantity of unfixed C is of the order of 0.8–1.2 CH_{50} units, the amount of complement fixation can be determined directly by addition of EA to the undiluted mixtures. Included in this category are the quantitative techniques (perhaps better described as semiquantitative) of Christiansen, of Maltaner and associates, of Stein and Van Ngu, and of others.

The introduction of Mayer's method permitted investigators to establish with precision the relations between antigen and antibody in the complement fixation reaction. By maintaining the antibody dose constant and varying the concentration of Ag, a CF curve is produced that notably resembles the curve of specific precipitation, clearly exhibiting a zone of inhibition by excess antigen (Fig. 7.15). However, when a fixed dose of Ag is added to a varying dose of immune serum, the curve changes and does not ex-

Fig. 7.15. Quantitative complement fixation studied by the macromethod of Mayer et al. in systems with constant levels of antibody (11.9 mg, 18.5 mg, and 29.4 mg) and variable amounts of antigen

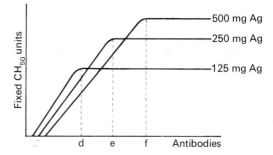

Fig. 7.16. Quantitative fixation of complement studied by the macromethod of Mayer et al. in systems with constant amounts of antigen (125 mg, 250 mg, and 500 mg) and variable amounts of antibody

hibit a zone of inhibition (Fig. 7.16). Still, in both cases the quantity of fixed C reaches a maximum that corresponds to the maximally reactive dose of antigen (in the tests with constant antiserum) or of serum (in the tests with constant antigen).
If we represent graphically the quantities of serum on the abscissa, and the number of units of complement fixed in the presence of maximally reactive doses of antigen on the ordinate, a sigmoid curve is obtained (Fig. 7.17). The fixation potency, expressed in terms of CF_{50} (being the dose of serum at which 50% of the complement units involved are fixed) is found at the linear portion of the curve.
In the semiquantitative techniques, the maximally reactive dose of antigen is not established for each dilution of antiserum;

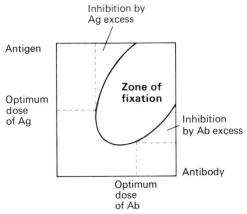

Fig. 7.18. Isofixation curve for the determination of the optimum concentration of antigen

Fig. 7.17. Sigmoidal curve of the number of units of complement fixed by varying quantities of antibody, in the presence of optimum amounts of antigen. Determination of CH_{50}

rather, a dose capable of reacting optimally with a series of serum dilutions is utilized. To establish this dose, it is necessary to determine the curve of isofixation through experiments of the "checkerboard" type, in which the antigen and the serum are varied in perpendicular directions. The optimum doses are indicated by the minimum quantities of antibody (or antigen) and can be visualized easily by inspection of the isofixation curve (Table 7.2 and Fig. 7.18).

Under the conditions of the semiquantitative test, Maltaner and his associates verified the direct proportionality between $K'sa$, *the number of units of C required for 50% hemolysis in the presence of serum plus antigen*, and $1/D$, *the inverse of the serum dilution*, which permitted expression of the fixative titer in terms of the angular coefficient (slope) of the line $K'sa = b'(1/D)$. Since $K'sa$ is calculated by dividing n, the number of units of C used in the test, by the correlation factor (f) corresponding to the percentage of lysis, then

$$b' = D \times (n/f), \qquad (1)$$

in which $f = (y/1 - y)^h$ and h is the slope verified for the titration of the complement in the presence of serum or of antigen alone.

Antibody µg N/ml	Antigen µg N/ml							
	0.001	0.012	0.04	0.12	0.36	1.10	3.33	1.00
3.3	1[a]	0	0	0	0	0	0	0
2.2	2	0	0	0	0	0	1	1
1.5	4	0	0	0	0	0	1	4
1.0	4	1	0	0	0	1	4	4
0.66	4	3	1	1	1	4	4	4
0.44	4	4	2	3	4	4	4	4
0.30	4	4	4	4	4	4	4	4

Table 7.2. Semiquantitative determination of the optimum antigen dose in the bovine serum albumin-rabbit antibovine serum albumin system in a test with five units of complement

[a] 0, 1, 2, 3, and 4 represent, respectively, 0, 25%, 50%, 75%, and 100% hemolysis

More precise experiments have shown, however, that the rigorously linear relation is that which is observed between $\log D$ and $\log(y/1-y)$, in accordance with the equation $\log D = \log T + h's \times \log y/1-$ in which $h's$ is the angular coefficient corresponding to the quantity of residual complement after the fixation reaction. From this equation, the following formula results for the calculation of fixative titer:

$$T = D \times (1/f). \qquad (2)$$

Obviously, if $h = h's$, formula (1) gives a value equal to that of formula (2) or a multiple thereof. For example, if a serum at a dilution of 1/25 in the presence of the optimum antigen dose and in a test with 6 units of complement, produces 75.5% hemolysis where h is equal to $h's = 0.2$, and $f = f = 1.25$, then the values of the titers calculated with the two formulas are:

$$b' = 25 \times 6/1.25 = 120,$$

$$T = 25 \times 1/1.25 = 20.$$

However, depending upon the number of units of C utilized in the test, the nature of the antigen or serum, and other factors, the value of $h's$ can differ considerably from that of h, imparting a corresponding difference to the calculation of fixative titer. In these cases, to avoid the calculation of new conversion factors, the titer can be determined graphically, as indicated in Fig. 7.19.

Mechanism of Complement Fixation. The mechanism of the fixation of complement is still obscure. Even the early immunologists sought to interpret it, with Ehrlich maintaining that complement fixation operates at the level of a special group (a complementophil group) of antibody binders (amboceptors), whereas Bordet attributed the phenomenon to the absorption properties of the antigen–antibody complex.

Modern immunologists, influenced by the works of Ishizaka and others, tend to favor the original point of view of Ehrlich, attributing primarily to the antibody the capacity to fix complement: (1) The immunoglobulins capable of fixing C in the presence of antigen also do so when aggregated by nonspecific means, such as by heat and by bisdiazobenzidine. (2) The binding property resides in the Fc fragment of the antibody molecule, because only this fragment becomes anticomplementary when aggregated, unlike the $F(ab')_2$ fragment. (3) When two immunoglobulins react, one an antigen and the other an antibody, C binding is observed only when the antibody immunoglobulin is capable of fixation – e.g., CF positive with rabbit anti-fowl gamma-globulin antibody, but not with bird anti-rabbit gamma-globulin, if rabbit or guinea pig serum is used as complement.

Relevant experimental data indicate, however, that simple aggregation is not sufficient to activate complement, and suggest that, in combining with the antigen, the antibody molecule exposes certain structures previously occluded in the C_H2 region of the

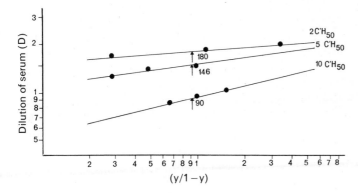

Fig. 7.19. Graphic determination of the fixation titer in the function of the curve $\log D$ versus $\log (y/1-y)$

Fig. 7.20. Mechanism of complement fixation by the antibody after its interaction with the specific antigen

Fc fragment, by a conformational mechanism comparable to the allosteric modification of enzyme molecules (Fig. 7.20).

In any case, electron microscopy shows that fixative capacity is associated with the formation of aggregates of four or more molecules of complete antibody, but not of Fab fragments (Fig. 7.21).

Effects of Complement Fixation on Cell Membranes. The fixation of components of

Fig. 7.21. Electron micrograph of antibody–hapten aggregates endowed with maximum capacity for complement fixation [Partial reproduction from Valentine RC, Green NN (1967) J Mol Biol 27:615

complement to the surfaces of cells gives rise to a series of manifestations that can be catalogued as follows:
1. Effects arising from fixation of C1 – C9
   (a) Immunocytolysis
   (b) Immunocytotoxicity
2. Effects arising from fixation of C1 – C3
   (a) Immunoadherence
   (b) Immunoconglutination.

Immunocytolysis

Even in the early days of immunology, it was observed that bacteria or red blood cells, "sensitized" by the specific antibody, were lysed upon the addition of complement. We have already referred in detail to the mechanism of specific hemolysis, i.e., the sequential action of the C1–C9 components of complement. In this section, we deal only with the phenomenon of specific bacteriolysis, first observed in vitro after the inoculation of cholera vibrios into the peritonium of immunized rabbits. Under these conditions, whereas in the control animals examination of the peritoneal exudate revealed the presence of *V. cholerae* with its typical morphology and mobility, in immunized rabbits the vibrios quickly lost their mobility and disintegrated into granules (Pfeiffer's phenomenon). The phenomenon can be studied conveniently in vitro by mixing bacteria, immune serum, and complement, and determining the number of viable bacteria (bactericidal effect) by distributing the suspension on an agar plate and counting the colonies that are formed. Generally speaking, we can say that gram-negative bacteria (e.g., *V. cholerae*, *S. typhosa*, *S. dysenteriae*, *E. coli*, *P. aeruginosa*) are lysed and destroyed, whereas the gram-positive (e.g., gram-positive cocci, *B. subtilis*) are inhibited in their growth without concomitant lysis. In both cases, however, the cytocidal effect depends upon the sequential action of the nine components of complement: Serum of rabbits deficient in C 6, for example, is incapable of exercising bactericidal action on *S. typhosa*.

With red blood cells, lysis appears to depend exclusively upon the initial formation of ultramicroscopic lesions on the cell membrane, with an initial increase in the permeability to substances of low molecular weight (entry of H_2O and Na, exit of K), followed by distention and rupture of the membrane and by permeability to substances of high molecular weight (e.g., hemoglobin). In bacteria, however, this condition is not sufficient, because alteration of the cell wall is also necessary.

In gram-negative bacteria rich in phospholipids and with thin cell walls (10 mμ or less), the combining action of antibody and complement leads to the formation of damaged and defenseless spheroplasts, susceptible to lysis; in gram-positive bacteria, however, that have thick cell walls (15–50 mμ) and are poor in lipids, conditions are not favorable to the disintegration of the cell walls and lysis does not occur, although the lesion of the cytoplasmic membrane can have a bactericidal effect. Two experimental facts support this interpretation: (1) *E. coli* spheroplasts and *B. subtilis* protoplasts are lysed by the action of specific antibody plus complement; and (2) bacteria resistant to the action of antibody plus complement undergo lysis when lysozyme is added, which by destroying the cell wall exposes the damaged protoplasts.

The lysozyme is probably not the only nonspecific adjuvant factor that operates in specific bacteriolysis. It is possible that the bactericidal actions of normal serum, though generally attributed to natural polyspecific antibodies, are actually caused by serum factors nonspecific for the effect produced by small levels of specific complement-binding and complement-activating antibodies. Also not to be excluded is the hypothesis relating to the activation of complement by serum factors not related to antibodies – or even as a result of properties of the bacterial surface itself.

It is pertinent to mention the serum factor called properdin (from Latin perdere "to destroy"), which was described originally as a protein capable of combining with constituents of the cell walls of different microorganisms (including the mixture of polysaccharides of the yeast cell wall, called zymosan). It also was thought to have a bactericidal effect in the presence of complement and Mg. Apparently not an antibody, it is like an antigen–antibody complex that causes the elective fixation of C 3, consuming practically no C 1, C 4, or C 2.

The existence of properdin has been confirmed by biochemical experiments utilizing chromatographic fractionation to separate a β-globulin with a molecular weight of 223,000 daltons, homogeneous under electrophoresis and ultracentrifugation, and incapable of reacting with antibodies against IgG, IgA, IgM, or their heavy and light chains. This protein exhibits reactions characteristic of properdin – in particular, the capacity to inactivate C 3 through prior combination with a serum proactivator (C 3 PA). Its operative mechanism therefore approximates that of endotoxins and that of the so-called thermolabile opsonin of pneumococcus, which activates C 3 by an alternative means independent of C 4 b 2 a.

The betalysins may also be mentioned among the nonspecific bactericidins of normal serum; their action, independent of complement, operates predominantly on gram-positive bacteria. Such substances are liberated only after the coagulation of the blood, and do not appear to exercise any important function in vivo.

Immunocytotoxicity

Immunocytoxicity describes antigen–antibody–complement interaction with the surface of a cell that does not result in cytolysis, but is accompanied by cytotoxicity activity, or structural alterations, and disturbances of cellular function (immobilization, increase in permeability, metabolic alterations).

The immobilization of *T. pallidum* (TPI test) by sera of patients with syphilis is an example of a reaction of this type. Mobile treponemas are mixed with the patient's serum and guinea pig complement. If the reaction is positive after incubation at 37 °C for 16–18 h, there is immobilization of the treponemas; there is no immobilization when normal serum is added or when complement is omitted. The long incubation time is necessary because the treponemas possess a coating of hyaluronic acid that impedes access of the antibody to the antigenic determinants (proteins) of the spirochete. The addition of lysozyme hastens the reaction.

An example of a cytotoxicity test that involves an increase in cellular permeability is the lymphocytotoxicity test, used currently to disclose histocompatibility antigens, with a view to selecting donors for tissue or organ grafts. A purified suspension of human lymphocytes is mixed with antiserum and complement (human, rabbit serum). After incubation at 37 °C, trypan blue (or eosin) is added. Under the microscope it can be seen that the injured cells have taken up the stain and appear blue (or dark red), whereas intact cell membranes do not allow the uptake of stain (microdye-exclusion test).

Experimental glomerulonephritis, induced by the inoculation of heterologous antikidney serum (Masugi's nephritis), furnishes an interesting example of direct immunocytotoxicity (reaction with antigens of the glomeruli) and indirect immunocytotoxicity (reaction with heterologous antigens fixed to the glomeruli). If rabbit anti-rat kidney serum is injected into a rat, intense, precocious proteinuria occurs (when the antiserum dose is sufficient), resulting from the cytotoxic action of the anti-kidney antibody upon antigens belonging to the basement membrane (BM) of the glomeruli. Upon ultramicroscopic examination, a uniform thickening of the BM may be clearly

ascertained, and immunofluorescence discloses the presence of rabbit immunoglobulin and thickening of the capillary lumen (mesangial pattern) along the endothelial face of this membrane. The role of complement in nephrotoxic nephritis is clearly indicated (1) by the absence of glomerular lesions in complement-depleted animals; and (2) by the incapacity of the pepsin fragment of the nephrotoxic antibody to produce immediate proteinuria caused by the complete complement-fixing antibody. If, however, a non-complement-fixing antibody, is injected instead of a complement-fixing antibody, the proteinuria does not develop immediately. This process occurs in the classic experiment in which goose anti-rabbit kidney serum is injected into a rabbit. Since the antibody is incapable of fixing complement, proteinuria appears only after the heterologous immunoglobulin is bound to the BM and subsequently provokes the formation of rabbit anti-goose immunoglobulin, which then binds complement and is responsible for the delayed proteinuria (indirect immunocytotoxicity).

Distinct from nephrotoxic nephritis, the nephritis produced by the deposition of irregular masses (lumpy-bumpy pattern) of antigen–antibody–complement complexes is readily disclosed by immunofluorescence of the reactants involved.

Another example of indirect immunocytotoxicity is provided by thrombocytopenic purpura, which develops in certain cases of allergy to drugs, e.g., in cases of hypersensitivity to allylisopropylacetylurea (Sedormid) or to quinidine. In these cases, the specific antibody reacts with the drug, which is fixed to the platelets; complement is activated through the antigen–antibody complex, resulting in thrombocytolysis and consequently thrombocytopenia. Lysis of platelets can be achieved in vitro by mixing the patient's serum with normal platelets and the drug, along with complement. The serum of the sensitized individual causes lysis of the platelets; lysis does not occur in control tubes containing normal serum to which the drug or complement has not been added.

Immunoadherence

Certain microorganisms, such as spirochetes and trypanosomes, when mixed with the specific antibody in a suspension of platelets and in the presence of complement, adhere to the platelets forming grains clearly evident by dark-field microscopic examination (Rieckenberg reaction). This phenomenon has been reinvestigated, and today it is called immunoadherence (IA) – the adhesion of antigen–antibody–complement complexes to the surfaces of the erythrocytes of primates[6] or to the platelets of other species, microscopically and macroscopically evidenced by the agglutination of the indicator particles.

Fig. 7.22. Immunocytoadherence (Original of B. Biozzi)

Analysis of the role of complement in IA has shown that only the C 1 and C 3 components are involved, with the critical part being played by fixed C 3; equal immunoadherence capacity is exhibited by the $\overline{EAC\,1,4,2,3}$; $\overline{EAC\,1,4,3}$; or $\overline{EAC\,4,3}$ complexes. Immunoadherence is an extremely sensitive serologic reaction that can be used for detecting minimal quantities of autoantibodies (e.g., in detecting levels of autoantibodies not disclosed by other reactions), or for the titration of C 3. In addition to its serologic value for C 3 titration and as an indicator for the complement binding reaction, an important role is attributed to immunoadherence in phagocytosis: Erythrocytes or bacteria, treated with specific antibodies, can bind complement, and the coated C 3 b particles adhere not only to erythrocytes but also to the receptors of the macrophages.

Immunocytoadherence. Biozzi and associates used this term to describe rosettes formed by erythrocytes around the lymphocytes of immunized animals (Fig. 7.22). Thus, for example, the lymphocytes of the spleens of

normal mice are capable only in small numbers of forming rosettes with sheep erythrocytes. If, however, mice are immunized with these erythrocytes, the number of rosettes increases gradually from the fourth day and in amounts paralleling the agglutination titer of the serum. The phenomenon is interpreted in terms of the formation of antibodies at the cellular level prior to their liberation by the lymphocytes that produced them. Interesting data have been obtained with this technique concerning the cytodynamics of the formation of antibodies.

Conglutination and Immunoconglutination

Conglutination is the active agglutination by a euglobulin[7] existing in bovine serum called conglutinin (K) of sensitized erythrocytes (E'A) that are coated with complement (C). Fresh horse serum is generally

---

6 In the case of human erythrocytes, the receptor is destroyed by neuraminidase

7 The conglutinins can be purified through adsorption by zymosan in the presence of Ca^{2+} and subsequent elution by EDTA. The result is a highly asymmetric molecule, 7.8 S, mol. wt. 750,000, not related to the gamma globulins, with an elevated level of glycine (18%). It is resistant to heating to 56 °C and to treatment with ammonium salts, mercaptoethanol, neuraminidase, and pepsin; however, it is easily destroyed by trypsin and by papain

used in the conglutination reaction in a dose sufficient to provide an adequate quantity of C 1, C 4, C 2, and C 3, in the absence of hemolysis. The critical component is C 3, which, when fixed (C 3 b), is under the influence of a serum β-globulin (mol. wt. 100,000), probably an enzyme: this is the conglutinogen-activating factor (KAF); which exposes the polysaccharide determinants, which in turn combine with K in the presence of Ca^{2+}, producing the conglutination phenomenon

$$EAC\,\overline{1,4,2,3\,b}+KAF+KCA^{2+}\ \rightarrow\ Con\text{-}glutination.$$

The conglutination reaction is important in serodiagnostics, since, like the specific hemolysis reaction, it serves as an indicator of free C in complement fixation tests (e.g., in the serodiagnosis of glanders).

Immunoconglutination is the agglutination of EAC $\overline{1,4,2,3\,b}$ by anti-non-gamma-autoantibodies of a specificity directed against determinants exposed on fixed C 4 and C 3. Such autoantibodies, called immunoconglutinins (IK), can be produced experimentally by the injection of bacteria that are sensitized (or else in vitro by a heteroantibody) and coated with complement (heterostimulated IK); they also are produced naturally, during infections, by microorganisms that coat the antibody and autologous complement (autostimulated IK).

A role in nonspecific resistance to infection has been attributed to the immunoconglutinins, which through an opsonizing process promote phagocytosis and intracellular digestion of bacteria by macrophages of the reticuloendothelial system.

Serologic Reactions in Vivo

Phagocytosis and Opsonization

Live cells have the capacity to engulf particles through an active process that involves the formation of hyaloplasmic membranes and bears the general term endocytosis: The term phagocytosis is used specifically for solid particles (from Greek *phag*, as in *phagein*, "to eat"), and pinocytosis is used with regard to the incorporation of liquids and the particles dissolved in them (from Greek *pin*, as in *pinein*, "to drink").

Whereas phagocytosis is characteristic of cells called phagocytes, pinocytosis is exhibited by all cells and probably constitutes a particular case of phagocytosis of inframicroscopic particles and macromolecules.

In both cases, the mechanism of engulfment is fundamentally identical. It is initiated by the adhesion of a particle to the cytoplasmic membrane, followed by invagination, which deepens little by little and ends by sequestration of the particle in a cytoplasmic vacuole. At the same time, re-formation of the cytoplasmic membrane proceeds at the point of invagination (Fig. 7.23). It was formerly believed that phagocytosis depended upon a purely physical mechanism, i.e., the interplay of the forces of surface tension. However, today it is known that this mechanism requires supplementary energy through relevant modifications of the metabolism of the phagocyte, represented by a conspicuous increase in anaerobic glycolysis of the polymorphonuclear leukocytes (see Chap. 11).

Phagocytosis, which in lower organisms represents the essential mechanism of nutrition (intracellular digestion), is also of fundamental importance for cleansing the organism (by scavenger cells) through the removal of waste products of internal origin

Fig. 7.23 a–d. Successive phases of phagocytosis. a Before engulfment, b cytoplasmic invagination, c formation of the phagocytic vacuole, d degranulation: evacuation of the enzymatic content of the lysosymes into the phagocytic vacuole

(e.g., dead cells or components of injured cells, denatured macromolecules), or through the elimination of foreign bodies, including microorganisms, regardless of their nature. As ingeniously recognized by Metchnikoff at the end of the last century, this latter process constitutes the basic defense mechanism against infections – in lower organisms as well as in the higher animals. In the latter, the digestive function becomes extracellular by means of enzymes situated in the gastrointestinal tract; however, some cells of mesenchymal origin still endure, scattered throughout the organism (fixed cells of the reticuloendothelial system) or accumulated at the sites of local inflammation, constituting an effective barrier to the penetration and dissemination of infectious agents, especially in immunized animals.

The Phagocytic Cells. In vertebrates, Metchnikoff distinguished two classes of phagocytes – microphages and macrophages. Microphages correspond to polymorphonuclear leukocytes of the blood, capable of phagocytosis (neutrophils and eosinophils), whereas macrophages are cells found throughout the organism and include (1) the monocytes of the blood; (2) the endothelial cells of the hepatic (Kupfer cells), splenic (red pulp), and lymphatic sinusoids; and (3) free phagocytes encountered in the tissues (e.g., in the milky spots of the omentum) and in inflammatory exudates (e.g., in peritoneal exudate and in pulmonary alveoli).

As vital staining methods advanced, it became possible to characterize the macrophage system better on the basis of a common physiologic property. This property is granulopexis, or the capacity of macrophages to capture electronegative-staining colloidal micelles (trypan blue, lithium-carmine, etc), or micelles of colloidal carbon, accumulating them in the form of granules in their cytoplasm.

For the group of cells endowed with the granulopexic function, Aschoff proposed the name reticuloendothelial system (RES).

This system includes:
1) The monocytes of the blood
2) The histiocytes of the tissues
3) the microglia of the central nervous system
4) The reticular cells (weakly active) of the lymphatic tissues
5) The endothelial cells (very active) that coat the lymphatic and blood sinusoids (liver, spleen, bone marrow, adrenals, and anterior pituitary).

The macrophages encountered in the inflammatory exudates are thought to originate from monocytes in the blood or from tissue histiocytes.

Quantitative Study of Phagocytosis of Inert Particles by the RES. It is possible to study quantitatively the phagocytosis of inert particles by the RES by injecting into the vein of an animal a known quantity of a suspension of uniform-sized particles, sufficiently large that they cannot be eliminated by the blood. Under these conditions, study of the elimination of the inoculated colloid with time (elimination curve) permits evaluation of the intensity of the phagocytic function exercised by the reticuloendothelial cells that enter into contact with the blood. The quantitative relationship between the concentration C, at a particular time t, and the initial concentration C_0 is expressed by the equation

$$C = C_0 \times 10^{-kt}.$$

From the preceding equation, the value of k can easily be calculated (the phagocytic or granulopexic index) by

$$k = \frac{(\log C_0 - \log C)}{t}, \text{ or } \frac{(\log C_1 - \log C_2)}{(t_2 - t_1)},$$

which measures the phagocytic efficiency of reticuloendothelial cells that enter into contact with the injected colloid (Fig. 7.24). The value of k is inversely proportional to the quantity of colloid injected (d), so that the product kd is essentially constant for each animal species. Thus, the kd product in

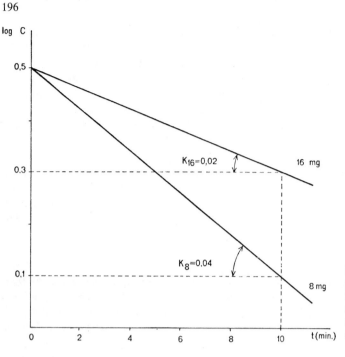

Fig. 7.24. Determination of the phagocytic index based upon the linear regression between the logarithm of the concentration of circulating carbon and the time elapsed

the rat equals 0.208 in tests performed with colloidal carbon, which is to say that for a dose of carbon equaling 8 mg/100 g, the value of k equals 0.208/8 or 0.026, and that for a double dose, k is two times smaller (0.013).

In repeated tests, the values of k for constant doses of colloid in the same animal species vary considerably, e.g., in rats injected with 8 mg/100 g of colloidal carbon, $k = 0.026 \pm 0.015$. This variation is not due to a corresponding variation in phagocytic activity, but to a variation in the weight of the active tissue, i.e., the hepatosplenic tissue (W_{fb}), in relation to the total weight of the animal (W_t). In numerous determinations, it was verified that the k values were inversely proportional to the cube of the W_t/W_{fb} ratio; thus, multiplying the ratio by the cube root of k, a new constant is obtained – α (corrected phagocytic index), which expresses the phagocytic activity as a function of the relative weight of the active tissue:[8]

$$(W_t/W_{fb})^3 \times K = \alpha^3,$$
$$\alpha = (W_t/W_{fb}) \times \sqrt[3]{k}$$

Unlike k, the α index is subject only to small variations ($\pm 10\%$), and it is effectively constant for any animal species, as illustrated by the 8 mg/100 g dose:

Index	Rat	Mouse	Rabbit
k	0.026	0.047	0.08
α	5.4	5.4	6.0

Quantitative Study of Phagocytosis of Bacteria by the RES. Applying the preceding method to the study of the elimination from the blood of bacteria labeled with radioactive isotopes, the identical quantitative relationship was confirmed. However, contrary to what occurred with the inert particles, the dose involved was not found to affect the value of the phagocytic index. This is easily understood when one considers that the

---

8 The active tissue is practically all represented by the hepatosplenic mass: After injection of colloidal carbon into mice, 90% can be recovered from the liver, 4% from the spleen

phagocytosis of bacteria (and not that of inert colloids) depends upon their interaction with serum components called opsonins, and therefore is subject to the influence of this limiting factor. Under these conditions, above a certain critical value of inoculum, the number of microorganisms phagocytosed corresponds to the maximum number that interacted with the limited level of opsonins available in the plasma of the animal involved.

Normal Opsonins and Immune Opsonins. It has long been known that the phagocytosis of microbes is facilitated by certain proteins existing in normal serum and, in a much more accentuated fashion, by specific antibodies against antigenic determinants of the microbial surfaces.

These substances are called opsonins (Greek *opsonein* "to soften food"), and the process is called opsonization; those in normal serum are called normal opsonins, whereas those in specific antisera are called immune opsonins.

Classically, immune opsonins (formerly called bacteriotropins) were distinguished from natural opsonins by their thermostability; the former remain active after being heated to 56 °C, whereas the latter are destroyed. This thermolability is explained by the fact that the normal opsonins require complement in order to be effective, whereas opsonization by specific antibodies, though it is enhanced by complement, is clearly evident in the absence of complement.

It is still not possible to define with precision the facilitating factors in normal serum phagocytosis; but we can relate them to the activation of the C 3 and C 5 components of complement through the mediation of natural antibodies in low titers or through a thermolabile serum factor (heat-labile factor or HLF) of a non-gamma-globulin nature.

The Role of Complement in Phagocytosis and the Mechanism of Ingestion. The action of complement in fostering phagocytosis can be evidenced clearly by in vitro and in vivo experiments. In the former, through study of the phagocytosis of sensitized erythrocytes (EA) treated with the various complement components, it has been verified that the phagocytosable complex corresponds to EAC 1,4,2,3, in which the effect of C 5 is minimal. Nevertheless, experiments with encapsulated pneumococci treated with fresh guinea pig serum evidenced participation, albeit to a lesser degree, of the C 5 component. With in vivo experiments, the role of complement in phagocytosis is clearly indicated by the retarded elimination of labeled bacteria from the serum of animals lacking complement.

The relevant role of C 3 can be interpreted as a function of the confirmed existence of receptors for $C\overline{3b}$ on the surfaces of polymorphonuclear cells and of monocytes, thereby assuring the initial stage of phagocytosis, i.e., the adhesion of the opsonized particle to the surface of the phagocyte.

The engulfment itself utilizes high affinity receptors for Fc on phagocytes. Following opsonic adherence through C 3 b, the Fc portion of the opsonizing IgG antibody moves along the Fc receptors acting like a zipper to sequester the particle in a phagocytic vacuole (phagosome), which in a later stage becomes a phagolysosome. The mechanism described above corresponds to the classical opsonization of humoral immunity and involves mainly polymorphonuclear leukocytes. Monocytes may also participate in this process, since they are equally provided with C 3 b and Fc receptors. However, the ingestion by macrophages is rather more associated with cellular immunity through the interaction with immune T lymphocytes, as described in a subsequent section (see Immune macrophages). Macrophages may also be armed with cytophilic antibodies or similar factors, e.g., the "specific macrophage arming factor" (SMAF) and thus be enabled to ingest the particle with or without previous opsonic adherence.

Determining Opsonin Concentrations. The classic methods for finding opsonin concentrations consist of comparing the average number (N') of bacteria phagocytized in a mixture of bacteria and leukocytes suspended in a medium containing the serum under study, with the value N, obtained with an identical mixture suspended in normal serum. The N'/N quotient represents the opsonization index of the serum in question. Thus, for instance, if in a counting of 50 leukocytes we encounter 120 phagocytized microorganisms in the suspension containing the patient's serum, and 200 in the suspension containing normal serum, we may conclude that the opsonization index of the patient's serum is 120/200 or 0.6, i.e., that the serum of the patient possesses 60% of normal opsonization power. A variant of this technique is the opsonocytophagic test, formerly used in the serodiagnosis of brucellosis. Today such tests have fallen into disuse, for they furnish no more diagnostic information than the simple direct or passive agglutination test.

For quantitative determination of the levels of opsonins in sera, the best method available is that based on the rapidity of elimination from the blood of bacteria labeled with radioactive isotopes. To avoid variations resulting from the level of natural opsonins in the experimental animals, a suspension of bacteria is injected and the initial k value is determined in the absence of the immune serum. Then the serum to be studied is injected and the new value of the phagocytic index, k', is determined. The difference, $k'-k$, permits calculation of the number of opsonizing units of the serum in question (Fig. 7.25). If we arbitrarily designate 0.01 as the value $k'-k$ for one opsonizing unit, we can evaluate the number of opsonizing units (OU) of any serum using the formula

$$OU/ml = 1/V \times D \times 100 \ (k'-k),$$

in which V and D represent, respectively, the volume and the inverse of the dilution of the serum injected. Thus, for example, if in the testing of a mouse we obtain a k value of 0.01 and k' equals 0.05, for the injection of 0.1 ml of the 1:500 dilution of a determined antiserum, we can conclude that the level of

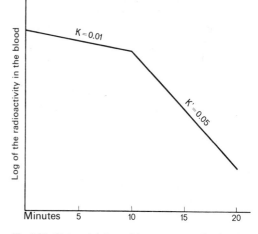

Fig. 7.25. Determination of immune opsonins by the velocity of elimination of *S. typhosa* labeled with [131]I. Biozzi et al., 1963

opsonizing units is equal to

$$1/0.1 \times 500 \times 100 \ (k'-k),$$
or 20,000 OU/ml .

The application of this method has indicated an impressive correlation between the specificity of the agglutination and that of the opsonizing activity in anti-salmonella sera. For example, different O variants of *S. typhimurium* (4,12; 1,4,12; 4,5,12; and 1,4,5,12) could be opsonized by the monospecific antiserum (anti-1,4,5 or 12) only if it possessed the respective antigenic determinants. The anti-H antibodies did not have any opsonizing power.

Postendocytic Phenomena: Intracellular Digestion. After the ingestion of opsonized particles, due to increased anaerobic glycolysis, strong acidity (pH 3–pH 6) develops at the level of the phagocytic vacuoles. Moreover, phase microscopy discloses that degranulation of the polymorphonuclear vesicles takes place around the vacuoles – the granules being lysosomes containing numerous enzymes, in particular, acid and alkaline phosphatases, ribonuclease, deoxyribonuclease, and β-glucuronidase. Electron microscopy reveals, in addition, that the vacuole membranes fuse with the membranes of the adjacent lysosomes, which empty their enzymatic contents directly into the site in which the phagocytosed bacteria are encountered. This occurs without exposure of the cytoplasm of the phagocyte, which is thus spared from the possible fatal effect of the enzymes.

Aside from the lysosomic enzymes mentioned, two substances must be specially mentioned that are also liberated by lysosomes and probably constitute important agents in intracellular digestion: lysozyme and phagocytin.

Lysozyme is an acetylamino-polysaccharidase which exists in relatively high concentrations in the polymorphonuclear leukocytes and acts synergically with antibody and complement in the lysis of gram-negative bacteria in vitro, possibly acting similarly in the phagocyte.

Phagocytin is a wide-spectrum, labile protein enzyme that acts upon gram-positive and gram-negative bacteria.

Many other bactericidal substances have been extracted from leukocytes (leukin, leukozymes, etc), but their role in postendocytic digestion is doubtful. The current view is that the intracellular bactericidal effect depends, as does the extracellular effect, upon antigen–antibody–complement interaction, and that the enzymes and other substances liberated by degranulation of lysosomes act only synergically.

Immunophagocytes. Phagocytosed bacteria are not always destroyed by intracellular digestion. Microorganisms such as *D.pneumoniae*, *S.pyogenes*, and *K.pneumoniae* perish rapidly (in 15–30 min) after their ingestion by polymorphonuclear leukocytes; other bacteria, e.g., *M.tuberculosis*, *B.abortus*, *L.monocytogenes*, and *S.typhimurium*, are not destroyed following engulfment but remain alive in a state of latency in the interior of the phagocyte for long periods. The prolonged immunity that develops in response to infection by the bacteria mentioned previously or to immunization with the respective live vaccines (BCG

vaccine against tuberculosis, live vaccines against bovine brucellosis) can be attributed to the persistence of such centers of latent or chronic infection. The mechanism by which this immunity develops is unknown. To explain the absence of multiplication of bacteria surviving in the interiors of the phagocytes, it was at first thought that the macrophages of the immunized animal transformed into cells specifically capable of destroying the infectious agent (immunomacrophages). Today it is known, however, that the resistance of the phagocytes is induced by the interaction of the antigen with sensitized lymphocytes, probably through the liberation of lymphokines capable of "activating" the macrophages, making them resistant to the intracellular multiplication of the infecting agent.

It should be noted, however, that although such induction results from a specific interaction, its expression is nonspecific: for example, macrophages of tuberculous animals, resistant to *M. tuberculosis*, also demonstrate resistance to unrelated bacteria such as *Brucella*, *Listeria monocytogenes*, and others.

It is also possible to produce in mice considerable resistance to infection by *S. typhimurium* by various treatments that substantially increase the value of the phagocytic index, k – such as via the injection of live BCG, of endotoxin, or of suspensions of killed *Corynebacterium parvum*.

Neutralization of Toxins

The bacterial exotoxins (diphtheria, tetanus, *Cl.perfringens*, botulin, and others) and the animal venoms (ophidic, arachnidic, scorpion, and others) are highly antigenic proteins that induce the formation of antibodies (antitoxins, antivenoms) capable of neutralizing the effects of the corresponding toxins. Discovered in 1890 by Behring and Kitasato, the antitoxins were the first known antibodies, for which relatively precise methods of titration have long been established.

200   Otto G. Bier

Unit of toxin	Antitoxin added	Mode of administration	Reaction observed
MLD	–	Subcutaneous	Death in 4 days
MRD[a]	–	Intradermal	Minimum erythematous reaction
L_o[b]	1 AU	Subcutaneous	Minimum edematous reaction
L_r	1 AU	Intradermal	Minimum erythematous reaction
L_t	1 AU	Subcutaneous	Death in 4 days
L_f	1 AU	In vitro	Optimal flocculation

Table 7.3. Units of measurement for the diphtheria toxin

[a] The MRD, minimum reactive dose, is about 250–500 times less than the MLD
[b] Examples of experimental values for the doses above in a toxic filtrate: $L_o = 0.18$ ml, $L_t = 0.21$ ml, $L_f = 0.155$ ml

In Vivo Determination of Antitoxin Concentration. The fundamental research in this domain was performed by Ehrlich with the Diphtheria toxin and antitoxin. To determine the neutralizing level of anti-diphtheria serum, Ehrlich initially used as a base that dose of antiserum capable of neutralizing a test dose based upon 100 minimum lethal doses (MLD). This former unit is called antitoxic unit (abbreviated AU); the latter (MLD) he defined as the minimum 100%-lethal dose (death in 4 days) for guinea pigs weighing 250 g.

The instability of the diphteria toxin and its progressive transformation into atoxic (toxoid) molecules made it impossible to fix a test dose in terms of MLD. Consequently, Ehrlich had to define it in terms of combination units, through the use of a standard antitoxin, which today is obtained from international reference laboratories such as the National Institutes of Health in the United States.

Practically, it has proved more expedient to read a point from a dose greater than L_o, rather than the neutralization point (L_o). Ehrlich adapted as a point of reference the toxin mixture + 1 AU, which kills a guinea pig in 4 days; to the quantity of toxin contained in such a mixture, he gave the name "lethal limit" (L_+). Later, Römer adopted another reference point close to L_o, corresponding to the mixture that produces minimum local erythema when 0.2 ml of the mixture is injected intradermally. He called this new reference dose L_r (reaction limit). The different units of measure of diphtheria toxin are described in Table 7.3; and Fig. 7.26 graphically presents the relationship of AU, L_o, L_r, and L_+ to one another.

The assay of an unknown antitoxin involves two successive determinations: (1) standardization of the toxin, or determination of the test dose (L_r or L_+) in the presence of 1 AU furnished by the standard antitoxin; and (2) assay of the antitoxin by mixing succes-

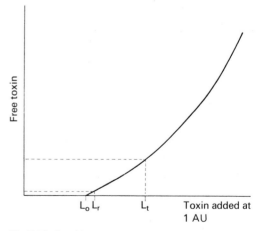

Fig. 7.26. Graphic presentation of the relationship between L_o, L_r, L_t, and AE

sive dilutions of the antiserum containing the previously standardized toxin.

Neutralization of Toxins and Precipitation. When the antitoxins were discovered, precipitation of the toxin–antitoxin (TA) complex was not observed, and the effect of the antibody was characterized only by its in vivo neutralizing power.

In 1922, it was recognized, however, that T and A, in optimum proportions, were capable of precipitation. This caused Ramon to develop an in vitro method for assaying antitoxins.

Quantitative studies of the reaction between T and A yielded curves similar to those obtained with other anti-protein precipitating systems, making it possible to observe a curve of the "horse type" or of the "rabbit type," depending on the origin of the antitoxic immunoglobulin.

In the bell-shaped curve observed in the quantitative study of precipitation of diphtheria toxin by horse antitoxin (Fig. 7.27), there is a maximum point corresponding to neutralization (L_o and L_f in close proximity), and a second point remote from the first that corresponds to the L_t dose.

Immunoglobulin Classes of Horse Antitoxin. Equine antitoxins belong to two subclasses of IgG: 1) On initial immunization, to a fast component (γ_2 or γ_1 mobility) termed IgG(T); and 2) on continued immunization, to slow (γ_2) IgG.

The two antibodies can be separated by successive chromatography on DEAE- and CM-cellulose. The γ_2-antitoxin gives the "rabbit type" of precipitin curve (see Fig. 7.30), whereas IgG(T) gives the bell curve characteristic of Ramon flocculating antibodies (Fig. 7.27).

In other species (cattle, sheep, rabbit, monkey, and man) antitoxin is always associated with the slow, IgG fraction.

Avidity of Antitoxins. Certain antitoxins dissociate easily from the TA complex and are called non-avid, in contrast to those that form firm combinations and are thus called avid. This is an important characteristic to be checked for in antitoxic sera, because satisfactory therapeutic results cannot be expected with the use of non-avid antitoxins. Initially it was observed that certain TA mixtures were innocuous when injected subcutaneously, but demonstrated toxicity upon intravenous inoculation. Later, when it was determined that the toxicity of an injected TA complex was dependent upon its concentration, this effect (no toxicity with subcutaneous, toxicity with intravenous injection) was found to result from the dilution of the TA complex.

Cinader proposed an index for measuring the avidity of antitoxins – the ratio

$$\frac{T/A}{T'/A'}$$

for the quantities of toxin and antitoxin required to constitute neutral mixtures with respect to two levels of toxin, T and T′, with T′ being less than T (for example ½ T). If the Cinader index is greater than 1, the antitoxin is considered non-avid, revealing a capacity to dissociate from the TA complex upon dilution.

Another important value in determining the avidity of antitoxins is the ratio of the in vi-

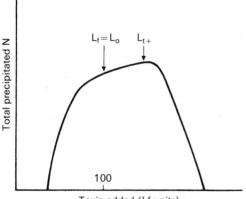

Fig. 7.27. Bell-shaped curve of the precipitation of diphtheria toxin by horse antitoxin, indicating the location of the points corresponding to Lf, L_o, and L_t

vo/in vitro concentrations, measured by the quotient

$$\frac{L_t}{L_f} \text{ or } \frac{L_r}{L_f}.$$

Antitoxin flocculates better than it neutralizes and consequently yields L_f values considerably lower than e.g.,

$$\frac{L_t}{L_f} = \frac{0.2}{0.1} = 2.$$

With avid antitoxins this ratio generally approaches a value of 1.

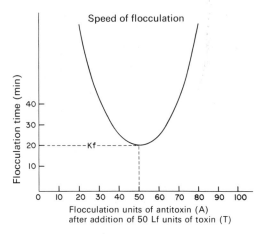

Fig. 7.28. Determination of K_f value

Flocculation. The minimal flocculation time, which corresponds to the complete neutralization of T by A, is called K_f and is inversely proportional to the concentrations of the participating reagents.[9] Thus, if T and A are in concentrated solutions, flocculation occurs rapidly. In fact, in adjacent tubes containing the optimal neutralizing mixture, flocculation occurs almost simultaneously. This prevents an exact determination of the tube corresponding to the flocculation optimum, which again indicates the value of K_f. On the other hand, if T and A are too dilute, only a light, late flocculation occurs, which cannot be clearly defined. Therefore it is necessary to use favorable concentrations, e.g., 2 ml of a 25 L_f/ml solution of toxin and variable amounts of antitoxin with about 50 flocculation units (Fig. 7.28).

Determination of the K_f value is of great practical importance, because it depends not only on the optimal T/A ratio, but also on the inherent properties of the reagents: (1) If a known serum is used, an increased K_f value, i.e., a slow flocculation, suggests an alteration in T. (2) When the same toxin is used, slow flocculation signifies minimal avidity. Purified T and A result in rapid flocculation.

Mechanism of Neutralization. The mechanism for neutralization of toxins by antitoxins remains obscure but admits of three distinct possibilities (Fig. 7.29): (1) The antitoxin may bind, through competitive inhibition, at the level of the T site responsible for the toxicity. (2) The antitoxin may act at a site near the active T region and hinder the toxic effect by a steric hindrance mechanism. (3) The antitoxin may act upon a distant site and impede toxicity by an allosteric mechanism. With anti-enzymes, which can be considered in the case of antitoxins, possibility (1) can be excluded because for a fixed quantity of antibody, inhibition of enzymatic activity is not influenced by the increase in the concentration of the substrate. It is not possible, however, to decide between hypotheses (2) and (3).

Some experimental support for interpretation (2) is supplied by the fact that total inhibition occurs only when both enzyme and substrate are of low molecular weight, e.g., lecithinase from *Cl. perfringens* (30,000) and lecithin (1,200), with no inhibition occurring when the enzyme is of high molecular weight and the substrate is of low molecular weight, as occurs with the galactosidase (800,000)-lactose (350) system. When the enzyme is small and the substrate is large, e.g., with ribonuclease (14,000) and RNA ($n \times 10^6$), inhibition is partial.

---

9 The variation of K_f as a function of the concentrations of T and A is expressed as the empirical equation $\log K_f = a - b \log(A+T)$

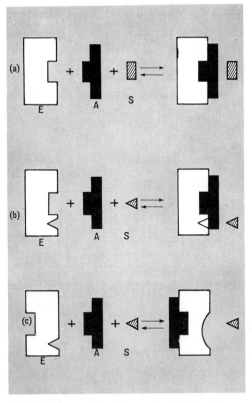

Fig. 7.29. Interpretation of the mechanism by which enzymes are neutralized by anti-enzymes (Original of O. G. Bier)

Protective Action of Antibacterial Sera

The antibacterial sera are capable of passively protecting laboratory animals by the action of opsonizing bactericidal anti-bodies or bacteria directed against surface antigens of the infecting microorganism. For example, anti-pneumococcus serum through its antibodies (carbohydrate S, type-specific) protects mice against pneumococcic infection by an alteration of the capsule, as evidenced by its swelling *(Quellung)*, which fosters the phagocytosis of virulent pneumococci.[10]

Examples of the same type are supplied by anti-*Hemophilus influenzae* serum, which also acts upon the capsular polysaccharide of the microorganism, and by anti-streptococ-cus serum, whose protective action is due to antibodies against the type-specific M protein of the beta-hemolytic streptococci.

In the case of intestinal bacteria (*V. cholerae*, *S. typhosa*, *S. dysenteriae*, and others), aside from their opsonizing action, antibodies with bactericidal action may play an important part, with or without bacteriolytic effect.

Early immunologists attributed to bacteriolysis (Pheiffer's phenomenon) the role of the fundamental mechanism of immunity, but today it is generally considered that the cytotoxic and cytolytic actions mediated by antibody and complement (C1–C9) contribute, overall, as synergic factors within the framework of a more fundamental mechanism represented by phagocytosis followed by intracellular digestion. According to this interpretation, the action of the antibody–complement system resides essentially in a lesion of the cell wall, which conditions the transformation of the gram-negative bacteria into spheroplasts that are either lysed extracellularly, or more frequently, are destroyed in the interiors of macrophages that phagocytose them.[11]

Antibacterial antibodies can be either IgG or IgM, the latter appearing to be more active, whether as opsonizing agents or as bacteriocidins.

Deeply situated antigens that are exposed by the rupture of the capsid, or coat, via the precipitation reaction or fixation by complement, do not appear to be related to the protective action. However, the surface antigens, associated with the sites responsible for the fixation of viral particles to the receptors of the sensitized cells, are considered of vital importance, because they stimulate the production of antibodies capable of impeding the multiplication of the virus and of neutralizing its pathogenic effect.

---

10 The antibody against somatic carbohydrate C lacks protective action

11 The bactericidal action exhibited by immune sera against *S. typhosa* or *S. typhimurium* notwithstanding, there is evidence that the immunity against these microorganisms is fundamentally cellular and that it lies in their inability to multiply in the interior of the macrophages of an immunized animal (see Chap. 6)

The mechanism for neutralization of viruses is exemplified by the much-studied model of the influenza virus (myxovirus), whose virion contains an internal group-specific S antigen associated with the nucleocapsid of the helical structure and an external V antigen, type-specific, associated with the coat or, more precisely, with the spicula that radiate from the surface of the viral particle. The V antigen is a glycoprotein and corresponds to hemagglutinin, being capable of establishing bridges between the virion and agglutinable erythrocytes. The formation of these bridges is assured by the presence, on the erythrocytic membrane, of a mucoprotein receptor with residual terminals of N-acetylneuraminic acid (sialic acid). Identical receptors are encountered on the surfaces of sensitized cells, and when free in the secretions they act as inhibitors.

In the presence of the anti-V antibody, the hemagglutinin is coated, and hemagglutination is inhibited. The hemagglutination-inhibition reaction can be considered the equivalent in vitro of the neutralization of the pathogenic effect in vivo, attributable to a blocking action of the antibody in relation to the fixation of the virus to the sensitized cells (target cells).

In practice, the in vivo neutralization test is performed by inoculation of a series of dilutions of serum with a constant number of viruses in tissue culture into a fertilized egg or into a sensitized animal, with 50% being adopted as a point of reference for the reading of the results. As with the T–A complex, the virus–antibody complex is reversible, dissociating upon dilution.

The anti-virus antibodies present in the immune sera can be either IgG or IgM immunoglobulins; in the secretions the predominant type is IgA, which is produced locally. Some authors contend that IgA antibodies play a part in immunization against influenza, which was practiced with success in the Soviet Union through nasal administration of attenuated virus. It is also possible that the high degree of immunity obtained in the oral vaccination against poliomyelitis with attenuated virus may be attributed to local production of antibodies capable of neutralizing the virus in the intestines before it reaches the blood.

Quantitative Study of the Antigen–Antibody Reaction

Quantitative Precipitation

Precipitation Curve. Quantitative study of the specific precipitation reaction, initiated in 1929 with the introduction of a precise analytical method by Heidelberger and his associates in the United States, constituted the starting point of modern immunochemistry.

Increasing quantities of specific antigen[12] are added to a series of tubes containing a constant quantity, say 1 ml, of rabbit anti-ovalbumin serum. After incubation at 0 °C for 24 h or more to allow complete precipitation, the tubes are centrifuged; the precipitates are washed with 0.15 M NaCl at 0 °C and quantitatively transferred to micro-Kjeldahl tubes to measure the content of protein nitrogen. Alternatively, any other method of measuring protein content can be used, such as colorimetric methods (biuret, Folin-Ciocalteu, and others) as well as ultraviolet absorption at 280 nm.

It has been verified under these conditions that the quantity of precipitate increases progressively with the quantity of antigen added until a maximum is reached, from which point the quantity begins to decline by virtue of the formation of soluble complexes due to antigen excess. Representative data from an experiment of this type are shown in Table 7.4 and in Fig. 7.30.

Figure 7.30 shows that the specific precipitation curve comprises three distinct segments: an initial ascending portion, a

---

12 Heidelberger and Kendall first used pneumococcal polysaccharide as antigen, which has the advantage that it does not interfere in the determination of the antibody protein as N. This problem has since been solved through the use of radioactively labeled antigens

Ag	Precipitate (Ag + Ab)	Ab	Weight ratio Ab/Ag	Molar ratio Ab/Ag	Test of the Supernatants
9	156	147	16.2	4	Antibody excess
40	526	486	12.2	3	Antibody excess
50	632	582	11.6	2.9	Antibody excess
74	794	720	9.7	2.4	Neither Ag nor Ab
82	830	748	9.1	2.3	Trace of Ag
90 (87)[b]	826	739	8.5	2.1	Antigen excess
98 (80)	820	731	8.2	2	Antigen excess
124 (87)	730	643	7.4	1.8	Antigen excess
307	106	–	–	–	Antigen excess
490	42	–	–	–	Antigen excess

Table 7.4. Quantitative data of specific precipitation in the ovalbumin-rabbit anti-ovalbumin system[a]

[a] Addition of increasing amounts of ovalbumin to 1 ml of serum. Values expressed in µg N

[b] The values in parentheses correspond to the quantities of antigen in the precipitates, calculated by subtracting from the total Ag the quantity measured in the supernatant in the presence of a calibrated antiserum. The Ab/Ag molar ratio was obtained by dividing the weight ratio by the quotient of the molecular weights of the antibody and the antigen $(160,000/40,000 = 4)$

plateau corresponding to the precipitation maximum, and a descending terminal segment. These three segments are clearly delineated by examination of the supernatant from each reaction tube after centrifugation of the specific precipitates. Such tests can be performed either by means of the ring test in the proper capillary tubes, or by gel precipitation as indicated in the figure. Under these conditions, one can demonstrate that the initial (ascending) portion and the terminal (descending) portion correspond, respec-

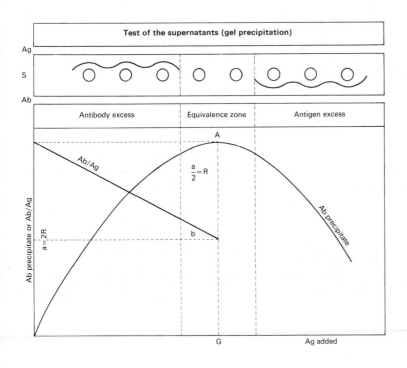

Fig. 7.30. Quantitative relationships in specific precipitation

tively, to antibody-excess and antigen-excess zones, whereas the plateau region has an excess of neither. The plateau region thus depicts an equivalence zone in which the antigen and antibody are in optimum proportions and are incorporated into the precipitate.

The curve just described exhibits only the suggestion of an inhibition zone in the area of antigen excess; since this fact is commonly observed with rabbit antisera, this type of curve is called "rabbit type" or "precipitin type." With anti-protein horse sera (e.g., against diphtheria toxin), the curve is different: it does not originate at 0 but rather from a positive abscissa value, and it has a characteristically bell-shaped form. Such antisera thus exhibit two inhibition zones, one for antibody excess and another for antigen excess. This type of curve is termed "horse type" or "flocculation type." In reality, horse antitoxin can exhibit both types of curves, depending upon the nature of the immunoglobulin with which it is associated – IgG (precipitin type) or IgGT (flocculation type).

Quantitative Relationships in Specific Precipitation. Figure 8.30 further shows that the antibody/antigen (Ab/Ag) weight ratio in the specific precipitates is a linear function of Ag, expressed by the equation

$$Ab/Ag = a - b(Ag), \qquad (1)$$

in which a (intersection with the ordinate axis) and b (slope of the line) are constants proper to each antiserum.
From eq. (1) we derive

$$Ab = a(Ag) - b(Ag^2), \qquad (2)$$

which permits calculation of the Ab value for each dose along the precipitation curve. In the example in Table 8.4, $a = 15.8$ and $b = 0.083$, so that the equation of the serum is

$$Ab = 15.8(Ag) - 0.083 \times Ag^2,$$

when Ag is expressed in µg N, or

$$Ab = 15.8(Ag) - 83 \times Ag^2$$

when Ag is expressed in mg N.
The absolute quantity of antibody in a serum corresponds to the value of Ab for the dose that maximally precipitates Ag. This dose can be calculated easily by the formula $A_{max} = a/2b$, which can be deduced from the relationship $b = R/Ag_{max}$ by taking into consideration the finding that a is approximately equal to 2 R (whereby $R = a/2$):

$$Ag_{max} = R/b = a/2 b.$$

Ab_{max} can be calculated from the equation

$$Ab_{max} = a(Ag_{max}) - b \times Ag_{max};$$

then, substituting $a/2 b$ for Ag_{max},

$$Ab_{max} = a(a/2\ b)\ -b(a^2/4\ b^2) = a^2/4\ b. \qquad (3)$$

Applying eq. (3) to the antiserum in the example, we obtain

$$Ab_{max} = \frac{(15.8)^2}{4 \times 0.083} = 752\,\mu gN,$$

which is in close accord with the experimental value of 748 µg N (Table 8.4), corresponding to a slight antigen excess.
In eq. (1), the constant a (which equals 2 R) denotes the degree of reactivity of the antibody, since evidently the greater the value of R, the greater is the quantity of Ab that combines with an equivalent quantity of Ag. The value of b depends not only on the quality, but also on the quantity of Ab, because b is equal to R^2/Ab_{max}. The latter ratio is calculated from $b = R/Ag_{max}$, substituting Ab_{max}/R for Ag_{max} (by definition, $R = Ab_{max}/Ag_{max}$, where $Ag_{max} = Ab_{max}/R$).
To compare the equations of various sera with respect to relative antibody qualities, it is necessary to eliminate the quantitative factor; this can be achieved by multiplying b by Ab_{max} to cancel out the denominator and make b equal to $R^2/1$.

Table 7.5. Molecular composition of the precipitate for different immune systems (rabbit antibody)

Antigen	Molecular weight	A = 2R	Molar ratio	
			Equivalence	Extreme antigen excess
Ribonuclease	14,000	33	1,5	3
Ovalbumin	40,000	20	2,5	5
Serum albumin	60,000	15	3	6
Gamma globulin	160,000	7	3,7	7

Let us consider, for example, two antisera whose equations are

I) $Ab = 21.4 \, Ag - 101 \, Ag^2$,

II) $Ab = 21.4 \, Ag - 167 \, Ag^2$.

The two sera are seemingly different, because for one of them $b = 101$ whereas for the other $b = 167$. However, if we reduce eqs. I and II to the level of 1 mg of antibody by multiplying each b value by the respective Ab_{max} (1.136 for I, and 0.685 for II), a single equation results, denoting the identity of the two antisera:

$Ab = 21.4 \, Ag - 114 \, Ag^2$.

The quantitive study of the specific precipitation reaction furthermore permits calculation of the molecular composition of the precipitates in the different zones of the precipitation curve. Thus, for example, in the ovalbumin-antiovalbumin system, the Ab/Ag ratio in the zone of extreme antigen excess is approximately equal to 5, whereas in the zone of extreme Ab excess, that figure is closer to 20. Since the molecular weights of the reagents involved are 40,000 and 160,000 daltons, the molar ratio of the complex in the extreme antibody-excess zone is

$$\frac{20/160,000}{1/40,000} = 5,$$

indicating an $AgAb_5$ complex. In the equivalence zone, the formula of the complex is $AgAb_{2.5}$, and in the antigen-excess zone it is $AgAb$ or Ag_2Ab.

The molecular weights of the antigens, the average a (or 2 R) values, and the respective molar ratios in the equivalence and extreme antigen-excess zones for different systems are shown in Table 7.5.

The molar Ab/Ag ratio in extreme Ag excess is frequently adopted as an estimate of the minimum number of determinants on the surface of the antigen molecule – as a measure of the valence of the Ag. However, this is a minimum estimate, for obviously there can be determinants incapable of uniting with the antibody because of steric hindrance; besides this, since the Ab is bivalent, a single antibody molecule can unite with two determinants of the same antigenic molecule.

Applications of the Precipitation Reaction: Qualitative Precipitation

The precipitation in liquid medium, in the form of the ring test, was introduced at the beginning of this century for the identification of blood stains in forensic investigations. Such identification was also useful for the discovery of hemophagocytic vectors.

The qualitative precipitation reaction is also used to diagnose infectious diseases, e.g., in the postmortem diagnosis of anthrax (Ascoli's reaction), and to identify bacteria, e.g., the Lancefield groups and the M-type streptococci. Today, precipitin reactions are used in the gel-precipitation form for antigenic analyses.

Quantitative Precipitation

Quantitative Assay of Antibodies. The absolute quantity of precipitins can be determined, in terms of milligrams of protein or of N per milliliter of antiserum, by means of the Heidelberger–Kendall method, or by analysis of the precipitate obtained through the addition, to a proper constant volume of antiserum, of a quantity of antigen slightly greater than the equivalence dose (see Table 8.4).

Even without analysis of the specific precipitates, it is possible to make an approximation of the level of precipitins by means of the so-called supernatants method, with its basis in the prior determination of the value of R, i.e., of the Ag/Ab ratio in the equivalence zone. Thus, for example, if to 1 ml of antiserum it is necessary to add 50 μg N ovalbumin so that a slight antigen excess remains in the supernatant – knowing that the value of R for the system involved is 10 – we could conclude that the antiserum contains approximately 500 μg of antibody (in N) per milliliter.

In the Heidelberger–Kendall method, the serum is maintained constant and the anti-gen is added in increasing quantitites to determine the maximum quantity of precipitate (slight Ag excess). However, one can determine comparatively the relative antibody content in different sera through the use of labeled antigens, (e.g., with ^{125}I or ^{131}I), thus determining the percentage of Ag incorporated into the specific precipitate. In the so-called P-80 method, the point of reference for the comparison is the dilution of serum corresponding to 80% incorporation (20% antigen excess in supernatant); this reference point generally is situated at the point of maximum precipitation.

In another method introduced by Farr for the assay of nonprecipitating antibodies,[13] the soluble complexes are precipitated by the addition to each tube of an equal volume of saturated ammonium sulfate solution,

---

13 It was formerly thought that the precipitating antibodies were univalent, but equilibrium dialysis experiments have shown that such antibodies can be of low or high affinity. Possibly, the high-affinity bivalent antibodies, when incapable of precipitation, possess an anomalous distribution of electric charges or other alterations that make a linkage with antigenic determinants impossible because of steric hindrance

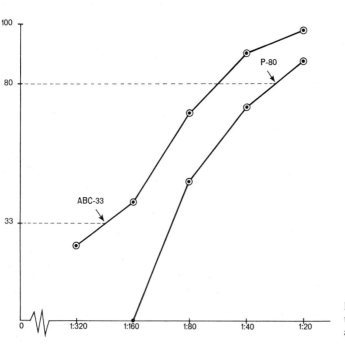

Fig. 7.31. Antibody concentrations measured by the ABC-33 and P-80 methods

and the precipitates are analyzed after careful washing to determine the percentage of fixed antigen (ABC method, antigen-binding capacity). The point of reference in this method was arbitrarily fixed at one-third of incorporation (ABC-33), which represents a considerable excess of antigens in the supernatant (two-thirds of the antigen added). In Fig. 7.31, the parallel results are depicted for the assay of an antiserum by the P-80 and ABC-33 methods.

Farr's method incontestably is of great interest in the study of nonprecipitating systems, but it requires rigorous standardization of experimental conditions and is limited by the fact that it can be applied only to systems in which the antigen is not precipitated by semisaturated ammonium sulfate, as in the anti-ovalbumin or anti-albumin systems.

Assay of Antigens. Quantitative precipitation can be utilized for assaying antigens, provided that a monospecific antiserum calibrated for the antigen in question, is available. An important application of this technique is the assay of gamma globulins in cerebrospinal fluid, of great importance in neurologic diseases – particularly in multiple sclerosis and neurosyphilis, formerly diagnosed by a nonspecific test (benzoin colloidal reaction).

Study of Cross-Reactions. Quantitative precipitation is also of special interest in the study of cross-reactions; it permits differentiation of those that are due to the existence of common antigenic determinants from those that result from the interaction of similar (but not identical) determinants and fairly well adapted antibodies.

The former case is exemplified by the reactions between chicken and duck ovalbumin, or between the S 3 and S 8 pneumococcic polysaccharides and their respective antisera. In this last example, which has been particularly well studied by Heidelberger and his associates, the cross-reaction is due to the existence in both of the polysaccharides of repeated units of cellobiuronic acid (1,4-glucuronoglucose or GnGl), in which S 3 is a linear polymer of GnGl, whereas S 8 is composed of alternate units of GnGl and of glucosyl-galactosyl (GlGa):

S 3 (GnGl)-(GnGl)-(GnGl)-(GnGl)-

S 8 (GnGl)-(GlGa)-(GnGl)-(GlGa)- .

Experimentation has confirmed what had been anticipated based upon the structure of the foregoing polysaccharides – that S 3, containing 100% GnGl residues per molecule, must precipitate better with anti-S 8 than does S 8 (only 50%) with anti-S 3.

The second type of cross-reaction embodies the reaction between similar antigenic determinants, e.g., m-azophenylsulfonate and m-azophenylarsonate, or 2,4-dinitrophenyl-lysyl and 2,4,6-trinitrobenzene.

In the case of common determinants, the heterologous reaction never reaches the maximum of the homologous reaction, with both curves exhibiting an equivalence zone clearly followed by an antigen-excess inhibition zone; however, if the cross-reaction occurs through similar determinants, the heterologous reaction curve can rise as high as that of the homologous reaction (when a sufficient quantity of antigen is added); however, it does not exhibit a distinct equivalence zone, and it forms soluble complexes only with difficulty because of the high degree of dissociation of the Ag-Ab complex.

Quantitative Inhibition of Specific Precipitation

Univalent antigens, incapable of precipitating, are nevertheless able to inhibit precipitation by the multivalent antigens. This inhibition can be studied quantitatively by mixing the antiserum first with an inhibitor and, second, with a multivalent antigen in a dose approximating equivalence. Thus, for example, if in the absence of inhibitor, the precipitation equaled 100 µg, whereas in the inhibitor's presence 80 µg was detected, we could say there was 20% inhibition. By comparing the inhibition percentages for different amounts of inhibitor, a dose corresponding to 50% inhibition can be determined and adopted for use in determining the relative potency of different inhibitors.

Three important applications are derived from quantitative inhibition of the Ag-Ab reaction.

1. *Determination of the size of the antibody-combining site.* From the pioneering work of Kabat with the human anti-dextran antibodies and dextran, it can be concluded that the "cavity," or combining site, of the antibody corresponds to a chain of six or seven glucose molecules. This conclusion resulted from inhibition experiments with different oligosaccharides of isomaltose (IM 2 to IM 7), in which it was verified that maximum inhibition was obtained with isomaltohexose (IM 6) or with isomaltoheptose (IM 7). For different antisera, the relative inhibitive powers of the different oligosaccharides were variable, and this gave rise to an important additional conclusion, namely, that there was a heterogeneous population of antibodies with "cavities" of diverse sizes up to a maximum corresponding to IM 6 or IM 7. Experiments performed with other systems confirmed the data initially obtained with the dextran-antidextran reaction, that is, the antibody-combining site was capable of accommodating, at a maximum, six to seven glucose molecules or five to seven amino acids, with dimensions corresponding approximately to $34 \times 17 \times 7$ Å. The study of the dextran-antidextran system permitted further interesting inferences concerning the combining energies of the different groups of antigenic determinants. Based upon the proportionality existing between inhibitory potency and combining energy (ΔF^0), it was possible to evaluate the percentage contribution of each glucose to the total combining energy of IM 6. Although the first glucose (from the nonreductive end) contributed 40%, and the first three 90%, the increase from that point on was minimal (2%–5%). The group that contributed the greatest percentage of the total combining energy of the antigenic determinant was termed the "immunodominant group."

2. *Determination of the structure of the antigenic determinant.* Quantitative inhibition is also an important method for determining the structure of the antigenic determinants. For example, the A, B, and H determinants of the substances of the AB0 blood-group system are inhibited, respectively, by N-acetyl-D-galactosamine (A), by D-galactose (B), and by D-fucose (H), indicating that these sugars are the immunodominant groups of the determinants in question. The structure of the A determinant was investigated further through quantitative inhibition with the following oligosaccharides obtained through acid or alkaline hydrolysis of the A substance:

α-D-GalNAc-(1- → 3)-β-D-Gal-(1- → 3)-D-GNAc

α-L-Fuc-(1-2)
|
α-D-GalNAc-(1- → 3)-β-D-Gal-(1- → 4)-β-D-GNAc-R;

in which GalNac = N-acetyl-D-galactosamine; Gal = galactose, GNAc = N-acetyl-D-glucosamine, Fuc = fucose, and R is a radical resulting from the reduction of galactose. The reduced pentasaccharide was shown to be a more potent inhibitor than the trisaccharide, and the results of the quantitative inhibition taken together have permitted elucidation of the structure of the A determinants.

In addition to inhibition of specific precipitation, cross-reactions also can be used for the study of the structure of antigenic determinants. Using cross-reactions with antisera capable of reacting with antigens of known structure, Heidelberger studied the reactions of numerous polysaccharides with different type-specific horse sera. He was thus able to draw a conclusion concerning the unknown structures of those substances. For example, cross-reactions with anti-S 2 could be due to residues of glucose, ramnose, or glucuronic acid; however, in the particular case of the reaction with acacia (gum arabic), it was possible to demonstrate that the reaction occurred with glucuronic acid, which otherwise constituted the immunodominant group of the S 2-anti-S 2 interaction. The anti-S 14 serum reacts with polyglucoses as well as with terminal residues of galactose, which condition the cross-reaction with the substances of the AB0 group system, as well as with certain gums and mucilages of vegetable origin.

3. *Radioimmunoassay.* This type of assay is extremely sensitive. It permits measurement of antigen quantities at the level of picograms, based upon the competitive action between an unlabeled antigen (Ag) and the same antigen (Ag^x) labeled with a radioactive isotope (usually ^{125}I) in the formation of immune complexes in the presence of a limited quantity of specific antibody (Ab), which is linked covalently to an insoluble matrix (e.g., particles of Sephadex), or in the form of an insoluble anti-Ab complex (co-precipitation double-antibody system).

In a hypothetical example, if to five molecules of bivalent antibody (10 combining sites) variable quantities of unlabeled antigen are first added, followed by a fixed dose of labeled antigen (10 molecules), the percentage of bound radioactivity (or the bound Ag^x/free Ag^x ratio) would decrease, as illustrated in Fig. 7.32 and in the graph of Fig. 7.33. Upon comparision with a reference curve obtained from an Ag solution of known concentration, one can determine, by the decrease in radioactivity, the quantity of antigen present in a solution of unknown concentration.

Radioimmunoassay has been used with excellent results in the detecting and assaying of peptides and hormones (steroids, insulin, growth hormone, ACTH, gonadotropin and chorionic gonadotropin, follicle-stimulating and luteinizing hormones, lactogenic, placental, and other hormones); of certain tumoral antigens (α-fetoprotein, carcinoembryonic antigen); of drugs (digoxin, morphine); of viral antigens (Hb); and of immunoglobulins (IgE).

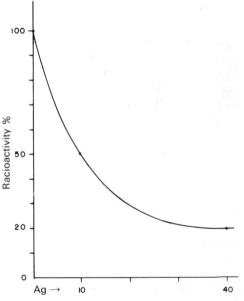

Fig. 7.33. Curve based upon the hypothetical example shown in Fig. 7.32: The drop in bound radioactivity due to the competitive action of Ag and Ag^x is approximately sigmoidal. When the antigen quantities are represented by logarithms along the abscissa, a straight line is obtained whose slope facilitates the calculation of the concentration of Ag in an unknown solution (once the standard curve is established)

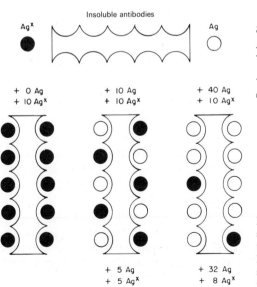

Fig. 7.32. Diagrammatic representation of the principle of the radioimmunoassay

Enzyme-linked Immunosorbent Assay (ELISA)

This method is in principle entirely analogous to direct or indirect immunofluorescence techniques. Instead of a fluorescent dye, an enzyme is conjugated to an antibody; horseradish peroxidase is most commonly used as enzyme, but virtually any enzyme can be employed as long as it is soluble, stable, and not present in biological fluids in quantities that would interfere with serum determinations. The test can be used to measure either antigen or antibody and is analogous to the radioallergosorbent test (RAST) (see p. 275). To measure antibody, antigen is fixed to a solid phase, incubated with test serum, and then reacted with enzyme-tagged anti-immunoglobulin. Enzyme activity adherent to the solid phase is measured spectrophotometrically, and then related to amount of antibody bound.

To measure antigen, antibody is bound to the solid phase, a test solution containing antigen is added, and then a second enzyme-labeled antibody is added. This test requires that at least two determinants are present on the antigen. Advantages of the enzyme immunoassay include sensitivity (ng/ml range), simplicity, stability of reagents, lack of radiation procedures, and that it is relatively inexpensive.

Quantitative Study of the Hapten–Antibody Reaction

The hapten–antibody reaction is a reversible reaction:

$$S + H \leftrightharpoons SH ,$$

whose association constant can be calculated by the law of mass action:

$$K = \frac{(SH)}{(S)(H)} ,$$

in which S represents the combining site of the antibody and H represents the hapten. If n represents, the valence of the antibody,

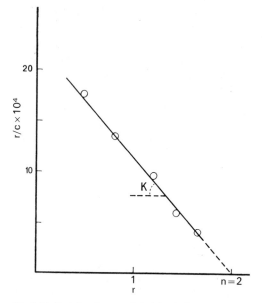

Fig. 7.34. Scatchard's equation (r/c vs. r)

r, the number of molecules of H bound per molecule of antibody, and c, the concentration of H, then

$$K = \frac{r}{(n-r)\,c} ,$$

for $r = SH$ and $(n-r)$ is equivalent to S. From the preceding equation,

$$r/c = K_n - K_r \text{ (Scatchard's equation) ,}$$

for the equation of the line that expresses the variation of r/c as a function of r in which K_n is the intersection with the ordinate and K is the slope (Fig. 7.34).

For the zero value of the ordinate, the intersection of the line with the abscissa corresponds to a value for r equal to n (for $r/c = 0$, $K_n = K_r$).

It thus becomes possible to calculate K and n if we know the values of r and c, which are obtained experimentally by special techniques (equilibrium dialysis, fluorescence quenching), described below.

Frequently, however, the variation r/c versus r is not linear in its full extension, so that the values for K are not uniform.[14] It is convenient, therefore, to measure the affinity of antibodies by expressing them as a function of a median value K_o (intrinsic association constant), which corresponds to the occupation of half of the sites S ($r=1$). This value can be calculated as K_o equals $1/c$, for if in Scatchard's equation we make n equal to 2 (bivalent antibody) and r equal to 1, we obtain

$$1/c = 2K - K = K^\circ .$$

The value of K° ($1/c$) can also be estimated graphically as the middle of the K_n intersect, or the r/c value corresponding to $r=1$.

Equilibrium Dialysis. One milliliter of purified antiserum (S) is placed in a small cellophane tube. The tube is closed with a knot and is placed inside a glass flask containing

---

14 To correct the effect of the heterogeneity of the antibodies in relation to the value of K, Sips' function (similar to Gauss's function) is used, which leads to the equation
$r/(n-r) = (K \times c)^a$,
in which a represents the index of heterogeneity. For $a=1$ (absence of heterogeneity), the preceding equation is transformed into Scatchard's equation

1 ml 0.15 M NaCl to which is added a known concentration of hapten (H). The mixture is agitated gently until the concentration of H in the exterior liquid reaches a constant value (equilibrium). The initial and final distributions of the molecules of hapten and antibody are illustrated in Fig. 7.35.

Where H is a colored compound, its concentration can be measured spectrophotometrically. Otherwise, one should use a solution of labeled hapten. The experiment should include controls for the nonspecific adsorption of the hapten on the normal gamma globulins.

Knowing the value for the free concentration of H (c), one can determine by subtraction how many moles of H have combined with the antibody and, consequently, r can then be calculated, where r equals the number of moles of H fixed per mole of antibody. Table 7.6 illustrates the simplified protocol of an experiment of this type.

If one supposes that the number of moles of H in the exterior phase of the tube in equilibrium is equal to 1.11×10^{-5}, then the quantity of free H in both sides is equal to 2.22×10^{-5} M. If tube 1 indicates nonspecific adsorption of 10% to the membrane,

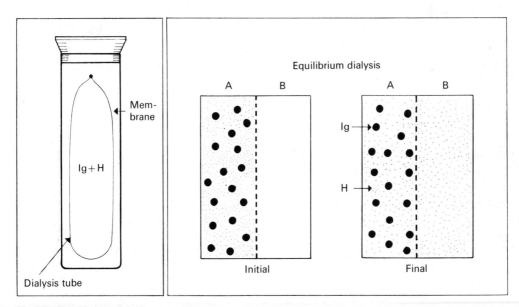

Fig. 7.35. Equilibrium dialysis

Table 7.6. Simplified protocol of an equilibrium dialysis experiment

Tube no.	Interior	Exterior
1	$0.15\,M$ NaCl	$5 \times 10^{-5}\,M$ H
2	4×10^{-5} S	$5 \times 10^{-5}\,M$ H

this value must be corrected by $(2.22 + 0.22) \times 10^{-5}$ or to 2.44×10^{-5}, and the quantity of H fixed by S can be estimated at $(5 - 2.44)$, i.e., at $2.56 \times 10^{-5}\,M$.

Since the total amount of antibody added is known $(4 \times 10^{-5}\,M)$, $r = 2.56/4 = 0.640$. K° $(1/c)$ is equal to the reciprocal of 2.44×10^{-5}, or $0.41 \times 10^{5}\,M$.

Fluorescence Quenching. The hapten–antibody reaction tends to extinguish part of the fluorescence that normally is exhibited by the immunoglobulin when irradiated with ultraviolet light (280 nm). This fluorescence quenching is due to residues of tryptophan found in the combining site of the antibody, which, when covered by the hapten, transmit to the latter the energy it has absorbed and that it should have emitted in the form of fluorescent light (330–350 nm).

The technique of fluorescence quenching is advantageous in that it can be performed rapidly and requires only tiny quantities of antiserum; however, to be applied to unknown systems, it must always be run in parallel with an equilibrium dialysis, which is the standard method.

Thermodynamics of the Hapten–Antibody Reaction. Energy is the capacity to produce work, whereas so-called free energy (F) is that which produces maximum work. The value of F cannot be measured in absolute terms; however, it is possible to measure the positive or negative variations of F that occur when there are transformations in a system. In exothermic reactions – those that liberate energy – F has a positive value; in endothermic reactions – the inverse – energy

must be furnished and F has a negative value.[15]

Free energy F is an exponential function of the association constant:

$$K^{\circ} = e^{-\Delta F/RT},$$

where

$$\Delta F^{\circ} = -RT \times \ln K^{\circ} = -4.57 \times T \times \log K^{\circ}.$$

For example, if the determination of K°, at the temperature of 25 °C (298 T) results in the value 1.57×10^{5}, the variation of free energy can be calculated as

$$\Delta F^{\circ} = -4.57 \times 298 \times \log(1.57 \times 10^{5}) = -7.09\ \text{kcal/mol}.$$

For different Ag–Ab systems, different values for $-\Delta F^{\circ}$ are encountered from 6 to 11 kcal/mol, corresponding to values for K° between 1×10^{4} and 1×10^{9}.

Intermolecular Forces in the Antigen–Antibody Reaction

The union of the antibody with the antigen, as with the union of an enzyme with the substrate, depends essentially upon the complementary adaptation of their tridimensional structures. This stereometric adaptation results in the mutual attraction of the opposed surfaces through short-reaching covalent forces that are inoperative between molecules not in sufficient proximity.

An analogous example is the glueing together of two fragments of a broken piece of china; after a layer of glue is brushed on the surface of each fragment, the two pieces

---

15 Free energy (F) represents merely one part of the total energy (enthalpy or H); the other part includes a degraded form of energy associated with the disorder of the system, called entropy (S): $\Delta H = \Delta F + T\Delta S$. To calculate the value of enthalpy (and, by subtraction, that of entropy), it is necessary to determine the association constants for two temperatures and to utilize Van t'Hoff's formula: $\Delta H = R \times T_1 \times T_2 \times \ln(K_2/K_1)/(T_2 - T_1)$

must be held closely fitted together for a period of time. In the antigen–antibody reaction, the glue is represented by attractive forces which operate at the level of the combining sites of the reagents, subject to the complementary adaptation of their surfaces. The following are the intermolecular forces that come together in the Ag–Ab union:

1. *Ionic or coulomb forces* result from the electrostatic attraction between ions of opposite charges, e.g., COO^- and NH_4^+.

2. *Polar attraction forces* occur between dipoles and between ions and dipoles. A particular case is represented by the hydrogen bond, in which H, linked covalently to an electronegative atom, is attracted by a pair of unshared electrons of another electronegative atom:

$$\ddot{:}F\ddot{:}H\longrightarrow \ddot{:}F\ddot{:} \quad \text{or} \quad F^-H^+\longrightarrow F^-.$$

Though they are weak (3–7 kcal/mole), the numerous hydrogen bridges between the NH and CO groups of peptide bonds play an important role in maintaining the secondary structure (alpha helix) of the proteins:

3. *Van der Waals forces* are the weakest forces (1–2 kcal/mol), operating only in a short radius of action, where the proximity of the molecules results in the induction of fluctuating charges originating from the attrac-

Table 7.7. Relative sensitivities of various immunologic techniques

Method	Vol. of serum used in test (ml)	Sensitivity Limit	
		µg N-Ab/ml	µg N-Ab
Specific precipitation			
Qualitative:			
Ring test	0.1	2 – 5	0.2 – 0.5
Gel diffusion			
Oudin	0.2	2 – 5	0.4 – 1.0
Ouchterlony	0.1	5 – 10	0.5 – 1.0
Preer	0.01	5 – 10	0.05 – 0.1
Quantitative:			
Micro-Kjeldhal			20 (20 – 100)
Mod. Markham			10 (10 – 100)
Biuret (550 nm)			20 (20 – 100)
Folin-Ciocalteu			2 (2 – 30)
(750 nm)			
UV absorption			5 (5 – 100)
(277 or 287 nm)			
Passive hemagglutination	0.1	0.03 – 0.06	0.003 – 0.006
Complement fixation	0.1	0.5 – 1.0	0.05 – 0.01
Diptheria toxin neutralization (Römer-Frazer test)	0.1	0.01 – 0.04	0.001 – 0.004
Passive cutaneous anaphylaxis (rabbit-antibody, guinea pig skin)	0.1		0.003 – 0.006
Radioimmunoassay; ELISA		µg-ng range	ng-pg range

tion exercised by the nucleus of one of the atoms upon the electrons of the external orbit of the other atom and vice versa. Also called London forces, these intermolecular forces do not appear to play an important role in the Ag–Ab union.

4. *Apolar or hydrophobic bonds* occur in aqueous solution between apolar groupings. They work by virtue of their property of excluding the ordered network of H_2O molecules that are interposed between the dissolved molecules, furthering the approximation of these to the action radius of short-reaching forces – Van der Waals forces in particular. The hydrophobic residues of certain amino acids (alanine, phenylalanine, leucine, isoleucine, tyrosine, tryptophan, methionine) play a relevant role in the tertiary structure of the proteins.

Comparative Sensitivities of Serologic Techniques

The various methods for detecting antibodies exhibit greatly differing sensitivities, as indicated in Table 7.7, in terms of the concentration or of the absolute quantity of antibody that the respective reactions are capable of disclosing.

The determination of the minimum quantity of antibody evidenced by a reaction depends upon the underlying practical conditions, or more specifically, upon the volume of serum utilized and the inherent peculiarities of the individual test. Thus, for example, passive hemagglutination is capable of detecting 0.003–0.006 µg N of antibody in tests that utilize 0.1 ml of serum.

In cutaneous anaphylaxis (PCA) however, in which 0.03 µg of Ab-N can be detected, a serum that contains 0.3 µg Ab-N does not exhibit the PCA reaction because of the blocking action of normal immunoglobulins.

With the radioimmunoassay, serum at a dilution up to 10^{-6} can be used, and antigens such as corticosterone can be measured with precision in amounts as small as 5 pg $(1.5 \times 10^{-14} M)$.

References

Ackroyd FF, Turk JL (eds) (1970) Immunological methods. Blackwell, Oxford

Arquembourg PC, et al. (1970) Primer of immunoelectrophoresis. Ann Arbor Humphrey, Ann Arbor/ Mich.

Barret JT (1970) Textbook of immunology. An introduction to immunochemistry and immunobiology. CV Mosby, St. Louis

Berson SA, Yalov R (1968) General principles of radioimmunoassay. Clin Chim Acta 22:51

Burrows W (1951) Endotoxin. Ann Rev Microbiol 5:181

Campbell DH et al. (1970) Methods in immunology (2nd ed). WA Benjamin, New York

Chase MW, Williams CA, jr (1971) Methods in immunology and immunochemistry, vols I and II. Academic Press, New York

Coombs RRA, et al. (1961) The serology of conglutination and its relation to disease. Blackwell, Oxford

Coons AH (1958) Fluorescent antibody methods. In: Danielli JF (ed) General cytochemical methods. Academic Press, New York

Crowle AJ (1961) Immunodiffusion. Academic Press, New York

Davis BD, et al. (1967) Microbiology (2nd ed) Chaps 12–18. Harper & Row (Hoeber), New York

Dubos RJ, Hirsch JG (eds) (1965) Bacterial and myotic infections of man, 4th ed. Lippincott, Philadelphia

Eisen HN (1964) Equilibrium dialysis for measurement of antibody-hapten affinities. Methods in Med Res Yearbook 10:16

Fahey JL, McKelvey EM (1965) Quantitative determination of serum immunoglobin in antibody agar plate. J Immunol 94:84

Furth R van, et al. (1972) The mononuclear phagocytic system, monocytes and their precursor cells. Bull WHO 46:845

Givol D (1970) Procedures for sensitive radioimmunoassay. Int Atom Energy Agency 1245:15/72

Grabar P, Burtin P (1960) L'analyse immunoeléctrophorétique. Masson, Paris

Heidelberger M (1947) Immunochemistry of antigens and antibodies. In: Cooke (ed) Allergy in theory and practice. Saunders, Philadelphia

Heidelberger M (1969) Quantitative absolute methods in the study of antigen-antibody reactions. Bact Rev 3:49

Holborrow EJ (ed) (1970) Standardization in immunofluorescence (2nd ed). Blackwell, Oxford

Kabat EA (1961) Kabat and Mayer's Exp Immunochemistry, 2nd ed, Chaps 1–12. CC Thomas, Springield/III.

Kabat EA (1971) Einführung in die Immunchemie und Immunbiologie. Springer, Berlin Heidelberg New York

Kabat EA (1976) Structural concepts in immunology and immunochemistry, 2nd ed. Holt, Rinehart & Winston, New York

Karush F (1962) Immunological specificity and molecular structure. Adv Immunol 2:1

Kwapinski JBG (1972) Methodology of immunochemical and immunological research. Wiley, Chochester

Nairn RC (1969) Fluorescent protein tracing. Livingstone, Edinburgh

Oakley CL (1954) Bacterial toxins. Ann Rev Microbiol 8:411

Osler AG (1968) Quantitative study of complement fixation. Bact Rev 20:166

Ouchterlony O (1958/1962) Diffusion-in-gel methods for immunological analysis. Progr Allergy 5:1/6:30

Oudin J (1952) Specific precipitation in gels and its application to immunochemical analysis. In: Methods in Med Res Yearbook 5:335

Pappenheimer A, Jr (1948) Proteins of pathogenic bacteria. Adv Protein Chem 1:69

Pinckard RN, Weir DM (1973) In: Weir DM (ed) Handbook of exp immunology, 2nd ed. Blackwell, Oxford

Prevot AR (1950) Hemolysines et antihemolysines bactériennes. Le Sang 21:565

Raynaud M (1959) Heterogeneity of diphtheria antitoxin. In: Mechanisms of hypersensitivity. Little, Brown and Co, Boston

Relyveld EH (1959) Toxine et antitoxine diphthériques. Etude immunologique. Harmann, Paris

Schmidt H (1931) Die Praxis der Auswertung von Toxinen und Antitoxinen. Gustav Fischer, Jena

Staub AM, Raynaud M (1971) Cours d'Immunologie générale et de Sérologie de l'Institut Pasteur. CDU, Paris

Thomas L (1954) The physiological disturbances produced by endotoxins. An Rev Physiol 16:467

Van Heyningen WE (1954) Toxic Proteins. In: Neurath, Bailey (eds) The Proteins, vol II. Academic Press, New York

Westphal O (1957) Pyrogens. In: Second Macy Conf on Polysaccharides in Biology. Macy Foundation, New York

Zwilling R (1977) Immunologisches Prakticum. Gustav Fischer, Stuttgart

Chapter 8   Blood Groups

OTTO G. BIER

Contents

The blood has always been regarded by man as an object of mystery and fascination – a vitalizing and rejuvenating element. Even ancient authors reported transferring the blood of animals, usually of sheep and dogs, to man. They noted that such transfusions invariably resulted in fever and hemoglobinuria, and terminated not infrequently in the death of the patient. Blundell (1818), who can be considered the father of the modern blood transfusion, recognized that when the recipient and the donor were of the same species, e.g., dog-to-dog or human-to-human transfusions, the tolerance was greater, although even then there were numerous accidents. The problem was not resolved until 1900, when Landsteiner, having discovered the blood groups of the AB0 system, interpreted the post-transfusion reactions in terms of an interaction between the red cells of the donor and isoantibodies (or more properly, alloantibodies) existing in the serum of the recipient. About 40 years later, with the discovery of the Rh system by Levine, it was demonstrated that even the transfusion of blood compatible for the AB0 system could give rise to transfusion reactions: These were attributable to anti-Rh alloantibodies contained in the serum of the recipient that had been induced by previous transfusions with Rh^+ red blood cells or by antigenic stimulation from fetal red blood cells during gestation. In addition to its importance in blood transfusions, we have already observed the practical importance of alloimmunization in the genesis of hemolytic disease in the newborn (erythroblastosis fetalis).

More recently, attention has been focused on the leukocyte groups, whose delineation is particularly important in connection with histocompatibility tests in organ transplantation and susceptibility for specific diseases (they are described in detail in Chaps. 6 and 9).

Erythrocytic Systems

AB0 System: Differentiation of Groups and Subgroups

By allowing the red blood cells of six individuals to react with each other, Landsteiner characterized at the outset three blood types – today called 0, A, and B. Some time later, after increasing the number of experiments, he identified a fourth group, AB. The reactions exhibited by these four blood groups are shown in Table 8.1.

Table 8.1. Reactions of erythrocytes with antisera against the AB0 blood group

Erythrocytes	Serum			
	0	A	B	AB
0	−	−	−	−
A	+	−	+	−
B	+	+	−	−
AB	+	+	+	−

Table 8.2. Differentiation of the subgroups A_1 and A_2

Erythrocyte	B Serum (Anti-A + A_1)		
	Not absorbed	Absorbed with A_1	Absorbed with A_2
A_1	+	−	+
A_2	+	−	−

These reactions are easily interpreted in light of Landsteiner's rule, i.e., antibodies never occur in an individual against red blood cells of his own blood group; they appear only in response to erythrocyte antigens from a different individual (alloimmunization). Thus, for example, 0 erythrocytes are nonagglutinable in any serum, yet the serum of 0 individuals agglutinates all erythrocytes with the exception of 0 red cells. In contrast, AB red cells are agglutinated by any serum except that of AB individuals, and sera from AB individuals are incapable of agglutinating red cells of any of the AB0 types. A red cells agglutinate in B serum, which is anti-A; similarly, B red cells agglutinate in A serum, which is anti-B.

In addition to the four classic groups of Landsteiner, subgroups of group A and group B are recognized – in particular the subgroups A_1 and A_2, which are differentiable by absorption tests. A_1 and A_2 red cells are agglutinated in the presence of nonabsorbed B serum; absorption with A_2 (weak A) only removes antibodies against A_2, but not against A_1 (Table 8.2).

It was thought in the beginning that 0 red cells did not contain agglutinogen (0 antigen or "ohne" antigen), but later it was recognized that they contain an agglutinogen now designated as H agglutinogen, which also occurs in A, B, and AB red cells, albeit in lesser quantities (it is most abundant in A_2 or A_2B red cells). Only rare individuals of the Bombay type do not posses H and consequently are able to form anti-H.

Reproduced in Table 8.3 are the reactions necessary for the typing of the AB0 system, including subgroups A_1 and A_2 and the Bombay type.

The following serve as anti-A_1 reagents: (1) about 80% of B sera, which contain anti-A + A_1, when absorbed with A_2 red cells (A antigen only); (2) plant hemagglutinin (lectin) extracted from *Dolichos bifloris* seeds.

For anti-H reagents, the following can be used: (1) certain bovine sera (weak); (2) eel serum *(Anguilla anguilla)*, which is capable of reacting in high dilutions (1:100–1:500); (3) serum of Bombay individuals (extremely rare); and (4) lectins of *Ulex europeus* and *Lotus tetragonolobus*.

Table 8.3. Typing of the AB0 system

Erythrocyte	Serum 0 (anti-A + A_1 + B)	Serum B (anti-A + A_1)	Serum A (anti-B)	Anti-A_1	Anti-H
A_1(A + A_1)	+	+	−	+	±
A_2(A)	+	+	−	−	+
B	+	−	+	−	±
A_1B	+	+	+	+	±
A_2B	+	+	+	−	+
0	−	−	−	−	+ +
Bombay	−	−	−	−	−

Genetics. The groups and subgroups of the AB0 system are hereditary characteristics that are determined, according to Bernstein's theory, by a combination of three alleles – 0, A, and B – with 0 being an amorphous recessive gene and the A and B genes being codominant. In accord with this scheme, the four classic groups (phenotypes) correspond to six genotypes: 00, A0, AA, B0, BB, and AB. With the further inclusion of subgroups A_1 and A_2, we must recognize ten genotypes corresponding to six phenotypes (Table 8.4).

Table 8.4. Genotypes of the AB0 system

Phenotype	Genotype	
	Homozygote	Heterozygote
0	00	
A_1	A_1A_1	A_1A_2, A_10
A_2	A_2A_2	A_20
B	BB	B0
A_1B	A_1B	
A_2B	A_2B	

The H antigen, present in all red cells (except the Bombay type), is not modified by the amorphous 0 gene; hence the phenotype 0 results. The structural genes A and B act upon H (more intensely in A_1 individuals than in A_2 individuals), converting them into A_1 and A_2 agglutinogens and yet leaving a certain quantity of H (incomplete conversion). Further details relating to the genetic control of the biosynthesis of these group substances are discussed below, in the treatment of the interrelations of the AB0 and Lewis systems.

Alloantibodies of the AB0 System. The alloantibodies of the AB0 system can be either natural or immune antibodies. The former occur in normal serum, usually in low titers; they probably appear in response to natural stimuli resulting from the ubiquity of the blood group substances, especially in the bacteria of the intestinal tract. For example,

chicks born and maintained in germ-free environments do not form hemagglutinins; yet they readily produce anti-B when *E. coli*, a carrier of B substance, is added to their diet. In man, agglutinogens exist on the red cells even at birth, but the natural hemagglutinins only begin to appear around the third month of life. These are of the IgM type (previously existing maternal agglutinins are of the IgG type, which are capable of crossing the placental barrier). Individuals exposed to natural antigenic stimuli evidently form antibodies only against antigens that do not exist on their own red cells (Landsteiner's rule) – in other words, against antigens for which tolerance has not developed during prenatal life.

Immune antibodies, particularly the anti-A_1 antibodies, develop in elevated titers in response to transfusion of incompatible blood (e.g., B into A, or A into 0); through heterospecific pregnancy (e.g., a B fetus in an A or 0 mother); through exposure to biologic products containing group substances (e.g., tetanus or diphtheria toxoids derived from cultures in peptonized mediums, or antitoxins purified through digestion with pepsin); and by the infection of purified group substances (Witebsky substances). Table 8.5 summarizes the most important characteristics in the differentiation of natural and immune alloantibodies.

Table 8.5. Characteristics differentiating natural and immune alloantibodies

Properties	Natural antibodies	Immune antibodies
Immunoglobulin Class	IgM or IgG	IgG
Agglutination in 0.9% saline[a]	+	Frequently
Hemolysis in presence of complement	–	+
Optimum temperature	20 °C	37 °C

[a] The problem of the so-called incomplete antibodies, which are incapable of agglutinating in saline solution yet are capable of agglutinating in colloidal medium, is discussed in relation to the antibodies of the Rh system

Lewis, Lutheran, and Secretory Systems: Differentiation and Genetic Interrelationships

In about 80% of all individuals, the substances A, B, and H are encountered only in red cells, whereas in the remaining 20%, blood group substances occur in mucous secretions (nonsecretor and secretor types). H-like substances have been demonstrated in secretions and in erythrocytes. These substances, termed Lewis (Le) substances, have two specificities, Le^a and Le^b. The former is encountered in secretions but not on erythrocytes, whereas the latter also occurs on the erythrocytes. In the nonsecretors, Le^b is absent whereas Le^a appears in the secretions as well as on the red cells (Table 8.6).

Also associated with secretions is the Lutheran system, which contains two antigenic specificities: Lu^a in nonsecretors, and Lu^b in secretors.

The genetics of the Lutheran system remains obscure, although the genetic interrelationships between the Lewis system and the secretory system have been clarified, largely due to the efforts of Ceppellini. The appearance of A, B, H, Le^a, and Le^b appear to result from the combined effect of four gene groups, which may act sequentially in the following order: Le-le (alleles for Lewis), Se-se (alleles for secretion), H-h, and O-A-B. The data summarized in Table 8.6 can be correctly interpreted only after a study of the chemistry of the group substances and of the genetic control of their biosynthesis. One

can quickly infer, however, that the Le^b specificity results from interaction between the H and Le genes in individuals of the secretor type and that a double dose of the "se" gene can inhibit this interaction. When the Le, Se, and H genes are present, the Le^b substance appears in elevated concentrations in the secretions and part is absorbed onto the red cells; Le^a also is formed, but only in quantities insufficient to absorb onto the red cells.

Chemistry and Biosynthesis of Group Substances

The substances responsible for the A, B, H, and Lewis specificities cannot easily be extracted from the red cells, because they occur in relatively small quantities and probably in association with lipids and proteins. For this reason, the chemical study of such substances has been conducted with materials isolated from body fluids: A, B, and H from secretors and Le^a from nonsecretors (see Table 8.6).

In human material, the level of group substances is particularly elevated in meconium, in amniotic fluid, and in the fluid of ovarian cysts. Appreciable quantities are also encountered in the saliva,[1] gastric juice, seminal fluid, urine, and blood serum. The

---

[1] Saliva from the A or B secretors inhibits the agglutination of the respective red cells by the corresponding antibodies: H saliva from H secretion inhibits the agglutination of O red cells by Ulex anti-H or eel serum

Table 8.6. Genetic interaction between the AB0, Lewis, and secretory systems

Secretion genes	Other genes	Erythrocytes				Secretion			
		A or B	H	Le^a	Le^b	A or B	H	Le^a	Le^b
Se	A or B H Le	+	+	−	+	+	+	+	++
sese		+	+	+	−	−	−	+	−
Se	00 H Le	−	+	−	+	−	+	+	++
sese		+	+	+	−	−	−	+	−
Se	A or B H lele	+	+	−	−	+	+	−	−
sese		+	+	−	−	−	−	−	−
Se or	A,B,0 hh Le	−	−	+	−	−	−	+	−
sese (Bombay)	A,B,0 hh lele	−	−	−	−	−	−	−	−

animal sources that furnish the highest yields of A, B, and H substances are the gastric mucosa of the horse and the pig.

Among the methods available for the isolation and purification of group substances, that of Morgan and King is most widely used. It consists essentially of extraction with 90% phenol followed by precipitation with ethanol. Under these conditions, products can be obtained that satisfy the chemical and immunologic criteria for purity, such as constant solubility, homogeneity under ultracentrifugation and electrophoresis, and total precipitation by the specific immune serum.

Chemical analysis shows that the group substances are glycoproteins formed by a peptide skeleton, rich in serine and threonine, to which a polysaccharide chain is attached. This chain is composed of two amino sugars (D-N-acetylglycosamine and D-N-acetylgalactosamine) and two sugars (D-galactose and L-fucose).

The manner in which the units of the polysaccharide chain are associated was investigated particularly by Morgan and by Kabat and his colleagues. Following diverse approaches, they concluded that the immunodominant groups in question were D-N-acetylgalactosamine (GaN) for substance A, D-galactose (Ga) for substance B, and L-fucose (Fu) for substances H and Le^a, depending upon the position of linkage (Fig. 8.1).

Little is known concerning the biosynthesis of the polysaccharide precursor – which among other properties exhibits cross-reactivity with type XIV pneumococcic polysaccharide – except for the verification of a close relationship to the antigen I, present in virtually all adult red cells and responsible for acquired hemolytic anemias, due to production of cryoagglutinins. In fact, the degradation of substances A, B, and H by combined treatment with periodate and borohydrate (Smith's degradation) exposes determinants capable of reacting with anti-I.

The H substance is synthesized under the influence of the H gene through the addition of α-L-fucose in a (1,2) bond, from the acetylgalactose terminal of the precursor. In individuals deprived of the H allele, i.e., those that are "h" homozygotes, no formation of H occurs. These are the extremely rare Bombay individuals.

In the biosynthesis of the group substances, the precursor is first subjected to the action of the glucosyltransferase controlled by the Le gene, which promotes the addition of α-L-fucose to the subterminal acetylglucosamine in a (1,4) linkage. In this way, the Le^a substance results. Next, the H substance is formed. In secretors, there is an additional interaction between Le and H, from which the Le^b specificity results. Ultimately, the O-A-B genes come into play: O, being an amorphous gene, does not modify the H substance; however, the glucosyltransferases controlled by the A and B genes cause binding of a (1,3)α-D-acetylgalactosamine (specificity A) and a (1,3) α-D-galactose (specificity B) to the D-galactose terminal.

Figure 8.1 shows that two precursors are possible: In the I chains, the linkage of the terminal galactose to the acetylglucosamine is (1,3); in the II chains, it is (1,4). The Lewis substances, which originate by the addition of L-fucose to the subterminal acetylglucosamine through a (1,4) linkage can ap-

Gene A Gene H   Gene Le

α-GaN   α-Fu   α-Fu
(1,3)\ |(1.,2) |(1,4)
      \ β-Ga(1,3) β-GN(1,3) β-Ga(1,3) β-GN(1,3) β-Ga(1,3) α-GaN.....P
       \   (1,4)
(1,3)/
α-Ga

Gene B

Fig. 8.1. Structure of the blood-group substances, including the genes that participate in the biosynthesis parently only be formed from the I chains, because in the II chains, position 4 is occupied.

MNSs and P Systems

Two factors, M and N, were found on the red cells of each ABO group. No alloagglutinins exist in the serum for these factors, and it is necessary for their identification to utilize properly absorbed rabbit antisera (e.g., to immunize with OM red cells and absorb with ON red cells to obtain a specific anti-M serum). To identify the N factor, one can also use the lectins extracted from the seeds of *Vicia graminea*.

For the MN system, one can differentiate three groups: M, N, and MN. Because the antigens are controlled by codominant genes, the absence of both factors is never observed.

Initially, the MN system appeared to be the simplest blood-group system, but later it was recognized that it is genetically associated with another system (Ss) and that there are numerous antigenic variants of M and N, in addition to other antigens linked to the system that are nonallelic to Ss. Among these antigens, we might cite the Hu (Hunter) and He (Henshaw) factors, relatively frequent in blacks; and the Gr (Graydon), Vw (Verweyst), Mi^a (Miltenberger), and U factors.

Considering, however, only the alleles N,M and Ss, and assuming that such genes form four gene complexes – MS, NS, Ms, and Ns – in the MNSs system, then nine phenotypes corresponding to ten genotypes are differentiated.

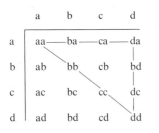

In the foregoing diagram, the genes MS, NS, Ms, and Ns are represented, respectively, by

a, b, c, and d. Of the ten genotypes included in the triangle on the right (the rest are duplicates), the genotype "bc" (encircled) will have an expression identical to that of the genotype "ad" (NSMs and MSNs), which reduces the number of phenotypes to nine: MS, Ms, MSs, NS, Ns, NSs, MNS, Mns, and MNSs.

The P system was discovered by a method similar to that utilized in the study of the MN system, which ultimately was characterized as analogous to A$_1$–A$_2$, with three principal types, P$_1$, P$_2$, and "p" – this last being incapable of reacting with the antisera that identify the first two. Such "p" individuals are extremely rare. Their sera contain anti-P + P$_1$ (anti-Tj^a or Jay) alloantibodies, which agglutinate the red cells of almost all individuals. Given the extreme rarity of "p" individuals, scattered all over the world, if one of these should require a transfusion, compatible blood might be obtained only through an international organization.

Rh System

In 1939 Levine encountered in the body of a mother who had delivered a stillborn child an irregular agglutinin capable of agglutinating the blood of about 85% of white donors in the United States. Shortly thereafter, Landsteiner and Wiener reported that a similar serum could be produced in rabbits by the injection of red cells from the *Macacus rhesus*. The relationship between the two observations was evident, and the new agglutinogen, for which Levine had encountered an alloantibody, came to be called Rh (from rhesus), because of its occurrence on the red cells of this primate species (Fig. 8.2).

Factors and Agglutinogens. The Rh system which at first appeared simple (85% Rh$^+$ individuals and 15% Rh$^-$ individuals), was later revealed to be highly complex because of the multiplicity of antigenic determinants and of their variants involved in the composition of the different types of agglutinogens. In addition to the original serum, two more alloantisera were soon encountered: one

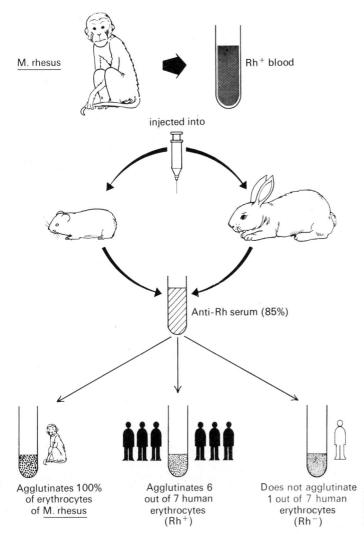

M. rhesus

Rh⁺ blood

injected into

Anti-Rh serum (85%)

Agglutinates 100%
of erythrocytes
of M. rhesus

Agglutinates 6
out of 7 human
erythrocytes
(Rh⁺)

Does not agglutinate
1 out of 7 human
erythrocytes
(Rh⁻)

Fig. 8.2. Protocol of experiments leading to the discovery of the Rh factor (Original of O. G. Bier)

from patients subjected to multiple transfusions, which agglutinated 70% of human red blood cells; and another from the mother of an infant with fetal erythroblastosis, which agglutinated the blood cells of 30% of all individuals. The three antisera represented distinct antigenic determinants, which Wiener designated, respectively, Rh_0, rh′, and rh″. Later, two antisera were encountered that exhibited reactions opposite to those of anti-rh′ and anti-rh″ sera and thus were designated anti-hr′ and anti-hr″. A third, postulated, antiserum, i.e., one that would react against anti-Rh_0, has not been discovered even though it is theoretically possible.

Thus, there are five antisera available for the determination of the principal factors of the Rh system; and with these, 32 (2^5) phenotypes can be identified. The determinants corresponding to these antisera, designated Rh_0, rh′, hr′, and hr″ by Wiener, are associated in groups of two or three to constitute the agglutinogens Rh_0, Rh_1, Rh_2, rh′, and rh″.

Differing interpretations of the hereditary mechanism of the Rh system induced Wiener in the United States, and Fisher and

Table 8.7. Nomenclature of the factors and agglutinogens of the Rh system

	Wiener	Fisher-Race
Factors	Rh_0	D
	rh'	C
	rh''	E
	hr'	c
	hr''	e
Agglutinogens	Rh_0	Dce
	Rh_1	DCe
	Rh_2	DcE
	Rh_2	DCE
	rh	−ce
	rh'	−Ce
	rh''	−cE
	rh^y	−CE

i.e., Rh^+, corresponds to a reactivity frequency of $2+54+14+15 = 85\%$. The anti-C serum (anti-Rh') corresponds to a reactivity frequency of $1.5+54+15 = 70.5\%$, and the anti-E serum to one of $0.5+14+15 = 29.5\%$.

Clinically, interest is limited merely to differentiation of the Rh^+ group through the use of anti-D serum. However, in anthropologic or forensic studies, differentiation of the different genotypes as well as that of the different phenotypes becomes relevant. Of particular importance in this respect is the differentiation of the homozygous and heterozygous types, achieved through the use of anti-hr (anti-c, anti-e) sera.

Race in England to adopt a different nomenclature for the factors, whereby Wiener's nomenclature has the disadvantage of using identical symbols for certain factors and agglutinogens (e.g., Rh_0, rh', and rh''), but the advantage of being easier to pronounce when dealing with the type designations (e.g., Rh_1, Rh_2, instead of DCe/DcE) (Table 8.7).

Differentiation of Types. If we consider only the three anti-Rh sera first discovered, i.e., the anti-D (85%), anti-C (70%), and anti-E (30%), we can differentiate 8 (2^3) types, as indicated in Table 8.8 – in which the reactivity percentages for each type encountered among white populations are also listed.

The data in Table 8.8 enable us to calculate the percentages corresponding to the reaction incidence of each of the antisera. Thus, the anti-D serum (anti-Rh_0), which reacts only with red cells of the group to the right,

Antigenic Variants. The Rh factors exhibit numerous antigenic variants (D^u, D^w, C^u, E^u, E^w, E^t, e^s, etc.) as well as compound antigens [G(CD), f(ce), V(ce^s), and others], which greatly increase the complexity of the system.

The D^u variant merits special mention. There is no specific antiserum at our disposal for this variant, but D^u erythrocytes react, albeit weakly, with anti-D, these reactions varying in intensity (strong D^u and weak D^u). Weak reactions require the antiglobulin test for their demonstration; in routine tests they can be falsely identified as Rh^-.

Genetics. Two genetic theories have been proposed for the Rh system. According to Wiener, there is a single locus with six codominant alleles, whereas Fisher theorizes three closely linked loci, each of them with a pair of codominant alleles: D-d, C-c, E-e.

Table 8.8. Typing of erythrocytes for the Rh antigen with anti-C, D, and E Sera

Serum	Rh-negative types				Rh-positive types			
Anti-D	−	−	−	−	+	+	+	+
Anti-C	−	+	−	+	−	+	−	+
Anti-E	−	−	+	+	−	−	+	+
Phenotypes								
Per Wiener	rh	rh'	rh''	rh'rh''	Rh_0	Rh_1	Rh_2	Rh_1Rh_2
Per Fisher-Race	cde	Cde	cdE	CdE	cDe	CDe	cDE	CDE
Percentages	13	1.5	0.5	−	2	54	14	15

The Fisher genes codify the appearance of the respective antigenic determinants, whereas the Wiener genes, termed r, r', r'', R_0, R_1, and R_2, would represent genetic complexes capable of codifying three factors. Wiener originally postulated six genes; however, the possible existence of eight genes came to be recognized; two more were discovered and termed R_z and R_y (agglutinogens Rh_z or CDE, and rh_y or CdE):

Leaving aside the R_z and r_y genes, the eight Rh phenotypes mentioned in Table 8.8 correspond to 21 genotypes $(6 \times 7/2)$ formed by six alleles:

Phenotype	Genotype
rh	rr
rh'	rr', r'r'
rh''	rr'', r''r''
rh' rh''	r' r''
Rh_0	R_0r, R_0R_0
Rh_1	R_0r, R_0R_1, R_1R_1, R_1r', R_1r
Rh_2	R_0r'', $R_0 R_2$, R_2R_2, R_2r'', R_2r
$Rh_1 Rh_2$	R_1R_2, R_1r'', R_2r'

With the Fisher-Race nomenclature, the designation of the genotypes becomes more complicated: dce/dce instead of rr; DCe/DcE instead of R_1R_2, etc.

We might mention, finally, that the divergencies between the theories of Wiener and of Fisher lack practical importance; from a theoretical point of view, whether to include one or three effects in a single gene is purely an academic question, since the real limits of the genes are unknown.

Rh Alloantibodies. Unlike the ABO system, the Rh system does not produce natural antibodies; anti-Rh is encountered only in the sera of Rh^- individuals immunized with Rh^+ red cells.

There are two anti-Rh varieties: (1) antibodies agglutinating in saline medium; and (2) antibodies capable of agglutinating only in colloidal medium, e.g., in diluents with high protein concentrations (compatible serum, bovine serum albumin).

It was thought originally that the nonagglutinating antibodies were incomplete antibodies, carrying only one combining site. However, this hypothesis was abandoned when it was recognized that such antibodies agglutinated erythrocytes in colloidal medium and that even in saline solution they were capable of agglutinating red cells previously treated with proteolytic enzymes (papain, bromelain, ficin). This gave rise to the suggestion that the incapacity for agglutination in saline medium could be attributed to the insufficient formation of a complex of divalent antibodies because the antigenic determinants were unfavorably localized on the erythrocyte surface, or because the electric charge of the red cells did not permit sufficient approximation of their surfaces. According to the first hypothesis, the enzymatic treatment would have the effect of exposing the inaccessible or recessed sites; in the second case, the colloidal diluent causes a reduction of the zetapotential of the erythrocytes, thus making agglutination possible. Zeta potential refers to the difference of electrostatic potential between the net charges of the erythrocytic membrane and of the surface of the ionic cloud that envelops the particle, separating it from the suspension medium. For agglutination to occur, it is necessary that the zeta potential fall to a critical level that permits sufficient approximation for the establishment of bridges between particles by the bivalent antibody.

Nonagglutinating antibodies can be demonstrated with the highly sensitive Coombs antiglobulin test. The test consists of adding an appropriate dilution of specific anti-human gamma-globulin serum to red cells previously incubated with the antiserum to be tested and then washed. The antiglobulin reacts with antigenic determinants of the Fc part of the fixed antibody, thus establishing the connecting bridges required for agglutination. In certain systems, such as Lewis, Kell, Kidd, and Xg^a, by virtue of the fixation of complement on the surface of the red cell, better results are obtained using anticomplement (anti-β1 C)-disclosing serum. The Rh antibodies further differ from normal ABO agglutinins in that they are more active at 37 °C than at room temperature (20 °C). Under these circumstances, the Rh-anti-Rh interaction proceeds in vitro under conditions similar to those in which they ex-

ercise their pathogenicity in vivo, i.e., in the presence of a high level of proteins and at 37 °C (warm agglutinins).

Other Erythrocytic Systems

Other erythrocytic systems should also be mentioned:

(1) Systems revealed by the Coombs test (with anti-nongamma or anticomplement). These include the Kell-Cellano (K-k), Duffy

Table 8.9. Differentiation of systems other than AB0 and Rh

System	Specific Antiserum			Phenotype	Genotype	%
MN	Anti-M	Anti-N				
	+	+		MN	MN	50.0
	+	−		MM	MM	25.0
	−	+		NN	NN	25.0
P	Anti-Tj^a	Anti-P$_1$				
	(P, P$_1$)					
	+	+		P$_1$		75.0
	+	−		P$_2$		25.0
Lewis	Anti-Le^a	Anti-Le^b	Secretion			
	−	+	+	Le(a$_-$b$_+$)		70.0
	+	−	−	Le(a$_+$b$_-$)		25.0
	−	−	+ ou −	Le(a$_-$b$_-$)		5.0
Lutheran	Anti-Lu^a	Anti-Lu^b				
	−	+		Lu(a$_-$b$_+$)	Lu^b Lu^b	92.0
	+	+		Lu(a$_+$b$_+$)	Lu^a Lu^a	7.9
	+	−		Lu(a$_+$b$_-$)	Lu^a Lu^a	0.1
Kell-Cellano	Anti-K	Anti-k				
	−	+		k	kk	90.0
	+	+		Kk	Kk	9.8
	+	−		K	KK	0.2
Duffy	Anti-Fy^a	Anti-Fy^b				
	+	−		Fy(a$_+$b$_-$)	Fy^a Fy^a	15.0
	−	+		Fy(a$_-$b$_+$)	Fy^b Fy^b	50.0
	+	+		Fy(a$_+$b$_+$)	Fy^a Fy^b	35.0
Kidd	Anti-Jk^a	Anti-Jk^b				
	+	+		Jk(a$_+$b$_+$)	Jk^a Jk^b	50.0
	+	−		Jk(a$_+$b$_-$)	Jk^a Jk^a	25.0
	−	+		Jk(a$_-$b$_+$)	Jk^b Jk^b	25.0
Xg	Anti-Xg^a					
	+			Xg(a$_-$)		85(1) 65(2)
	−			Xg(a$_+$)		15 35
Diego	Anti-Di^a					
	+			Di(a$_+$)		36(3)
						8 − 12(4)

(1) Women. (2) Men. (3) South-American Indians. (4) Japanese.

(Fy^a, Fy^b), Kidd (Jk^a, Jk^b), and Diego (Di^a, Di^b) systems.

(2) System I. Antigen I exists on almost all adult human red cells. It can be demonstrated with anti-I produced by the rare I-negative individuals (about 1 in 5,000). In the newborn, the reaction with anti-I is weak or absent, since the antigen develops during the first 2 years of life.

(3) System Xg. This system carries only one Xg^a antigen, which occurs more frequently in women (about 65%) than in men (about 25%) and appears to depend upon a gene linked to the X chromosome. The two phenotypes are Xg(a+) and Xg(a−).

(4) Public and private groups. These designations include certain extremely frequent antigens (Vel, Yt^a, Go^b, Gy^a) and some extremely rare antigens (Levay, Becker, Ven, Yt$_b$, and many others).

Data relating to systems other than ABO and Rh are summarized in Table 8.9.

Practical Applications of Immunohematology

Blood Groups and Transfusion

Transfusions without prior determination of the blood type may not be performed: Incompatibility between the sera of the donor and that of the recipient could result in severe shock. In addition to the benign reactions due to pyrogen release, the immediate and grave consequences of the transfusion of incompatible blood consist essentially of chills, precordial oppression, lumbar and abdominal pains, prickling sensations in the limbs, dyspnea, intravascular cyanosis of the face, hemoglobinuria, and renal complications sometimes resulting in fatal anuria. This incompatibility is caused principally by the transferred red cells, since the natural agglutinins in the plasma of the donor are diluted in the blood volume of the recipient. Furthermore, the anti-A and anti-B agglutinins involved bind in large part to the substances existing in the fluids and tissues of the recipient. In light of this concept,

O individuals were long considered universal donors, in contrast to AB types, who were thought incapable of donating blood to any other group, yet able to receive from all (universal recipients). A and B individuals can receive from their own types, but are able to donate only to their respective types or to AB types.

It is known today, however, that type O blood is not universally compatible and can be dangerous: it can exhibit elevated titers of anti-A and anti-B, even though these can be neutralized by the addition of group substances; furthermore, danger arises by virtue of potential incompatibility with respect to other systems – above all, the Rh system. Rh$^-$ individuals repeatedly subjected to transfusions of Rh$^+$ blood or Rh$^-$ women who have borne Rh$^+$ fetuses can acquire high titers of Rh antibodies, generally of the incomplete type, and thus can exhibit grave reactions to the transfusion of Rh$^+$ blood. Even if type O Rh$^-$ blood is used, or Rh$^-$ blood of the same ABO group, a reaction can occur resulting from incompatibility relating to other systems. For this reason, in addition to determining the blood types of the recipient and the donor, it is advisable to perform cross-matching tests for compatibility – i.e., between the red cells of the donor and the serum of the recipient. The test should be carried out in colloidal medium and, if possible, a Coombs test also should be done to detect rare sensitivities to the Kell, Kidd, Duffy, and MNSs factors, among others.

Blood Groups and Maternal–Fetal Incompatibility

Antibodies from the maternal serum can cross the placenta and lyse the red cells of the fetus. This is observed principally when there is maternal–fetal incompatibility in relation to the Rh system, i.e., when the mother is Rh$^-$ and the fetus (father) is Rh$^+$. The limiting factors involved are primarily the following: (1) the genotype of the father (if homozygous Rh$^+$, RR, the fetus is Rh$^+$

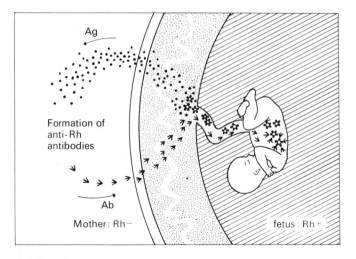

Fetus: Rh+ labels within figure: Ag, Formation of anti-Rh antibodies, Ab, Mother: Rh−, fetus: Rh+

Fig. 8.3. Pathogenesis of fetal erythroblastosis due to Rh incompatibility

in 100% of cases; if heterozygous Rh^+, Rr, only in 50%); (2) the quantity of fetal red cells that manage to enter the maternal organism; and (3) the capacity of the mother to form the harmful alloantibody. In successive pregnancies, a booster (secondary stimulus) effect evidently occurs, which leads to more rapid and intense production of the alloantibody, thus increasing the possibility of injury to the fetus.

Of great value in diagnosing hemolytic disease of the newborn is the direct Coombs test, which consists of adding antiglobulin to red cells washed from the blood of the umbilical cord to detect sensitization in vivo of the fetal red cells. The test is also run during the pregnancy to determine the presence of maternal anti-Rh, with an eye toward taking measures designed to mitigate or to impede the appearance of fetal disease, either in the first parturition or in subsequent pregnancies.

Such measures include (1) exchange transfusion, or substitution of compatible serum for the bulk of the newborn's blood, laden as it is with harmful antibodies and toxic products resulting from red-cell destruction; and (2) prophylaxis for subsequent pregnancies with anti-D gamma globulin, administered within 24–48 h post partum.

Prophylaxis with anti-D gamma globulin has yielded excellent practical results, e.g., 0.17% anti-Rh production in treated

mothers as against 12.7% in the control group – nearly 75 times less.

The small quantity of antibody required (about 300 µg) suggests that what occurs is not a total masking of the antigenic determinants of the fetal red cells, but rather a suppression of antibody synthesis by inhibition of the proliferation of the lymphoid cells involved in the formation of anti-D (feedback inhibition).

Blood Groups and Autoimmune Hemolytic Anemia

Autoimmune hemolytic anemias can be classified into two groups: (1) "cold" anemias, associated with antibodies that act at 4 °C, and (2) "warm" anemias, due to antibodies reacting at 37 °C.

The first group includes the following diseases: (a) the classic paroxysmal cold anemia of Donath and Landsteiner[2], formerly common, associated with syphilitic infection and characterized by a diphasic reaction: fixation of the autohemolysin at 4 °C and lysis by complement at 37 °C; (b) the rapidly reversible hemolytic anemia observed in a certain percentage of primary

---

2 This is not to be confused with paroxysmal nocturnal hemoglobinuria, apparently associated with a defect of the erythrocytic membrane, which becomes particularly vulnerable to complement, without sensitization by antibodies (reactive hemolysis by C 567)

atypical pneumonia cases caused by *Myco-plasma pneumoniae*; and (c) hemolytic anemia related to the Ii system.

The antibody involved in these anemias is of the IgM type and binds complement; red cells from patients generally are positive in the direct antiglobulin test using either anti-gamma or anti-nongamma (anti-β-1 C).

In the group of "warm" autoimmune hemolytic anemias, we mention only those produced by anti-e of the IgG type.

Blood Groups and Forensic Medicine

The individuality of the blood as revealed by determination of the blood groups is considerable; as such, numerous forensic applications are possible. Considering just 6 ABO groups, 9 MNS groups, 2 P groups, and the 18 Rh types differentiated by the anti-D, -C, -E, -c, and -e, we already have $6 \times 9 \times 2 \times 18$, or 1,944 different types. By computing further the remaining factors and variants of the erythrocytic groups, the serum allotypes, and the leukocytic groups, serologic individualization increases to millions of types, approximating the diversity of fingerprints. However, the methodologic complexity inherent in differentiation militates against a use as widespread as that of fingerprints.

Aside from being utilized in the identification of blood stains, saliva, or sperm, and in investigations relating to the possibility of exchanged newborns, the determination of blood groups has been particularly useful for the exclusion of paternity (Table 8.10).

Table 8.10. Exclusion of paternity by the AB0 system

Child	Mother	Excluded father
0	0	AB
	A	AB
	B	AB
A	0	0, B
	B	0, B
AB	A	0, A
	B	0, B
	AB	0

Exclusion rests on the following principles: (1) A factor or agglutinogen not present in at least one of the parents is never encountered in their child. (2) The child can, however, lack a factor or agglutinogen present in one or both of the parents. (3) A type O man cannot father AB children or vice versa. (4) An N father cannot produce an M child or vice versa.

The following examples illustrate the importance of determining the erythrocytic groups in the exclusion of paternity, using only the ABO system.

1) *A man of group A_1 is alleged to be the father of two children, types O and A_2; the mother belongs to group O.*
Result: The possible genotypes of the father are A_1A_1, A_1A_2, and A_1O. In the first possibility, he could not be the father of either of the two children; in the second, he could be the father only of child A_2 and not child O; and in the third, he could be the father only of child O and not child A_2. The only possible conclusion, therefore, is that the accused man is conclusively not the father of one of the children; the test does not allow determination as to which one.

2) *A man of group O is alleged to be the father of two children, types O and A_2; the mother belongs to group A_1.*
Result: The only possible genotype for the A_1 mother of an O child is A_1O; the genotype of the A_2 child must therefore be A_2O. Since the father does not have the A_2 gene that appears in the child, the child can only have been fathered by another man. The paternity of the man accused in relation to child A_2 therefore can be excluded.

3) *The Rh system is of service in solving cases that cannot be resolved relying solely on the ABO and MN systems.* For example: A_1/MN/Rh_1 is alleged to have fathered a child A_1/M/Rh_2 with woman A_1/MN/rh. Exclusion, impossible by ABO and MN analysis, can be found in the fact that the man possesses factor C, absent in both mother and child; and also lacks factor E, absent in the mother but present in the child.

The probability of exclusion with ABO and MN was just 30%, but increased to 62% after the introduction of Ss, Rh, Kell, Lutheran, Duffy, and Kidd.

The occurrence of extremely rare factors, as well as the association of rare factors in the man and in the child but not in the mother, would suggest paternity.

Anthropologic Applications of Immunohematology

Considerable differences have been found in relation to the incidence of blood groups in different populations. For example, the Basques are characterized by a high percentage of Rh$^+$ (30%) and a low incidence of groups B, C^w, and Fy^a. Blacks exhibit high

Table 8.11. Approximate percentage incidence of the groups of six erythrocytic systems in Brazilian populations

Groups	Whites	Blacks	Indians[a]
0	45	49	100
A	41	25	0
B	10	22	0
AB	4	4	0
M	30		49–80
N	20		1–9
MN	50		19–42
P$_+$	75	97	89
P$_-$	25	3	11
Rh$_+$	85	90	100
Rh$_-$	15	10	0
Di (a$_+$)	0		30–45
Di (a$_-$)	100		55–70
Fy (a$_+$)	65	35	40–75
Fy (a$_-$)	35	65	26–60

[a] Data refer to Indians of the Amazonian group of the Imbelloni classification, which includes four important linguistic groups: The Yalhoama, who dominate the forests of the Orinoco to the Alto Rio Negro, and the Makú, Tukáno, and Tariáno groups, who inhabit the Uapés River basin on the frontier with Columbia and the forests between the Rio Negro and the Japurá. Also included in the Amazonian group are the Indians of the central altiplano (high land), e.g., the Xavantes of Mato Grosso. The Parque Nacional de Xingu shelters about 1000 Indians of different tribes

percentages of B (20%–25%), unlike the Eskimos and Australian aborigines who exhibit an increased frequency of A ($>50\%$). These differences admit of interesting speculations, although most are disputable. It was imagined, for example, that the ancestral human race was of type O and that the A and B genes emerged later, by mutation, first in Australia and Greenland and later in Central Asia and in Africa. Migrations would subsequently have determined the degree of intermixture of genes and the phenotype percentages observed in different countries. However, this theory encountered a serious drawback because A and B specificities appear in the anthropoid monkeys. Another interesting example is provided by the Diego factor (Di^a), encountered exclusively in Mongoloids and Brazilian Indians, appearing frequently in the latter.

Table 8.11 summarizes the approximate percentages represented by the different groups among six erythrocytic systems in white, black, or Brazilian Indian populations.[3]

Analysis of Table 8.11 reveals that the percentages of the different blood groups in white Brazilian populations does not differ significantly from those observed in whites (Caucasians) of other continents (Europe, North America), and that the blacks exhibit figures resembling those of African blacks, yet with evidence of intermixture. In addition to the high incidence of B and the low incidence of Fy^a, the prominent feature is the frequency of Sutter and V factors in blacks and their near nonexistence in other races. Additional characteristics of blacks are elevated frequencies of R$_o$ and D^u, as well as of rare factors of the MNSs system, such as Hunter and Henshaw.

The Indians exhibit genetic markers that surely indicate racial purity, such as the ab-

---

3 The Indian population of Brazil is calculated at about a thousandth of the general population, i.e., at approximately 100,000 for a population of 100 million. Only close to 40,000 retain their primitive culture in small, isolated populations, mostly in the virgin forests of the amazonian basin and the central highland (Mato Grosso, Goias)

sence of the following antigens that have been sought but never encountered in them: A_2, Kell, Lewis (a), Berrian (Be), Henshaw (He), Lutheran (Lu^b), Sutter (Js^a), V of the Rh system, Verweyst (V^w) of the MN system, and Wright (Wr). Pure Indians are almost always O and Rh^+ (100% in the case of Brazilian Indians) and exhibit elevated frequencies of R^2 (DcE), Se, M, and Diego.

References

Amos DB, Ward FE (1975) Immunogenetics of the HL-A system. Physiol Rev 5:271

Boyd WC (1963) The lectins: Their present status. Vox Sang (Basel) 8:1

Fisher RA (1947) The rhesus factor. Am Sci 35:95

Kabat EA (1956) Blood group substances, their chemistry and immunochemistry. Academic, New York

Kabat EA (1976) Structural concepts in immunology and immunochemistry. Holt, Rinehart & Winston, New York

Levine P (1951) A brief review of the newer blood factors. Trans NY Acad Sci Sect II 13:205

Marcus DM (1969) The ABO and Lewis blood group system. Immunochemistry, genetics, and relation to disease. N Engl J Med 280:994

Mollison PL (1967) Blood transfusion in clinical medicine. Blackwell, Oxford

Morgan WTJ (1960) Croonian lecture: A contribution to human biochemical genetics. Proc Roy Soc B 151:308

Post RH, et al. (1968) Tabulations of phenotype and gene frequencies for 11 different genetic systems studied in the American Indian. In: Biomedical challenges presented by the Indian. PAHO/WHO, Washington

Prokop O, Uhlenbruck G (1969) Human blood and serum groups. McLauren, London

Race R R, Sanger R (1968) Blood groups in man, 5th edn. Blackwell, Oxford

Schiff F, Boyd WC (1942) Blood grouping technic. Interscience, New York

Springer GF (1971) Blood-group and Forrsman-antigenic-determinants shared between microbes and mammalian cells. Prog Allergy 15:19

Watkins W (1966) Blood group substances. Science 152:172

Wiener AS (1946) Blood groups and blood transfusion. C C Thomas, Springfield, Ill.

Wiener AS, Wexler IB (1958) Heredity of the blood groups. Grune & Strattan, New York

Witebsky E (1932) Die Blutgruppenlehre unter besonderer Berücksichtigung physiologisch-serologischer Fragestellungen. Ergebn Physiol 34:271

Zmijewski CM (1968) Immunohematology. Appleton-Century-Crofts, New York

Chapter 9 Transplantation

Dietrich Götze and Ivan Mota

Contents

Terminology

Transplantation is defined as the transfer of living cells, tissues, or organs from one site to another in the same individual (*syngeneic* transplantation) or from one individual to another – of the same (*allogeneic* transplantation) or another (*xenogeneic* transplantation) species. The terminology used to characterize the genetic relationship between recipient and donor was presented in Table 4.1 (see pp. 132). If a transplant is transferred to the same site, i.e., to its normal anatomic location, it is termed an *orthotopic* graft; if it is implanted in a location other than its normal one, it is termed a *heterotopic* graft. The fate of the graft is determined by the genetic relationship between donor and recipient. Grafts exchanged between genetically identical individuals are *accepted*. Grafts exchanged between genetically different individuals are *rejected*, i.e., they are destroyed. Rejection is the result of a specific immune response to histocompatibility antigens. Under certain conditions, the recipient can be rendered incapable of reacting to the transplant, a state called *immunologic tolerance* (see Chap. 5). If the capacity for an immunologic reaction is suppressed by circulating antibodies ("blocking antibodies"), one speaks of *enhancement*.

If only the recipient is capable of a reaction, one speaks of a host-versus-graft reaction; however, if the graft consists of immunocompetent cells – or contains such cells – there is a graft-versus-host reaction. The former is the case with organ transplants such as skin, kidney, heart, liver, etc.; the latter occurs after transplantation of bone marrow, spleen, lymph node, or thymus cells.

The structures responsible for the transplantation reaction are controlled by histocompatibility genes. These include those that control 1) erythrocyte alloantigens, 2) lymphocyte alloantigens, and 3) transplantation antigens. This subdivision is based on the methods of their identification. Erythrocyte alloantigens are demonstrated primarily by agglutination (see Chap. 7, p. 177), lymphocyte antigens primarily by the lymphocytoxicity test, and transplantation antigens by tissue (skin) and tumor grafts.

Approximately 60 such genes (or loci) are known in the mouse, of which a little more than half belong to the third category. On the basis of the strength of the induced immune response, one can divide the H genes into two groups: 1) those that cause an acute reaction, in vivo and in vitro (major histocompatibility complex, MHC), and 2) those that cause a delayed, chronic reaction (minor histocompatibility genes, non-MHC). In addition to the different forms of reactivity in relation to a graft, there are additional characteristics that differentiate the two groups: 1) The MHC is extremely polymorphic, with more than 50 alleles in the mouse (also in man, see Tables 6.4 and 6.8) in comparison to the non-MHC genes, in which a maximum of three alleles are known. 2) The MHC is closely linked with genes that control the immune response. 3) The MHC plays a decisive role in the graft-versus-host reaction and the mixed lymphocyte reaction. 4) It is much more difficult to induce tolerance to MHC antigens than to non-MHC antigens. 5) Immunosuppression is more effective for non-MHC antigen differences than for MHC-antigen differences.

In man, two groups of histocompatibility genes can be distinguished: genes that control 1) lymphocyte alloantigens (HLA = MHC) and 2) blood-group antigens (AB0, P).

In general, MHC antigens cause acute rejection of transplanted organs or tissue, such as skin, heart, bone marrow, kidney, and liver. Two organs appear to be exceptions to this rule. Cases of kidney transplant have been described in which the transplanted kidney was accepted despite different MHC antigens between the recipient and the donor; in many of these cases, however, the skin of the kidney donor was normally rejected, without affecting the function of the transplanted kidney. Such occurrences are observed regularly in experimental kidney transplants in the rat and dog. This phenomenon may be dependent upon "enhancing" (blocking) antibodies.

The second organ that deviates from this rule is the liver. In experiments in pigs, an unexpectedly large number of animals that received a liver allograft survived for a long period even without immunosuppressive therapy. However, not only did the liver transplant survive longer (and here the liver transplant differs from the kidney transplant), but organs from the same donor animal that were simultaneously or later transplanted (skin, kidney, heart) were protected from normal rejection (also in pigs, these organs were immediately rejected by untreated animals). However, animals that tolerated skin or kidney transplants after liver transplantation normally rejected grafts from a second, different donor. This tolerance can also be achieved through intraperitoneal or intraportal injection of liver extract. The basis of this protective effect is not yet understood, but perhaps the liver releases antigens in a tolerogenic form.

Transplantation Reactions

Host-Versus-Graft Reaction

The sequence of the host-versus-graft reaction of a skin graft between allogenic mice can be summarized as follows: The transplant first appears pale; after 2–4 days, the transferred skin becomes vascularized and appears pink. A difference between allo- and autografts is visible after 4–7 days: With an autograft, the pink color (circulation) remains and epithelialization of the grafted area progresses; the graft is integrated into the skin of the recipient (hair growth occurs after about 12 days). The allograft, on the other hand, turns cyanotic and later necrotic, and falls off after 10–12 days (rejection).

Histologically, around the fifth day, one can observe in the allografts perivascular infiltration by mononuclear cells (lymphocytes, histiocytes), an increase in mitoses in the basal layer of the epidermis, and a little later, vascular thrombosis – a microscopic index of rejection that precedes macroscopic rejection.

The time of rejection is determined by four principal factors: the quantity of tissue engrafted, the immunogenicity of the transplantation antigen of the donor, the degree of genetic difference between the donor and the receptor, and the immune status of the recipient.

In recipients that receive a second graft from the same donor, the rejection, instead of taking 10–12 days (first set rejection) occurs in 5–7 days (second set rejection). In hyperimmunized animals that have antibodies in their blood against the transplantation antigens of the donor, the rejection is even more rapid and proceeds before the graft has had time to vascularize (white graft rejection).

Graft-Versus-Host Reaction

Such a reaction is caused by immunocompetent cells implanted in a recipient that itself is not immunologically reactive. This is the case 1) when a newborn is the recipient and the result is runt disease, or 2) when an adult recipient is rendered immunologically non-reactive by immunosuppression (accidental, therapeutic or experimental chemotherapy or radiation), or by existing immune deficiency diseases (primary, Chap. 12, or secondary, by the presence of neoplastic processes or treatment with immunosuppressives), or finally 3) by the transplantation of immunologically competent homozygous parental cells in F_1 hybrids. The syndrome caused by the reactions of the transplanted cells is called secondary disease (the primary disease is one of those named above) or "wasting" syndrome or disease.

The graft-versus-host (GVH) reaction can be studied experimentally by three principal methods:

1. *Lethally irradiated* (900 r) *adult animals* (e.g., mouse) receive, 1 day after irradiation, several million lymphoid cells intravenously. If spleen, lymph node, or thymus cells are injected, a GVH reaction occurs between the 8th and 20th days and the animals die, whereas control animals (which are lethally

irradiated but receive syngenic cells) survive; animals that are irradiated but receive no cells die between the 5th and 9th day. If bone-marrow cells are transferred, a GVH first occurs after the 20th day and exhibits a protracted course.

2. *The splenomegaly test according to Simonson*, whereby newborn F_1 mice (less than 24 h old) are injected intraperitoneally with several million spleen cells from an allogeneic (parental) donor. The animals are killed 10 days later; their body (B_{exp}) and spleen (S_{exp}) weights are measured and compared to those of the control animals (which received syngeneic cells):

$$\frac{S_{exp}/B_{exp}}{S_{con}/B_{con}} = \text{spleen index (SI)}.$$

Depending upon the standard deviation of the ratio S_c/B_c, a GVH reaction is positive with values of $SI > 1.0$ or > 1.3.

3. *The local lymph node weight test according to Ford* whereby F_1 animals or animals treated with anti-lymphocytic globulin and lethally irradiated (stimulator) receive 20×10^6 cells of a parental (or allogenic) donor (responder) in the foot pad; as a control, syngenic cells are injected in the other foot pad. Five days later, the popliteal lymph nodes are removed, freed from fat tissue, washed in acetone, and dried overnight. The next day the lymph nodes are weighed. Depending on the standard deviation, a quotient (stimulation index) of ≥ 2.0 between the weight of the allogenically stimulated and the syngenically stimulated lymph nodes indicate a positive GVH.

Genetics of Rejection

Host-Versus-Graft Reaction

The genetics of histocompatibility in general has been described in Chap. 6. Here, we shall give a more detailed picture. The most important genes which induce a graft reaction (rejection) are those of the major histocom-

Table 9.1. Survival time of skin grafts exchanged between siblings as a function of the HLA genotype[a]

Recipient genotype	Donor with HLA genotype			
	1 B/D[a]	2 A/D	3 B/D	4 A/C
1 B/D	∞[c]	14	22	13
2 A/D	14	∞	13	13
3 B/D	20	16	∞	13
4 A/C	12	14	13	∞

[a] Used with kind permission of Ceppellini R (1968). The genetic basis of transplantation. In: Rapaport FT and Dausset J (eds) Human transplantation. Grune and Stratton, New York
[b] A/B are the paternal genotypes, C/D, the maternal genotypes.
[c] Autotransplant.

Table 9.2. Skin graft survival times for differences for individual loci of the major histocompatibility complex in the mouse and in man

MHC locus difference between recipient and donor	Average survival time in days
Mouse	
−	∞
Non-H-2	Between 25 and >200
H-2K	<11
H-2I-A	10–14
H-2I-E	18–>200
H-2S	>200
H-2G	?
H-2D	<16
B. Man[a]	
−	∞
Non-HLA	$\geqq$16
HLA-A	14
HLA-B	13,3
HLA-D	11,5
HLA-A, HLA-B and HLA-D	10

[a] From van Rood JJ et al. (1975) LD typing by serology. IV. Description of a new locus with three alleles. In: Kissmeyer-Nielsen F (ed) Histocompatibility testing 1975. Munksgaard, Copenhagen, pp. 629–636; and Dausset J et al. (1970) Skin allograft survival in 238 human subjects: Role of specific relationships at four gene sites of the first and second HL-A loci. In: Terasaki PI (ed) Histocompatibility testing 1970. Munksgaard, Copenhagen, pp. 381–397

patibility complex, MHC (Table 9.1). Disparity in MHC alleles between recipient and donor leads to an acute reaction; differences in several of the MHC linked loci have a cumulative effect on the speed of the reaction (Table 9.2). (The fact that skin grafts exchanged between HLA identical individuals are also rejected eventually is due to various non-HLA allelic differences which are not linked to the HLA complex and, therefore, are inherited independently of these.)

Among the MHC genes in the mouse, differences for the K, D, and I alleles cause rejection reactions (Table 9.2). The I region appears to harbor at least two histocompatibility genes, one that is identical with or closely linked to the I-A locus, and the other located between the I-A and S locus. The former is a strong histocompatibility gene, the latter a weak one. Disparity for the S locus does not cause graft rejection.

In man, differences for individual HLA loci lead to an accelerated rejection, i.e., HLA-A, B, and D represent strong histocompatibility genes (whether HLA-C is a histocompatibility gene has not yet been determined). The survival time of skin grafts with HLA-D differences shows a direct correlation to the magnitude of the stimulation between donor and recipient (Fig. 9.1).

Graft-Versus-Host Reaction

A graft-versus-host (GVH) reaction is caused by differences in MHC alleles as well as in *non-HLA* alleles between recipient and donor. The time course and severity of a GVH in combinations differing for minor histocompatibility alleles depends upon the "strength" of the minor locus(i) in question, and upon the number of injected cells, the route of administration, and the preimmunization. In general, the strength of the reaction parallels that of the HVG reaction for the same H-gene differences. With individual minor-H-gene differences, the reaction is delayed and is in most cases chronic, even if spleen cells have been injected.

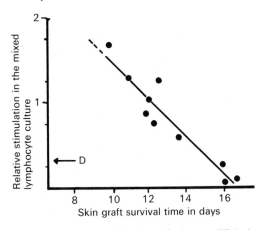

Fig. 9.1. Survival times for skin grafts between HLA-A and B identical, HLA-D different donor–recipient pairs (Summarized from Koch CT et al., 1973). The relative importance of matching for the MLC versus HLA loci in organ transplantation. In: Dausset J and Colombani J (eds) (1972) Histocompatibility testing, Munksgaard, Copenhagen; pp 521–524; and Thorby E, Jorgensen F (1973) Skin graft survival time and MLC response in four HLA seroidentical unrelated combinations, ibid, pp 525–526

When there are differences for MHC genes between recipient and donor, there is always an acute graft reaction after injection of lymphoid cells. This leads acutely to death when spleen, lymph node, thymus, or peripheral blood cells are injected. However, a chronic course is displayed if bone-marrow cells are transferred. Clearly, the strongest reaction occurs with differences for the I genes; but also differences for K or D alleles cause an acute reaction. Within the I region, several loci have been identified that can elicit a graft-versus-host reaction and that appear to be identical to those that cause an MLR in vitro.

Mechanism of Graft Rejection

Graft rejection is a complex process, and the mechanism that leads to rejection can be different for different organs, e.g., for skin, kidney, or bone marrow (lymphoid tissue). The process can be differentiated into three principal phases: recognition, proliferation and differentiation, and destruction. The recognition and destruction phases occur directly on the graft, whereas proliferation and differentiation phases take place in the regional lymph nodes that drain the graft bed.

Recognition Phase

Immediately after transplantation, antigen from the donor organ is shed into the systemic circulation of the recipient, or resides on the cells of the vascular endothelium of the graft; they are exposed to the recipient's immune cells in the circulation. The effector component of the immune response consists of lymhocytes, macrophages, and polymorphonuclear cells, each with an individual role to play but in many instances either cooperating with or suppressing one or another component of the system.

The recognition of the alloantigens is achieved by T lymphocytes which have the characteristics of T helper cells ($Ly\text{-}1^{+}2^{-}3^{-}$). Receptors of T cells could be demonstrated, using specific anti-idiotypic antibodies, to have specificity for alloantigens. The question is not yet answered whether or not these T cells possess a second receptor unit for *self* (shared antigens) in order to recognize the alloantigen in association with self. The antigens are either recognized by T cells passing through the graft, or after being "collected" by macrophages in the graft or out of the tissue fluid (lymph), and presented to T cells in the lymph node (macrophage–T cell cooperation).

Proliferation and Differentiation

After contact and recognition of the antigen(s), the lymphocytes apparently return – if they have recognized the antigen(s) as cells passing through the graft – to the regional lymph nodes, proliferate, and stimulate additional effector precursor cells, such as T effector cells and B lymphocytes. The majority of the newly sensitized cells leave the lymph node and via the blood reach the graft where they directly or with the help of other systems (K cells – see below, polymorphonuclear leukocytes, specific antibodies with or without complement) destroy the graft. A certain number of lymphocytes remain in the circulation as memory cells .

Destruction Phase

The destruction of the graft is effected by several pathways, every one of which may act alone or in combination:
1) Activated T killer cells (with the characteristic markers Ly-1$^-$2$^+$3$^+$) bind via specific cell-bound receptors to the cells of the graft and lyse them; T cells also release factors, such as macrophage migration inhibition factor (MIF) which accelerate the rate of mononuclear cell infiltration.
2) Activated B lymphocytes differentiate to plasma cells and produce antibodies specific for the graft's antigens; they may bind directly and activate complement which then attracts polymorphonuclear leukocytes (PMN). Disruption of PMN causes the release of lysosomes and proteolytic enzymes with resulting destruction of graft tissue. Vasoactive peptides cause vasospasm, which slows blood flow and facilitates accumulation of both PMN and monocytes, and thereby produces diffuse ischemic changes. Accumulation of platelets also occurs, with resulting activation of clotting mechanisms and the formation of thrombi.
3) Recently, a type of lymphocyte has been identified – K lymphocytes – which recognize humoral antibodies (IgG) against specific donor antigens, react with the Fc portion, and destroy the target cells to which they are attached. This system is known as antibody-dependent, cell-mediated cytotoxicity (ADCC) (see Chap. 2, pp. 43 and 56).
The first of the three outlined pathways appears to be the primary mechanism of graft destruction in unsensitized recipients, in which the two latter mechanisms come into play only to complete the rejection. In sensitized recipients (sensitized by preimmunization, e.g., blood transfusion or pregnancy), all three mechanisms may contribute equally to the graft's destruction.

Individual phases can be studied in in vitro experiments: the mixed lymphocyte culture reaction appears to represent an in vitro equivalent of the recognition and proliferation phases. The destruction phase can be studied in the form of a primary or secondary response in vitro using the cell-mediated lympholytic reaction (CML).

Mixed Lymphocyte Culture

The principles of the mixed lymphocyte culture (MLC) reaction were discussed on pp. 142. Only the reaction partner and the possible mechanism are briefly discussed here.

Reaction Partner

Stimulator. In the one-way reaction, the cell whose proliferation is blocked by treatment with mitomycin C or by irradiation (2,500–5,000 r) is termed the stimulator. To stimulate the untreated cell, the stimulator must be alive and able to be metabolically active; RNA or protein synthesis inhibitors or germicidal ultraviolet irradiation cause a loss of stimulating ability.
Lymphatic cells exhibit good stimulation, however, stimulation can also be observed with epidermal cells but not with kidney cells. Of the lymphoid cells, primarily B cells appear to cause stimulation; although, stimulation by T cells and macrophages has also been demonstrated. In addition to B lymphocytes, T lymphocytes also stimulate, depending upon the genetic differences for certain I-subregions between responder and stimulator.

Responder Cell. It is generally agreed that the cells in a MLC that proliferate in response to a stimulus are T cells (Thy-1$^+$ cells). With the additional T-cell markers Ly-1, 2, and 3, it was shown in the mouse that the transforming cells are derived from Ly-1$^+$,2$^+$,3$^+$ cells and that among the proliferating cells, Ly-1^+, 2^-, 3^- as well as Ly-1^-, 2^+, 3^+, cells are found.

The following findings in the mouse were obtained from selection experiments (i.e., pretreatment of the responder cell population with anti-Ly-1 or anti-Ly-2,3 serum plus complement): Responder T cells stimulated by K or D molecules exhibit primarily the markers Ly-2 and Ly-3; responder cells stimulated by I molecules are composed of both T-cell populations. These findings by Cantor and Boyse, and results obtained from studies by Wagner and colleagues, suggest the following: After contact with allogeneic cells differing for the H-2 K, D, and I molecules, T precursor cells (Ly-1^+, 2^+, 3^+) are stimulated by the I molecules to differentiate to T helper cells (Ly-1^+, 2^-, 3^-), and by the K and D molecules to differentiate to T effector cells (Ly-1^-, 2^+, 3^+). The generated T helper cells augment the production of T effector cells reacting specifically with K or D molecules, and initiate the formation of T effector cells reacting specifically with I molecules (T–T cell interaction) (see also below, CML). At the same time, T helper cells also affect B cells and bring about their differentiation into antibody-secreting plasma cells (T–B cell interaction). If there is no difference between the responder cell population and the stimulator cell population for I-gene-controlled molecules, the antigen apparently must first be processed by macrophages before it is in the position to bring about the formation of T helper cells (macrophage-T cell cooperation).

Whether T helper cells and T effector cells derive from the same T precursor cells or whether both types of cells originate from different precursor cells that develop before contact with the antigen, i.e., independently of the antigen, from common precursor cells, is still unknown.

Specificity of MLR

Although it is generally accepted that the T-cell response to antigens is clonal like that of B cells, there is as yet no direct proof. This does not mean that no specificity can be shown. Selection experiments have indicated that stimulated cells in a specific allogenic combination react specifically:

1) *Negative selection:* One obtains negatively selected cells by injecting lymphocyte cultures at the time of maximal proliferation into previously lethally irradiated animals of a strain from which the stimulator cells are derived; a few hours later, the ductus thoracicus is drained; it contains only those responder cells that were not stimulated in the allogenic culture because the stimulating cells were absorbed in the host.

2) *Positive selection.* Positively selected cells are obtained by injecting proliferating cells of an MLC into syngenic (to the responder), thymectomized, lethally irradiated animals that have been reconstituted with anti-Thy-1 serum plus complement treated bone marrow (B animals). The cells can be "parked" in such animals for weeks.

Positively and negatively selected cells can also be obtained by an in vitro process: If cells in the proliferative phase are separated in a serum gradient at 1 g (1 g velocity sedimentation), two cell populations are obtained: One consists of lymphoblasts, the other of lymphocytes. Lymphoblasts are the positively selected cells, whereas the lymphocyte fraction contains the nonstimulated (negatively selected) cells. Both cell fractions can be maintained in culture for weeks and can be used to test their reactivity to allogenic cells. Negatively selected cells no longer react to allogenic cells that originate from the donor used for the first stimulation; their ability to react to other allogenic donors is, however, in no way influenced. Positively selected cells react much faster and more vigorously to cells of donors used for the first stimulation. However, they also react (in various degrees) to cells that are unrelated to the original cells, which can be explained by the considerable cross-reactions exhibited by alloantigens.

Immunologic specificity can also be demonstrated by specific tolerance: Lymphocytes of tolerant rats do not react to cell antigens of the strain used to induce tolerance, but they react with a normal proliferative response to "third party" stimulator cells.

Furthermore, it has been shown that antibodies against receptors that recognize the alloantigens of the specific stimulator can destroy these lymphocytes, and the remaining cell population no longer shows reactivity against these stimulator cells; however, it can react unimpaired against cells of other allogenic donors.

Number of Allogenic Reactive Cells

The number of cells in the allogenic MLR has been calculated to be about 3%–6% of the T cells used. Different methods are employed for this calculation, including the following: Hydroxyurea in appropriate concentrations (10^{-2}–10^{-3}) leaves blast formation untouched but can reversibly block DNA synthesis. This substance can be used to arrest the reacting cells in the blast stage. By counting the blasts at the time of maximal transformation, one can easily calculate the number of stimulated cells.

The percentage of cells that react to an allogenic stimulus is, at first glance, high. Assuming that only two or three antigenic determinants per haplotype lead to stimulation, one must conclude that not more than about 20–50 different determinants occur in one species. This is, however, obviously not the case. It appears, therefore, that allogenic stimulation occurs via a large number of determinants, whereby unrelated haplotypes share a large though variable number of determinants. This would also explain why there is a clear proliferative response of positively selected cells toward third-party stimulator cells. This hypothesis is also substantiated by the linear proportionality of the relative reactivity due to the presence of 0, 1, or 2 HLA-D antigen differences (Fig. 9.2) between the responder and the stimulator.

Genetics of MLC Reactivity

In allogenic combinations in man, the capacity to stimulate is almost entirely linked to the *HLA-D* locus; weak stimulations have been observed for differences of the *HLA-A* and *HLA-B* loci. These are possibly caused by genes located between the *HLA-A* and *HLB-B* that control weak lymphocyte-activating determinants (LD_2 locus).

In the mouse, variations in individual non-MHC histocompatibility genes between responder and stimulator lead in some cases to stimulation (*H-1*, *H-3*, and *H-4*), whereas in other cases no stimulation is observed (*H-7*, *H-8*, *H-9*, and *H-Y*). Differences for several non-MHC genes in general lead to stimulation. The *H-2* haplotype also influences the reactivity in the MLC. Thus, the reaction against non-MHC determinants is strong in the presence of the *H-2*[a] haplotype; however, the difference for the same non-MHC determinants causes weak stimulation in the presence of almost all other *H-2* haplotypes, particularly the *H-2*[b] haplotype.

Relatively strong stimulation has been described in cases of differences in the Thy-1 locus; in comparison, the Ly antigens 1 and 2 and the TLa antigen apparently lead to no stimulation. Festenstein described a locus

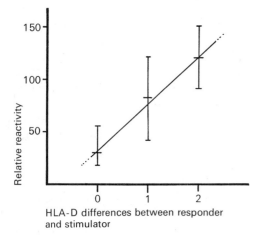

Fig. 9.2. Reactivity in the mixed lymphocyte culture between unrelated cells that differ in the 0, 1, or 2 HLA-D determinants (From Thosby E et al., 1975). Human MLC activation determinants. In: Kissmeyer-Nielson F (ed) (1975) Histocompatibility testing 1975. Munksgaard, Copenhagen; pp 502–208

(M) with four alleles, M_1, M_2, M_3, and M_4, which is not linked to genes of the H-2 complex but causes stimulation that is comparable in strength to that observed with H-2 disparity. (An M locus disparity leads neither to an HVG nor to a GVH reaction, and M-locus-controlled determinants cannot be serologically demonstrated but are apparently expressed on B lymphocytes.)

H-2 disparity leads to strong stimulation in the MLC. In the MLC, disparity in the I region clearly causes the strongest reactions, primarily dependent upon determinants controlled from I-A genes. However, also the I-E region controls determinants that lead to clear but weak reactions. A disparity for K and D antigens also causes stimulations which are, however, clearly weaker.

Other findings support the supposition that the lymphocyte-activating structures are identical with Ia antigens (in the mouse) or B-cell-specific HLA-D linked antigens in man: 1) The tissue distribution of Ia antigens is the same as that of the stimulating antigens. 2) The stimulation can be inhibited by antisera that react specifically with Ia antigens. Finally 3), the gene loci that control stimulation in the MLR, are found in all species examined thus far on the same chromosome region as that which controls the Ia antigen (or Ia-like antigens).

The ability of lymphocytes to react in xenogeneic combinations was also tested. In certain combinations, stimulation reaches the magnitude of HLA-D or H-2 disparate allogenic combinations; however, reactivity appears to decrease as the phylogenetic relationship becomes more and more distant.

Cell-Mediated Cytotoxicity

Cell-mediated cytotoxicity can occur in two ways: 1) through direct interaction between target cells and specific sensitized lymphocytes in the absence of antibodies and complement (cell-mediated cytolysis, CML) and 2) through antibody-dependent, cell-mediated cytotoxicity (or lysis) (ADCC).

Direct Cell-Mediated Cytolysis. Cell-mediated, antibody-independent cell lysis (CML) can be considered as the effector phase of MLR. Lymphocytes stimulated by alloantigens in vitro or in vivo lyse cells of the same donor when they are offered to them as target cells. Culture cell lines, mitogen-stimulated lymphoblasts (LPS, PHA or con A) or macrophages are suitable target cells in vitro. The destruction of the target cells is usually measured by the release of ^{51}Cr, with which the target cells were previously labeled.

Sensitized or nonsensitized lymphocytes are co-cultivated with stimulator cells for 5 days; then the activated lymphocytes are added to ^{51}Cr-labeled target cells in different proportions to the number of effector cells. The cell mixture is incubated for 6–16 h at 37 °C, and after removal of the cells by centrifugation, the radioactivity in the supernatant is measured. The specific lysis is given as a percentage of the maximum release of radioactivity (measured by lysis with water or NP 40) after subtraction of the spontaneous release.

In this reaction in the mouse, the effector cell is an Ly 2^+, 3^+-T cell. For the destruction of the target cell, neither B cells nor macrophages need be present. The effector cells are either still in the blast stage or have, after stimulation, already transformed back into small lymphocytes. Upon a second contact with the antigen (e.g., 10–30 days), effector cells need not go through a proliferative phase; they are completely effective lytically. However, it appears that effector cells are short-lived, because one no longer observes lysis when primary stimulated cells come into renewed contact with the antigen after a few weeks, although an accelerated proliferative response can still be seen; this proliferative response is probably dependent on T helper cells (Ly-1$^+$), which accordingly survive longer. Direct contact between effector cells and target cells is required for lysis.

Specificity and Genetics. From studies of families with children who exhibit recombinant *HLA* haplotypes, the following results were obtained:

1) *Responder-stimulator combinations which differ* for HLA-A, HLA-B, and HLA-D, show a good proliferative reaction, and generate cytotoxic effector cells that specifically destroy target cells carrying the same *HLA* haplotype as the stimulator; likewise, target cells that have only the HLA-A and/or HLA-B antigens in common with the stimulator cell are destroyed. Target cells that share the HLA-D determinants with the target cell but whose HLA-A and HLA-B antigens differ from those of the stimulator cell are not destroyed.

2) *Responder-stimulator combinations which are identical* for HLA-A and HLA-B antigens, but differ for HLA-D determinants, exhibit a good proliferative reaction but no formation of effector cells, i.e., target cells that are identical with the stimulator cells are not destroyed.

3) *Responder-stimulator combinations which differ* only for the HLA-A and/or HLA-B antigen, but not for HLA-D determinants, show no or only a weak proliferative reaction and no cytotoxic effector cells; i.e., target cells with HLA-A or HLA-B antigens identical to those of the stimulator cells are not destroyed.

From these findings one can conclude that (1) for the induction of cytotoxic effector cells, the stimulator cell population must differ for the HLA-A and/or HLA-B antigens as well as for the HLA-D determinants from the responder cell population, and (2) the specificity for the effector cells produced is only directed against the HLA-A and HLA-B antigens of the stimulator cells, not against HLA-D determinants.

Further studies have shown that for the formation of specific anti-HLA-A or anti-HLA-B effector cells, the A or B antigen on the one hand and HLA-D determinants on the other need not be present on the same stimulator cells; rather, the latter (or the former) could be offered through a third cell. In principle, these results can be substantiated by studies with cells from unrelated donors. However, one finds here – in contrast to families in which phenotypic identity signifies also genotypic identity – a more or less strongly expressed cross-reactivity, i.e., effector cells that are induced against specific HLA-A or HLA-B antigens of a stimulator cell usually lyse not only target cells that have the HLA-A or HLA-B antigens of the stimulator cells, but also target cells that carry other HLA-A or HLA-B antigens. These findings are explained by the high cross-reactivity of the HLA antigen known from serologic studies.

In the mouse, it has been found that all three loci, *K*, *D*, and *I*, can independently of each other induce a proliferative response as well as effector cell generation with specificity for K, D, and I molecules. It could be shown that the effectivity for the induction of K or D antigen-specific effector cells is significantly increased if, in addition to the K or D molecule disparity, a difference for *I* loci controlled determinants exists, i.e., in the proliferative reaction, Ly-1$^+$ (helper) cells as well as Ly-2$^+$, 3$^+$ (effector) cells are generated; the former enhance the recruitment of the latter (see above, MLR).

The different results obtained in studying man and the mouse might be explained on methodological grounds: In man, PHA stimulated cells are generally used as target cells; these cells do not express readily detectable DR antigens. In mice, usually LPS or ConA stimulated cells serve as target cells which express Ia antigens; if PHA target cells are employed, Ia-antigen-specific effector cells cannot be easily detected.

Antibody-Dependent Cell-Mediated Cytotoxicity. In addition to direct, cell-mediated cytolysis, another type of cell-mediated lysis can be observed, particularly in man: antibody-dependent, cell-mediated lysis (lymphocyte antibody lympholytic interaction, LALI, or antibody-dependent, cell-mediated cytotoxicity, ADCC). Human lymphocytes that are not specifically sensitized have the capacity to lyse target cells such as chicken erythrocytes, sheep fibroblast monolayers, Chang liver cells, a human liver-cell line, human erythrocytes, when these are charged with a xenogeneic or allogeneic antibody that reacts specifically with determinants of the target cell. For cell lysis to occur, the antibody must be complete, i.e., without the Fc fragment, no lysis occurs. Complement is not necessary for the reaction. Different mononuclear cells apparently can be used as effector cells, whereby different target cells from different effector cells are lysed:

1) *K cells* (killer cells) are nonadherent, nonphagocytic cells that exhibit neither B- or T-cell characteristics (Ig$^-$, Thy-1$^-$) and have the appearance of small to medium-sized lymphocytes. K cells carry receptors for the Fc fragment of immunoglobulin as well as for C3b and C3d. K cells lyse human lymphocytes that are coated with anti-HLA antibodies, chicken erythrocytes but not human erythrocytes, numerous cell lines, and some tumor cells, if they are sensitized with corresponding antibodies.

2) *B cells* also appear able to lyse coated chicken erythrocytes.

3) *Macrophages and monocytes* can lyse different sensitized target cells.

In addition to the cells mentioned here, other cells can affect sensitized target cells cytolytically, including fetal liver cells, lymphoid human cell lines, and long-term, nonlymphoid mouse culture tumor-cell lines.

It is not known whether this reaction plays a role in vivo, but there are a large number of K cells in mononuclear infiltrates of transplanted kidneys in patients who exhibit a chronic rejection reaction. There is also experimental evidence that this type of antibody-dependent cell-mediated cytotoxicity may play a role in virus infections and in certain types of neoplasms (melanoma, virus-induced and methylcholanthrene-induced tumors).

Specific Absence of Reaction Against Allogenic Tissue

Enhancement. Under certain conditions, allogeneic tissue, after it is transferred, induces no rejection reaction. One such situation will be discussed in detail below: specific immunologic tolerance. This form of lack of reaction is maintained by a cellular mechanism. Another form of the specific lack of reaction is enhancement. Enhancement can be transferred by serum and leads to prolonged or permanent survival of a tissue (or tumor) graft that normally would be rejected.

Enhancement can be achieved through active or passive immunization. The mechanism of immunologic enhancement is still unclear; however, it appears that antibodies that are not cytotoxic (i.e., cannot activate complement) bind with alloantigens on the surface and thus prevent the induction of a specific cellular immune response (afferent enhancement) or, by covering the alloantigen, obscuring the target for the cytotoxic killer cell (efferent enhancement).

In the rat, the preferred animal model in enhancement studies, it is also observed that during the production of alloantisera by repeated injection of lymphatic cells the recipient produces antibodies directed against idiotypes of its own anti-alloantigen antibodies (auto-anti-idiotype antibodies). Thus, antibodies with the specificity for this alloantigen disappear from the serum, as do probably also lymphocytes with the receptors that possess these idiotypes. The result of this reaction is also a specific lack of reaction to corresponding allogeneic tissue, a state in which the border between enhancement and tolerance begins to disappear.

Immunotolerance. Immunotolerance is a state of immunologic inactivity that is specific in regard to antigens or cells that, in normal animals, would induce an immune response. The most notable example of immunologic tolerance is the incapacity of the organism to be stimulated by its own constituents, even though these elicit immunogenic activity when transferred to other organisms. To explain this phenomenon, Ehrlich postulated the existence of a mechanism that he named "horror autotoxicus," by virtue of which the organism was incapable of producing antibodies against its own antigenic constituents.

The first clarifications regarding the phenomenon of immunotolerance originated from what could be classified as an experiment of nature: When dizygotic bovine twins occur, there is an anastomosis of the placental vessels. Each twin is born possessing not only red cells belonging to its own blood group, but also those of the sibling. Curiously, such red cells do not behave as antigens, that is to say, they are not recognized as foreign. Such twins possess a state of acquired immunologic tolerance which has been called chimerism [in Greek mythology, the chimera (Lat. *chimaera*, Gr. *chimaira*) was a fabulous monster with a lion's head, a goat's body, and a serpent's tail]. On the basis of these observations, made by Owen in 1945, Burnet and Fenner sought to explain why the organism did not form antibodies against its own constituents. They suggested that during embryologic development the organism "learned" to recognize its own constituents and thus predicted that if an embryo were injected with an antigenic substance, the organism would, as an adult, become tolerant to that particular antigen. The theory of Burnet and Fenner encouraged Medawar and his collaborators in England to extend the experiments of Owen, showing that dizygotic bovine twins failed to reject skin grafted between them, yet rejected in normal fashion grafts from other siblings.

The prediction of Burnet and Fenner was thus verified; corroboration followed by the Hašek group in Czechoslovakia. By joining in developing chicken embryos the chorioallantoid membranes, which are extremely rich in blood vessels, Hašek and his colleagues achieved an intense interchange of cells between the embryos (parabiosis). Under these circumstances, after hatching, neither bird was capable of producing antibodies against the antigens of its partner or of rejecting grafts of its skin.

In the experiments of Medawar, schematized in Fig. 9.3, embryos of strain A mice were injected on the 17th day of fetal life with a suspension of cells obtained from strain CBA mice[1]. Two months after birth, the strain A mice, having received skin from the strain CBA mice, were unable to reject such grafts, which remained viable for the entire life of the recipient animal. Meanwhile, these same animals retained the capacity to reject, in a normal period of time (10–14 days), grafts from other donors. This state of tolerance could be abolished by transfer of lymphoid cells from a normal strain A mouse, or from an animal of the

---

1 The cells of the lymph nodes and spleen are more efficient in inducing tolerance than those of the thymus or bone marrow

Fig. 9.3. Induction of immunologic tolerance (Medawar's experimental procedure). Embryos or newborn strain A mice are injected with spleen cells from strain CBA mice; the donor cells are not rejected because the immune system of the recipient is still undeveloped. Subsequently adult strain A mice, whose lymphocytes have acquired tolerance to the H antigen of strain CBA mice, accept skin grafts from them

Cell donor (CBA)

Spleen cells

Injection into embryos (A)

or

Injection into newborn mice (A)

Skin donor (CBA)

Skin graft (CBA) accepted by adult mouse (A)

same strain, immunized by previous contact with cells of the CBA strain. The breaking of tolerance required a longer period of time and a much greater number of cells in the first case. These observations demonstrate that tolerance represents an inherent form of reaction of the immune response and that the graft maintains its immunogenicity in the tolerant animal.

The prediction of Burnet and Fenner was corroborated by numerous immunologists, who demonstrated, soon after the experiments of Medawar and Hašek, that the injection of numerous antigens into neonate animals produced a state of specific immunologic tolerance that persisted for a limited time (months or years) and disappeared gradually. A state of permanent tolerance nevertheless could be obtained by repeated injections of the same antigen. To maintain such a state of tolerance, the constant presence of the antigen appears to be indispensable.

In all species, there exists a period in fetal or postnatal life in which tolerance can easily be induced. The existence of this period, called "the period of tolerization," should not be seen as implying the existence of a period outside of which tolerance cannot be induced. Actually, contrary to what initially was maintained, it is possible to make even adult animals tolerant to allografts. To realize this possibility, however, it is necessary to repeatedly inject large numbers of the donor's cells into the recipient, or to maintain the two animals united by parabiosis for a determined period before performing the graft. The degree of genetic difference between the donor and the recipient determines the magnitude and the duration of contact with the donor antigens required to render the recipient tolerant.

Tolerance to "dead" antigens may be established with large or small doses. Tolerance for large doses, or "high-dose tolerance," requires quantities of antigens several times greater than those normally necessary to induce a perceptible immune response. Tolerance for small doses, or "low-dose tolerance," requires the continuous or repeated injection of quantities of antigen considerably smaller than those necessary to induce high-dose tolerance. The tolerogenic capacity of antigens is highly variable; however, generally speaking, weak antigens, i.e., poorly immunogenic antigens, are highly tolerogenic whereas strong antigens are poorly tolerogenic.

The induction of tolerance in adult animals is facilitated by diverse treatments that temporarily diminish the immunologic reactivity of the animal. Through the use of antimetabolic substances such as cortisone, X-rays, antilymphocytic serum, depletion of the lymphocytes by lymphatic drainage, etc., it is possible to achieve tolerance using a quantity of antigen that normally would induce an immune response. With certain antigens, such as serum proteins, it is possible to induce tolerance in adult animals using highly soluble *antigens*, which through ultracentrifugation, are rendered aggregate-free.

Animals that are already sensitized against an antigen and therefore have memory cells, can be made tolerant to this antigen only with great difficulty. In such cases, contact even with an extremely small quantity of a weak antigen stimulates a vigorous immune response, and it has not been possible to induce low-dose tolerance under such conditions. In special circumstances (e.g., in animals that have received an immunosuppressive agent and when large doses of a weak antigen are used), it is possible to induce high-dose tolerance even after a primary response.

It should be noted that immunologic tolerance may be partial as well as total. In the former condition, only part of the cellular population is rendered tolerant. Every time the lymphoid system enters into contact with an antigen, two alternatives are presented to each cell whose specificity is directed against this antigen: Either the cell proliferates, or it is blocked. In the first case, an immune response occurs, whereas in the second, tolerance results. It should further be noted that at the cellular level, cellular activation and tolerance are opposed phenomena; in the organism as a whole, the two phenomena may occur simultaneously, the dominance of one or the other depending upon conditions not yet understood.

As we have noted, two types of immunocompetent cells evolve during the response of the organism to a large number of antigens. One of these, the B lymphocyte, possesses on its membrane receptors for antigens similar to those of serum antibodies – these being direct precursors of the plasma cells. The activation of these cells requires, or is greatly accentuated by, the cooperation of one other cellular type, which itself is incapable of producing or of differentiating into cells forming antibodies: T helper cells. Studies regarding the mechanism of tolerance have demonstrated that both cellular types can be involved in this phenomenon. Thus, tolerance can, in comparison to thymus-dependent antigens, be determined by the absence of either a T-cell or a B-cell response. It was shown that T and B cells can be made tolerant, but that the induction mechanism, the duration, and the loss of tolerance are different for both cell types.

If T and B cells from animals tolerant to human γ-globulin are administered at various intervals, after induction of tolerance, to irradiated, syngeneic mice and the capacity of recipients to produce antibodies is then tested, it can be shown that T-cell tolerance can be induced with low doses of antigen and that it occurs more quickly (24 h in contrast to 15–20 days in B cells) and lasts longer (> 100 days) than B-cell (~ 45 days) tolerance. The findings suggest that natural tolerance to self-antigen is probably dependent upon T cells.

For thymus-dependent antigens, B- or T-cell tolerance is sufficient to make the entire organism tolerant. Because the threshold of tolerance for T cells is considerably lower than for B cells it is difficult in vivo to obtain exclusive tolerance for B lymphocytes, at least with protein antigens. However, this difficulty can be circumvented through the use of haptens conjugated to molecules that do not stimulate T cells. For example, specific tolerance of B cells for haptens has been produced by the introduction into the organism of haptenic groups conjugated to nonimmunogenic synthetic copolymers, to autologous proteins, or even to syngeneic erythrocytes.

Mechanisms of Tolerance. From the experimental data available, it appears unlikely that clonal deletion ("forbidden clones"), i.e., tolerance resulting from the elimination of lymphocyte clones specific for the tolerogen, as proposed by Burnet, is the underlying mechanism to induce and maintain tolerance. It has been demonstrated that lymphocytes can be sensitized against syngeneic tissue under appropriate conditions (e.g. in vitro) indicating that immune cells specifically reacting with self-determinants are not eliminated but present in normal animals; however, they appear to be inactivated or suppressed.

On the basis of experimental data, several mechanisms have been proposed for the induction and maintenance of tolerance which either result in the prevention of T-helper-cell activation, or the predominant activation of T suppressor cells:
(1) small amounts of soluble antigens which may interact with antibody and surface receptors, thereby preventing cooperation of macrophages, T helper cells and B cells;
(2) large amount of soluble antigen, which lead to activation of T suppressor cells: high dose-tolerance (see above) induction is accompanied by an increase in DNA synthesis in thymocytes which proliferate and differentiate to T suppressor cells; (3) antibodies especially in small quantities have been shown to be immunosuppressive (see p. 334, anti-D antibodies in preventing fetal erythroblastosis); it is thought that antibodies prevent interaction of the sensitizing antigens with host lymphocytes by (a) forming soluble (antigen excess) complexes and, therefore, preventing the formation of stimulating aggregates on macrophages (B cells), and/or (b) covering antigens so that they cannot be recognized by T cells, and/or (c) acting as feedback inhibitors blocking the activation of suppressor cells

specific for B cells or antigen specific T helper cells, or causing the formation of anti-idiotypic antibodies (see Chap. 6); and (4) antibody-antigen complexes, the effects of which are discussed in more detail in Chap. 10 (pp. 282–287).

It is now recognized that each individual possesses very low levels of autoantibodies in the serum, and the presence of T suppressor cells, preferrentially in thymus and spleen, has been ample demonstrated: after transfer of thymocytes from mice tolerant to sheep red blood cells (SRBC) into normal mice the formation of anti-SRBC antibodies is blocked in the recipient. Mice treated with anti-T cell serum show an enhanced antibody response to pneumococcal polysaccharide; this augmented response can be abrogated by reconstitution with thymocytes. Experiments with carrier-hapten conjugates suggest that the T suppressor cell effect is mediated through carrier recognition like that of T helper cells; thus, thymocytes of carrier-tolerant mice suppressed the anti-hapten response after transfer to normal mice; however, when hapten-tolerant T cells are transferred to normal mice, B cells are able (allowed) to produce anti-hapten antibodies.

Thus, it appears that tolerance is the result of an actively maintained balance between help and suppression and requires the continuous presence of low levels of antigen and antibodies.

Organ Transplantation

The transfer of tissue and organs from one individual to another is not a discovery of our time. In the Middle Ages, attempts were made to heal wounded surfaces with skin grafts (Tagliacozzi). As early as 1800, Baroni carried out successful autografts on sheep. Paul Bert in 1860 described the different behavior of auto- and allografts. The first kidney transplants were carried out around 1900 by Carrel and Guthrie in cats. In different places, attempts were made to treat uremia with xenogenic kidney transplants. The biologic factors responsible for the failures remained unknown until the studies of Little, Loeb, Gorer, and Snell produced the first evidence of an immunologic rejection process. Medawar and his colleagues then carried out a series of classic experiments (1944–1946) that served as the basis for the progress in transplantation immunity observed today. The successful series of clinical kidney transplants between identical twins by Murray and Merril in Boston (1955) gave clinical transplantation a lasting impetus.

Today it is known that the prerequisite of a successful tissue graft is histogenetic conformity between recipient and donor. The methods of choice are the serologic typing of lymphocytes (HLA-A, HLA-B, HLA-C, and HLA-DR antigens) and erythrocytes (AB0 and P blood groups) and the mixed lymphocyte culture reaction for determination of histogenetic relationship.

Serologic Typing

Although clinical findings clearly indicate that the degree of serotypic identity and the graft survival time are directly proportional, there is the limitation that serotyping for unrelated pairs does not permit a prediction concerning the fate of the graft. The following factors support this statement: (1) antigens still unknown; (2) cross-reactions; (3) different individual reactions to HLA antisera and HLA antigens; and (4) the fact that serotyping encompasses only some of the structures responsible for the immunologic reaction.

Serotyping has a completely different value for family members in the phenotype and genotype are identical and whom the limitations just described play almost no role.

Cellular Typing

The MLC reaction has achieved a particular significance for compatibility testing because it can uncover differences for the major histocompatibility complex that cannot as yet be serologically recorded: HLA-D. In contrast to serologic typing, in which testing is based on identity, in cellular typing, differences between donor and recipient are uncovered. If stimulation by the donor cells is weak or nonexistent, then the graft function is usually good. The disadvantage of this method is that 5 days are necessary before the results are available, so that, in general, it can be carried out only for bone marrow grafts and organs from living donors. An accelerated but not yet routinely used modification of the MLR is the PLT (primary lymphocyte typing) test. In this test, specifically sensitized lymphocytes are used as reference cells. The cells are stimulated only by lymphocytes that possess determinants identical to those used for the first stimulation. The secondary proliferation occurs after 24 h. Cross-reactions represent a certain uncertainty factor, as does the fact that donor and recipient cells are not tested in direct contact with one another, but in relation to a third cell.

Clinical Organ Transplantation

Organ transplantation is an ideal therapy for many pathological conditions. However, histogenetic matching is only one of several factors that have to date prevented widespread application of most organ transplantations. Organ transplantation is, with few exceptions, still in its pioneer stages. Therefore, we shall restrict the discussion here to transplantation of kidneys and bone marrow, where substantial progress has been made in the last decade, and the thymus because of the theoretical importance.

Kidneys

The kidney was the first internal organ whose transplantation was attempted. The large number of patients who died from uremia was the stimulus for these attempts. The primary diseases are chronic glomerulonephritis and pyelonephritis, diabetic nephropathies, cystic kidneys, malignant hypertonia, and amyloidosis. Because he-

modialysis now offers the anephric patient an alternative treatment, transplantation is no longer urgently indicated in all cases of terminal kidney failure. However, absolute indications include progression of uremic complications, hypertension, and the side effects of dialysis such as osteoporosis and polyneuritis. Patients with antibodies against the glomerular basal membrane are not suitable recipients for a graft because they often experience recurrence of the glomerulonephritis that necessitated the transplant in the first place.

Patients should be taken into a transplantation program early, because a graft as a last resort, i.e., when dialysis is no longer effective, represents a worse prognosis that an early transplant. In other words, it should be decided early whether a graft or dialysis should be used.

The large number of successful kidney transplantations – in contrast to most other organ transplantations – results partially from the organ's relative resistance to ischemia. This and the development of nationally and internationally organized exchange systems (Eurotransplant) and efficient conservation methods over recent years permit large-scale use of cadaver kidneys for implantation into the best-matching (AB0, HLA) patient. In addition, the kidney is the only organ (except bone marrow) that can be obtained from living donors.

Suitable donors are people killed in accidents and victims of subarachnoid hemorrhage or heart infarcts. Kidneys from living donors should only be considered if there is histogenetic identity. Kidneys from living donors who are identical for one haplotype (parents, siblings) and that show only minimal stimulation in the MLC reaction provide approximately the same chance of survival as kidneys from unrelated serotypic- and *HLA-D*-identical donors.

In general, the kidney is implanted heterotopically in the fossa iliaca. Immediately after the vessels are unclamped, the transplanted kidney becomes pink and achieves its normal turgor. When the kidney is not damaged, urine production begins immediately.

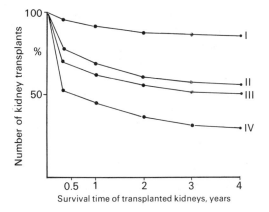

Fig. 9.4. Survival time of kidney transplant in relation to tissue compatibility between recipient and donor. *I*, Transplants from HLA-identical siblings; *II*, transplants from one haplotype-identical siblings; *III*, transplants from HLA-identical, unrelated donors; *VI*, transplants from HLA-different, unrelated donors. [From Hors et al. (1974) France-transplant: kidney transplantation as guide for bone marrow grafting. Transplant Proc 6:421]

Even though the chances of survival appeared slim (in 1963, only 6 of 176 people receiving a transplant survived longer than a year) in the early years of allogenic kidney transplantation, the chances of survival have increased considerably in the last 15 years. Today, the chances of survival for the recipient of an HLA-identical kidney from a relative is over 90% after 1 year and 85% after 4 years, those of recipients of an HLA-identical, unrelated kidney greater than 60% after 1 year and ca. 50% after 4 years (Fig. 9.4). Most deaths occur in the first 6 months. The survival rate of patients (not of the kidney) is today increased through (1) early removal of the graft when rejection occurs, with subsequent hemodialysis (or a second graft) and (2) reduced immunosuppressive treatment (see Chap. 14), which renders the recipient less sensitive to infection.

A hyperacute rejection reaction is rarely observed: When it does occur, immediately after resumption of blood flow, the kidney is irreversibly damaged due to intravascular thromboses. It is thought that circulating antibodies were present even before the transplant.

Acute rejection reaction is expressed as a decrease in bodily functions, swelling, pain, fever, tachycardia, general malaise, lymphocytosis, thrombopenia, lymphocyturia, and increase in blood pressure. An immediate, intensified treatment with immunosuppressives can render the rejection reaction milder or cause it to stop.

Chronic rejection reactions are first manifested clinically as proteinuria. There is progressive obliteration of the vascular lumina and thus decreased renal perfusion. Tertiary hyperparathyroidism with bone dystrophy can occur as a result of disturbance in kidney function.

Specific complications accompanying kidney transplants include recurrence of glomerulonephritis in the transplanted kidney and metabolic disturbances. Immediately after transplantation, there can be intense diuresis and hypokalemia that result in severe dehydration and sometimes lead to shock or even death of the patient. Whereas secondary hyperparathyroidism is found in almost all patients with chronic kidney failure, after successful transplantation the parathyroidial function usually normalizes again – if not, a parathyroidectomy is necessary. Osseous alterations in children with hyperparathyroidism usually do not, in the case of a kidney transplant, re-form. Skeletal alterations and growth disturbances are therefore frequent causes of invalidism in young kidney transplant recipients. Heterotopic implantation of the kidney in the pelvis in general is not a contraindication for a pregnancy. The influence of immunosuppressive substances on the pregnancy and/or the fetus is not yet completely clear; normal children have been borne by recipients of kidney transplants undergoing immunosuppressive treatment. The immunosuppressives azathioprine and prednisolone do not appear to have any damaging influence on spermatozoa. Donor kidneys should not be obtained from patients with malignant disease, because tumor cells present in the transplanted kidney may be transferred, and the recipient dies from metastases. The infectious diseases that can be transferred from donor to recipient include in particular viral hepatitis and histoplasmosis. Thrombocytopenic purpura and hypersensitivity reaction also can be transferred.

Thymus. The effects of neonatal thymectomy were cured experimentally by thymus implant. As a result, thymus transplants were performed in patients with immunologic insufficiency syndrome (see Chap. 12). A thymus implant is considered for patients suffering from decreased or failed thymus function, i.e., those with Di George's syndrome and Swiss-type agammaglobulin anemia. In some cases, considerable improvement was achieved after transplantation of a histogenetically almost identical thymus, in some cases combined with bone marrow transplant. In one case with an isolated T-cell defect, clear improvement was achieved by implantation of a fetal thymus. A possible alternative is the administration of purified thymus hormone (thymosin, see Chap. 1). In patients with primary (thymus aplasia) or secondary (lymphatic leukemia and other neoplasms) immune insufficiency, noticeable improvement in immunologic capacity was achieved by administration of a thymosin fraction (from calf thymus). However, it appears that long-term therapy is necessary to maintain this effect. In contrast, one patient with combined immune deficiency exhibited no improvement of immunologic function after administration of thymosin. This finding may indicate that in certain cases of immune deficiency later steps in differentiation are not disturbed and that developmental disturbances exist at the level of the lymphopoietic stem cells or prolymphocytes.

Bone Marrow Transplant

In contrast to organ transplants, bone marrow transplants consist of the transfer of immunocompetent cells or their precursors. If the recipient and donor are not identical histogenetically, the transplant can lead to a further complication: the graft-versus-host reaction. Therefore bone marrow transplant assumes a particular place among the organ transplants.

Cases for bone marrow transplants include immune-deficiency diseases, aplastic anemia and severe hemoglobulinopathies, leukemias, and radiation damage. According to results thus far, identical twins (syngenic transplant) or HLA-A, HLA-B, HLA-C, and HLA-D identical siblings (allogenic transplantation) are acceptable as donors.

Recipients of syngenic bone marrow do not need any pretreatment with immunosuppressives (however, they may undergo cytoreductive treatment); the same is true for patients with severe, combined (total) immune deficiency who are recipients of syngenic or allogenic bone marrow. All other recipients of allogenic bone marrow must be pretreated with immunosuppressives in order for the bone marrow to be "taken." Patients with aplastic anemia are usually pretreated with cyclophosphamide, 50 mg/kg/day on each of 4 days followed 36 h later by the marrow infusion.

Acute leukemia is pretreated with chemotherapeutic (antileukemic) and total-body irradiation:

Six and five days before irradiation, patients receive 60 mg/kg cyclophosphamide in addition to antileukemic treatment. Irradiation is applied as total-body irradiation with 1,000 rad from two opposing sources (^{60}C, two sources are necessary to achieve homogenous irradiation).

With the donor under narcosis, the bone marrow is taken from the iliac crest by multiple aspirations, usually 400–800 ml. Using filtration through a sieve, a single-cell suspension is produced. The number of cells transferred intravenously can vary between 10^8 and 10^9 per kg. In the presence of severe immunodeficiency, purified stem cells in small but repeated doses might be infused. Whether the purification of stem cells is necessary and advantageous for the success of a bone marrow transplant is strongly affirmed by some (van Bekkum) but questioned by others.

The acceptance of a transplant is evident from the fast increase in the numbers of granulocytes, reticulocytes, and thrombocytes in the blood between the 10 th and 30 th day after transplantation. Chimerism, i.e., the survival of the donor's cells, can be verified by the presence of donor blood group markers, immunoglobulin allotypes, blood cell enzyme allotypes, or chromosomal markers (sex chromosome).

Acute graft versus host reactions are characterized by hepatomegaly with increase in transaminase level and jaundice, intestinal disturbances, decreased in blood cell counts, and erythematous eruptions. Chronic graft-versus-host reactions cause autoimmune-like symptoms, i.e., scleroderma-like skin alterations (see p. 395), sicca-syndrome (see p. 390), and chronic aggressive hepatitis (see p. 385).

Prophylactic immunosuppressive therapy post-transplantation consists of administration of corticosteroid, cyclophosphamide, methotrexate, or cyclosporine A for the first 100 days; with the occurrence of an acute graft-versus-host reaction, corticosteroid doses are increased and anti-lymphocyte serum (or gamma globulin) is additionally administered. In cases of chronic graft-versus-host reactions, a long-term therapy with steroids and azathioprine is necessary. Whether a germ-free environment (gnotobiotic unit, lamina flow) is an advantage for the survival of the patient after transplantation, except for the presence of immunodeficiency, is not yet clear.

The prognosis of bone marrow transplantation has improved considerably since the first operations at the end of the 1960 s. In most transplant centers, up to 80% of patients with aplastic anemia who had received syngeneic bone marrow had been cured. Patients with aplastic anemia who had received transfusions prior to the marrow graft of allogeneic, HLA-identical do-

nors, and were conditioned for engraftment by the administration of cyclophosphamide recovered to about 50%. In contrast, about 95% of the patients who had never received blood transfusion have been cured under the same regimen.

The prognosis for leukemia is not as good as for aplastic anemia. In the Seattle group, 37% of leukemic patients pretreated with cyclophosphamide and total body irradiation (TBI), and who had received syngeneic (identical twins) bone marrow, survived in remission more than 7 years following transplantation.

After allogeneic (HLA-identical) bone marrow transplantation, approximately 25% of those with acute lymphatic leukemia (ALL), and about 17% of those with acute myeloic leukemia (AML) survived more than 2 years. More than half of patients with acute myeloic or lymphatic leukemia who had received a bone marrow graft during remission showed long-term survial.

The causes of death in bone marrow transplantation in the presence of aplastic anemia or leukemia are rejection reactions, graft-versus-host reactions, infections (general, and specific as cytomegalovirus and pneumocystis carinii), recurrent leukemia (but not aplasia!), and immunodeficiency (humoral as well as cellular, of unknown etiology).

Of 14 patients in the Minnesota Group (Good) with severe immunodeficiency (autosomal recessive, sex-linked immunodeficiency and Swiss-type agammaglobulinemia) who received bone marrow transplants, five survived more than 2 years; of these, three patients were able to lead a normal life for 3, 4, and 5 years, respectively. In most cases, the cause of death was a combination of graft-versus-host reaction and infection (sepsis).

Blood Transfusion

Repeated transfusion leads to the formation of leukagglutinating and lymphocytotoxic anti-HLA antibodies. The presence of such antibodies in polytransfused patients can lead to nonhemolytic, febrile, and urticaria-accompanying reactions. However, there is no absolute correlation between antibody titer and the intensity of the reaction.

To prevent such reactions with antileukocytic antibodies patients can receive leukocyte- and platelet-free blood. In this way, the numbers of leukocytes and thrombocytes are sharply reduced by mechanical methods.

Thrombocyte Transfusion. In patients who have antibodies against HLA antigens – even when clinically no transfusion reaction occurs – the survival time of leukocytes and thrombocytes is sharply reduced because they are destroyed and eliminated. Antibodies against platelet-specific antigens (Zw, Ko, and Pl^e) in general play a minimal role in this reaction, although severe cases of incompatibility with the Pl^A system due to the presence of anti-Pl antibodies have been observed.

It is therefore advantageous for patients who need regular platelet transfusions to use HLA-identical, at best related, donors.

Leukocyte Transfusion. Leukocyte transfusions are used primarily as preventive or curative measures for infection in severe aplasia or agranulocytosis. Because the survival time of granulocytes and monocytes is short (half-life less then 6 h), the transfusion must be repeated frequently at short intervals in order to be effective. Also in these cases donors should be HLA-typed and only those who are most similar to the recipient should be chosen. Whether alloantigens are significant on neutrophilic leukocytes (NA, NB, and the 9 system) is unknown. However, it is known that neutropenia in a newborn can result from maternal antibodies against NA or NB.

For a more detailed description of erythrocyte and plasma transfusions, see Chap. 8.

References

Albert E, Götze D (1977) The major histocompatibility system in man. In: Götze D (ed) The organisation of the major histocompatibility system in man and animals. Springer, Berlin Heidelberg New York, p 7

Burnet FM (1969) Self and non-self. Cambridge University Press, Cambridge

Cantor H, Boyse EA (1975) Functional subclasses of T lymphocytes bearing different Ly antigen. I. The generation of functionally distinct T cell subclasses is a differentiative process independent of antigens. J Exp Med 141:1376

Cantor H, Boyse EA (1975) Functional subclasses of T lymphocytes bearing different Ly antigens. II. Cooperation between subclasses of Ly$^+$ cells in generation of killer cell activity. J Exp Med 141:1390

Dresser DW, Mitchison NA (1968) The mechanism of immunological paralysis. Adv Immunol 8:129

Eisen HN (1974) Immunology. In: Introduction to molecular and cellular principles of the immune response. Harper and Row, New York

Feldman M, Nossal GJ (1972) Tolerance enhancement and the regulation between T cells, B cells and macrophages. Transplant rev 13:3

Floersheim GL (1971) Transplantationbiologie. Springer, Berlin Heidelberg New York

Götze D (ed) (1977) The major histocompatibility system in man and animals. Springer, Berlin Heidelberg New York

Gold P (1971) Organ transplantation. In: Freedman SO (ed) Clinical immunology. Harper and Row, New York, pp 419–464

Hašek MA, et al. (1962) Mechanisms of immunological tolerance. Pub House Czechoslovac Acad Sci, Prag

Heimpel H, Gordon-Smith EC, Heit W, Kubanck B (eds) (1979) Aplastic anemia. Springer, Berlin Heidelberg New York

Howard J, Mitchison NA (1975) Immunological tolerance. Prog Allergy 18:43

Klein J (1975) the biology of the mouse histocompatibility-2 complex. Springer, Berlin Heidelberg New York

Landy M, Braun W (eds) (1969) Immunological tolerance. A reassessment of mechanisms of the immune response. Academic, New York

MacLennan ICM, Harding B (1974) Workshop report: Non-T cytoxicity in vitro. In: Brent L, Holborow J (eds) Progress in immunology II, vol 3. North-Holland, Amsterdam, pp 347–350

Medawar PB (1961) Immunological tolerance. Nobel lecture. Nature 189:14

Nossal GJV (1971) Recent advances in immunological tolerance. In: Prog Immunol Academic, New York, p 666

Rood J van, van Leeuwen A, Termijtelen A, Kuening JJ (1976) B cell antibodies, Ia-like determinants, and their relation to MLC determinants in man. Transplant Rev 30:122

Santos GW, Elfenbein GJ, Tutschka PJ (1979) Bone marrow transplantation. Transplant Proc 11:182

Snell GD, Dausset J, Nathenson S (1976) Histocompatibility. Academic, New York

Thomas ED, Storb R, Clift RA, Fefer A, Johnson EL, Neiman PE, Lerner KG, Glucksberg H, Buckner D (1975) Bone marrow transplantation. Part I. N Engl J Med 292:832; ibid Part II. N Engl J Med 292:895

Voisin G (1971) Immunological facilitation, a broadening of the concept of the enhancement phenomenon. Prog Allergy 15:328

Weigle WO (1973) Immunological unresponsiveness. Adv Immunol 16:61

Chapter 10   Hypersensitivity

Ivan Mota

Contents

Hypersensitivity

Since it was established that an initial contact of the organism with certain infectious-toxic or noxious agents may result in the production of antibodies which protect the individual by lysing, neutralizing, or eliminating the foreign substance, numerous observations have indicated that the immunologic reaction does not always benefit the organism, and the organism is often damaged as s result. This type of harmful reaction is called an allergic or hypersensitivity reaction. The organism, tissue, or cell capable of exhibiting a hypersensitivity reaction is said to be sensitized. The allergic reactions, being immunologic reactions, are extremely specific, with the sensitized organism reacting exclusively with the antigenic determinant used for immunization or a similar structure. Hypersensitivity reactions are separated into two different types according to the time that elapses between the contact of the sensitized organism with the antigen and the macroscopic observation of the allergic phenomenon. Thus, whereas the so-called immediate hypersensitivity reactions require only minutes or perhaps a few hours to appear, delayed hypersensitivity reactions develop only after many hours. Today, although this criterion of the reaction time remains valid for classification of hypersensitivity reactions, it is understood that more important differences separate the two types. Thus, whereas reactions of the immediate type include all the reactions reproducible by various types of antibodies present in the serum – and which consequently can be transferred from one individual to another by antiserum – reactions of the delayed type depend upon sensitized cells and, therefore, are not transferable by antisera, but only by cells. The transfer of an immune state by cells is called adoptive immunization because the recipient organism adopts the cells of the donor that confer upon it the immunity acquired in another organism. The phenomenon of transferring a hypersensitivity state by cells is termed adoptive sensitization. Adoptive immunity as well as adoptive sensitization are possible only between isogenic individuals. Notably, whereas delayed hypersensitivity is transferable only by cells, immediate hypersensitivity is transferable either by antibodies or by cells.

Classification

The following scheme summarizes the classification of various types of hypersensitivity. Immediate hypersensitivity reactions include anaphylaxis, cytotoxic reactions, and the reactions due to antigen–antibody complexes. In all types of immediate hypersensitivity, an antigen–antibody reaction occurs, resulting in alterations in the tissues. In anaphylaxis, the antibody bound to the cells provokes cell alterations when it reacts with an antigen; in cytotoxic reactions, it is the antigen that is associated with the cells. In reactions due to antigen–antibody complexes, neither the antigen nor the antibody is associated with the cells; the reaction occurs in the extracellular fluid. In addition, whereas

the last two reactions depend upon the presence of complement, the anaphylactic reactions proceed without activation of this system. Evidence indicates that in almost all these reactions, the response of the organism is due to the action of substances formed or liberated by the tissues through the antigen–antibody reaction. These substances, which usually possess intense pharmacologic activity, are called pharmacologic mediators. Diverse active substances are also produced in the delayed hypersensitivity reaction.

Hypersensitivity reactions	Immediate or Humoral	Anaphylaxis (type I) Cytotoxic reactions (type II) Reactions by antigen-antibody complexes (type III)
	Delayed or Cellular	Due to tuberculin or other proteins, infectious germs. Due to purified proteins. Due to simple chemical substances (contact dermatitis, type IV)

Anaphylaxis (Type I)

In an animal, the first injection of a nontoxic antigen (sensitizing dose) does not cause any reaction; however, after an interval of 2–3 weeks (sensitizing period), a second dose of the same antigen produces a violent reaction (symptomatically diverse depending upon the animal involved), which frequently is fatal. This phenomenon was observed for the first time by Portier and Richet (1902), who were investigating the toxic effect of extracts from the *Actiniaria* (sea anemone). Portier and Richet named this phenomenon anaphylaxis to indicate a status contrary to that of immunity (*ana*, against; and *phylaxis*, protection). Anaphylaxis later was observed in many laboratories where horse serum and other antigenic mixtures were injected into guinea pigs for experimental purposes, and in human beings injected with antisera for treatment of infectious diseases. Anaphylaxis can appear either as a general phenomenon, affecting the entire organism,

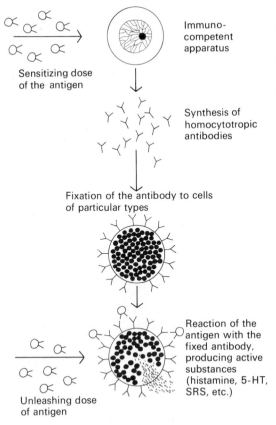

Sensitizing dose
of the antigen

Immuno-
competent
apparatus

Synthesis of
homocytotropic
antibodies

Fixation of the antibody to cells
of particular types

Reaction of the
antigen with the
fixed antibody,
producing active
substances
(histamine, 5-HT,
SRS, etc.)

Unleashing dose
of antigen

Fig. 10.1. Mechanism of the anaphylactic reaction

as always occurs when the antigen is injected intravenously, or as a localized phenomenon such as occurs when the antigen is injected extravascularly – e.g., intradermally or sub-cutaneously. The former is called systemic anaphylaxis, whereas the latter is termed local anaphylaxis. In either of these situations, the presence of the antigen, the specific antibody, and the cellular element to which the antibody is fixed are indispensable. The reaction between the antigen and the antibody results in a response of the target cell, i.e., the cell to which the antibody is fixed, which gives rise to the formation or liberation of mediators (Fig. 10.1). A summary of the symptomatology of systemic anaphylaxis, or anaphylactic shock, in different animal species is found in Table 10.1. The symptomatology of anaphylactic shock, although different for each species, results from a spasm of the smooth musculature, from an increase in capillary permeability, from an alteration in the distribution of the circulatory volume of the blood, or from a combination of these factors.

In this chapter, we first examine anaphylaxis in the guinea pig and then in man. In the interpretation of the latter is included a summation of thoughts obtained from clinical and experimental observations.

Anaphylaxis in the Guinea Pig

The guinea pig has been the species of choice for the study of anaphylactic phenomena due to the facility with which it becomes sensitized and the intensity with which it reacts

Table 10.1. Characteristics of anaphylaxis in different species

Species	Shock organ	Active substances liberated	Principal symptoms
Man	Lung + larynx	Histamine, kinins, SRS	Edema of the bronchia and larynx; emphysema
Dog	Hepatic veins	Histamine, kinins, SRS	Hepatic congestion; hemorrhage of intestinal mucosa
Guinea pig	Lung	Histamine, kinins, SRS	Emphysema
Rabbit	Pulmonary, circulation	Histamine, serotonin, SRS	Obstruction of the pulmonary capillaries by micro-thrombi of platelets and leukocytes. Failure of the right ventricle. Congestion of the abdominal organs
Rat	Intestines	Histamine, serotonin, SRS	Circulatory collapse, intestinal hemorrhage
Mouse	Intestines	Histamine, serotonin, SRS	Circulatory collapse, Intestinal hemorrhage

to a second contact with the antigen. This species can be sensitized by any means of administration of the sensitizing dose, even by inhalation of an aerosol containing the antigen. A few weeks later, further contact with the same antigen, particularly intravenously, provokes intense symptomatology, characterized by severe puritis in the muzzle, contractions in the masticatory muscles, sneezing, spasmodic coughing, intense dyspnea, relaxation of sphincters with elimination of feces and urine, and in the final phase prostration with violent contractions of the respiratory muscles. The violence of the shock produces the death of the animal within a matter of minutes as a consequence of asphyxia resulting from constriction of the smooth musculature of the bronchia and bronchioli. Postmortem examination discloses lung emphysema due to retention of air in the alveoli from expiratory difficulties. The predominance of pulmonary alterations and of death by respiratory insufficiency characterizes the lung as the "shock organ" in the guinea pig. At an early date Dale (1920) attributed anaphylactic phenomena in the guinea pig. He noted the essential similarity between anaphylactic shock in this species and the shock produced by the injection of histamine. Histamine liberated from sensitized tissues by the antigen was later obtained from the livers of dogs and the isolated lung of the guinea pig. These were the first demonstrations of the existence of a mediator in anaphylactic reactions. Acute anaphylaxis in the guinea pig appears to be due exclusively to the action of histamine, to which the smooth musculature of this species is extremely sensitive.

Protracted Shock. In contrast to the efficiency of the intravenous mode, sensitized animals in which the antigen is injected subcutaneously or intraperitoneally frequently do not exhibit acute respiratory symptoms, but present a different clinical picture. Protracted shock, as this manifestation is called, is characterized by prostration, hypothermia, and hypotension, with death occurring

many hours after the animal is subjected to the second dose of the antigen. Upon postmortem examination, the emphysema characteristic of acute anaphylaxis is not observed, but hemorrhagic lesions are visible on the intestines. The nature and mechanism of this type of shock are unknown.

Passive Anaphylaxis. Shortly after recognition of anaphylaxis as an immunologic phenomenon, its transmission to an unsensitized animal by antisera obtained from actively sensitized animals was observed, thus demonstrating the dependence of this phenomenon upon the antibodies existing in the serum. Passive sensitization was extremely useful in the study of anaphylactic phenomena, for it permitted their study with known quantities of homologous antibodies or with different classes, subclasses, and fragments of antibodies. All the phenomena of anaphylaxis obtained in the actively sensitized animal are also reproducible after passive sensitization. A primary insight resulting from the study of passive anaphylaxis was recognition of the existence of the so-called latent or sensitization period.

Sensitization Period. After the injection of the sensitizing dose of antibody, it is usually necessary that a given period of time elapses before administration of a second antigen dose produces an anaphylactic reaction. The interval between the application of the antibody and that of the antigen is called the latent or sensitization period. What happens during this period? This question remains without a definitive answer despite numerous attempts to provide one. This necessary interval suggests the existence of a process of fixation of the antibody to special receptors existing in certain types of cells of the tissues. Supportive of this idea is the fact that certain types of antibodies require a long sensitization period for the antigen to provoke an anaphylactic reaction of maximum intensity.

The necessity for fixation of the antibody to obtain an anaphylactic reaction is a possible explanation for the observation that antibodies of a certain animal species are not always capable of transmitting sensitivity to another species. For example, the guinea pig can be passively sensitized by rabbit, monkey, and human antibodies, but not by horse, goat, cattle, chicken, or rat antibodies. The nature of the receptors existing on the cells for fixation of the antibodies is unknown, but they are probably located on the mastocytes and basophilic leukocytes.

Experiments in which the quantity of antiserum was varied and the sensitization period was constant have demonstrated a direct relationship between the quantity of antibody used for the sensitization and production of an anaphylactic reaction of maximum intensity, thus demonstrating the existence of an optimum antibody dose above which the effects are not modified. These experiments have also shown that, by increasing the quantity of antibody, one can reduce the sensitization period practically to zero when the quantity of antibody injected reaches levels far above the optimum dose for a sensitization period of 48 h. The anaphylaxis obtained under these conditions, i.e., with a large quantity of antibody and without a sensitization period, exhibits a clinical picture similar to the anaphylaxis obtained with small amounts of antibody after the sensitization period. It is called anaphylaxis by aggregation.

Passive Cutaneous Anaphylaxis. One of the simplest and most elegant techniques for the study of anaphylaxis is passive cutaneous anaphylaxis (PCA), which consists of sensitizing a small area of skin by intradermal injection of antiserum and, after an adequate sensitization period, injecting the antigen intravenously together with a dye such as Evans blue to facilitate reading of the reaction. The antigen rapidly reaches the sensitized site, reacts with the antibody and, by a mechanism to be discussed subsequently, produces an increase in local capillary permeability evidenced by the blue stain taken on by the area (Fig. 10.2). Passive cutaneous anaphylaxis also can be obtained by injecting the antibody into the blood, consequently, all of the animal's skin is sensitized. In this case, after an appropriate period of sensitization, the antigen is injected into the skin at any location.

Fig. 10.2. Passive cutaneous anaphylaxis (*PCA*) in rats induced with reaginic antibody (IgE): *C* PCA in untreated control animal; *B* PCA in animal previously treated with serotonin inhibitor (diethylamide of D-bromolysergic acid (BOL-148); *M* PCA in animal treated with antihistamine (mepyramine); *MB* PCA in animal treated with BOL-148 and mepyramine. The necessity for the simultaneous presence of histamine and serotonin inhibitors to completely abolish the reaction indicates that these two mediators are responsible for the increase in capillary permeability that occurs in PCA of the rat induced with reaginic antibody. Mota I (1963) Life Sci 12:917

Inverse Passive Cutaneous Anaphylaxis. Inverse passive cutaneous anaphylaxis (IPCA) is produced when, instead of the antibody, the antigen is first injected into the skin and, after a sensitization period, the antibody is injected into the blood. The reaction is called inverse because of the inversion of the order of injection. It should be noted that IPCA is possible only when the antigen is a gamma globulin of a species whose antibody is capable of sensitizing the recipient species by direct PCA. Thus the guinea pig can be prepared for IPCA by using as antigen rabbit gamma globulin that is injected into the skin; there it is fixed to the cellular receptors as if it were an antibody. Later, upon reacting with the anti-rabbit gamma-globulin antibody injected intravenously, it produces a local anaphylactic reaction. However, if horse gamma globulin is used as antigen (which does not sensitize the guinea pig when used as antibody), subsequent injection of anti-equine gamma globulin does not produce anaphylaxis. This is explained by the apparent incapacity of the equine gamma globulin to attach to the cellular receptors of the guinea pig.

Homocytotropic and Heterocytotropic Antibodies. So-called homocytotropic antibody is capable of sensitizing the same species that produced it (it may or may not be capable of sensitizing another species), whereas heterocytotropic antibody is incapable of sensitizing the same species that produced it, but is capable of sensitizing another species. Studies with anti-DNP and anti-picryl antibodies produced by hyperimmunized guinea pigs demonstrated the existence in this species of two populations of IgG possessing the same specificity, but differing in electrophoretic mobility. The population of antibodies migrating more rapidly was designated IgG_1 and the slower one IgG_2. When the biologic activity of these subclasses was analyzed, it was shown that whereas the IgG_1 antibodies were capable of passively sensitizing the guinea pig, the IgG_2 were incapable of doing so, but were capable of sensitizing another species such as the mouse. IgG_1 and IgG_2 of the guinea pig are typical examples of homocytotropic and heterocytotropic antibodies, respectively. The homocytotropic antibodies appear capable of attaching only to homologous cellular receptors (or those of a closely related species), whereas the heterocytotropic antibodies do not have this capacity. The activity of the heterocytotropic antibodies is not clearly understood, but it is attributed hypothetically to the fact that these antibodies have molecular configurations capable of adapting to the cellular receptors of other species.

Among the homocytotropic antibodies, two types are distinguished (type I and type II) which are present in almost all species studied and are easily differentiable by their physicochemical and biologic properties (Table 10.2). Type I homocytotropic antibodies are characterized by high serum levels; by being resistant to heat (50 °C) and to treatment with mercaptoethanol followed by alkylation; by crossing the placental barrier; by exhibiting a short optimum sensitization period (2–4 h); and by persisting in the skin after passive sensitization for a maximum period of 24–72 h. The known type I antibodies are subclasses of IgG. The 7S IgG_1 immunoglobulin of the guinea pig is a typical example of this group. Type II homocytotropic antibodies are characterized by appearing in unusually low serum levels; by being destroyed by heat treatment and mercaptoethanol followed by alkylation; by not crossing the placental barrier; by possessing an optimum sensitization period of 48–72 h; and by persisting in the skin for many days after sensitization (>30). Some of the type II antibodies, such as the reaginic antibodies in man, rabbit, guinea pig, rat, and mouse (and perhaps also in other species) belong to a distinct class of antibodies, IgE. One peculiarity of IgE antibodies is the fact that they appear in elevated levels in the sera of individuals who are carriers of parasitic infection, particularly helminths (see p. 326). This contrasts with the modest levels obtained when the dead parasites or antigens extracted from them are injected into the organism – even when rein-

Table 10.2. Characteristics of the homocytotropic antibodies

	Human[a] Type		Guinea pig[b] Type		Rat Type		Mouse Type		Dog Type	Rabbit Type	
	I	II	I	II	I	II	I	II	I	I	II
Immunoglobulin	IgG (?)	IgE	IgG	IgE	IgG$_2$	IgE	IgG	IgE	IgE	IgG	IgE
Electrophoretic mobility		$\gamma_{1/2}$	$\gamma_{1/2}$	?	$\gamma_{1/2}$	$\gamma_{1/2}$	$\gamma_{1/2}$	$\gamma_{1/2}$	$\gamma_{1/2}$	$\gamma_{1/2}$	$\gamma_{1/2}$
Sedimentation coefficient		7S	7S	?	?	7S	7S	?	7S		
Complement fixation	0	0	?	+	0	0	?	?	+		0
Thermolability	+	0	+	0	+	0	+	+	0	0	0
Persistence in the skin	28 d	2–4 d	45 d	24 h	31 d	24 h	15 d	15 d	?		17 d
Optimum sensitization period	48 h	4–6 h	48 h	2–4 h	48–72 h	1–3 h	72 h		24–48 h	48 h	72 h
Transfer across placental barrier	0	+	?	?	0	?	?	?	?	?	?
Quantity present in the serum	Traces	+ + + +	Traces	+ + + +	Traces	+ + + +	Traces	+ + + +	Traces	Traces	+ + + +

[a] The existence of a type I homocytotropic antibody is probable, although not definite. Various works indicate the existence of a homocytotropic antibody belonging to IgG. In the dog, a type I homocytotropic antibody has not yet been identified

[b] Apparently, more than one type I homocytotropic antibody exists in the guinea pig

forced with an adjuvant. For example, high levels of reaginic antibodies directed against antigenic components of *S. mansoni* are encountered in individuals with schistosomiasis, as well as in monkeys and rabbits experimentally infected with this helminth. In contrast, single or repeated injections of extracts of the adult worm or of cercariae induce them only in modest levels. The reason for this difference is not known.

Antibody Fixation and Cellular Receptors. The existence of a sensitization period in anaphylaxis suggests the necessity for the occurrence of a union or fixation between the antibody molecule and cellular receptors. The existence of the latter, of which little is known, is inferred from experiments in which specific fixation of antibody molecules to the cell membrane has been observed. In man and higher primates, the fixation of IgE molecules on basophilic leukocytes and mastocytes is practically specific, because other classes of antibodies such as IgG are bound to these same cells by a factor of 100 less than the number of IgE molecules fixed. With the use of ^{125}I-labeled IgE, the number of receptors for IgE on the surface of basophils has been calculated to be 30,000–90,000. The observation that the IgE molecules fixed to the cell can be dissociated from the receptors (at pH 4) without injuring them indicates that the union between the IgE molecules and the receptors is reversible and not covalent. Various methods have been used to isolate these receptors, and it is possible that their chemical structure will soon be elucidated.

Present understanding of that part of the antibody molecule responsible for fixation to the cell receptor is incomplete. However, PCA experiments with antibody fragments obtained by enzymatic degradation yielded some information concerning the part of the antibody molecule responsible for the union. It appears that the capacity of the guinea pig IgG$_1$ antibody to attach to tissues and the inability of the IgG$_2$ of the same species to do the same depends upon differences in the structure of these molecules. Guinea pig IgG$_1$ and IgG$_2$ antibodies possess identical Fab and Fd fragments, yet differ in the antigenic properties of the Fcagment. It is possible, therefore, that the Fc-fragment of the IgG_1 possesses a molecular configuration that permits its fixation to the cellular receptors – a configuration lacking in the IgG_2. The importance of the Fc fragment in the fixation of antibody to the tissues was demonstrated using the PCA and IPCA techniques. In experiments in which guinea pigs were sensitized with whole (control) antibodies or with Fab and univalent 5S fragments obtained from the same antibody through papain digestion, the second injection of antigen produced PCA only in the locations sensitized with the whole molecule or with the fragment containing the Fc part. The same results were obtained with IPCA (Fig. 10.3). In these experiments, guinea pigs were first injected intradermally with the Fab and Fc fragments obtained from rabbit antibodies and subsequently were given an intravenous injection of anti-rabbit gamma globulin. The antigen–antibody reaction

produced an anaphylactic reaction only at the site injected with the Fc fragment capable of binding to the cellular receptors. The experiments pointed definitively to the Fc fragment as being responsible for this fixation.

The Fc fragments of IgG and IgE include $C_\gamma 2$, $C_\gamma 3$, and $C_\varepsilon 2$, and $C_\varepsilon 3$ and $C_\varepsilon 4$ domains, respectively. When subjected to different processes of enzymatic digestion, the Fc fragment can be cleaved into smaller fragments composed of either the C-terminal portion, corresponding roughly to $C_\gamma 3$ (in the case of IgG) and to $C_\varepsilon 3$ and $C_\varepsilon 4$ (in the case of IgE), or corresponding to the N-terminal portion of $C_\gamma 2$ and $C_\varepsilon 2$. Subsequent experiments investigating the function of the subfragments of immunoglobulin produced from Fc pieces suggest that the entire Fc region is necessary for antibody fixation. It should be remembered that the anaphylactic reaction is a complex phenomenon, and even when it appears that the entire Fc region must be intact in order to be bound, it does not mean that every domain takes part in the fixation.

These notions and the fact that the primary structure of the ε chain is fully known notwithstanding, the molecular basis of antibody cytotropism is not yet understood. Still, it is accepted that fixation of an IgE molecule to the mastocyte membrane involves at least two fixation sites localized on $C_\varepsilon 3$ and $C_\varepsilon 4$. These two fixation sites differ in localization and cellular specificity. The primary sites, binding only to the mastocyte and basophil receptors, function only as recognition units and are localized in $C_\varepsilon 4$. There are, furthermore, secondary, nonspecific binding sites that bind to receptors of different cells and are possibly localized on $C_\varepsilon 3$ as well as on $C_\varepsilon 4$. These findings may signify that the binding site for the mast cell membrane differs from a second site that is necessary for the secretion of mediator.

Ab or fragment used for sensitization   PCA

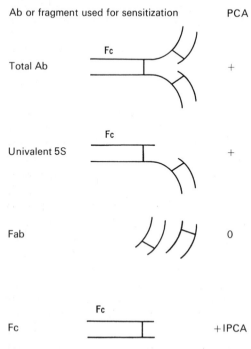

Fig. 10.3. Efficiency of the univalent 5S, Fab, and Fc fragments in inducing direct or inverse passive cutaneous anaphylaxis

Valence of the Antigen and Antibody in Anaphylactic Reactions. The use of antibodies and antigens of known valence in PCA experiments led to the conclusion that whereas the antigen must be at least bivalent, the antibody can be monovalent, although two molecules of antibody must be involved in the reaction. This conclusion is based on experiments in which the efficiency of monovalent, divalent, or multivalent haptens in producing anaphylaxis was studied, verifying that the univalent haptens were incapable of producing PCA whereas equimolar solutions of divalent or multivalent haptens demonstrated equal efficiency for production of PCA. In other experiments with the same system, researchers studied the capacity of a monovalent hybrid hapten containing one BPO grouping (benzylpenicilloil) and one DNP grouping to produce PCA reactions in guinea pigs sensitized with anti-BPO or with anti-DNP, or with anti-BPO and anti-DNP simultaneously. Only immunization with monovalent hybrid hapten in animals simultaneously sensitized with anti-BPO and anti-DNP led to a PCA reaction. It was also shown that monovalent fragments such as the 5 S fragment or artificially prepared monovalent antibodies are capable of producing anaphylaxis when bound to the target cell. It is accepted, then, that at least two conditions need to be satisfied for an anaphylactic reaction to occur: (1) fixation of the antibody by the Fc piece to the cellular receptors; (2) reaction of the fixed antibody with bi- or multivalent antigens to form a complex involving two or more antibody molecules. Apparently, it is sufficient that the antigen molecule forms a bridge to unite the two active sites of two antibody molecules bound to the tissues (Fig. 10.4).

Mechanism of Anaphylaxis

Pharmacologic Mediators. The term mediator is applied to substances liberated directly or indirectly as a consequence of antigen–antibody combination that are responsible for the various manifestations of immediate hypersensitivity. Some of the mediators exist preformed in the cells; some are formed in the cells during the hypersensitivity reaction,

Fig. 10.4 a, b. Activation of target cell (mastocytes or basophilic leukocytes) through formation of bridges between 2 IgE molecules **a** through the specific antigen that binds to the antibodies found on the cell membrane, or **b** through anti-antibodies that react with the cell-membrane-bound IgE molecules

whereas others are formed by the activation of humoral enzymatic systems. Mediators can be liberated from the cells by cytotoxic mechanisms and by noncytotoxic mechanisms. In cytotoxic liberation, irreversible lesions of the cellular membrane occur along with loss of control of cellular permeability, which leads to the loss to the external medium of the mediator and other cell constituents. Cytotoxic liberation results generally from the lytic action of the terminal components of the complement system activated in the classic or the alternate manner (see Chap. 5). With anaphylactic (nontoxic) liberation, selective passage of the mediator(s) to the exterior occurs without either irreversible lesions in the cellular membrane or the death of the cell. Noncytotoxic liberation probably involves a mechanism equal or similar to that of secretion (see Table 10.3).

Histamine. Histamine, a product of the decarboxylation of histidine, which is widely distributed in nature, is located in mammalian tissue primarily in the granules of the mastocytes. In the blood of some species such as man, histamine is localized in the leukocytes, particularly in basophils,

Table 10.3. Mediators for anaphylactic ilactious

Mediators	Origin	Identifying properties
Histamine	Mastocytes	Contracts guinea pig ileum
	Basophils	Does not contract rat uterus
	Platelets	Inhibited by the antihistamines
Serotonin	Enterochromaffin cells	Contracts guinea pig ileum and rat uterus
	Mastocytes	
	Platelets	Inhibited by lysergic acid
Lys-Arg-Pro-Pro-Gly-Phe-Ser-Pro-Phe-Arg Bradykinin	Plasma α-globulin	Contracts guinea pig ileum and rat uterus. Inhibited neither by lysergic acid nor by antihistamines
Slow-reacting substance (SRS)	Mastocytes Polymorphonuclear cells?	Contracts guinea pig ilusm. Does *not* contract rat uterus
(Unknown structure)	Others?	Not inhibited by antihistamines
Prostaglandins	?	Contracts rat stomach and colon; Contracts chicken rectum
ECF–A	Mastocytes	Chemotactic for eosinophils

whereas in rabbit blood it is also found in the platelets. Histamine causes contraction of the smooth muscle of the intestine and uterus of the guinea pig; of the bronchi in man, guinea pig, dog, and cat; and of the smooth muscle of the veins and arterioles of various species; in addition, it causes vasodilation and increasing permeability of the capillaries. In anaphylactic reactions, histamine is liberated from the tissues of numerous species and, in some of them such as the guinea pig, the intravenous injection of histamine reproduces a clinical picture similar to that of anaphylactic shock. The histamine liberated from the tissues of various species for the most part originates from the mastocytes, the basophilic leukocytes, and/or the platelets. The importance of histamine as a mediator of anaphylaxis depends upon the species considered and particularly upon the sensitivity of its smooth muscle to this substance. Thus, histamine is the most important mediator in anaphylactic shock of the guinea pig, contributes considerably to hypotension in anaphylactic shock of the dog, and appears to be responsible for certain phenomena of anaphylaxis in man, such as edema of the glottis and urticaria. In other species such as the rat and mouse, its role in anaphylaxis appears minor.

Serotonin. Serotonin (5-hydroxytryptamine) results from the decarboxylation of tryptophan after introduction of an –OH group in the indole ring. In most species, it is encountered principally in the intestinal mucosa, in the brain, and in the platelets. In the rat and mouse, it also is localized in mastocyte granules. This substance is liberated, during anaphylaxis, by the platelets of rabbit blood and by the mastocytes of rat and mouse tissue. In the mouse, it also appears to originate from the argentaffin cells of the intestinal tract: Serotonin produces contraction of smooth muscle and augments capillary permeability in many species. There is no evidence indicating its participation in the anaphylactic phenomena in man and in the guinea pig. It appears to play a more important role in the rat and mouse, due to the greater sensitivity of their tissues to this substance. It has been suggested that the simultaneous action of serotonin and histamine is of fundamental importance in the anaphylactic shock of the mouse.

Bradykinin. The kinins or kallidins, which are better known as bradykinin or kallidin II, originate from precursors or kininogens (α-globulins) existing in the plasma, under the influence of enzymes called kallikreins:
(1) Bradykininogen + kallikrein $\rightarrow$ lysylbradykinin
   (decapeptide) or kallidin I
(2) Lysylbradykinin + aminopeptidase $\rightarrow$ bradykinin
   (nonapeptide) or kallidin II.
Bradykinin produces contraction of the smooth musculature, increases capillary permeability, and has a greater vasodilatory action than any other known substance. Experimental data suggest its participation in anaphylactic phenomena. It has been detected during anaphylactic shock in the blood of various species, and a diminution of bradykininogen occurs in the plasma of the rabbit and dog during anaphylaxis.

Slow-Reacting Substance. This substance, usually called SRS, is characterized by the ability to cause gradual contraction of the smooth musculature of various species. It is an acid substance, soluble in water, dialyzable, and of unknown chemical nature. Unlike histamine and serotinin, it does not preexist in the tissues, but is formed during anaphylaxis. It was detected initially in the perfusion fluid of the isolated lungs of sensitized guinea pigs – and later in the lungs of man, rabbit, and monkey. Human bronchi are extremely sensitive to the action of SRS, unlike guinea pig bronchi. SRS has been detected together with histamine in the perfusion fluid from lungs of asthmatic patients after the addition of antigen to which the patients have been sensitized. It is possible that SRS plays an important role in human asthma, contributing to the contraction of the bronchi.

Eosinophilotactic Factor of Anaphylaxis. It has been observed that a factor capable of specifically attracting eosinophils appears in the tissues of human or other species in anaphylactic reactions mediated by IgE. The liberation of this factor is independent of the complement system. Eosinophilotactic factor of anaphylaxis (ECF-A) exists preformed in the tissues and, at least in the rat, is associated with the mastocyte granules. It is possible that the old observation of an infiltration of eosinophils into the tissues after an allergic reaction may be explained by the presence of this factor (see also p. 302).

Prostaglandins. Prostaglandins are cyclic fatty acids containing 20 carbon atoms derived from unsaturated fatty acids such as arachidonic acid. These substances affect the adenyl cyclase in various tissues, diminishing the concentration of cyclic AMP of the adipose cells and augmenting the concentration of this compound in the lungs, diaphragm, spleen, and kidneys. Prostaglandins are liberated from guinea pig lungs during anaphylaxis in vitro. Prostaglandins effect increased permeability of the venules and relaxation of the bronchial musculature; they are probably involved in anaphylaxis. Prostaglandins also have an anti-inflammatory effect and can inhibit histamine liberation under certain conditions. Their role as mediators of anaphylaxis is not understood.

Heparin. To these pharmacologic mediators one might add heparin, the acid mucopolysaccharide responsible for the metachromatic coloration of the mastocyte granules, which is liberated during anaphylactic shock in the dog. Its only known effect in this species is to inhibit the coagulation of the blood, which does not appear to have an important role in the pathogenesis of anaphylaxis in other species.

Cells Involved in Anaphylaxis. The target cells of anaphylaxis, or those that exhibit morphologic or biochemical alterations following an anaphylactic reaction, include mastocytes, leukocytes, and platelets.

Mastocytes. The mastocytes are cells of the connective tissue characterized by an extreme abundance of granules that totally fill the cytoplasm, frequently to the point of impeding the visibility of the nucleus. These granules are composed principally of glycoproteins; they stain metachromatically due to their mucopolysaccharide sulfate content.

In the majority of species, the mastocytes are extremely rich in histamine and heparine and, in the rat and mouse, are also rich in serotonin. The histamine present in the mastocytes is synthesized from histidine through an enzyme, histidinodecarboxylase, whereas serotonin is synthesized from tryptophan through the activity of 5-hydroxytryptophanodecarboxylase. All of these substances are found in the cytoplasmic granules of the mastocytes (see also pp. 8 and 325).

Morphologic alterations of the mastocytes have been described in active anaphylaxis in man, monkey, dog, guinea pig, pig, rat, and mouse (Fig. 10.5). In the guinea pig and rat, the agents that inhibit the liberation of histamine simultaneously inhibit the morpho-

Fig. 10.5 a–d. Morphologic alterations of the mastocytes in anaphylaxis. **a** Mastocytes in the skin of unsensitized rats injected with ovalbumin. Note the distinct outlines of these cells and the absence of extracellular granules. **b** Mastocytes in the skin of rats sensitized to ovalbumin after intravenous injection of the antigen. Note the considerable extrusion of the granules and the imprecise outline of the cells. **c** Normal appearance of the mastocytes in the guinea pig mesentery. Note the cytoplasm totally filled with granules that conceal the nucleus. **d** Mastocytes of the mesentery of a sensitized guinea pig after contact with the same antigen. Note the disappearance of most of the granules, leaving the nucleus visible. There is no extrusion of the granules as occurs in the rat. Mota I (1953) Tese de Livre-Docenica, Universidade de Sao Paulo; Mota I, Vugman I (1956) Nature 177:427; Mota I (1959) J Physiol 147:425

logic alterations of the mastocytes. These alterations were attributed to the presence of certain types of hypothetical antibodies bound to the cellular membrane of the mastocytes, which, upon reacting with the specific antigen, caused the cellular reaction, together with activation and liberation of substances of intense pharmacologic activity. Experiments with guinea pig mesentery demonstrated the possibility of passive sensitization of the mastocytes in vitro, with this sensitization followed by specific alterations of these cells provoked by subsequent contact with the specific antigen. The suggestion that the lesions of the mastocytes resulted from an antigen–antibody reaction at the level of the cell itself was reinforced by the observation that such cells were capable of responding to the antigen with morphologic alterations and liberation of active substances even when isolated. These experiments were performed with mastocytes collected from animals actively sensitized or after passive sensitization in vitro. In the rat, these alterations could be followed microscopically by phase contrast and were described as a "bubbling" of the surface of the cell accompanied by extrusion of the cytoplasmic granules (Fig. 10.6). Observed with an electron microscope after an anaphylactic reaction, the mastocyte membrane exhibited protrusions or spherical projections from the cellular membrane, measuring about 200 Å in diameter, whose nature and significance remain unknown. It is possible that these projections represent vestiges of canals in the cellular membrane through which the granules are expelled to the exterior. In this respect, the expulsion of the mastocyte granules may be a particular case of

Fig. 10.6 a–d. Response to antigen by mastocytes isolated from the abdominal cavities of rats actively sensitized to ovalbumin. a and b The appearance of the isolated mastocytes under the phase-contrast microscope (a, before the addition of antigen; b, after the addition of antigen). The *arrows* indicate vacuolization in the cytoplasm. c and d Appearance of the mastocytes isolated after fixation and staining (c, before the antigen; d, after the antigen). Mota I, Dias da Silva W (1960) Nature 186:245

exosmosis, i.e., the process by which particles are eliminated by the cell to the exterior. According to this line of thinking, the reaction of the antigen with the antibody fixed to the cell membrane initiates modifications of the cell membrane, causing it to invaginate. The invaginated part melts together with the granule membrane, forming a passage through which it is carried to the exterior. The first step in the mechanism that gives rise to the liberation of mediator (after the reaction of the antigen with the antibody molecule bound to the cell) may take place at the level of the cellular membrane.

The response of sensitized mastocytes to the antigen requires metabolically active cells maintained at physiologic temperature. For the cellular response to occur, Ca^{2+} and a thermolabile factor of unknown nature are indispensable. In addition to histamine, other mediators such as serotonin, SRS, and ECF-A also originate from the mastocytes in the anaphylactic reactions mediated by IgE. In the guinea pig, for example, the anaphylactic liberation of histamine is always accompanied by the formation of SRS, and all the conditions that inhibit the liberation of histamine simultaneously suppress the formation of SRS. In the rat, the IgE-induced anaphylactic reaction and the formation of SRS require the presence of mastocytes. Compound 48–80, a chemical liberator of histamine with selective effect upon the mastocytes, also induces the formation of SRS when added to a suspension of these cells. Thus, it appears that SRS also originates from the mastocytes, although these cells certainly do not comprise the only source of this substance.

Fixation of the antibody molecule to the mastocyte membrane was suggested after the first observations were made of degranulation of these cells induced by the antigen in the rat. This possibility was reinforced by the subsequent observation that rat mastocytes were capable of responding to the antigen even when isolated. The specificity and constancy of the anaphylactic alterations of the mastocytes in various species suggest the existence of receptors for IgE and other anaphylactic antibodies on the cellular membrane of these and other target cells. In vitro sensitization experiments with rat mastocytes and homologous IgE and IgG_2 antibodies have shown that there is competitive inhibition between these antibodies and suggests that they either bind to receptors of the same type or to dissimilar receptors situated so close to one another that the fixation of one of the antibodies impedes the fixation of the other. The nature of these receptors remains unknown.

Basophils. The polymorphonuclear cells of various species, including the human, are rich in histamine, which is localized principally in the basophils (50%–85%) and, in lesser quantities, in the neutrophils and eosinophils. Basophils are myeloid cells that otherwise are extremely similar to mastocytes, with both cell types possessing metachromatic granules rich in heparin and histamine (see also pp. 8 and 326). Addition of extremely small quantities of specific antigen (10^{-6} µg protein) to a suspension of sensitized leukocytes produces liberation of histamine without visible morphologic alterations of these cells. This type of reaction depends upon the reaginic antibody and does not depend upon complement. Greater quantities of antigen produce visible alterations of these cells.

It is now recognized that the basophils are the cells responsible for the histamine liberated by the antigen from leukocyte suspensions taken from atopic patients. This conclusion implies that basophils, in the same manner as mastocytes, must bind IgE molecules exclusively or preferentially. Actually, the addition of anti-IgE to a suspension of human leukocytes produces liberation of histamine and degranulation of the basophils. Moreover, autoradiography of human leukocytes previously incubated with anti-IgE labeled with ^{125}I has revealed localization of the IgE exclusively in the basophils. The presence of IgE in these cells also has been confirmed by electron microscopy. With the use of myeloma IgE labeled with ^{125}I, the number of receptors for this antibody on the membrane of the basophils was calculated to be 30,000–90,000 per cell.

The anaphylactic liberation of histamine by human leukocytes is used as a test to detect and study the sensitivity of allergic patients. For this purpose, the patient's leukocytes can be incubated directly with antigen, or normal leukocytes can be incubated with the allergic patient's serum and later transferred to the specific antigen. In both cases, the positivity and intensity of the reaction are measured through the liberation of histamine. The antibodies responsible for the sensitization of leukocytes in the human and rabbit are homocytotropic antibodies of the IgE class. As with mastocytes, in order for the cellular response to proceed, the leukocytes must be metabolically intact, and both Mg^{2+} and Ca^{2+} ions must be present.

Platelets. Platelets are particles originating from the cytoplasm of megakaryocytes (see p. 12). Platelets contain organelles such as mitochondria, microtubules, lysosomes, and granules of unknown nature. When lysed, platelets liberate diverse substances including adenosine diphosphate (ADP), adenosine triphosphate (ATP), epinephrine, histamine, and lysosomal enzymes. The platelets do not synthesize the histamine and serotonin found within them; they are accumulated by an unknown mechanism. Contrary to what occurs with leukocytes and mastocytes, the liberation of active substances from the platelets does not depend upon an antigen–antibody reaction on the surface of these cells, since the platelets are incapable of fixing antibodies of any kind. Certainly, platelets of all species thus far studied are activated through antigen–antibody complexes or through immunoglobulin aggregates. In some species, though not all, complement is necessary for the activation of the platelets. For example, complement is necessary for the activation of rabbit platelets through antigen–antibody complexes; human platelets are also activated in the absence of complement.

In the human, as well as in several other species, platelets are activated mainly by two mechanisms: (1) a secretory mechanism initiated by the adherence of Fc pieces of antibodies that have bound antigen to the platelets; if an antibody binds an antigen or if an immunoglobulin aggregation results, conformational changes occur in the Fc pieces which permit adherence to the platelet; and (2) an indirect reaction that is induced originally by an antigen–antibody reaction on the surface of the leukocytes; platelet-activating substances are liberated as a result of this reaction.

This mechanism was first demonstrated in experiments in which rabbit blood cells were added to (1) unsensitized platelets, (2) sensitized leukocytes, or (3) unsensitized platelets plus an equal quantity of the sensitized leukocytes present in (2). The amount of histamine liberated in (3) was much greater than that in (2), whereas none was liberated in (1). The leukocyte responsible for this phenomenon is the basophil sensitized with IgE. The cell is activated by the fixation of antigen to the IgE antibodies on the membrane and, in addition to histamine, it liberates a soluble factor that can activate platelets, called platelet-activating factor (PAF). Chemically, it is a phospholipid l-0-alkyl-2-acetyl-sn-glycosyl-3-phosphorylcholine with the length of the alkyl chain mainly C_{16} and C_{18} (Fig. 10.7). PAF has also been demonstrated in other species, and can be obtained from human mast cells. PAF causes aggregation of platelets.

Fig. 10.7. Chemical structure of platelet-activating factor (PAF)

The activation of platelets requires Ca^{2+}, uses energy, and is influenced by 3′,5′-AMP. Microtubules and microfilaments appear to play a role in the platelet-secretion mechanism. Platelet activation may play a significant role in the deposit of antigen–antibody complexes on the vascular wall. Basophils and/or mast cells sensitized with IgE lead to activation of platelets and this together with increase in permeability during an anaphylactic reaction appears to make possible or at least facilitate the deposit of complexes in the tissue.

Eosinophils. Despite numerous investigations, the role of eosinophils in allergic inflammatory reactions has not yet been fully elucidated (see p. 326). About 25% of human eosinophils possess IgE molecules on their membranes and respond to the specific antigen or to an anti-IgE serum with liberation of prostaglandins, which inhibit the anaphylactic liberation of histamine by the mastocytes. A possible function of the eosinophils, therefore, is the modulation of allergic inflammatory reactions. Thus, since the prostaglandins are also potent bronchodilators, eosinophils of the respiratory tract in asthmatics could have the double function of impeding the liberation of histamine and impeding the constriction of the bronchial tree.

Antibodies Involved in Anaphylaxis. In all species studied, both homocytotropic antibodies (IgG and IgE) are present in the serum of sensitized animals; however, the importance of the contribution of each in the allergic reaction is difficult to evaluate. Homocytotropic antibodies of the IgG class (type I) are usually resistant to heat and to treatment with mercaptoethanol, reaching high concentrations in the serum, and are demonstrable in the skin after passive sensitization for a short time (24–48 h). Homocytotropic antibodies of the IgE class (type II), in contrast, are sensitive to heat and to mercaptoethanol, are present in serum in low concentration, and persist in the skin after passive sensitization for a long time (30–40 days) (see also p. 325). Data suggest that the type of mediator liberated depends upon the type of antibody bound to the cells. This implies that the anaphylactic phenomena, although possibly symptomatically similar, can be caused by intrinsically

different mechanisms. A summary of the antibodies involved in anaphylaxis along with their characteristics is given in Table 10.2.

Biochemistry of Antigen-Induced Liberation of Mediators. The sequence of the biochemical events that follow cell activation immediately after the complexing of membrane-bound antibodies is unknown. However, some of the biochemical reactions are known from experiments in which the anaphylactic liberation of mediators in the presence of specific enzyme inhibitors and in the presence or absence of specific ions was examined. These experiments showed that at least five sequential steps occur between antigenic stimulation and liberation of mediator: (1) calcium-dependent activation of serine esterase; (2) autocatalytic activation of this esterase; (3) an energy-consuming process; (4) a second calcium-dependent reaction; and (5) a $3',5'$-AMP-inhibitory phase. Thus, no mediator is liberated when the antigen comes in contact with sensitized cells in the presence of diisopropylfluorophosphate (DFP irreversibly phosphorylizes serine residues in the active region of the serine esterase), although complete liberation of mediator occurs if DFP is removed before it comes in contact with the antigen. This signifies that the activation of a proesterase is necessary for liberation of mediator. Furthermore, if contact with the antigen occurs in the presence of DFP and if the cells are then washed and transferred to a DFP-free medium, liberation of mediator occurs in inverse proportion to the length of time of antigen contact in the presence of DFP. Because DFP irreversibly inactivates serine esterase, these results indicate that mediator liberation after removal of DFP reflects the continual activation of the remaining proesterase following contact with the antigen. On the other hand, the inactivation of the esterase is blocked by DFP when the DFP-containing buffer lacks calcium ions during antigen contact. In this case, the complete liberation of histamine occurs when the cells are transferred to a DFP-free buffer after antigen contact. These results indicate that without Ca^{2+}, the antigen cannot activate proesterase to DFP-sensitive esterase. Once activated, the esterase activates itself auto-catalytically and probably affects the substrate, in that an inhibitory protein is split off.

An energy-dependent step follows proesterase activation, which requires glucose and which is inhibited through 2-deoxyglucose (2-DG). The next step requires Ca^{2+} and can be inhibited by EDTA; EDTA prevents the suppression of the 2-DG-mediated inhibition by glucose of the anaphylactic liberation of mediator, although 2-DG does not prevent the cancellation of EDTA inhibition of liberation of mediator through Ca^{2+}. Catecholamines also block the suppression of EDTA inhibition of liberation of mediator through Ca^{2+}, which suggests that the site of the inhibitory effect by increasing concentrations of 3',5'-AMP occurs simultaneously with or subsequent to the second Ca^{2+}-requiring step.

Apparently, the complexing of IgE molecules on the mast-cell membrane causes the transport of extracellular Ca^{2+} to the site of a proesterase that is converted to a chymotrypsin-like serine esterase. An energy-consuming process follows that may be related to the function of a contractile protein, because dense bands of microfilaments around the mast-cell granula during degranulation were observed. These findings agree with information that suggests a relationship between the Ca^{2+} influx, the relative concentration of 3',5'-AMP, the direction of the microtubules, and their function. The five biochemical steps of the anaphylactic liberation of mediators are shown schematically in Fig. 10.8.

Anaphylactoid Phenomena. In numerous situations artificially created in the laboratory, anaphylactic syndromes are observed similar to those classically obtained after introduction of antigen into a sensitized animal. These include Forssman shock and the shock induced by anaphylatoxin.

Forssman Shock. The Forssman antigen is a heterophilic antigen, i.e., it belongs to a group of antigenic substances of similar specificities, present in cells of widely different species. In 1911, Forssman observed that the immunization of rabbits with extracts from the kidney of a guinea pig induced the production of antibodies that also reacted with sheep erythrocytes. This phenomenon is explained by the presence on sheep erythrocytes of antigenic determinants similar to those encountered on the cells of the guinea pig. Antibodies formed against the Forssman antigen are called Forssman antibodies. Forssman shock is obtained by injecting intravenously into the guinea pig, which produces a clinically acute symptomatology resembling anaphylactic shock. Postmortem examination, however, reveals lungs with minimal emphysema, but with severe edema and hemorrhage. The Forssman antigen occurs in the tissues of the guinea pig in particularly high concentrations on the endothelial cells of the blood vessels. Neither liberation of histamine nor alteration of the mastocytes occurs in this type of reaction. Forssman shock is the result of a typical cytotoxic reaction and as such requires complement.

Anaphylatoxin-induced Shock. In 1910, Friedberger demonstrated that serum or

Fig. 10.8. Reaction chain of the liberation of anaphylactic mediators

plasma of the guinea pig incubated with antigen–antibody complexes in vitro and then centrifuged and injected intravenously into guinea pigs produced a shock closely resembling that of anaphylaxis. This indicated the formation of an anaphylatoxic substance by contact of the antigen–antibody complex with components of the serum. Friedberger named this substance anaphylatoxin. Many years later, it was verified that anaphylatoxin acted via the liberation of histamine and that, as in anaphylaxis, the histamine liberated by anaphylatoxin also originated from the mastocytes, which, upon contact with the anaphylatoxin, exhibited lesions identical to those produced by the antigen in the anaphylactic reactions. The liberation of histamine provided the explanation for the extreme similarity between the shock produced by anaphylatoxin and anaphylactic shock. Anaphylatoxin was also capable of contracting a isolated guinea pig ileum. Diverse substances such as agar, dextran, kaolin, and others, when incubated with serum or fresh plasma, also activate anaphylatoxin. An important observation made at an early date by Friedberger is that the heating of the serum or plasma to 56 °C destroys its capacity to form anaphylatoxin – a detail that later suggested the necessity of the thermolabile components of complement in the mechanism of the formation of anaphylatoxin. Subsequenty, it was shown that anaphylatoxin involves cleavage products of the complement system – specifically C3 and C5 (see Chap. 5).

Anaphylactic Phenomena in Man

Acute Anaphylaxis. Acute anaphylaxis in man is a rare though serious accident with possible fatal consequences. When serotherapy was at its zenith, acute anaphylaxis was usually produced by serum. Currently, it is produced more commonly by drugs, especially penicillin. The majority of drugs possess small molecules that require a covalent bond with tissue proteins in order to become capable of inducing an immunogenic response, as occurs, for example, with penicillin. Penicillic acid, which forms spontaneously in neutral penicillin solutions, is extremely active in the formation of a large number of derivatives with the amine and sulfhydryl groups from proteins. These derivatives behave as foreign substances, inducing the formation of antibodies directed against the haptenic penicillin group. Aside from penicillin, the most frequent causes of anaphylaxis in man are the bites of some insects (particularly bee stings), skin tests with antigens, and occasionally, heterologous serum. The symptoms appear some minutes after contact with the antigen; they consist of headache, precordial pain, sensation of heat, generalized pruritus, urticaria, apnea, hypothermia, and hypotension. Less frequently, the response is characterized by acute circulatory collapse. In fatal cases, autopsy reveals edema of the upper respiratory passage mucosae, particularly edema of the epiglottis, which could be the immediate cause of death.

Local Anaphylaxis. More frequently, anaphylaxis is evidenced by localized phenomena produced by contact of the antigen with specific organs or tissues. For example, anaphylaxis can be localized in the skin in the form of eczema or urticaria; in the respiratory apparatus, as with allergy to pollen or bronchial asthma; in the digestive tract with various functional perturbations due to the sensitization of the individual to certain foods, etc.

Atopy. Most people can be actively sensitized so as to exhibit typical anaphylactic symptoms when in contact with the antigen. However, there are certain individuals who are sensitized easily, even spontaneously, to a great number of environmental antigens, such as pollen, dust, dye, plants, and fungi. This facility in certain individuals to become allergic, termed atopy (Greek *uncommonness*), is familial and probably genetically controlled.

Tests for Detecting and Measuring IgE

Prausnitz-Küstner Test. In 1921, Prausnitz and Küstner described the test that today bears their names, commonly referred to as the PK test. This test, similar to the passive cutaneous anaphylaxis test, consists of injecting intradermally 0.1 ml of whole or diluted serum from an allergic individual into an unsensitized individual and, after about 24 h, injecting the antigen into the same site. A positive test produces local itching and formation of a papule surrounded by a zone of erythema. The reaction reaches a maximum within 10 min, persists for about 20 min, and gradually disappears. The antibody responsible for the Prausnitz-Küstner reaction was found at an early date to be thermolabile, losing its activity after heating to 56 °C for several hours; later, its sensitivity to reduction by sulfhydryl agents, such as 2-mercaptoethanol, followed by alkylation, was observed. The quantity of IgE present in the serum of an allergic patient is indicated by the highest dilution of serum still capable of producing a PK reaction.

Liberation of Histamine. The addition of the specific allergen to a suspension of leukocytes obtained from an allergic patient liberates histamine which can be measured biologically or chemically. The quantity of histamine liberated is usually proportional to the degree of atopy exhibited by the patient and to the level of IgE in his serum.

Leukocyte Sensitization Test. Leukocytes obtained from nonallergic individuals are incubated with serum from an allergic patient and then washed and resuspended with the specific allergen. The quantity of histamine liberated is generally proportional to the quantity of IgE antibodies present in the serum.

Radioallergosorbent Test. This test, abbreviated RAST, is based on the absorption of IgE antibody by the insolubilized specific antigen and in the subsequent determination of the quantity of IgE antibody absorbed. In practice, the antigen is first combined by covalent linkage with particles of an insoluble substance (cellulose or activated Sepharose), and this combination is then added to the serum of the patient in a quantity that represents an antigen excess. After the particles are washed, the amount of absorbed IgE is determined with labeled anti-IgE antibody (Fig. 10.9).

Radioimmunodiffusion. IgE also can be measured by the Mancini technique using specific anti-IgE antibody labeled with ^{125}I. The labeled anti-IgE antibody is suspended in agar in which, after solidification, wells are made into which is placed the serum of the subject whose IgE level is to be determined. Forty-eight hours later, the agar plate is washed, dried, and covered with a photographic film. After several days, the film is developed, and the diameters of the rings that appear are measured. With the help of a standard curve, one can determine the concentration of the IgE.

Biologic Activity of Human Reagin. Being a homocytotropic antibody, the human reagin (IgE), aside from sensitizing homologous tissues, is also capable of sensitizing tissues of the higher primates. Experiments with

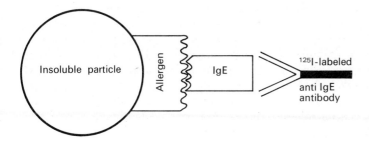

Fig. 10.9. Radioallergosorbent test

rhesus monkeys have demonstrated that reactions similar to the PK reaction can be induced in the skin of this species with human sera obtained from atopic patients and that the sera lose this capacity after heating to 56 °C. It was also verified that segments of rhesus ileum could be passively sensitized with human reagin, producing Schultz-Dale reactions when placed in contact with the antigen. Neither cutaneous anaphylaxis (PK) nor the intestinal (Schultz-Dale) anaphylaxis could be reproduced with human antibodies of any other class of immunoglobulin. The anaphylactic phenomena produced in the tissues of the rhesus monkey with human reagin are accompanied by liberation of histamine. Skin sections from the rhesus monkeys sensitized with human IgE and treated with fluorescent antigen revealed selective fixation of human IgE in the mastocytes of these species. In addition, human reagin is capable of binding to homologous basophilic leukocytes. Morphologic alterations of the mastocytes were observed after incubation with lactic proteins of the mesentery of a patient sensitized to milk; furthermore, the passive sensitization of human lung by incubation in vitro with human reagin and subsequent contact with the specific antigen also resulted in morphologic alterations of the mastocytes, along with liberation of histamine and SRS.

In the passive cutaneous anaphylactic reactions of the guinea pig, homologous Ig and the Ig of certain other species blocked homologous sensitization by the IgG antibody. This blockage has been explained as being due to competition between the antibody and the nonspecific gamma globulin for the cellular receptors. It has been verified that nonspecific human IgE also blocks the binding of IgE antibody in the PK test (competitive inhibition at the cellular receptor level).

Effect of Heating and Alkylation-Reduction on the Cytotropic Activity of the IgE Antibody.

One characteristic of the IgE antibody is that its cytotropic activity is destroyed by heating or by reduction and alkalization of the disulfide bridges: The capacity of the molecule to attach to the mastocyte and basophil membranes disappears when the antibody is heated to 56 °C, or when it is treated with a reducing agent (mercaptoethanol) and alkylated. Studies of the alteration of the circular dichroism spectrum of the IgE molecule and its fragments (Fab', Fc'', and Fc) indicate that only the two terminal domains of the molecule ($C_\varepsilon 3$ and $C_\varepsilon 4$) undergo irreversible alterations after heating to 56 °C. These results are in accordance with earlier observations indicating that, after heating, the IgE lost the skin-sensitizing property without loss of the ability to combine with the antigen. This same phenomenon occurred after reduction and alkylation of the molecule. The disulfide bridges responsible for the cytotropic properties are found between the Fd- and the hinge region of the heavy chains. Cleavage at this point considerably diminishes the cytotropic property of the molecule, but the capacity for fixation is totally lost only when one of the disulfide bonds between the ε chains of the N-terminal portion of the Fc fragment is cleaved.

Inverse Prausnitz-Küstner Reaction.

Since individuals not recognizably allergic possess IgE, it was hoped that this type of immunoglobulin might be found under normal conditions in the target cells of normal organisms. Actually, an intradermal injection of specific antibody against IgE produces an inverse Prausnitz-Küstner (PK) reaction. The minimum quantity of antibody capable of producing inverse PK is of the order of 10^{-5} μg N. The sensitivity of the skin to anti-IgE depends upon the quantity of IgE present in the skin. An allergic patient with an elevated concentration of IgE in the serum responds to 10^{-8} μg N of anti-IgE, whereas patients with agammaglobulinemia cannot respond to 10^{-3} μg N of anti-IgE. Specific antibodies against IgG, IgA, IgM, and IgD do not produce any reaction when injected into the skin of the normal individual. F(ab')$_2$ fragments obtained from anti-IgE antibody also are capable of producing inverse PK, whereas the Fab fragment is not. These results suggest the necessity of bivalence for the induction of inverse PK and that the union of two molecules of IgE bound to the tissues is necessary to induce cellular damage (see Fig. 10.4). The fact that an inverse PK test also can be induced by the $F(ab')_2$ indicates that complement is not involved.

Mechanism of Immunotherapy in Atopic Diseases. If a sensitized guinea pig is injected repeatedly with small quantities of antigen insufficient to cause death by anaphylaxis, the animal becomes desensitized; it loses, for as long as several days, reactivity to an antigen dose that in other conditions would be fatal. It is thought that the small, repeated doses of antigen exhaust the antibodies existing in the organism, thus impeding the shock that otherwise would be induced. The desensitization – or better, hyposensitization – is frequently used to render an atopic patient tolerant of a substance to which he is allergic (immunotherapy). In man, however, immunotherapy is attributed to the formation of so-called blocking antibodies. These can be detected and measured in the serum of allergic patients after prior heating of the serum to destroy the reaginic antibody. Different quantities of inactivated serum are mixed with constant quantities of antigen, and these mixtures are injected into previously sensitized skin locations on a healthy volunteer. The blocking antibody, if present, blocks the PK reaction, and the richer the serum of the patient is in blocking antibody, the less the quantity necessary to block the reaction. Atopic patients are commonly treated with injections of increasing doses of antigen, beginning with extremely small quantities, at proper intervals in order to avoid a possible systemic anaphylactic reaction. This treatment gives rise to the synthesis of blocking antibody. It is believed that these are nonanaphylactic antibodies which, although directed against the same antigen, do not possess the capacity of combining with the cells. However, the binding of the allergen via the blocking antibodies in the serum cannot always be correlated with improvement of the patient's symptoms.

IgE and IgG levels in sera from patients suffering from hay fever, in whom immunotherapy was being carried out, were examined. Immediately after the start of treatment, IgG and IgE levels rose noticeably, but the rise in IgG was much more pronounced. After long-term immunotherapy, the concentration of IgE antibodies decreased, whereas the IgG concentration continued to rise. Furthermore, there was no IgE secondary response in patients undergoing immunotherapy, which is normally observed in hay-fever sufferers during the hay-fever season. However, the increase in the concentration of IgG antibodies following immunotherapy cannot be entirely responsible for the repression of the IgE secondary response following immunotherapy.

Experiments in mice indicate that decreased IgE synthesis after repeated administration of antigen is dependent upon repression of the T-cell helper function, probably through the appearance of T suppressor cells. The positive effect of immunotherapy on increased production of blocking antibodies has also been attributed to suppressor T cells.

Control of Anaphylactic Reactions at the Cellular Level. Anaphylactic phenomena can be blocked or attenuated by drugs that generally act by antagonizing the pharmacologic action of mediators or by impeding their formation and liberation. For example, antihistamines act by inhibition through competition, i.e., by blocking the pharmacologic action of the histamine at the receptor level. Numerous compounds with antihistaminic activity have been used in the treatment of allergies. Although these compounds may be effective in certain anaphylactic syndromes such as urticaria, they are relatively inefficient in other cases such as bronchial asthma – possibly because other mediators are implicated in these situations. In cutaneous anaphylaxis of the rat and mouse, it has been observed that the simultaneous application of an antihistamine and an antagonist of serotonin has a cumulative effect, with the use of the two drugs abolishing the reaction totally, whereas the use of either drug singly produces only partial eradication of the reaction. In addition to inhibiting the action of histamine, the antihistamines, depending upon their concentration, not only can impede the anaphylactic liberation of histamine but, when used in excess, can actually produce the liberation of histamine. Diethylcarbazamine citrate (Hetrazan), a drug used as an anthelmintic agent, has a beneficial effect when used in asthmatic patients. Experiments with rat and monkey tissues have shown that this substance impeded the formation of SRS and histamine induced by the antigen–antibody reaction in anaphylaxis. Another substance, used clinically in asthma therapy, is sodium chromoglycate. This compound inhibits the anaphylactic liberation of histamine. Both of these drugs act subsequent to the antigen–antibody interaction. The inhibitory effect of chromoglycate appears to vary according to the type of antibody involved in the reaction and the tissue type or animal species used in the test. For example, PCA reactions induced by IgE in the rat are completely eradicated by chromoglycate, whereas the same reactions induced by the same type of antibody in the mouse are not affected by this compound. The operative mechanism of both compounds is unknown.

The principal symptoms of anaphylaxis are due to vasodilation and to contraction of smooth muscle. Thus, compounds with pharmacologic activity contrary to these effects are used in the prevention of experimental and asthmatic anaphylaxis. Beta-adrenergic substances such as epinephrine and isoprenaline, which possess a strong bronchodilator effect, are beneficial in the treatment of anaphylaxis, particularly in guinea-pig anaphylaxis and human respiratory asthma, in which death is due to a respiratory deficit. In addition, the β-adrenergic compounds possibly owe their efficiency to their capacity to inhibit the liberation or formation of mediators through modulation of the level of $3',5'$-cyclic adenosine mono-

phosphate (cAMP). The cAMP molecule is formed intracellularly from ATP by the action of an enzyme, adenyl cyclase encountered in the cellular membrane. Under normal conditions, the transformation of ATP into cAMP proceeds slowly. However, when a hormone is liberated into the blood, the hormone, acting as a primary messenger, binds to specific receptors on the cellular membrane and in this fashion augments the activity of adenyl cyclase, consequently accelerating the transformation of ATP into cAMP. This compound then acts as a second messenger, activating processes of synthesis and cellular secretion. For example, in hepatocytes, the augmentation of the reaction ATP $\rightarrow$ cAMP results in the conversion of glycogen into glycose. In the cells of the adrenal medulla, it results in the synthesis and secretion of the steroid hormones.

In various other conditions, however, an increase in the concentration of cAMP results in inhibition of the secretory mechanism. This appears to occur via the liberation of mediators of anaphylaxis. Normally, the level of cAMP depends on an equilibrium between the activity of the α- and β-receptors of the mastocytes (or basophils). Thus, stimulation of the β-receptors results in an increase of cAMP and in a consequent diminution of the enzymatic system responsible for the liberation of the mediators. Stimulation of the α-receptors produces a decrease of cAMP and an increase in activity of the enzymatic system. Thus, production and liberation of the mediators can be controlled with substances that stimulate or block the α- and β-receptors. Epinephrine and isoprenaline, which stimulate the β-receptors, cause an increase in cAMP levels and a decrease in the liberation of the mediators, whereas norepinephrine, which stimulates the α-receptors, has the opposite effect. Substances such as methyl-xanthines, which inhibit the action of phosphodiesterase (an enzyme that normally transforms $3',5'$-AMP into $5'$-AMP), also diminish the liberation of the mediators by causing an increase in cAMP. Some of the prostaglandins are capable of increasing the intracellular level of cAMP and thus function as inhibitors of histamine liberation.

It has been shown that acetylcholine and carbamylcholine, in extremely small concentrations, enhance the anaphylactic liberation of mediators, independent of the 3′,5′-AMP cell level. There is evidence that the cholinergic receptor in the cell membrane is guanyl cyclase, which is activated through cholinergic substances and which transforms guanosyltriphosphate (GTP) into 3′,5′-guanosylmonophosphate (3′,5′-GMP). In mast cells and basophils, intracellular increase of 3′,5′-GMP levels leads to an increase in the liberation of mediators. This liberation can be specifically inhibited with atropine. 3′,5′-GMP is transformed into its inactive form, 5′-GMP, through a phosphodiesterase. Phosphodiesterase can be competitively inhibited by methyl-xanthine. Methyl-xanthines are much more effective on adenylphosphodiesterases than on guanyldiphosphodiesterases, which probably explains the previously discussed influence of methyl-xanthine on the 3′,5′-AMP system. The liberation of mediators from mast cells and basophils is apparently dependent upon equilibrium of the intracellular concentration of 3′,5′-AMP and 3′,5′-GMP.

Fig. 10.10. Schematic representation of liberation of mediator (H), and the effect of different medications on the progression of this reaction. The anaphylactic reaction activates an enzyme system (X→XA→Y→Z) on the mast cell membrane that is responsible for the liberation of the mediator and whose activity appears to be controlled through the opposing effects of 3′,5′-AMP and 3′,5′-GMP (Yin-Yang hypothesis of biologic control). An increase in 3′,5′-AMP inhibits liberation of mediator, whereas a decrease in 3′,5′-AMP enhances liberation. Intracellular levels of 3′,5′-AMP can be increased through β-adrenergic substances like epinephrine and isoprenaline, (PGE₁), which activate adenylcyclases, or through methyl-xanthines (theophylline), which inhibit phosphodiesterase activity. Decrease in the 3′,5′-AMP level through α-adrenergic substances or through an increase of 3′,5′-GMP through cholinergic stimulation, enhances mediator liberation. Colchicine, which causes dissociation of microtubules, inhibits mediator liberation, whereas heavy water (D₂₀), which causes aggregation of microtubules, increases mediator liberation

Microtubules are organelles that play a role in the cellular secretion mechanism. Apparently, they are important in the mechanism of mediator liberation. Study of the function of the microtubules has been facilitated by the use of drugs that specifically alter these structures. Colchicine, which binds to the subunits of the microtubules, producing dissociation and disappearance of these structures, inhibits the degranulation of the mastocytes and the anaphylactic liberation of the histamines from these cells and basophils. On the other hand, deuterium oxide induces the aggregation of the microtubule subunits, and in this way enhances the liberation of histamine. Figure 10.10 schematically summarizes the regulatory mechanisms of anaphylaxis.

Control of IgE Production. The induction of IgE antibody production depends primarily upon the manner in which the antigen is presented to the organism (dose, route of administration, adjuvant) and upon the genetic constitution of the individual. Since these conditions differ substantially from those that lead to the production of IgG and IgM antibodies, it is believed that the IgE antibody has a specific mechanism controlling its production at the cellular level. Studies of IgE production under experimental conditions indicate that B cells and T cells must cooperate in the production of this antibody, that the B-IgE cells (B-cell precursors of the IgE-producing cells) appear more sensitive than do the B-IgG cells to the auxiliary and suppressor effects of T cells, and that these effects are mediated by soluble substances.

Genetic Control of IgE Production. For years, it has been known that allergies are familial, which suggests genetic control. Furthermore, inbred strains of mice differ in their ability to form IgE, an indication that their sensitivity to allergic phenomena, like human atopy, is genetically controlled. Experiments with inbred strains indicated that two gene loci control the production of IgE;

findings from human population studies suggest a similar genetic control.

The ability to react to an antigen is controlled by numerous autosomal-dominant genes (Ir gene), a few of which are linked to the major histocompatibility complex. In addition to the ability to form antibodies against specific antigenic determinants, the IgE system also has "IgE genes" which control the ability to form IgE. Thus, the extent of IgE formation in response to an allergen is controlled primarily by the Ir gene; however, the subsequent continuous formation of IgE appears to be controlled by such "IgE genes."

Control of Anaphylactic Reactions in the Atopic Individual. The intensity of the anaphylactic reaction in the atopic individual depends, in addition to the nature and quantity of the antibody involved, upon other factors such as reactivity of the target cell, response of the anatomic structures sensitive to the mediators, and control of the autonomic nervous system. The reactivity of the target cells, such as mastocytes and basophils, appears to depend upon an equilibrium between the adrenergic α- and β-receptors that control the activities of the enzymes responsible for the formation and liberation of the mediators.

The intensity of the smooth-muscle response (as well as that of other structures) to the mediators also depends upon the equilibrium between their adrenergic α- and β-receptors. Stimulation of the α-receptors causes a diminution of $3',5'$-cyclic AMP, which enhances the contraction of the smooth muscle of the respiratory apparatus. Stimulation of the β-receptors produces an increase of cAMP that results in the opposite effect, i.e., relaxation of the smooth muscle and consequently bronchodilation.

In this way, β-adrenergic substances such as epinephrine and isoprenaline increase intracellular levels of cAMP through activation of β-adrenergic receptors, thereby inhibiting liberation of mediator and smooth-muscle contraction. For this reason, they have a favorable effect on bronchial asthma.

Methyl-xanthines such as theophyllin exert a synergistically favorable effect when used together with epinephrine because they inhibit phosphodiesterases, thereby causing an increase in cAMP. Norepinephrine has the opposite effect because it causes a reduction in cAMP concentration by the activation of α-adrenergic receptors, which results in increased liberation of mediator and contraction of smooth musculature. Furthermore, equilibrium between the cAMP and $3'$-$5'$-GMP systems, helps maintain homeostatic control of cell activity. This stimulation with acetylcholine causes an increase in $3',5'$-GMP, which leads to increased liberation of mediator as well as to intensified contraction of smooth musculature. The effect of cholinergic stimulation is blocked by atropine.

Atopic individuals exhibit excessive irritability of the smooth muscle of the bronchial tree and of other sectors of the organism due to blockage of the response of the β_α-adrenergic receptors. It is thought that atopic individuals lack the normal equilibrium between the α- and β-adrenergic receptors, which might also account for the therapeutic efficiency of drugs such as catecholamines, theophylline, and the corticosteroids, which enhance the effect of epinephrine and the β-receptors.

Cytotoxic Reactions (Type II)

Complement-Dependent Antibody Reactions

Cytotoxic reactions are those in which the antibody combines with an antigen present in the tissues – either in the cells or in extracellular structures. The antigen can be a natural constituent of the tissues or it can be artificially bound to the cell surface. Transfusion reactions due to blood incompatibility, in which there is lysis of erythrocytes by antibodies against the ABO and other systems, are a good example of the cytotoxic reaction in which the antigen is a natural constituent of the cells. On the other hand, the lysis of platelets in purpura, induced by Sedormid or other drugs, exemplifies a cytotoxic reaction in which the antigen is not a natural component of the tissues. This type of cytotoxic reaction is due to the fact that numerous drugs are capable of binding to the cell surface, inducing the formation of antibodies that lyse the cells. Nephrotoxic nephritis, which results from antibodies against antigens present in the basement membrane of the renal glomerulus, represents a cytotoxic reaction in which the antibody combines with an extracellular structure. In most of these reactions, for there to be lesions of the tissues, fixation and activation of the complement system (see Chap. 5) are necessary.

Complement-Independent Antibody-Reactions

There are situations in which the binding of antibodies to cell structures results not in damage of the cell, but in stimulation of the specific function this cell exerts. An example of that is the so-called long-acting thyroid stimulator (LATS), an antibody reacting with antigenic structures at or near the TSH (thyroid-stimulating hormone) receptor; this results in an activation of the adenylcyclase in the cell membrane, the resulting cyclic AMP stimulates thyroid cells. A similar situation exists in lymphocyte stimulation. Small lymphocytes with immunoglobulin as antigen receptors are either stimulated by the binding of antigen or by binding of an anti-Ig (anti-idiotype, anti-allotype) antibody.

Blocking antibody is an example of the reverse situation. Thus, IgG antibodies to an allergen may competitively inhibit the binding of that antigen with IgE antibodies and thereby block the release of vasoactive amines; or, antibodies which mask histocompatibility antigens on tissue cells permit them to escape rejection; or, antibodies against tumor specific antigens prevent lymphocytes cytotoxic for those cells to damage the tumor, and therefore permit continued growth of tumor cells.

Another mode of complement-independent action of antibodies is the antibody-dependent cell-mediated cytotoxicity (ADCC), described in detail in Chaps. 2 (p. 43), 9 (p. 244), and 11 (p. 327).

Reactions by Antigen-Antibody Complexes (Type III)

Another type of immediate hypersensitivity reaction associated with complement activation is that of *vasculitis* mediated by antigen-antibody complexes (Fig. 10.11). Such forms of vasculitis occur when elevated concentrations of antigen–antibody complexes are formed in vivo, fix to walls of the arterioles, and then activate the complement system, generating chemotactic factors for leukocytes. Local types of vasculitis can be of great severity, producing localized hemorrhages and necrosis when the antigen is injected locally into an organism possessing a large quantity of circulating antibodies (Ar-

thus reaction). There are also generalized forms of vasculitis, frequently involving the glomeruli (glomerulonephritis) observed when an organism is subjected to a dose of antigen sufficiently great that antigens are still present in the circulation at the time when antibodies begin to form. Large quantities of antigen–antibody complexes are formed in the blood, exceeding the clearing capacity of the reticuloendothelial system and localizing in the arteriolar networks throughout the organism. This type of phenomenon is common in persons injected with animal sera for the prophylaxis or treatment of infections (tetanus, diphtheria antisera) generating a syndrome called "serum sickness", but has also been recognized as a cause of many immunopathological effects in infectious, and autoimmune diseases (Table 10.4, and p. 373).

Methods for Detection of Immune Complexes

The fact that numerous test have been described in the last past years to detect circu-

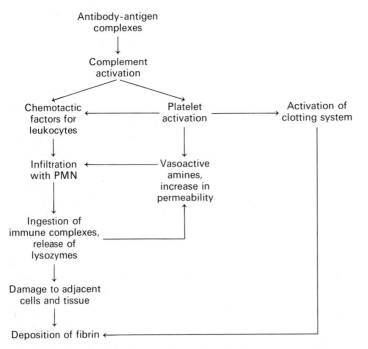

Fig. 10.11. Pathogenesis of inflammatory lesions due to immune complexes

Table 10.4. Diseases associated with immune complexes

Infections	
bacterial:	meningococcal (arthritis, vasculitis), gonorrheal, streptococcal (endocarditis, glomerulonephritis), lepromatous leprosy, syphilis (glomerulonephritis) staphylococcal (shunt nephritis)
viral:	Dengue hemorrhagic fever, cytomegalovirus, hepatitis, infectious mononucleosis, subacute sclerosing panencephalitis, mumps, variola, varicella, adeno- and echovirus infections
parasitic:	malaria (nephropathy), trypanosomiasis, schistosomiasis (mesangia of glomeruli), toxoplasmosis (glomerulonephritis) leishmaniasis, filariasis
Autoimmune diseases	rheumatoid arthritis (RF-IgG/M-IgG complexes), Felty's syndrom (RF-IgG-IgG complexes), systemic lupus erythematodes (antinuclear-antibodies and RF-IgM complexes), Sjögren syndrom (RF-IgM and other complexes), systemic sclerosis (RF and cryoglobulins), Hashimoto's thyroiditis
Other diseases	Crohn's disease (with extraintestinal manifestations), cystic fibrosis (secondary due to chronic and recurrent bacterial infections), sarcoidosis (in granulomas), multiple sclerosis (brain, kidney), myasthenia gravis, atopic diseases (IgE complexes), pemphigus (skin, autoantibody complexes), celiac disease, serum sickness, penicillamine nephropathy

lating immune complexes indicates that no single test is sufficient for all situations. Since the identity of the antigens is generally unknown particularly in the human, specific detection of the antigen is not possible – with some exceptions: nucleic acid antigen in systemic lupus erythematosus, drugs in drug sensitivity, and HB_sAg in some cases of polyarteritis nodosa.

Microcomplement Consumption Test. Presumptive evidence for the presence of immune complexes in sera is obtained by assessing the consumption of a standard amount of complement (C) added to heat-inactivated serum samples. Residual C activity is measured by the degree of lysis of IgM antibody-sensitized sheep red blood cells. Disadvantages of this test are that the serum samples have to be heat-inactivated, which may create immunoglobulin aggregates, and that not all human immunoglob-

ulin classes activate complement (e.g. IgG_4), or they activate complement preferentially via the alternate pathway (IgE, IgA).

C1q Solid Phase Radioimmune Assay. C1q is adsorbed on plastic polystyrene tubes. The samples are incubated in the coated tube, then washed out. The amount of immune complexes bound to C1q is estimated by binding of radiolabeled or enzyme-linked anti-immunoglobulin antibodies or by binding of radiolabeled aggregated IgG onto free C1q. The sensitivity of the test is 1–10 µg Anti-Human-Gamma globulin (AHG) per ml.

Conglutinin Radioimmune Assay. Conglutinin is an unusual protein (mw 750,000) which occurs naturally in cattle serum (see p. 193). It has strong affinity for immune complex-fixed C3 fragment; it is not an immunoglobulin. Conglutinin produces strong agglutination of sheep red blood cells coated with IgM antibodies and C. The binding of conglutinin to immune complexes is complement and Ca^{2+} dependent and appears to be specific for the inactivated form $C3bi$ of $C3b$. The assay is performed by placing serum samples in microtiter plates coated with conglutinin; the amount of bound IgG is then quantitated with a radiolabeled or enzyme-linked anti-IgG antibody. The sensitivity is in the order of 5–10 µg AHG per ml.

Platelet Aggregation Test. Platelets aggregate after their surface Fc-receptors interact with IgG-type immune complexes or aggregates. The test is sensitive (5–10 µg AHG per ml) but can give false positive results due to materials other than immune complexes (antiplatelet-antibodies, myxoviruses, enzymes).

Macrophage Inhibition Test. Immune complexes can be phagocytosed in vitro by macrophages. This is used in a *phagocytosis inhibition test.* Guinea pig peritoneal macrophages are incubated with the sample to be tested and with radiolabeled aggregated IgG. The presence of immune complexes in the sample is revealed by a decrease in the uptake of radioactivity by the cells compared to a control where incubation takes place with labeled aggregates alone.

Raji Cell Assay. B cells have surface receptors for C3 through which they can bind complement-fixing immune complexes. Cells of the cultured B-type lymphoblastoid cell line Raji possess high affinity C3 receptors but lack surface immunoglobulins. Immune complexes bound to their surface can thus be estimated by secondary fixation of radiolabeled anti-Ig antibodies. The sensitivity of the test is 6–12 µg AHG per ml. Another cell line which is used in a similar way, is the cultured L1210 murine leukemia cell, which binds immune complexes via Fc receptors with high affinity for the Fc portion of aggregated IgG.

Arthus Reaction.

Shortly after the discovery of anaphylaxis, Arthus described another immunologic phenomenon dependent upon an antigen-antibody reaction; however, fundamental differences were noted between the mechanism of this reaction and that of anaphylactic reactions. Arthus observed that rabbits repeatedly inoculated intradermally with heterologous serum exhibited a local inflammatory reaction characterized by edema, erythema, hemorrhage, and in the more intense lesions, by necrosis.

The Arthus reaction can be elicited in practically any species with any antigen. It is distinguished from the anaphylactic reaction by many characteristics: (1) The anaphylactic reaction is rapid and transitory, whereas the Arthus reaction develops slowly, requiring hours to reach its maximum and hours or days to disappear. (2) Whereas in anaphylaxis the antibody involved is found fixed to the tissues and the reactions can proceed in the absence of circulating antibody, in the Arthus reaction binding of the antibody to the tissues is not necessary (hence absence of the latent period), and the reaction does not proceed in the absence of circulating antibody. (3) The type of antibody also is different in the two reactions in that the Arthus reaction requires precipitating antibody, whereas anaphylaxis does not. Furthermore, in the guinea pig, the IgG_1 antibody is highly efficient in producing anaphylaxis but inefficient in producing the Arthus reaction – with the contrary occurring with the IgG_2 antibody. This difference appears to relate to the fact that IgG_2 is capable of fixing complement whereas IgG_1 is not. IgG_1 induces an anaphylactic reaction effectively, but is hardly in a position to induce an Arthus reaction. There appears to be an interaction between IgG_1 and IgG_2 in the active Arthus reaction. (4) The Arthus reaction requires complement, which does not appear to be necessary in anaphylaxis (Fig. 10.12). (5) The Arthus reaction requires enormous quantities of antibody – about 10 mg when injected intravenously in-

Fig. 10.12. Effect of decomplementation on the Arthus reaction

to rabbits and 0.1 mg when injected locally. In contrast, for a local anaphylactic reaction, fractions of micrograms (0.02 μg) are sufficient. (6) Polymorphonuclear leukocytes are necessary for the Arthus reaction. Depletion of circulating polymorphonuclear cells reduces or suppresses the Arthus reaction but does not modify the anaphylactic reaction. (7) The Arthus reaction is characterized by formation and precipitation of antigen–antibody complexes in the affected vessels, which does not occur in anaphylaxis. (8) In anaphylaxis, the principal phenomenon is increase in capillary permeability; the Arthus reaction is much more complex, involving edema (generally intense), hemorrhage, cellular infiltration and, in more severe reactions, ischemia with necrosis and loss of tissue in the area affected. (9) The passive Arthus reaction does not require a period of sensitization as does the anaphylactic reaction.

Pathogenesis. Tissue modifications occurring in the Arthus reaction are the same as those occurring in the phenomenon of inflammation. Microscopic observations made with a transparent chamber adapted to the ear of an immunized rabbit have shown that the first modifications visible after contact with the antigen consist of constriction of arterioles, with decrease in blood flow, adherence of the polymorphs and

platelets to the vessel walls, with formation of small clots, diapedesis of the leukocytes, and passage of plasma and erythrocytes to the interstitium . After several hours, edema and polymorphonuclear cell infiltration predominate. In more intense cases, there is ischemia due to thrombosis, producing necrosis of the affected tissues. Hemorrhage is a consequence of lesions of the blood vessels. It has been demonstrated by immunofluorescence that the first phenomenon to occur during the Arthus reaction is the deposition of antigen–antibody complexes. However, the formation of antigen–antibody complexes alone is not sufficient to produce the Arthus phenomenon. In fact, even given the formation of complexes, the reaction does not develop if the animal has previously been decomplemented (e.g., by injection of aggregated gamma globulin) or if it has been rendered leukopenic by the injection of antipolymorphonuclear serum. Thus the Arthus reaction depends upon the following sequence of phenomena: (1) deposition of antigen–antibody complexes on the walls of the small vessels, between the endothelium and the basement membrane; (2) complement fixation; (3) having fixed complement, the complexes become chemotactic, provoking the migration of leukocytes to the site of the reaction; and (4) phagocytosis of the antigen–antibody complex and liberation of the lysosomal enzymes that aggravate the vasculitis, producing focal necrosis and other inflammatory alterations. The sequela just described is the principle pathogenic mechanism unterlying the development of autoimmune diseases (see p. 373).

Serum Sickness

From the beginning of this century until about 1940, various types of infections were treated with injection of relatively large volumes of heterologous antisera. After 1 or 2 weeks, patients subjected to this treatment generally exhibited a typical syndrome consisting of adenopathy, fever, erythematous or urticarial eruptions, and pain in the joints. This syndrome came to be known as serum sickness. Today, although serotherapy is not frequently used, the same syndrome may be produced by allergic reactions to penicillin or other drugs. The lesions generally disappear in a few days. In rare fatal cases, autopsy discloses vascular lesions resembling those observed in the Arthus reaction. The syndrome is easily reproduced experimentally, and its pathogenic mechanism is well known.

Pathogenesis. In essence, serum sickness depends upon antigen–antibody interaction in the circulatory system, with formation of antigen–antibody complexes in the presence of antigen excess.

Experimental serum sickness is produced only with antigens capable of remaining in the circulation for long periods, such as the plasma proteins. These, when heterologous, are removed from the circulation by an elimination process that occurs in three successive stages. In an initial stage, 50% of the foreign protein disappears from the circulation within 24 h as a result of the passage of the protein to the extravascular spaces. The second step is represented by a constant decrease that follows an exponential curve; i.e., a constant aliquot is eliminated in a unit of time. This phase, which appears to repre-

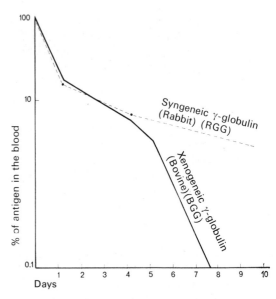

Fig. 10.13. Elimination curve of a xenogeneic protein (bovine gamma globulin) and a syngeneic (or allogeneic) protein (rabbit gamma globulin) in a normal rabbit injected with ^{131}I-labeled proteins

sent the elimination of foreign protein by normal catabolic processes, lasts 6–7 days. This stage is followed by a third stage, sudden and accelerated, called the immune elimination phase. This phase results from the production of antibody against the foreign protein, giving rise to the formation of antigen–antibody complexes that are rapidly sequestered from the circulation by the activity of the reticuloendothelial system. The elimination curves of ^{131}I – labeled syngeneic and xenogeneic gamma globulins (bovine) injected in normal rabbits can be seen in Fig. 10.13. The complexes formed initially are small and originate in extreme antigen excess. These complexes of the Ag_2Ab type do not fix complement and can endure for a long time in the circulation. The size of the complexes or their antibody content increases proportionally to the increase in the quantity of antibodies produced. The complexes are of the Ag_3–Ab_2 type, fix complement efficiently, and are rapidly removed from the circulation. At this point, the exudative and inflammatory lesions of serum sickness are established in the tissues, particularly in the heart, arteries, joints, and kidneys. The glomerulonephritis is caused by the deposition of large quantities of antigen–antibody complexes on the epithelial side of the basement membrane. The events subsequent to deposition, include fixation of the complement components, production of chemotactic factors, attraction of leukocytes, liberation of proteolytic enzymes, and lesions of the endothelium, which cause the destruction of the glomerulus. A chronic form of glomerulonephritis can be produced experimentally by repeated injections of small quantities of antigen into an immunized animal or by injection of preformed antigen–antibody complexes. This type of mechanism occurs in glomerulonephritis associated with diseases such as diabetes mellitus (insulin-anti-insulin), thyroiditis (thyroglobulin-antithyroglobulin), and lupus erythematosus (DNA-anti-DNA) in which the individual produces antibodies against his own tissues. The lesions existing in these diseases are due primarily to the presence of complexes in the tissues (see Chap. 13). Such complexes are capable of activating C 1, giving rise to the production of fibrinolysin, anaphylatoxin, and vasoactive oligopeptides such as bradykinin. The role of these substances in the establishment of serum sickness lesions has not yet definitely been proved. After the complete elimination of the complexes, the lesions disappear rapidly and the recuperation of the tissues is as complete as possible. The dependency of the antigen–antibody complexes, the participation of complement, and the similarity of the histologic lesions raise the inference that serum sickness is a type of systemic Arthus reaction. In this case, the same dose of the substance injected would serve initially as immunogen and later as antigen. However, since the immune response is complex, homocytotropic antibodies are also formed and are possibly responsible for some lesions of the anaphylactic type, such as urticaria. Serum sickness is considered a mixed syndrome in which phenomena common to the Arthus reaction and the anaphylactic reaction coexist.

Cell-Mediated Reaction (Delayed Hypersensitivity, Type IV)

Delayed hypersensitivity reactions appear 12–24 h (or even several days) after contact with the antigen and are transferrable by sensitized lymphoid cells (adoptive sensitivity), but not by the antibodies.

Delayed hypersensitivity reactions include not only the classic tuberculin reaction and similar reactions observed with other microbial infections, viral or parasitic, but also reactions such as contact hypersensitivity, and delayed hypersensitivity to purified proteins or to protein-hapten conjugates, to certain autoallergic diseases (e.g., experimental autoallergic encephalomyelitis), and to the allograft rejection reaction.

Reaction to Tuberculin

The prototype of the delayed reaction is the reaction to tuberculin, exhibited by an individual sensitized to *Mycobacterium tuberculosis*. Koch observed that tuberculous guinea pigs inoculated with live tuberculosis bacilli responded with a local inflammatory reaction much more rapidly and intensely than did noninfected guinea pigs (Koch's phenomenon). Subsequently, it was verified that the same phenomenon could be reproduced by injection of tuberculin or of a filtrate of heated, concentrated *Mycobacterium tuberculosis* cultures. Currently, the proteins present in tuberculin are precipitated with ammonium sulfate and the product, known as PPD (purified protein derivative), is used in place of the tuberculin. When a sensitized individual is injected intradermally with tuberculin or PPD, no modification is observed at the site. After about 6–10 h, a small firm papule appears at the site, accompanied by erythema. This papule grows slowly, becoming considerably larger during the next 24–72 h, and then disappears slowly over several days. In the more intense reactions, hemorrhaging and necrosis can occur. A positive tuberculin test indicates that the individual has or has had a *Mycobacterium tuberculosis* infection.

In human beings the reaction can be obtained with extremely small quantities of PPD (of the order of 0.02 µg), whereas guinea pigs require larger quantities (0.5 µg) for an appreciable reaction. In rats and mice, the reactions are much weaker and sometimes require microscopic examination to identify the response. In man, the tuberculin reaction also can be provoked by percutaneous application, i.e., by direct application to the skin of pieces of filter paper (or other tissue) imbedded with tuberculin (patch test). The percutaneous reaction is not possible in the guinea pig, which does not possess sweat glands. It is positive in man only in the areas of the skin that contain sweat glands. The antigen may penetrate the skin through the ducts of these glands.

Systemic Reaction to Tuberculin

In sensitized persons or guinea pigs, the injection of relatively large quantities of tuberculin can provoke a generalized reaction, tuberculin shock. In the guinea pig, tuberculin shock is characterized by prostration and hypothermia, which appears within 2–3 h and can cause death. In extremely sensitive individuals, intradermal inoculation of tuberculin can produce, after a few hours, indisposition, headache, and prostration, and rarely death. If the individual is tuberculous, the inflammatory process in the pulmonary lesions or other locations can be exacerbated. Similar systemic reactions can be provoked with other antigens obtained from infectious agents in sensitized individuals. For this reason, it is advisable in performing the tuberculin test (Mantoux test) always to use only small quantities of tuberculin or PPD.

Delayed Reaction to Proteins

Delayed hypersensitivity reactions to simple proteins such as ovalbumin and serum albumin can be obtained using special sensitization methods. The method used initially was to inject the protein directly into the lesions of tuberculous guinea pigs. Currently, the more common method is the intradermal injection of small quantities of protein (of the order of micrograms) emulsified in complete Freund's adjuvant or of small quantities of antigen in the form of antigen–antibody complexes obtained in antibody excess.

Contact Sensitivity

Many natural substances and relatively simple chemical products are responsible for an allergic illness commonly encountered in patients – so-called contact dermatitis. The reaction typically is of the delayed type and, in this case, the sensitizing and unleashing doses are applied in the same fashion by contact with the skin. A great variety of substances can be responsible for the ailment; among the most common are certain plants, such as the primrose, cotton seed, citrus fruits, tomatoes; diverse drugs; and other commonly used chemical products (herbicides, insecticides, dyes, and cosmetics). These substances have two characteristics in common: They are nonimmunogenic, and they easily form conjugates with proteins. It is believed that such substances penetrate the epidermis and combine with the tissue proteins, which then become recognized as foreign. On many occasions an isolated contact with these substances is sufficient to establish contact sensitivity, whereas in other cases more frequent contact is necessary to obtain the same effect. About a week after the sensitizing dose, contact between any region of the skin and the antigen provokes, after 10–12 h, erythematous papules, which later transform into small blisters that burst, leaving erythematous areas without epidermis. Later still, there is extensive formation of crusts along with hyperkeratosis. In the guinea pig, the same reaction is observed, but without the formation of blisters. At the site of the reaction, the dermis is invaded by inflammatory mononuclear cells – especially around the blood vessels and the sweat glands. This cellular infiltrate is indistinguishable from those observed in other types of delayed reactions.

Many of the substances that cause contact dermatitis in man are also capable of producing contact hypersensitivity in the guinea pig. Of these, picryl chloride, dinitrofluorobenzene, and dinitrochlorobenzene are most often used. As with the delayed hypersensitivity reaction, contact hypersensitivity is more specific than the serologic reactions. For example, guinea pigs sensitized with 2,4,6-trinitrochlororbenzene (picryl chloride) react with this substance, yet they do not react with 2-4-dinitrochlorobenzene. In this case, the specificity conferred by the carrier protein is important, a phenomenon to be discussed more extensively later.

Transfer of Delayed Hypersensitivity

Numerous attempts at passive transfer of the delayed reactions by antisera have consistently failed. On the other hand, viable lymphoid cells obtained from sensitized guinea pigs conferred upon normal recipients the capacity to respond to the antigen with the typical delayed reaction, as indicated in Fig. 10.14. Transfer by cells is termed adoptive sensitivity. Adoptive sensitivity persists only while the transferred cells survive in the recipient. If the adoptive sensitivity occurs between genetically different individuals, the sensitivity is of short duration (about a week), but if occuring in syngeneic animals it persists for a long time. Dead lymphoid cells or lymphoid cells with damaged mechanisms for protein synthesis do not produce adoptive sensitivity. It should not be forgotten that adoptive sensitivity also transfers immediate hypersensitivity that is dependent upon the transfer of antibody-forming cells or those involved in the production of antibodies.

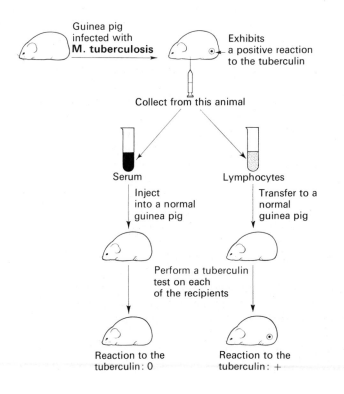

Fig. 10.14. Transfer of cellular or delayed hypersensitivity

Transfer Factor. Whereas in laboratory animals, adoptive sensitivity has been obtained only with viable lymphoid cells, Lawrence observed that the sensitivity of the tuberculin type in man can be transferred by means of extracts of leukocytes obtained from sensitized individuals. The retarded reaction appears in the recipients a few hours after the intradermal injection of the leukocytic extract, although it usually requires 2–3 days for maximum sensitivity. Sensitivity thus conferred persists for years and can be transferred in series, i.e., the cells of the first recipient are capable of transferring sensitivity to a second and from this to a third recipient, suggesting that the factor is capable of self-replication. The active component of these extracts is called the transfer factor; it can be liberated from lymphocytes incubated with the antigen. The material is stable, dialysable, and has an absorption spectrum in the nucleic acid zone, but is not inactivated by ribonuclease or by deoxyribonuclease. The nature and operative mechanism of transfer factor are unknown.

The Effector Cell in Delayed Hypersensitivity

The fact that the capacity to transfer delayed hypersensitivity is limited to lymphoid cells, together with the observation that at the site of delayed reactions there exists an infiltration of cells morphologically similar to lymphocytes, suggested that the cells transferred were totally responsible for the cellular infiltration of delayed hypersensitivity. However, transfer experiments with sensitized cells labeled with tritiated thymidine showed that these cells constituted only 5%–10% of the cells present at the site of the reaction. Moreover, when the cells of the recipient were labeled beforehand with tritiated thymidine, 80%–95% of the cells present in the infiltrate were labeled cells. Thus, it became clear that the transferred cells modified the behavior of the cells of the recipient, conditioning them to migrate to the locality of the reaction. Experiments with animals whose lymphoid and myeloid tissues had been destroyed by irradiation demonstrated that the local inflammatory reaction site in delayed hypersensitivity was comprised almost exclusively of macrophages originating from the bone marrow. In these experiments irradiated animals, incapable of exhibiting a delayed reaction to tuberculin, were divided into four groups, inoculated respectively as follows: (1) bone marrow cells of sensitized donors; (2) bone marrow cells of nonsensitized donors; (3) lymph node cells of sensitized donors; and (4) bone marrow cells of nonsensitized donors plus lymph node cells of sensitized donors. The results of these experiments are illustrated in Fig. 10.15. The animals of group (1) developed delayed reactions similar to those found in the nonirradiated control group. At the reaction site there was intense infiltration by mononuclear cells, many of which appeared to be lymphocytes. Delayed reactions with cellular infiltration identical to these were ob-

Recipient irradiated and inoculated with

		Delayed Reaction
(1)	Cells from the bone marrow of sensitized donor	+
(2)	Cells from the bone marrow of unsensitized donor	0
(3)	Lymph node cells from sensitized donor	0
(4)	Bone marrow cells from unsensitized donor plus lymph node cells from sensitized donor	+

Fig. 10.15. Protocol of experiment showing cooperation between cells of the bone marrow and lymph node cells in the establishment of delayed reactions

tained in the animals of group (4), but not in the animals of groups (2) and (3), which did not react to the tuberculin tests. These results demonstrated that the cells of the lymph nodes as well as of the bone marrow are capable of migrating to reaction sites. Apparently, the lymphoid cells condition the macrophages of the bone marrow, inducing them to migrate to the reaction site, thus showing the existence of cooperation between the bone marrow cells and the lymphocytes. The exact mechanism by which the macrophages accumulate in the site of the reaction is not known.

Interaction in Vitro of the Antigen with Sensitized Lymphoid Cells. Many types of tests have been developed to detect delayed reactions in vitro. One most often used is inhibition of macrophage migration by specific antigen. In performing this test, capillary tubes open at one end and filled with cells obtained from abdominal cavity exudates from sensitized animals (such exudates, produced experimentally by intraperitoneal injection of mineral oil, contain a large proportion of lymphocytes and macrophages) are immersed in culture medium in special chambers. Usually, two preparations of this type are made, but only one of them receives the antigen to be tested. Then the chambers are incubated at 37 °C for 24–48 h. Microscopic observation after this period demonstrates that in the control preparation the macrophages migrate to the exterior of the open end of the capillary tube, invading the culture medium, whereas in the preparation to which the antigen was added, this macrophage migration does not occur (Fig. 10.16). This inhibition of migration is specific, being produced only by the antigen capable of inducing a delayed reaction in the animal from which the cells were obtained. Cells of a nonsensitized animal do not respond to the antigen in the manner. If cells from nonsensitized animals are mixed with cells (1% is sufficient) from sensitized animals, the former become responsive to the antigen as if they also had come from sensitized animals. This transfer of sensitization

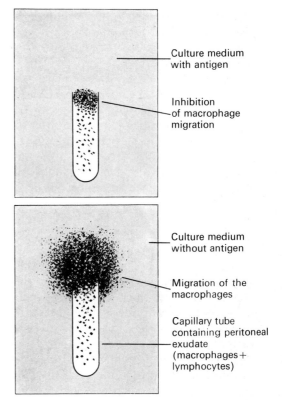

Fig. 10.16. Macrophage inhibition test

requires live cells; dead cells or cellular extracts are ineffective. Moreover, sensitized cells only transfer the capacity for inhibition to nonsensitized cells when they are capable of synthesizing proteins, since the phenomenon is inhibited by mitomycin C. Studies with pure lymphocyte and macrophage suspensions have demonstrated that it is the lymphocyte that possesses the immunologic information necessary for transmission to the macrophage of the capacity to be inhibited by the antigen. The fact that only 1% of sensitized lymphocytes are sufficient to transfer the property of antigen inhibition to a population of normal macrophages suggests that the inhibition does not result from direct cell-to-cell interaction. Various experiments have demonstrated that lymphocytes sensitized and incubated with antigen synthesize and liberate into the ambient medium a soluble substance of unknown nature, which has been named macrophage inhibitory factor, or MIF. The substance is dialysable, thermoresistant, is not destroyed by treatment with ribonuclease or deoxyribonuclease, but is destroyed by proteolytic enzymes. Its operative mechanism is unknown. The test for inhibition of macrophage migration has also been attempted with human cells. The addition of antigen to lymphocytes obtained from the peripheral blood of patients with delayed hypersensitivity liberates a factor inhibitive of the migration of both human and guinea pig macrophages. This observation suggests that the MIF is not species-specific. Aside from MIF, other substances may be produced upon contact between sensitized lymphocytes and antigen: These are collectively termed lymphokines. For example, in the supernatant of cultures of sensitized lymphocytes stimulated by the antigen, there is a factor that possesses a chemotactic effect on macrophages. Moreover, intradermal injection of MIF into nonsensitized animals induces the appearance of a local reaction resembling delayed hypersensitivity. The various lymphokines and their activities are summarized in Table 10.5. Whether or not each of these activities corresponds to a specific substance has not yet been established.

Table 10.5. Properties of the lymphokines

Lymphokine	Biologic activity
Macrophage activation factor	Augments motility and the phagocytosis of macrophages
Skin reactive factor	Produces inflammation in the skin
Chemotactic factor for macrophages	Attracts macrophages
Chemotactic factor for lymphocytes	Attracts lymphocytes
Chemotactic factor for neutrophils	Attracts neutrophils
Chemotactic factor for eosinophils	Attracts eosinophils
Mitogenic factor	Induces lymphocyte transformation (blast transformation)
Lymphotoxin	Destroys cells in a fashion identical to that of sensitized lymphocytes
Macrophage inhibitory factor (MIF)	Impedes migration of the macrophages in vitro
Macrophage aggregation factor	Causes aggregation of the macrophages
Transfer factor	Transfers human cellular hypersensitivity

Mechanism of Target-Cell Destruction

Histologically, the delayed hypersensitivity reaction is characterized by accumulation of inflammatory cells in the site where the antigen was inoculated, initially represented by polymorphonuclear cells, but later by mononuclear cells, with lymphocytes and macrophages predominating. Microscopically, one can observe the formation of perivascular islets of mononuclear cells resembling large lymphocytes, monocytes, or macrophages. These are the cells responsible for the local inflammatory phenomena. It is not known for sure by which mechanism these cells cause destruction of the tissues upon reacting with the antigen. Histologic studies suggest a direct destructive effect of the sensitized lymphocytes upon the cells that contain the antigen. Once activated by

the specific antigen, the lymphocytes are called effector cells or killer cells that destroy the target cell.

In general, it is thought that cell destruction during the delayed hypersensitivity reaction occurs through at least three mechanisms (Fig. 10.16).

(1) Contact lysis. Sensitized T cells come in direct contact with target cells and destroy them, although the exact procedure is unknown. If sensitized lymphocytes are mixed in in vitro culture with target cells, they adhere to the target cells by fine cytoplasmic protuberances, the "uropods." By electron-microscopic examination, one can observe wide areas of surface contact with narrow interstices between the lymphocytes and target-cell membrane, with long, fine projections from the cell surface and microvilli and microtubules in the cytoplasm in the area of the contact side. Some time after cell contact, the target cell swells, stops moving, and

Fig. 10.17 a–d. Sequence of a delayed hypersensitivity reaction. **a** The antigen encounters the sensitized lymphocytes in a venule and produces MIF. **b** The MIF alters the endothelium of the vessel and causes monocytes to cling to it. The monocytes acquire the characteristics of tissue macrophages. **c, d** The activated macrophages liberate enzymes, attack the vessel walls, and invade the local parenchyma, i.e., in this case, the myelin sheath in experimental encephalomyelitis [Adapted from Tomasi TB (1971) The Gamma Globulin A: a first line of defense. In: Immunobiology (eds Good and Fisher), p. 83. Sinauer Ass., Inc., Stamford, Conn.]

lyses. The recognition and adherence to the target cell probably occur via killer-cell receptors. If killer cells are added to a mixture of cells containing only one type against which they are sensitized, only the specific target cell is lysed, which suggests that lysis occurs because of a specific mechanism and does not depend on the liberation of a soluble, cytotoxic factor. Because a linear relationship exists between the number of added lymphocytes and the number of lysed target cells, one can postulate a reaction of the "one-hit" type.

(2) Lymphotoxin-mediated destruction. Sensitized lymphocytes, activated by a specific antigen, or nonsensitized lymphocytes, nonspecifically stimulated by mitogens, liberate a toxic substance (lymphotoxin) that kills cells. In these cases, the reaction with the antigen of the target cell is specific, but the destruction is nonspecific.

(3) Antibody-dependent cell-mediated cytotoxicity (see Chaps. 2 and 9). In this case, lymphocytes can destroy cells that have antibodies bound to their surfaces. However, the active cells are not only lymphocytes, but adherent cells, probably B cells, macrophages, or K cells (adherent lymphoid cells of unknown origin), which have surface receptors for immunoglobulin-Fc fragments. Complement plays no role in this reaction.

Antigen Recognition by Killer T Cells

Although it is accepted that T cells recognize antigens specifically and react with them, little is known about the recognition mechanism. Experimental results suggest that antigen recognition by T cells is probably dependent upon membrane alterations that occur after reaction of the antigens with specific receptors on other cells (B cells, macrophages). For example, if DNP lymphocytes (viable lymphocytes whose surfaces were conjugated with dinitrophenyl groups) are injected into syngeneic mice, T cells are formed (killer cells) that lyse DNP lymphocytes specifically but are inca-

pable of lysing normal (nonconjugated) lymphocytes. These cells are also incapable of lysing allogenic DNP lymphocytes that possess major histocompatibility antigens different from those of the killer cells. Studies of the membrane proteins of DNP lymphocytes showed that not only histocompatibility antigens but almost all membrane proteins are dinitrophenylized. The results could mean that the immune response against DNP lymphocytes is directed only against DNP–H-2 (major histocompatibility complex in the mouse)-conjugated proteins. This would explain why cells that differ only in their MHC proteins can form different antigenic conformations. It is possible that T cells do not even recognize isolated antigens, but rather that they are only activated if antigens together with MHC proteins are present on the cell surface. Furthermore, there is evidence that T helper cells can cooperate with B cells only when the latter carry *Ir*-gene products that the T helper cell recognized upon initial contact with the antigen.

The recognition of target cells by killer cells appears to proceed in a similar manner. For killer cells to recognize the target antigen, they must likewise be formed with the same antigen on their surface that was present on the stimulator cell that led to the differentiation of the killer cell. Thus, it appears that T cells require two different receptor specificities in order to recognize two different structures, either on the cooperating cell or on the target cell (see Chap. 6).

Jones-Mote Reaction

Under certain experimental conditions, a form of delayed cutaneous hypersensitivity can be obtained with characteristics that differentiate it from a typical delayed reaction. This reaction is called the Jones-Mote reaction and is characterized by the presence of an infiltration of basophilic leukocytes with cell infiltrate. The reaction is exhibited as a discrete area of erythema that persists for about 24 h and then quickly disappears; it is always of moderate intensity and never produces necrosis. The Jones-Mote reaction appears in guinea pigs in the course of daily intradermal injections of protein antigens – appearing 1 or 2 days before the appearance of the Arthus reaction and then immediately disappearing. The Jones-Mote reaction also occurs in guinea pigs immunized with proteins in incomplete Freund's adjuvant; in this case, it occurs some days before the appearance of the classic delayed reaction. The significance of this type of delayed reaction is not known.

References

Austen KF, Wassermann SI, Goetzl EJ (1987) Mast cell derived mediators: Structural and functional diversity and regulation of expression. In: Johansson SGO, Strandberg K and Uvnas B (eds). Molecular and biological aspects of the acute allergic reaction. Plenum Press New York

Bennich H e Bahr-Lindstrom (1974) Structure of immunoglobulin E (IgE). Prog Immunol 1:49

Becker EL (1971) Nature and classification of the acute allergic reaction. Adv Immunol 13:267

Braun W, Lichtensein NW, Parker CW (eds) (1974) Cyclic AMP, cell growth and the immune response. Springer, Berlin Heidelberg New York

Capron A, Dessaint JP, Capron M (1975). Specific IgE antibodies in immune adherence of normal macrophages to Schistosoma mansoni schistosomules. Nature 253:474

Coombs RRA, Gell PGH (1975) Classification of allergic reactions responsible for clinical hypersensitivity and disease. In: Gell PGH, Coombs RRA, Lachmann PJ (eds) Clinical aspects of immunology. Blackwell, Oxford

Gupta S, Good RA (eds) (1979) Cellular, molecular, and clinical aspects of allergic disorders. Plenum, New York

Ishizaka K (1976) Cellular events in the IgE antibody response. Adv Immunol 23:1

Johansson SGO, Foucard T, Dannaeus A (1974) IgE in human disease. Prog Immunol 4:61

Kaliner M, Austen KF (1973) A sequence of biochemical events in the antigen-induced release of chemical mediators from sensitized human lung tissue. J Exp Med 138:1077

Katz DH (1978) The allergic phenotype: Manifestation of "Allergic Breakthrough" and imbalance in normal damping of IgE antibody production. Immunol Rev 41:77

Kay AB (1980) Dinamics, role and function of eosinophils. In: Advances in Allergology and Applied Immunology. Oehling, Glazer, Mathov and Arbesman (eds). Pergamon Press, Oxford

Leslie RGQ, Alexander MD (1979) Cytophilic antibodies. Curr Top Microbiol Immunol 88:25

Mota I, Catty D (1974) Biological actions of anaphylactic antibodies. Prog Immunol 4:306

Ovary Z, Saluk PH, Quijada L, Lamm M (1976) Biologic activities of rabbit immunoglobulin relation to domains of the Fc region. J Immunol 116:1265

Stanworth DR (1974) The role of the antibody in immunological cell triggering processes. Haematologia (Basel) 8:299

Tada T (1975) Regulation of reaginic antibody formation in animals. Prog Allergy 19:122

Takatsu K, Ishizaka T, Ishizaka K (1975) Biologic significance of disulfide bonds in human IgE molecules. J Immunol 114:1838

Taurog JD, Fewtrell C, Becker EL (1979). IgE mediated triggering of rat basophil leukemia cells: Lack of evidence for serine esterase activation. J. Immunol. 122:2150

Theofilopoulos AN, Dixon FJ (1979) The biology and detection of immune complexes. Adv Immunol 28:89

Trotter CM, Orr TSC (1973) A fine structure study of some cellular components in allergic reactions. I. Degranulation of human mast cells in allergic asthma and perennial rhinitis. Clin Allergy 3:411

Chapter 11 Immunity

Dietrich Götze and Wilmar Dias da Silva

Contents

Mechanisms of Immunity

The resistance to infections is based on several defense lines erected at different levels of specificity: natural or nonspecific immunity, and adaptive, acquired, or specific immunity.

In simplified terms, natural resistance refers to the ability of an individual to resist infections through normal body functions. Natural resistance does not include resistance resulting from a previous exposure to the pathogenic organism or its toxic products; this is adaptive resistance. Natural resistance relies on nonadaptive or normal activities of an organism that are always present. On the other hand, natural resistance and adaptive immunity are intimately connected and operate together; deficiencies on either part will result in a marked increase in frequency and severity of infections (see Chap. 12).

Natural Immunity

The first lines of defense are skin and mucosa. They are not a mere physical barrier: desquamation and other forms of epithelial cell turnover at body surfaces remove large numbers of adherent microbes; in addition, it is known that lactic acid in sweat and unsaturated fatty acids from sebaceous glands are microbiocidal: skin and mucosa produce chemical disinfectants. Salivary glycolipids prevent attachment of potentially cariogenic bacteria to oral epithelial cell surfaces. Saliva and milk contain a lactoperoxidase-$SCN-H_2O_2$ system that possesses antibacterial activity. Mucosal tissue produces a gelatinous-like bioadhesive slime; microorganisms impinging on this film are caught and swept away by the cilial activity of the cell layer beneath the mucous film. Nasal mucus, tears, saliva, and also urine contain lysozyme (muramidase, see below) in high concentration, which cleaves a β-1,4-glycosidic bond that unites N-acetylglucosamine and muramic acid, a substrate accessible in the cell wall of gram-positive bacteria (in gram-negative bacteria, the enzyme substrate is also present, but shielded from the enzyme by lipid). In the stomach, a very acid (pH 1.0) environment is not favorable for the growth of microorganisms. Bile acids are excreted as glycine and taurine conjugates and are deconjugated by intestinal anaerobes. Deconjugated intestinal bile salts are inhibitory for a number of microorganisms (e.g., *Cl. perfringens*, lactobacilli, enterococci). The small and large intestines are heavily colonized with the normal flora, basically noninvasive bacteria, which, however, produce certain acid end products and antibiotic-like substances. In addition, almost all secretions contain (preformed, natural) antibodies, which are produced in response to many different, continuously present bacterial antigens, primarily of the intestinal flora.

Acidity of skin and vaginal secretions retards local colonization by potential pathogens. Spermine, a polyamine present in prostatic secretions, is a potent inhibitor of gram-positive microorganisms. Seminal fluid also possesses potent bactericidal activity.

Intact skin is not easily penetrated. For many pathogens, the first step in initiating infections is attachment to epithelial or mucosal cell surfaces. This is in part a function of the microbial surface, e.g., pili of *gonococci*, *shigellae sp.*, *vibrios*. Many viruses have surface components which allow them to attach to specific cell membrane receptors, e.g., influenza agglutinin attaches specifically to N-acetylneuraminic acid residues on cell membranes; human cells have receptors for poliovirus. Attachment by itself need not be followed by penetration of the microbe into the cell; thus, *Mycoplasma pneumoniae*, *C. diphtheriae*, and *B. pertussis* remain on the epithelial surface. Other penetrate into epithelial cells, stay there (e.g., shigellae), and do not spread further. Staying inside cells, particularly in those which do not have bactericidal systems (which phagocytes possess), protects the microorganisms from antibodies (and antibiotics), and very often from ingestion and killing by phagocytes (see below).

The host defense against these activities is manifold: (a) the above-mentioned "chemical factory" of outer and inner dermis may prevent effective attachment; (b) rapid turnover of the outer cell layer sweeps away attached or even penetrated microbes; (c) antibodies at the local mucosal level play a significant role in the interference with possible infections. The antibody response at mucosal surfaces is mediated primarily by secretory IgA. Mucosal immunity appears to be highly localized: elevated antibody titers in salivary secretions may not be associated with similar activity in the tears. This local activity is also suggested by the anatomical situation, i.e., the high number of lymphoid nodules of the tonsillary ring of Waldeyer, of the ileum (Peyer patches), and the diffuse lymphoid tissue in the lamina propria of the trachea, small intestine, and vaginal mucosa, all of which are directly fed by capillary lymph vessels coming from the mucosal surface.

It appears that secretory IgA has major importance in protection from many virus infections (e.g., poliomyelitis) by neutralizing infectious microbes on the mucosal surface. Of course, some microorganisms have developed mechanisms to prevent the action of IgA: thus, *N. onorrhoeae* and *N. meningotidis* possess IgA proteolytic activity in vitro, cleaving and so inactivating IgA. This game of effect and countereffect played by invaded and invading participants is the essence of resistance and susceptibility (see below).

Pathogens successfully penetrating these barriers will be confronted with the internal armour of defense. The polymorphonuclear (PMN) leukocytes are generally considered to be the first to fight against bacterial invasions, reflecting the fact that these cells are the first to arrive at the scene. The PMN is thus the hallmark of the acute inflammatory process. If the bacterial invasion is sufficiently strong such that the PMN are unable to cope with the swarms of invaders, the second in line, the macrophages, will take over, giving rise to the condition of chronic inflammation. The third line of defense, the adaptive immunity, becomes established only after lymphocytes have been stimulated and activated by "activated and antigen-presenting" macrophages (Fig. 11.1).

Polymorphonuclear cells and macrophages have been termed "professional" phagocytes, because their membranes possess specialized receptors for the Fc portion of IgG

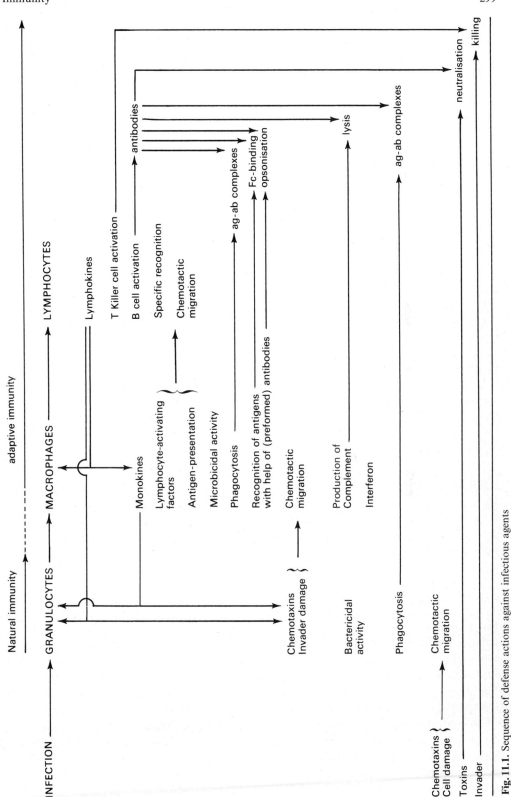

Fig. 11.1. Sequence of defense actions against infectious agents

molecules (IgG$_1$ and IgG$_3$ subclasses in man), and for activated C3. Nonprofessional or facultative phagocytes include endothelial cells, epithelial cells, fibroblasts, and other cells which will ingest microorganisms under specialized conditions but which do not possess receptors for IgG and C3.

Polymorphonuclear cells are concerned principally with the destruction of microorganisms which rely upon the evasion of phagocytosis for survival, i.e., extracellular pathogens; their prototype is the pneumococcus. Mononuclear cells are concerned with the control of microorganisms which are able to survive intracellular residence and against which neutrophils are ineffective.

Natural immunity does not only rely on the activity of the two phagocytic cell systems but is supported by factorial systems present in the blood. These are the pool of so-called natural or *preformed antibodies*, the *complement systems*, and certain proteins such as *betalysin, lysozyme*, and *C-reactive protein*.

Natural or *preformed antibodies* are actually not "natural" but have been formed by specifically stimulated antibody-secreting cells. We do not know their specificity in terms of which particular material induced their formation. They are formed primarily against microbial antigens of the intestinal flora and other "commensal" microorganisms, and against any other microbes which happen to come in close contact with the immune system, but are not necessarily pathogenic. Animals which have been delivered by caesarean section into a germ-free environment, and further raised under germ-free conditions, have a less well-developed immune system; the immunoglobulin synthesis is drastically reduced in comparison to animals raised conventionally. The factors and activities of the *complement system* have been described in detail in Chap. 5.

Betalysin is a highly reactive heat-stable cationic protein; it is released from platelets and destroys nonenzymatically the cell membrane of gram-positive microorganisms, except pneumococci. The characteristics and mechanisms of action of lysozyme, which is present in serum in a concentration of 1–2 µg/ml, will be discussed below.

C-reactive protein (CRP) is a nonimmunoglobulin acute-phase protein which appears in increased amounts in sera during infection and tissue damage; it is synthesized in the liver and released into the blood. CRP forms calcium-dependent precipitating complexes with somatic C-polysaccharide of pneumococcus, and of several other bacteria and fungi; it induces increased (random) migration of leukocytes, promotes phagocytosis, and activates complement through the classical pathway.

Polymorphonuclear Cells

After infection, PMN cells detect the pathogen and migrate out of the blood stream and into the tissue area where the intrusion occurred. This sequence of events involves an *increase in the permeability* of the capillary wall, *migration* through the endothelial gap of the vessel, and directed movement of the cell toward the pathogen in the tissue (*chemotaxis*). The initial "trigger mechanisms" that initiate these changes are not known with certainty but probably the bacterial surface and bacteria-produced substances are the activating components.

Migration

Permeability. Alteration in vascular permeability after the onset of the acute bacterial infection has a biphasic character; the initial phase of increased permeability begins immediately and lasts for no more than 1 h. A delayed second phase starts after about 2 h and reaches a peak after 4–6 h before subsiding. The first increase is almost certainly due to a release of histamine (serotonin in mice and rats) from basophils and mast cells. The mediators of the delayed permeability response are not identified with certainty, but kinins appear to be the most likely candidates; they are generated as indicated in Fig. 11.2. Possible other mediators are prostaglandins and the slow-reacting substance (see p. 267).

Migration. Concomitant with increased permeability, neutrophils adhere to the endothelium of blood vessels, extend pseudopodia, and penetrate the endothelium at or near the cell junction. The signal for adherence and emigration of cells has not been documented but it is assumed that the cells are responding to some type of chemotactic stimulus (see below). The cell movement is due to microfilaments and microtubules. The microfilaments are composed of contractile proteins; actin, myosin, and actin-binding protein have been demonstrated in neutrophils and macrophages. The actin in leukocytes is capable of reversible polymerization which is thought to underlie cellular locomotion. Also, microtubules have been implicated in the normal process of directed cell movement.

Chemotaxis. Substances with chemotactic activity have been collected from bacterial growth culture supernatants in which they have been released; these are peptides containing hydrophobic N-formylmethionin at the amino terminus, and lipids. In contrast to mammalian proteins, bacterial protein synthesis is universally initiated by incorporation of N-formylmethionin and as such is bacterial specific and a possible candidate for the "recognition molecule" to which phagocytes can respond. Perturbations of cell membranes lead to the mobilization from membrane phospholipids of the prostaglandin precursor arachidonic acid; oxidized compounds of this acid, HHT (12-L-hydroxy-5,8,10-Heptadecatrienoic acid) and HETE (12-L-hydroxy-5,8,10,14-eicosatetraenoic acid) are potent chemotactic factors for both eosinophils and neutrophils. Other chemotactic factors, generated by the interaction of bacteria with host components, derive from the activation by immune complexes of the classical, and by bac-

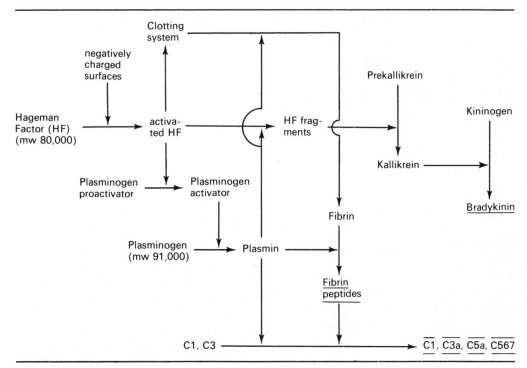

Underlined substances possess chemotactic activity

Fig. 11.2. Generation of chemotactic substances by the combined action of clotting and the complement system terial polysaccharides of the alternative, complement pathway, as well as from activation by negatively charged surfaces of Hageman factor of the clotting system (see Fig. 11.2). Stimulated host cells, e.g., mast cells, release chemotactic factors for neutrophils and eosinophils. The eosinophil chemotactic factor (ECF-A) is a family of 300–500 mol. wt. peptides. ECF-A extracted from human lung was extensively purified and was shown to contain two acid tetrapeptides of amino-acid sequence Ala-Gly-Ser-Glu and Val-Gly-Ser-Glu. Both highly purified ECF-A were maximally chemotactic for eosinophils at concentrations of 10^{-7} to $10^{-6} M$. Analysis of analogues of the tetrapeptides revealed that a hydrophobic amino terminus is required for interaction with the eosinophil, while an anionic carboxy terminus is required for chemotactic activation.

The mechanism whereby the various factors (summarized in Table 11.1) elicit a directed migration of the cell is obscure. It has been demonstrated that chemotactic factors cause activation of an esterase that contains a serine residue at its active site. Cells that have previously been incubated with serine inhibitors are unable to respond chemotactically to either complement components or bacterial factors. Likewise, once the serine esterase has been completely activated, the neutrophil is no longer capable of further chemotaxis. One might expect increased activation of the enzyme as it comes closer to the source of chemotactic factors. Once the neutrophil has made its way from the site of origin in the bone marrow to the area in the tissue where bacterial infiltration has occurred, the cell begins to phagocytoze or ingest viable microbes with subsequent destruction of the microorganism within the cell. This process consists of several stages: opsonization, adherence of neutrophils to bacteria, and ingestion.

Phagocytosis

Opsonization. The rate and extent of phagocytosis depends on a number of factors, particularly the nature of the particle. Not all bacteria are equally susceptible to phagocytosis; cells have special difficulty in ingesting encapsulated organisms. To counter this

Table 11.1. Chemotactic factors for human eosinophil and neutrophil polymorphonuclear leukocytes[a]

Chemotactic factor	Source	Structural characteristics
C5a	Classical and alternative complement pathways	17,000 mol. wt. basic protein
C$\overline{567}$	Classical and alternative complement pathways	435,000 mol. wt. protein complex
Fibrinopeptides and fibrin fragments	Coagulation and fibrinolytic pathways	30,000–50,000 mol. wt. 1,000 mol. wt. proteins and peptides
Plasma kallikrein	Kinin-generating pathway	108,000 mol. wt. α-globulin
C$\overline{3bB}$	Alternative complement pathway	234,000 mol. wt. protein complex
Bacterial soluble factors	Bacterial culture supernatants	300–1,000 mol. wt. peptides
Eosinophil chemotactic factor of anaphylaxis (ECF-A)	Mast cells	300–500 mol. wt. peptides
Histamine	Mast cells and basophils	111 mol. wt. amine
Crysta-induced chemotactic factor	Neutrophil lysosomes	8,400 mol. wt. glycoprotein
Lymphokines	Lymphocytes	12,500–60,000 mol. wt. proteins
Bacterial lipids	Bacterial culture supernatants	lipoproteins and lipids
HHT	Arachidonic acid cyclooxygenase pathway	280 mol. wt.
HETE	Arachidonic acid lipooxygenase pathway	330 mol. wt.

[a] After Valone FH (1980) Modulation of human neutrophil and eosinophil polymorphnuclear leukocyte chemotaxis: An analytical review. Clin Immunol Immunopathol 15:52

"armor coat" higher organisms have developed serum factors, opsonins, that attach to the bacteria and thus render them susceptible to phagocytosis. Two general classes of opsonins are known to exist (see also p. 197): (a) heat labile, derived from the complement system, involving activated components C 1, C 4, C 2, and C 3; and (b) heat stable, in serum of animals previously exposed to bacteria (immune opsonins). These are antibodies, primarily of the IgG_1 and IgG_3 subclasses.

A third factor stimulating phagocytosis was recently described and called "tuftsin" – because it was discovered at Tufts University in Boston. It is not really an opsonin but activates neutrophils to increased phagocytosis. Tuftsin is a tetrapeptide (threonine-lysine-proline-arginine) cleaved from gamma globulins (leukokinin) by the combined action of two proteolytic enzymes, one present in the spleen, and the other localized in the membrane of neutrophils (leukokininase (see p. 360).

Adherence is a prerequisite of subsequent ingestion but is not, in itself, sufficient. For example, mycoplasma adheres to human or rabbit neutrophils and this interaction leads to alterations of the metabolism in a manner similar to that observed with phagocytosis of particles, and yet no ingestion occurs. The adherence is thought to be mediated by receptors (Fc, complement), and appears to act as a trigger mechanism to initiate the biochemical events that accompany phagocytosis and bacterial killing by the cell. Concurrent with the attachment of a particle to the cell is a marked stimulation of the cellular metabolism including increase in oxidative metabolism and in lysosomal enzyme secretion.

Ingestion. Immediately following the attachment of the bacteria to the neutrophil under normal conditions, the phagocyte extends pseudopodia around the particle, eventually meeting and fusing to form the phagocytic vacuole (phagosome); the lining of the phagosome, therefore, is inverted plasma membrane. The phagosome buds off from the cell periphery and moves centripetally, apparently through the mediation of microtubules. The ingestion proceeds more readily if the particle is more hydrophobic than the membrane of the neutrophil; opsonization increases hydrophobicity. Parallel to these events, the phagocytic cells show an increased rate of glycolysis, a decrease in pH within phagocytic vacuoles – probably due to lactic acid accumulated as a result of increased glycolysis – and an increased turnover of lipids. The increased metabolism of lysophospholipids is of special interest since these compounds have detergent-like properties. Neutrophils possess a phospholipase-A activity that can remove a fatty acid from a phospholipid to yield the corresponding lysophospholipid. The presence of such enzymes in the plasma membrane may explain the turnover of membrane-lipid fatty acids and indicate the mechanism by which the cells reseal themselves. It has been suggested that membrane fusion might be facilitated by the presence of lysophospholipids in the membrane leading to the formation of micellar structures allowing fusion.

Bactericidal Activity

After ingestion, killing of bacteria depends upon two factors: *degranulation* of lysosomal constituents into the phagocytic vacuole, formation of phagolysosomes, and an alteration in oxygen metabolism referred to as *"respiratory burst."*

Degranulation proceeds by an unknown mechanism. At first, the specific granules with an optimal activity at neutral pH, containing lysozyme, lactoferrin, collagenase, and alkaline phosphatase, fuse with the phagosome. Only then, azurophilic granules (lysosomes) operating optimally at an acid pH and containing lysozyme, myeloperoxidase, acid hydrolases, neutral proteases, cationic proteins with bactericidal activity, and NADPH-oxidase, fuse with the phagosome; the activation of each type of granule is independent of the other. The net effect is that the contents of the various granules are brought into direct contact with the ingested particle. Frequently, the process of degranulation begins before the phagocytic vacuole is completely sealed; this results in the extrusion of granule constituents outside of the cell. This extrusion is selective, as only lysosomal enzymes accumulate in the medium during phagocytosis while cytoplasmic enzymes such as lactate dehydrogenase do not. This release of hydrolytic enzymes to the exterior of the cell may be responsible for much of the tissue damage that accompanies acute inflammation.

Oxygen-dependent Bactericidy. Concomitant with the ingestion and formation of phagolysosomes alterations in the oxidative metabolism, respiratory burst occurs. Cells that are unable to mount a normal respiratory burst show defective ability to kill many strains of bacteria; it appears, therefore, that these metabolic changes are necessary for the bactericidal activity. The respiratory burst is characterized by a marked increase in oxygen consumption which is cyanide independent, and therefore, mitochondrial-enzyme independent; an increase of glucose oxidation (via hexosemonophosphate shunt); and generation of high amounts of H_2O_2, and of highly reactive hydroperoxy radical (HO_2^-) and superoxide anions (O_2^-). The described appearance of chemiluminescence during phagocytosis is a reflection of superoxide anion generation since superoxide dismutase (SOD)[1] inhibits this chemiluminescence. Another reaction employed for the estimation of phagocytic activity, the reduction of nitroblue tetrazolium dye (NBT) to the insoluble blue formazan during phagocytosis, also shows an absolute requirement for oxygen and is inhibited by the addition of SOD; this reaction also reflects the formation of superoxide (see p. 343).

---

1 Two molecules of superoxide anions interact in a dismutation (or disproportionation) reaction to form oxygen and H_2O_2: $O_2^- + O_2^- + 2 H^+ \rightarrow H_2O_2 + O_2$. This reaction is catalyzed by the enzyme superoxide dismutase

Since H_2O_2 can penetrate into the cytoplasm, the presence of catalase and coupled glutathione is important for its extra-vacuolar destruction. Similarly, superoxide dismutase may function to protect the cell cytoplasm from superoxide anions.

The biochemical basis of the respiratory burst is the initial activation of NADPH-oxidase. NADPH is generated by the hexosemonophosphate shunt (Fig. 11.3). In this reaction, superoxide anions occur as intermediates and can spontaneously give rise to singlet oxygen ($^1O_2$).

A large number of mechanisms have been considered to explain the actual killing of microbes by neutrophils. It is clear that multiple interlocking microbicidal systems are present, providing considerable redundancy in host defense mechanisms. The antimicrobial mechanisms of human neutrophils may be divided into two general categories: oxygen dependent and oxygen independent (Table 11.2).

Table 11.2. Microbicidal mechanisms and substances operating in neutrophils

Oxygen dependent
Peroxidase dependent: oxidizable cofactors (halides)
Peroxidase independent: H_2O_2, free radical forms of oxygen
Oxygen independent
Lysozyme
Lactoferrin
Hydrolytic enzymes
Hydrolysases
Cationic proteins
Nuclear histones

The oxidative mechanisms of killing may be divided into those which are myeloperoxidase (MPO) mediated, and those which are not. Peroxidase-mediated processes are: iodination, formation of hypochloride (OCl^-) or Cl_2 with subsequent formation of hypochlorous acid, and singlet oxygen generation (Fig. 11.3).

The myeloperoxidase, present in the azurophilic granules, catalyzes optimally at an acid pH, a condition which is met in the pha-

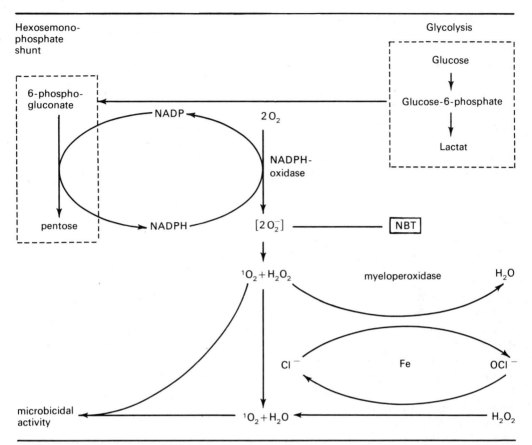

Fig. 11.3. Oxidative metabolism for the generation of H_2O_2, and its action with microbicidal mechanisms in polymorphonuclear cells

gocytic vacuole. In the presence of iodide (present in the serum in a concentration of $< 1\ \mu g/100\ ml$) or T_3 and T_4 which are membrane bound both to neutrophils and bacteria, microbial damage may occur through direct iodination of bacterial proteins, oxidation of sulfhydryl groups of enzymes or lipid peroxidation. Covalent attachment of activated iodide to tyrosine residues of external proteins of bacteria disrupts the protein's structure and results in alteration in permeability that causes the death of the microorganism.

Activated chloride might damage microorganisms by a number of mechanisms: oxidation of sulfhydryl groups, with enzyme inactivation; formation of aldehyde, which is known to be bactericidal,

and chloramine formation. Chloramines are amines, amides, or imides containing an N-chloro substituent; they are unstable in water, and release chlorine. It is thought that this reaction results in cleavage of proteins. Singlet oxygen is generated as a metastable oxygen intermediate during peroxide generation (see Fig. 11.3). It can react with compounds at areas of high electronic density such as unsaturated carbon-to-carbon bonds, to form oxygenation products

A number of individuals have been identified whose leukocytes carbonyl products contain no MPO. The bactericidal activity of MPO-deficient leukocytes is characterized by a lag period, but the killing of most ingested microorganisms is eventually complete. Thus, MPO is required for optimal microbicidal activity but its absence from phagocytes is not totally disabling. Obviously, there are MPO-independent oxygen-requiring mechanisms for the destruction of invading pathogens. These are the generation of hydrogen peroxide itself, and the formation of free radical forms of oxygen, superoxide anion, and hydroxyl radicals resulting from the interaction of superoxide and hydrogen peroxide (Haber-Weiss cycle)

$$O_2^- + H_2O_2 \rightarrow OH + OH^- + O_2 \,.$$

It has been demonstrated that this reaction occurs in human neutrophils during phagocytosis and that superoxide in combination with H_2O_2 results in products highly toxic to a number of bacterial species.

Oxygen-Independent Bactericidy. The preponderance of evidence suggests a major role for oxidative processes in the neutrophilic killing of most bacteria. Most studies suggest that H_2O_2 derived from dismutation of O_2 is the lethal species rather than the superoxide itself. In addition to these oxygen-dependent processes, nonoxidative microbicidal mechanisms are of obvious importance because certain microorganisms can clearly be killed by neutrophils under anaerobic conditions.

The simplest nonoxidative mechanism involves the decrease in pH (~ 4.5) that occurs within the phagocytic vacuole: some bacteria are very sensitive to acid (e.g., pneumococci); furthermore, a low pH provides optimal conditions for a variety of enzymes. *Lysozyme* was the first antibacterial substance to be discovered in leukocytes. It is a cationic (pI ~ 11), low molecular weight (14,000 daltons) protein consisting of a single polypeptide chain of 129 amino acids. Its substrate is the peptidoglycan portion of the bacterial cell wall (see p. 297).

Lactoferrin is a large protein (77,000 daltons) that is contained entirely within the specific granules of the cells. It may exert an antimicrobial function by binding and withholding iron required as an essential nutrient by the bacteria ingested, thus suppressing bacterial growth.

Some *hydrolytic enzymes* with different pH optima, e.g., alkaline phosphatase (pH optimum ~ 10), proteases, esterases (pH optimum ~ 7), are highly active in digestion of elastin, a particularly refractory substrate for proteolysis. Hydrolases, e.g., acid phosphatase, nucleases, a wide variety of carbohydrases, proteases, phospholipases, β-glucuronidase, neuraminidase, and aryl-sulfatase are released from azurophilic granules in large numbers. Cationic proteins are also released from azurophilic granules, also called "phagocytin" and "leukin." They bind to bacteria within the phagosome and damage microbial membrane barriers. Nuclear histones are substances which are released into surrounding tissue by death and autolysis of cells. They have a direct antimicrobial activity.

The intracellular killing of viable particles takes only a few minutes. Shortly after the microbes are digested, the membrane of vacuoles disintegrates and their contents are released into the cytoplasm causing the self-digestion (autolysis) of the neutrophil.

Macrophages

The mononuclear phagocyte system has its origin in the bone marrow monoblast and promonocyte (see p. 8). Only the intermediate stage cell, the monocyte, is ordinarily encountered in the circulation. Not nearly as much is known about macrophages as about neutrophils. Work with mononuclear cells is still in a more descriptive phase and biochemistry of these cells has been less precisely correlated with their antimicrobial and immunologic functions. The reasons for this deficiency lie in the fact that mononuclear phagocytes are functionally much more heterogeneous than granulocytes; unlike polymorphonuclear cells which are end cells and die when they have left the circulation, monocytes live for long periods (months, in man) and continue to differentiate after they have left the marrow, enter the tissue, and come under the influence of phagocytable particles and of lymphocytes. They cannot easily be obtained in bulk.

In general, it appears that mononuclear phagocytes ingest and kill microbes with mechanisms similar, or perhaps in some instances identical to those employed by PMN. They show less locomotion, they are sensitive to chemotactic factors which are different from those active for neutrophils. Chemotaxins for macrophages are C3a and C5a, C567 as well as lymphokines released by lymphocytes. They do not contain bactericidal cationic proteins and the MPO-peroxide-halide system as do neutrophils. On the other hand, macrophages are able to divide, produce a variety of active compounds involved in the immune response, including lymphocyte-activating factor(s) (interleukin-I) (see p. 161), monokines (Table 11.3), and can be activated by lymphocytes. After phagocytosis of

Table 11.3. Secretory products of macrophages, monokines

Regulator substances
    Interleukin 1 (lymphocyte activating factor, LAF)[a]
    Inhibitor of lymphocyte proliferation
    Colony-stimulating factor
    α_2-macroglobulin
    Prostaglandins
Effector substances
    Complement components: C2, C4, (C5?)
    Interferon
    Pyrogen
    Cytolytic, cytotoxic, cytostatic factors
Enzymes
    Acid hydrolases
    Neutral proteases
        Plasminogen activator
        Collagenase
        Elastase
    Lysozyme (muramidase)

---

[a] Acronyms are: MP, mitogenic protein; HP-1, helper peak-1; TRF-III, T cell replacing factor; TRF$_M$, T cell replacing factor from macrophages; BAF, B cell activating factor: BDF, B cell differentiation factor

microbial materials, processed immunogenic substances are presented to neighboring T lymphocytes; those which possess receptors for the presented antigenic determinants are stimulated. Stimulated T lymphocytes, in turn, release factors (lymphokines) that activate macrophages but also other T cells and B lymphocytes. Activated macrophages develop increased phagocytic and digestive power; they show increased attachment to and spreading on surfaces, a greater than normal number of lysosomes and mitochondria, an increased metabolic activity, and they are larger than normal macrophages.

Activated macrophages are not encountered in all stages of an infection. They occur rather late and reach a maximal concentration at a certain stage of the infection which depends upon species and number of infecting microorganisms. For instance, infection with *Listeria monocytogenes* causes an early appearance of activated macrophages in contrast to infections with *brucellae* in which activated macrophages appear much later. Macrophages are activated by immunological mechanisms; that can be demonstrated by adoptive transfer studies. Peritoneal cells of mice which have recovered from a sublethal infection of *L. monocytogenes* and which are therefore resistant to this organism are able to transfer this resistance to normal noninfected mice. Resistance cannot be transferred by serum from resistant mice. Parallel to the transferred resistance a delayed hypersensitivity to *L. monocytogenes* develops.

The activation of macrophages by lymphokines follows an immunologically specific interaction between lymphocytes and microbial antigens (presented by macrophages), but the expression of this reactivity is nonspecific against a wide range of microorganisms. Thus, macrophages activated by *M. tuberculosis* also show increased ability to digest and destroy other intracellular bacteria such as *L. monocytogenes* and protozoa such as leishmania. These and similar findings indicate that the acquired cellular resistance involves a heightened

nonspecific microbicidal power of macrophages; this declines with increasing time after immunization perhaps parallel with the
decline in amounts of persisting microbial
antigen. Nonspecific resistance can be specifically recalled by the reexposure of the
original pathogen. In persistent infections
such as tuberculosis, macrophages can remain activated for longer periods, probably
because of the continued expression of antigen.

Macrophages are also activated during the
course of certain virus infections, particularly those in which macrophages are themselves infected, and can express this reactivity against unrelated microorganisms. For
instance, when mice are infected with ec-
tromelia virus and 6 days later injected intravenously with listeria, the spleen macrophages show an increased ability to ingest
and destroy the bacteria. Less is known
about macrophage activation in protozoal
infections: in a resistant host, leishmania
parasites are destroyed after phagocytosis
by activated macrophages, and unrelated
microorganisms such as listeria are also killed. Nonactivated macrophages, in contrast,
generally support the growth of both leishmania and listeria. Mice primarily infected
with protozoa *Toxoplasma gondii* or *Bes-
noitia jellisoni* become resistant to *L. monocytogenes*, *S. typhimurium*, and the fungus
Cryptococcus neoformans. There is some evidence that activated macrophages in the
presence of antibodies (to promote phagocytosis) give protective immunity in malaria;
they ingest erythrocytes more extensively
than normal macrophages.

Not much is known about the reactivity to
metazoan parasites because of the enormous
diversity in their structure, behavior, and
habitat. But it appears that in cases of
Litomosoides carinii infection macrophages
are the major effector cell. After development from infective larvae, the adult worms
reside in the pleural cavity and give rise to
microfilariae that enter the blood stream.
The termination of microfilaremia (onset of
latency) is associated with adhesion of
mononuclear cells to microfilariae in the

pleural cavity. In vitro, cells from animals
with latent infections were found not to adhere to microfilariae, but cells from normal
or latent-infected animals adhered strongly
in the presence of serum from latent-infected
animals. Adherence is followed by death of
the microfilariae. Furthermore, treatment of
animals with antimacrophage serum led to
the breakdown of latency.

In shistosomia infection, granuloma form
around eggs in the lung; they contain macrophages but also lymphocytes and eosinophils. The relative roles of each cell type in
egg destruction is not known, but eosinophils from infected animals are the most potent effectors of egg destruction in vitro (see
p. 326).

The way in which activated macrophages exert their microbicidal activity is almost unknown. Increased phagocytosis per se is an
inadequate explanation because intracellular killing does not necessarily follow phagocytosis. Actually, many pathogens "seek"
phagocytosis to grow and multiply
(Table 11.4). Phagolysosome formation
with discharge of the content of lysosomes
into phagosomes as described for PMN certainly contributes a great deal to the microbicidal activity. However, there is other evi-

Table 11.4. Microorganisms that multiply in macrophages

Protozoa	Leishmania
	Trypanosomes
	Toxoplasma
Fungi	Cryptococcus neoformans
	Coccidia
	Candida albicans
	Histoplasma capsulatum
Bacteria	M. tuberculosis
	M. leprae
	L. monocytogenes
	Brucellae
Rickettsia	R. rickettsi
	R. prowazeki
Viruses	Psittacoses
	Herpes-type viruses
	Measles
	Arbovirus (Dengue)
	Poxvirus
	Lymphochoriomeningitis

dence indicating that microbicidal activity cannot be explained solely on the basis of lysosome activity. There is a lack of correlation between antimicrobial activity and lysosomal content of activated macrophages; by electron microscopy studies it could be observed that in rabbit alveolar macrophages infected with several bacteria (*L. monocytogenes, S. typhi, S. aureus*) there was no fusion of large electron-dense, lysosome-like bodies with the phagosome, but there was fusion of smaller vesicles with the phagosomes. The bacteria rapidly showed signs of damage. Around the phagosomes there was the appearance of nonmembrane-bound granular or fibrillar dense material, which also appeared in the phagosomes.

Interaction of Microorganisms with Phagocytes

Pathogens successfully interfere with the antimicrobial activities of polymorpho- and mononuclear cells. As pointed out above, the sequence of events in natural resistance after penetration of the outer surface by microbes starts with the migration out of the circulation attracted by chemotaxins of granulocytes and macrophages to the site of invasion; they attach to the microorganisms, ingest, and kill them. Disturbance of any of these events results in a less efficient or even no reaction of leukocytes against invaders.

The most straightforward antiphagocytic approach of microorganisms is to kill phagocytes. This is, indeed, the case in infections with pathogenic streptococci which release hemolysins (streptolysines). As the name indicates, these substances lyse red blood cells, but have even more profound effects on phagocytes. Within a few minutes of addition of streptolysin 0 to polymorphonuclear cells, their granules "explode" and their content is discharged into the cytoplasm with resulting autolysis. Some pathogenic staphylococci also release various hemolysins. In addition, staphylococci also produce a nonlytic leukocidin; this protein acts on the leukocyte membrane and causes discharge of the lysosomal content into the

cytoplasm. *L. monocytogenes* releases similar toxins. In general, polymorphonuclear cells are more sensitive to these toxins than macrophages, possibly because their lysosomes are more easily discharged. In addition to the lytic activity, streptolysin in low concentrations has been shown to suppress chemotaxis.

A prerequisite for phagocytosis is adherence or adsorption of the microbe to the surface of phagocytes. *Mycoplasma hominis* prevents in some unknown manner adsorption to the polymorph surface. Streptococci possess on their surface M proteins which are responsible for their attachment to the surface of epithelial cells in sites of infection, yet they do not adhere to macrophages. Under the electron microscope, these proteins are identifiable as a fine hairy layer on the outer surface. It has been suggested that this coat permits the bacteria to slither off the surface of macrophages. Similarly, pneumococci, but also *Hemophilus influenza* and *Klebsiella pneumonia* owe their resistance to phagocytosis to their polysaccharide capsule; these bacteria are readily phagocytozed when decapsulated by hyaluronidase. The cell walls of gram-negative bacteria contain a lipopolysaccharide complex (endotoxin) with the somatic (0) antigen in the polysaccharide side chain (see p. 179). This structure causes inhibition of phagocytosis; gram-negative bacteria lacking this antigen are normally phagocytozed. Anthrax and plague bacteria possess a thin acidic polysaccharide capsule which causes inhibition of phagocytosis. All these microbes are readily phagocytozed when they are coated with antibodies, except *Staphylococcus aureus*. These bacteria possess a Protein A that attaches to the Fc portion of IgG and, therefore, prevents binding of the Fc portion, and thus the opsonized bacteria, to the Fc receptor on phagocytes. They may attach, however, to macrophages by the C 3 b receptor.

There are microbial parasites that do not mind being phagocytozed but then start to interfere with the normal killing and digestive processes. Actually, phagosomes can be seen as a cordon of forts protecting their "residents" from any attack from the outside, i.e., antibody, complement, toxins, phagocytic cells, cytotoxic cells, if by some means the formation of phagolysosomes is prevented or the discharged content inactivated. This strategy is indeed applied by some microorganisms which multiply in phagocytic phagosomes and eventually kill the macrophage (Table 11.4). *Mycobacterium tuberculosis* produces sulfatides that inhibit fusion of phagosomes and lysosomes. *Toxoplasma gondii, Aspergillus flavus, psittacosis chlamydia,* and *staphylococcus aureus* are all phagocytozed but have developed mechanisms that prevent fusion; nothing is known about these mechanisms. Another way around the antimicrobial activity is resistance to killing, of which we know almost nothing. It is, however, likely to depend on the nature of the outer surface of microorganisms, and the production of lytic enzyme inhibitors. Thus the outer surface of *Mycobacterium lepraemurium* contains waxes which are not readily digested by lysosomal enzymes; these bacteria grow in phagocytic vacuoles even after extensive fusion with lysosomes.

Viruses fuse with the cell membrane and enter the cytoplasm. If they are trapped in phagosomes, the membrane of which is derived from the plasma membrane, they also reach the cytoplasm by fusion, usually before lysosomes have fused. In case of reoviruses, exposure to lysosomal enzymes is necessary to "uncoat" the virus particle and thus help the virus to multiply.

Adaptive Immunity

One of the most important properties of the macrophage is its mediator function linking the natural and adaptive parts of the immune system. The carriers of specific immunity, the lymphocytes, do (almost) nothing on their own unless being told by macrophages. Highly purified populations of committed lymphocytes do not respond to antigens, nor do purified normal lymphocytes respond to allogeneic cells in mixed lympho-

Table 11.5. Lymphocyte mediators, lymphokines

Mediators affecting macrophages
  Migration inhibition factor (MIF)
  Macrophage activating factor (MAF, indistinguishable from MIF)
  Chemotactic factors for macrophages

Mediators affecting polymorphnuclear leukocytes
  Chemotacting factors
  Leukocyte inhibitory factor (LIF)
  Eosinophil stimulation promoter (ESP)

Mediators affecting lymphocytes
  Interleukin 2[a]
  B cell suppressing factor

Mediators affecting other cells
  Lymphotoxin (LT)
  Osteoclast activating factor (OAF)
  Collagen-producing factor
  Colony-stimulating factor (CSF)
  Interferon
  Immunoglobulin binding factor (IBF, probably identical to IgG-Fc receptor on T cells)
Procoagulant (tissue factor)

[a] Acronyms are: TSF, thymocyte stimulating factor; TMF, thymocyte mitogenic factor; TCGF, T cell growth factor; Co-stimulator; KHF, killer cell helper factor; SCIF, secondary cytotoxic T cell-inducing factor

cyte reaction or to unspecific mitogens. Without being told (stimulated) they do not produce lymphokines either.

The reactivity of committed lymphocytes to antigen requires the presentation by macrophages of processed antigen to them suitably associated with class I (Ia) molecules of the MHC (see p. 160), and the stimulation by a factor, interleukin-I, produced by macrophages. The first lymphocytes activated in this process are T helper cells, possessing receptors which can bind the antigen in association with Ia molecules. These cells then activate, in turn, B lymphocytes, T suppressor cells, and cytotoxic T lymphocytes,[2] which proliferate and differentiate to effector and memory cells. The activation of these effec-

2 It is not known with certainty whether macrophages and/or T helper cells are needed to generate cytotoxic T cells in cases of virus or allogeneic (transplantation) infections; it might be that cytotoxic T cells are able to recognize the viral or allo-antigen in association with class I molecules directly. T helper cells certainly augment the recruitment of cytotoxic T cells

Table 11.6. Physicochemical properties of lymphokines

Property	Lymphokine				
	MIF[a]	CTF[a, b]	$\alpha-$LT[a, c]	LMF[a]	IBF[d]
Molecular weight	23,000–55,000	12,000	75,000–100,000	20,000–50,000	140,000–300,000
Sensitivity to chymotrypsin/ trypsin	Sensible	Sensible	Stable?	Sensible	Sensible
neuraminidase	Resistant	Resistant	Resistant	Resistant	Sensible
Temperature (56 °C, 30 min)	Stable	Stable	Stable	Stable	Labile
Isoelectric point (Ip)	4–6	10.1; 5.6	6.8–8.0	6.5–7.5	6.3
Electrophoretic mobility	Albumin	Albumin	α_2, β-globulin	–	–
Buoyant density (CsCl)	Protein	–	–	–	–

MIF, migration inhibition factor; CTF, chemotactic factor; LT, lymphotoxin; LMF, lymphocyte mitogenic factor; IBF, immunoglobulin binding factor
[a] From human
[b] Monocyte/macrophage chemotactic factor
[c] Two smaller components found in addition to $\alpha-$LT: $\beta-$LT, with a molecular weight of approximately 45,000, and $\gamma-$LT with a molecular weight of 10,000–15,000. These are not distinct substances but heterogeneous groups of unstable compounds
[d] From mice.

tor cells requires the presence and binding of antigen by the interacting cells as well as the action of factor(s), lymphokines (Table 11.5), which are produced by lymphocytes. These factors, in turn, regulate the activity of macrophages and polymorphonuclear cells but also that of other lymphocytes.

Most of these factors are not, or not well, characterized, and it is not clear whether the numerous functional effects which distinguish them are caused by many distinct products or by only few substances displaying several effects depending upon the experimental conditions (Table 11.6).

Immune Response to Infections

In the immune response to infections usually all parts of the defense system participate, i.e., the natural and the adaptive system.

However, since the natural system does not confer immunity (or only in a very restricted sense), i.e., specific resistance to repeated infections by the same pathogen, the term immune response refers primarily to the response of T and B lymphocytes against infectious agents. For practical reasons, these two parts of the immune response are distinguished as humoral (antibody-mediated) and cellular (cell-mediated) immunity. Both types of the immune response are only efficient when adequately supported by the two other important adjuncts, the complement systems and the polymorphonuclear-monocyte systems.

The participation of the two arms of the specific immunity is revealed by several activities: antibodies enhance phagocytosis due to opsinization; they neutralize microbial toxins; they neutralize viruses; they form immune complexes with subsequent activation of the complement system resulting in lysis of microorganisms and cells, and the

Table 11.7. Tests for detection of antibodies in infectious diseases (see Chap. 7)

Test	Antigen	Positive result	Microorganisms
In vitro			
Hemagglutination inhibition	Hemagglutinin on the surface of viruses	Inhibition of agglutination	Rubella, influenza, mumps, measles, variola, vaccinia, arbor encephalitis, adeno- and rheoviruses
Hemagglutination	Microbial antigens adsorbed to erythrocyte surface	Agglutination	Rhinoviruses, serum hepatitis (HB$_s$Ag) brucellosis, leptospirosis, leprosy, typhus (Felix reaction), infectious mononucleosis (Paul-Bunnel), toxoplasmosis, American trypanosomiasis, schistosomiasis, malaria, amebiasis, tuberculosis, metazoa
Hemolysis	Streptolysin – anti-streptolysine.	Inhibition of erythrolysis	Streptococcal infections
Latex test	Microbial antigen adsorbed to latex	Agglutination	Serum hepatitis B(HB$_s$Ag), leptospirosis, echinococcosis
Complement fixation	Microbial antigen reacts with antibody and fixes complement	Complement depletion	Most microorganisms
Precipitation, agglutination, gel diffusion	Antigen on surface of microbe, soluble microbial antigen	Visible agglutination or precipitation, precipitin line in gel	Salmonella (Widal), brucella, diphtheria (Elek), leptospirosis, histoplasmosis, aspergillosis
Immobilization	Antigen on locomotor organ (flagellum, cilium)	Inhibition of mobility	Treponema pallidum (TPI)
Immunofluorescence antibody test	Antigen on microorganism or antigen formed in infected cells	Binding of fluorescein labeled antibody (direct) or labeled anti-Ig (indirect)	T. pallidum, respiratory syncytial virus, malaria, leishmaniasis, trypanosomiasis, toxoplasmosis, trichinosis, filariasis, schistosomiasis
Radioimmune assay, ELISA	Microbial antigen	Binding of radiolabeled or enzyme bound antibody	Serum hepatitis (HB$_s$Ag)
Capsular swelling	Capsules on surface of bacteria	Swelling of capsule	Pneumococcus Klebsiella
Immunelectrophoresis	Soluble antigen	Precipitin line	Amebiasis, echinococcosis
Flocculation	Antigen (cardiolipin) adsorbed to surface of cholesterol crystals	Agglutination	T. pallidum (VDRL), trichinosis, echinococcosis, schistosomiasis
Methylene blue	Microorganism	Antibody and C cause loss of affinity of cytoplasm for methylene blue	Toxoplasmosis (Sabin-Feldman)
In vivo			
Intradermal (immediate hypersensitivity)	Toxin, microbial extract	Erythematous induration within 24–48 h	Streptococcus (Dick), diphtheria (Schick), lymphogr. venereum (Frei), Echinococcosis (Casoni), filariasis, schistosomiasis, trichinosis
Neutralization	Virus; multiplication in experimental animal or cell culture	Antibody inhibits multiplication and prevents pathologic lesions or death	Most viruses

liberation of kinins; they render microbes nonmotile and inhibit their growth by coating them. The ways in which antibodies can be detected and assayed have been described in detail in Chap. 7 and are briefly summarized in Table 11.7.

It is, however, not sufficient for the diagnosis of a present infection to demonstrate that antibodies against a certain infectious agent are in the serum; such antibodies could have been the result of an earlier infection a long time ago. Usually, the activity must have a certain strength above a "normal" threshold, and must increase with time in order to indicate an ongoing infection. Antibodies do not appear immediately after beginning of an infection, but only after a few days or even weeks; thus, antibodies against the H agglutinins and Vi agglutinins in typhoid infections appear rather late (Fig. 11.4). In other infectious diseases, antibodies appear only after the disease is resolved (cutaneous leishmaniasis, see below). Thus, in many cases, the determination of antibody formation is not helpful in the early diagnosis of an infection, but usually extremely valuable in the assessment of the development of protective immunity – or its failure to develop.

Cell-mediated immunity might be detected by several means: In vivo, by the induction

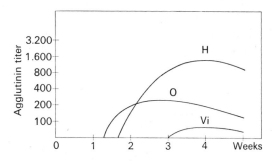

Fig. 11.4. Appearance of the anti-O, anti-H, and anti-Vi agglutinins during untreated typhoid fever [Adapted from Faure M et al. (1964) Les réactions sérologiques, 2éme ed. Albert de Visscher, Paris]

of inflammation and mononuclear cell infiltration by application of antigen into skin (see p. 287, tuberculin test). In vitro, by the proliferative response (incorporation of tritiated thymidin) of lymphocytes after exposure to the antigen; migration inhibition of macrophages (see p. 291); migration of macrophages and polymorphonuclear cells through millipore filters due to chemotactic factors; and destruction of cells bearing microbial antigens (e.g., virus) on their surface by cytolytic T lymphocytes, measured by the release of ^{51}Cr incorporated previously in the target cells (Table 11.8).

Test system	Outcome
In vitro	
Lymphocyte stimulation	^{3}H-thymidine incorporation of sensitized lymphocytes
Migration inhibition	Inhibition of macrophage migration (see Fig. 10.16)
Chemotaxis	Migration of macrophages into millipore filter (Boyden's chamber, see Fig. 5.8)
Blastogenic factor	Transformation of normal lymphocytes
Lymphotoxin	Cytotoxicity for certain cultered cells
Interferon	Protection of cells against virus infections
Cell-mediated cytotoxicity	Destruction of cells bearing antigens, e.g., viral antigens or haptens on the cell surface
In vivo	
Skin reactive factor	Induction of delayed hypersensitivity in guinea pig skin
DTH skin test	Delayed type hypersensitivity after injection of antigen (e.g., PPD, lepromin, parasite antigens)

Table 11.8. Test system for assaying cell-mediated immunity

The delayed hypersensitivity reaction in the skin does not become positive until several weeks in infections such as tuberculosis, brucellosis, and leishmaniasis, but after smallpox vaccination it is positive within 1 week. If the individual has been previously exposed to the antigen, the response takes a shorter time to develop, i.e., 1 or 2 days.

Special Aspects of Bacterial Infections

Bacteria owe their pathogenicity to two basic properties: invasiveness and toxicity. The invasiveness causes lesions at the areas of entry and metastases thereof; the formation of toxins leads to damages in areas far from the point of entry, sometimes systemic. Some bacteria are particularly invasive, e.g., pneumococcus and *B. anthracis;* others are pathogenic primarily because of toxin formation such as the diphtheria bacillus, *Clostridium tetani*, *Clostridium botulinum*, and the clostridia of gas gangrene. Frequently, invasive and toxicogenic properties are found together, e.g., in the case of *Staphylococcus* and *Streptococcus pyogenes*. The properties and effects of bacterial exotoxins are summarized in Table 11.9.

There are two mechanisms that lead to immunity in bacterial infections: the destruction of the microorganisms by lysis or phagocytosis-facilitating antibodies (antibacterial immunity), and the neutralization of toxins (antitoxic immunity). The mechanisms by which bacteriolysis and phagocytosis occur have been described in detail above. It is sufficient to indicate that the destruction of microorganisms inside the phagocytes takes place through distinct processes depending upon whether the bacteria in question are capable of multiplying outside the cell, e.g., pneumococcus, streptococci, and *B. anthracis*, or inside the macrophages, e.g., *M. tuberculosis*, *brucellae*, and *L. monocytogenes*. In the former case, the bacteria are opsonized by circulating antibodies acting together with $C1$ to $C5$ complement components. In the latter case, immunity is not mediated by circulating antibodies, but

rather by sensitized lymphocytes which, upon being stimulated by the antigen, liberate a chemotactic factor which attracts macrophages, and a macrophage-activating factor. Antibacterial immunity mediated by cells depends upon mechanisms described as delayed hypersensitivity (Chap. 10, pp. 287–294). In diseases such as tuberculosis, brucellosis, and others in which the organisms persist inside the macrophages, allergy and immunity not uncommonly develop parallel.

Antitoxic immunity depends upon the formation of antibodies (antitoxins) capable of neutralizing the bacterial exotoxins. The mechanisms for the neutralization of exotoxins have been described in Chap. 7 (pp. 199–204).

Special Aspects of Viral Infections

The kind of immunity which develops after viral infections depends to a large extent upon the way a virus spreads and replicates. At the cellular level, three types of viral transmission have been defined: (1) extracellular, infectious virions are released from the cell to spread in the extracellular space, and infect new cells; (2) intercellular, the virus spreads from cell to cell through desmosomes of intercellular bridges without contact with the extracellular milieu. The surfaces of infected cells often contain viral antigens (e.g., herpes virus); and (3) nuclear, the viral genome is latent or incorporated into the host genome and is passed from parent cells to progeny during mitosis (e.g., C type oncornaviruses). The first two modes are also called horizontal transmission, the latter is called vertical transmission.

It is obvious that antibodies are most efficient in the first mode; and they may be able to act in the two other forms if viral antigen is expressed on the surface of infected cells; here, cell-mediated immunity might be most efficient.

At the level of the host, two general types of viral spread are distinguished: (a) local, the viral infection is largely confined to a mu-

Table 11.9. Bacterial toxins and their properties

Microorganism	Disease	Toxin	Mol. wt.	Action	Symptoms	Toxicity[a] LD_{50} (kg)/ml
Bacillus anthracis	Gas gangrene	Complex of toxins		Chelating agents, increase in vascular permeability	Edema, hemorrhagia	
Bordatella pertussis	Whooping cough	Toxin	82,000	Ciliary damage	Necrosis of epithelial cells, leukocyte infiltration	
Clostridium botulinum	Botulism	8 type-specific neuro-toxins	Type A 70,000	Blocks release of acetylcholine	Neurotoxic signs, paralysis	20×10^6 (M)
Clostridium tetani	Tetanus	Tetanospasmin	67,000	Blocks action of inhibitory neurons	Overaction of motor neurons, muscle spasm	6×10^6 (M)
Clostridium welchii (perfringens)	Gas gangrene	α-toxin enterotoxin	90,000	Lecithinase Activates adenyl cyclase and raises cAMP levels	Loss of water and electrolytes, block of Na resorption; diarrhea	
Corynebact. diphtheriae	Diphtheria	Toxin	62,000	Inhibits cell protein synthesis	Cell necrosis, nerve paralysis	3.5×10^3 (GP)
Escherichia coli	Dysentery	Enterotoxin	24,000	Activation of adenyl cyclase, raises cAMP level	Diarrhea	
Shigella dysenteriae	Dysentery	Entero- and neurotoxin		Activation of adenyl cyclase Vascular endothelial damage (brain)	Diarrhea Neurological disturbance	1.2×10^6 (R)
Staphylococcus aureus	Scalded skin syndrome food poisoning	α-hemolysine, enterotoxin	$3 \times 10,000$ 40,000	Cytotoxic, acts on cell membrane Acts on the vomiting center in the brain	Necrosis of site of infection, Systemic toxic nausea, vomiting, diarrhea	
Streptococcus pyogenes	Scarlet fever	erythrogenic toxin	29,000	Vasodilatation	Scarlet fever rash	
		Streptolysine leukocidin streptokinase	60,000	Lysis of phagocytes and erythrocytes Lysis of fibrin	Phagocytolytic, hemolytic Promotes spread of bacteria in tissue	
Vibrio cholerae	Cholera	Enterotoxin	2 subunits A: 27,000 B: 14,000	Attaches to ganglioside receptors on epithelial cells Activates adenylcyclase and raises cAMP level	Water and electrolyte loss, block of Na resorption; diarrhea	

[a] M, mouse; GP, guinea pig; R, rat

cosal surface or organ (e.g., rhinoviruses on respiratory epithelium); and (b) systemic, either primarily when viruses are inoculated directly into the blood stream with subsequent organ dissemination (arbovirus, hepatitis B virus), or secondary, when the viral infection and replication initially occur on a mucosal surface and invasion into the blood stream or the tissue occurs afterwards (e.g., poliomyelitis, mumps).

The first type of infection elicits predominantly a humoral response whereby local plasma cells produce IgA, and immunity is not long lasting. The immune response to the second group of infections involves both humoral and cellular reactions; immunity is strong and long lasting; the predominantly produced antibodies are of the IgG type. IgA antibodies are, however, also produced which interfere with virus implantation at the site of entry (respiratory system, intestinal mucosa).

Antibodies probably constitute one of the more important mechanisms of host resistance to viral infections, but in most cases they appear to play no role in recovery from established infections. The following virus-antibody reactions have been identified in vitro and they presumably operate also in vivo. (1) Complement-independent neutralization by specific antibodies to virus coat protein (arbovirus, enterovirus, pox, herpes, and arena viruses); the antibodies prevent cellular adsorption and penetration of the virus. The exact mechanism of neutralization is unclear but probably it involves changes in surface structure configurations since only a few antibody molecules per virion are sufficient for neutralization. Of course, the reaction is only possible if the virus spreads extracellularly. (2) Complement-dependent neutralization. "Natural" IgM and early immune antibodies to several viruses enveloped with an outer lipoprotein coat neutralize virus more efficiently in the presence than in the absence of complement components (e.g., rubella, herpes, Newcastle disease virus). Complement may participate in neutralization in several ways: it stabilizes virus-antibody complexes, it causes lysis of enveloped viruses by mechanisms analogous to bacterio- or cytolysis, it prevents attachment of the virus to susceptible cells, and it promotes uptake of the virus by polymorphonuclear and mononuclear phagocytes. Complement-dependent host cell lysis may occur in cases in which viral antigen is expressed on the surface of infected cells (e.g., herpes virus, myxovirus).

Cell-mediated immunity can be demonstrated in many virus infections. Thus, macrophages are important in preventing spread of viruses from primary sites of infections to highly susceptible cells (e.g., hepatitis virus, herpes virus); they play an important role in collaboration with lymphocytes in controlling pox virus, herpes virus, measle, and cytomegalovirus infections. The antiviral mechanisms may include: lymphocyte cytotoxicity mediated by cytolytic T cells recognizing viral antigens expressed on the virus envelope (e.g., myxo-, paramyxo-, rhabdo-, arena-, togaviruses which mature by budding from the cell surface) or the surface of infected cells (e.g., pox and herpes virus), or with the help of cytophilic antibodies to which killer cells attach (see pp. 43 and 244) and release of lymphokines of which some are toxic (LT, see p. 311), others attract macrophages and polymorphonuclear cells, and still others which interfere with virus propagation and replication such as interferons.

Interferons are a family of low molecular weight proteins (20–35,000) discovered by Isaacs and Lindenmann in 1957, which are produced by a number of cells including lymphocytes, epithelial cells, and macrophages, fibroblasts in response to a variety of infectious agents (viruses, rickettsiae, protozoae) as well as bacterial endotoxins (lipopolysaccharide; Bru-Pel, an ether-extractable component of *Brucellae*), double-stranded RNAs, synthetic anion polymers, polynucleotides, but also the antibiotic kanamycin. Interferons are able to inhibit the growth of viruses and of other intracellular microorganisms such as *plasmodium berghei* and *toxoplasma gondii*, and also the multiplication of a number of normal cells

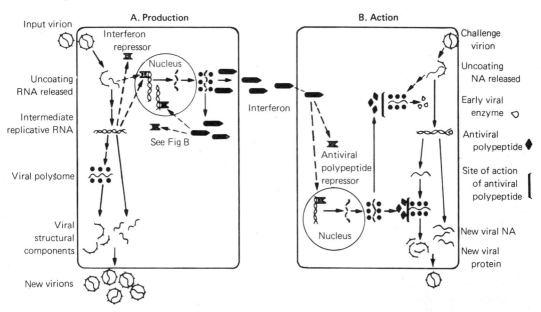

Fig. 11.5. Summary of our understanding of the formation (A) and effector mechanism (B) of interferon. The virus penetrates the cell membrane, and its RNA is liberated; the uncoated RNA, or more probably, the intermediate replicative double-stranded RNA induces de-repression of the interferon repressor. The binding of the de-repressor to the host's DNA induces the formation of mRNA for interferon. The newly formed interferons are released and reach neighboring cells, in which they bind the repressor for the antiviral protein; this leads to the formation of antiviral protein, which inhibits the production of viral proteins (enzymes and structural proteins) at the level of polyribosomes [reproduced with kind permission from Grossberg (1972) N Engl J Med 287:79]

(e.g., embryo fibroblast, hemopoietic cells). Their chemical properties are not well elucidated; however, they can be divided into two groups known as type I ("classical") and type II ("immune") interferons. Those produced by cells infected with viruses or treated with double-stranded RNA are termed classical or type I interferons, and those produced by stimulation with mitogen and antigen of reticuloendothelial cells are termed immune or type II interferons. Although both types share antiviral activity, they differ in their physical properties, e.g., type I, but not type II, interferons are stable at pH 2, and also in their biological properties. In particular, type II interferons appear to have a higher anticellular activity than antiviral activity.

Interferons are formed within hours after infection. Combination of interferon with the cell membrane of cells stimulates production of a protein which binds to ribosomes and inhibits by an unknown mechanism the translation of viral (but not host) messenger RNA. This process requires the presence of double-stranded RNA which is formed as a by-product of virus infections and implies that the effects on protein synthesis will only occur in cells which have already been infected (Fig. 11.5). It therefore does not matter that protein synthesis ceases, and the requirement for double-stranded RNA means that the uninfected cells will be unaffected by interferons, an excellent mechanism for ensuring the nontoxicity of an otherwise very potent agent. Interferons are highly host specific, but not virus specific. Interferons have an important function in resistance toward intracellular parasites, particularly at the onset of an infection at which time the immune response is just starting (Fig. 11.6).

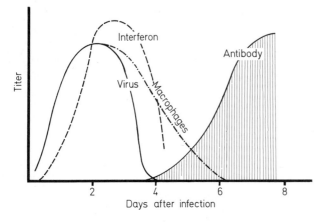

Fig. 11.6. Appearance of interferon, macrophages, and antibodies in virus infections; also shown is the increase of the virus load at the beginning of the infection. With increasing amounts of interferon produced, the virus titer decreases

Escape from Immune Defense Mechanisms. There are a number of viruses which have developed the ability to evade the immune defense mechanisms of the infected host or which interfere with the immune response in such a way that it becomes ineffective in eliminating or controlling the infection. This happens in cases when infections occur at inaccessible sites, when viruses reside within cells and do not express viral proteins in the membrane, or when they are able to change their antigenic makeup, or when they are able to avoid the induction of an immune response.

Some viruses are shed to the exterior via saliva (herpes, cytomegalovirus, rabies in vampire bats), milk (cytomegalovirus in man), or urine (polyoma virus in man). Others are only formed on the lumenal surface of cells or in the keratosquamous layer of epidermis (human wart virus), and there is no way in which lymphocytes or antibodies can reach these sites and eliminate the infections.

Herpes simplex or varicella virus persistently infect dorsal root ganglion cells, Epstein-Barr (EB) virus resides in circulating lymphocytes. Herpes and measles virus spread progressively from cell to cell, and are protected in this way from the action of immune cells or antibodies.

Another major way to escape the immune reaction is antigenic variation. Influenza and human rhinoviruses, and foot-and-mouth disease virus develop variants outside the host. Influenza B virus shows repeated small antigenic changes over the years (antigenic drift). A given individual can be reinfected later in life by an antigenic variant that has been gradually generated in other groups of individuals. Influenza A shows in addition to slight variations drastic antigenic changes (antigenic shift) in intervals of 10–15 years. The major antigenic changes involve one or both of the surface components of the virus, either hemagglutinin (H) or neuraminidase (N). New variants are thought to develop by recombination of nonhuman and existing human viruses when they infect a host at the same time (Fig. 11.7). Thus, in 1976 a new variant of influenza appeared with the neuraminidase of the 1946 pandemic strain combined with the hemagglutinin from pig influenza virus (Hsw 1 N 1) (Table 11.10). Whenever a new major variant appeared, major global outbreaks of flu occurred, since a large proportion of the population had not been exposed to such a virus and was, therefore, highly susceptible. Thus, antibodies against A_2, the pandemic strain appearing in 1957 (Asian flu) could be found only in individuals who had experienced the 1889 epidemic.

Table 11.10. Pandemic influenza A virus strains

Pandemic	Influenza A virus strain[a]	
1889	?	$(A_2?)$
1918/1919	H_0N_1	(A_0)
1933	H_0N_0	$(PR-8)$
1946	H_1N_1	(A_1)
1957	H_2N_2	$(A_2$, Asian flu)
1968	H_3N_2	(Hong Kong flu)
1976	Hsw_1N_1	(swine flu)

[a] Old designation in parentheses

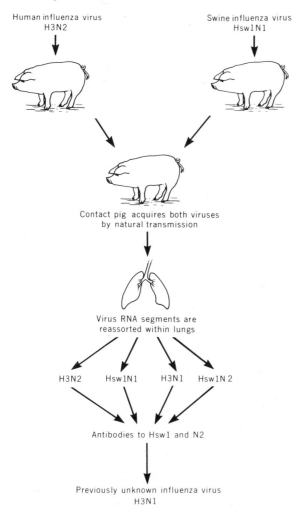

Human influenza virus
H3N2

Swine influenza virus
Hsw1N1

Contact pig acquires both viruses
by natural transmission

Virus RNA segments are
reassorted within lungs

H3N2   Hsw1N1   H3N1   Hsw1N 2

Antibodies to Hsw1 and N2

Previously unknown influenza virus
H3N1

Fig. 11.7. Experiment by Webster demonstrating recombination of human and swine influenza viruses to produce a virus with a new combination of hemagglutinin and neuraminidase antigens. The "new" virus was also shown to be pathogenic and transmissible in a stable form [reproduced from E. J. Shillitoe and F. Rapp (1979) Virus induced cell surface antigens and cell-mediated immune responses. Springer Sem. Immunopathol 2:237]

The simplest way for an agent to achieve a progressive infection is to elicit *no* immune response at all. There is indeed a group of viral microorganisms that multiply, persist, and spread in the infected host, giving pathological changes only after very long incubation periods. These microorganisms multiply in the brain and cause a neurological disease that is always fatal. To this group of "slow viruses" infections belong scrapie, transmissable mink encephalopathy, and in man, Kuru and Creutzfeld-Jacob disease. Scrapie has been best studied, and no indication for antibodies or cell-mediated responses after infection has been found. In mice, neonatal thymectomy or thymectomy, lethal irradiation, and reconstitution with fetal liver cells (T lymphocyte depletion) had no effect on the incubation period or pathology of scrapie. The infection neither induces nor is susceptible to the action of interferons. Other persistent viruses like lymphochoriomeningitis and leukemia virus in mice and human adenoviruses do not induce the production of interferon in spite of continued multiplication of virus. Presumably, infected cells do not recognize the virus nucleic acid as foreign.

Special Aspects of Protozoal and Metazoal Infections

Protozoa (plasmodia, amebia, leishmania, toxoplasma, and trypanosoma) and metazoa (trematedes, cestodes, and nematodes) are highly complex organisms; they represent a mosaic of antigens; their life cycle may consist of many different morphological forms, possibly bearing different antigenic structures; and they may be present simultaneously or sequentially within the same host. Therefore, immune responses to parasites have diverse manifestations, which are, additionally, modified ·by interactions of the parasite. In general, there are four possible results of immunological host-parasite interactions: (1) development of immunity with complete protection to reinfection (cutaneous leishmaniasis), (2) exaggerated hypersensitivity causing an immune disease (tropical eosinophil syndrome in filariasis, hepatic granulomae in schistosomiasis, antibody-mediated anaphylactic shock of a ruptured hydatid cyst), (3) absence of an effective immune response (malignant or diffuse cutaneous and mucocutaneous leishmaniasis, primary amebic meningoencephalitis, African trypanosomiasis, American trypanosomiasis), and (4) a balanced "immunity" which prevents large numbers of parasites from overwhelming the host but the response is generally ineffective at eliminating parasites (as in the majority of protozoan and metazoan infections).

Quite certainly, the last, "homeostatic" situation has to be the most favored by the parasite since it will secure its survival, and indeed, one key feature of most protozoan and metazoan infections is their chronicity. A number of mechanisms are invented by parasites to achieve this stage of "adaptive tolerance": anatomical inaccessibility, seclusion into host cells, antigenic variation, molecular masking, interference with the host's immune response such as inhibition of macrophage function, polyclonal B cell stimulation, induction of T suppressor cells, and immunosuppression (see p. 328). Resistance to homologous parasitic reestablishment is often seen in already parasitized individuals. The term "concomitant immunity" has been used to describe this situation, where parasitized hosts are already highly or completely resistant to reinfestation or reinfection with

the same parasite (e.g., schistosomiasis, fascioliasis). This type of immunity, in which *establishing* parasites are susceptible to immune responses which are ineffective against *established* parasites, has also been termed nonsterilizing immunity or premunition.

For some parasitic infections (e.g., malaria, filariasis), residents of endemic regions show less severe disease symptoms and the progression of the pathology is slower than in "immigrants." This suggests that there must be a modulating influence on the pathogenesis of infections in endemic areas, the source of which may extend back even into intrauterine, prenatal immunologic experience of the host: maternal-fetal transfer of (partially) protective IgG antibodies, infections at times at which the immune system or parts of it have not acquired complete maturity. Depending upon the stage of the development of the immune system and the presence of antibodies, the first encounter with a pathogenic parasite may direct the course of the disease in future infections: strong reactions with elimination of the parasite and subsequent immunity (cutaneous leishmaniasis) to weak, inadequate, or no reaction with extensive pathological effects (diffuse cutaneous leishmaniasis) to the same parasite in different individuals. Also in filariasis, various clusters of immunologic responses to the same parasite can be observed: immunologic hyperresponsiveness in tropical eosinophilia syndrome at the one extreme and asymptomatic microfilaremia at the other extreme; between these two lie states characterized by lymphatic inflammation and/or damage.

Protozoal Infections. In general, both the humoral and the cellular immune system, finely tuned, are needed to control the infection. In most cases, chronicity and pathogenesis of the parasite infection appear to be the result of an inadequate or impaired macrophage (*L. donovani* and *braziliensis*, *T. gondii* infections, *Tr. cruzi*), T cell (*Plasmodium*, *L. donovani* and *braziliensis*, *T. gambiense* and *rhodesiense* infections) and/or B cell response (*L. donovani* infections), which is most probably due to interference of the parasite with the activity of the immune system (see below).

The antibody response to parasites has captured most of the attention in the past, whereas the cellular immune response to parasites has just started to be explored and not much detailed knowledge is available for most of the parasitic diseases at the present time. From experiments in mice with parasites, which are "natural" to these animals (Table 11.11), it has been demonstrated that athymic nude (T cell deficient) mice develop a more severe picture of these diseases: parasite burdens are higher, infections persist longer, resistance to reinfections are not seen, or the mice are killed by infections which are not lethal in normal mice. The importance of cell-mediated immune responses in leishmaniasis is very clearly demonstrated by the fact that in cutaneous leishmaniasis an early and strong cellular reaction with almost no antibody present confers healing and sterile immunity, whereas visceral leish-

Table 11.11. „Natural" protozoan and metazoan parasites of mice

Plasmodium yoelii
Babesia microti
Leishmania tropica
Trypanosoma musculi
Giardia muris
Mesocestoides corti
Taenia taeniformis
Hexamita muris
Hymenolepsis nana
Nematospiroides dubius
Aspicularis tetrapetra
Syphacia obvelata

maniasis (a generally fatal disease if not treated) is characterized by a conspicuous absence of any cellular reaction; in animals, T cell depletion (neonatal thymectomy, ALS treatment, see p. 402) leads to a prolonged course of infections with *L. tropica*, which, in normal animals, is self-healing. Most of the aggravations appear due to a lack of T helper cell activity. Thus, in filariasis blast transformation in vitro is observed in the case of lymphocytes from young children exposed to the nematode, but this response is then "damped down" in chronic infections. The T cell dependency has been demonstrated to extend to macrophage activation, eosinophil activation in metazoan infections, and IgG response as well as fibrotic encapsulation, all of which are T helper cell functions. Delayed type hypersensitivity (skin test) in human parasitic infections is found in amebiasis, cutaneous leishmaniasis, *Tr. cruzi* infections (although only in the late stages), toxoplasmosis, schistosomiasis, echinococcosis, trichinosis, but not in malaria, diffuse cutaneous and mucocutaneous leishmaniasis, and *Tr. brucei* infections. Evidence for the presence of cytotoxic T cells against cells harboring parasites (malaria, toxoplasma, leishmania, *Tr. cruzi*) or parasites *(schistosoma)* has been found in mice: *Leishmania enriettii* infected macrophages are susceptible to lysis by T cells; splenocytes from *Tr. cruzi* infected mice were found to destroy infected fibroblasts in vitro. It is, however, not at all clear whether or not these mechanisms also operate in vivo.

Activated (by T cells) macrophages play an important role in controlling parasitic infections, and their effectiveness is impaired in malaria, toxoplasmosis, *L. donovani* and *braziliensis*, and *Tr. cruzi* and *brucei* infections. Unspecific activation of macrophages (e.g., by BCG) renders mice resistant to otherwise fatal infections of *Plasmodium winckii;* activated macrophages release mediators which produce degeneration of parasites within circulating erythrocytes; the mechanism of this effect is unknown. In toxoplasma infections, lymphokines are released which inhibit toxoplasma replication in macrophages; it has been demonstrated that the lymphokine interacts with a trypsin and neuraminidase sensitive receptor on the surface of macrophages. In addition, activated macrophages synthesize proteins which inhibit toxoplasma replication within their parasitic vacuole. In immunologically impaired individuals infected with toxoplasma parasites, there appears to be an impaired activation of macrophages by lymphocytes. On the other hand, blood forms of *Tr. cruzi* possess an antiphagocytic substance on their surface; removal of this substance by trypsin treatment in vitro renders them phagocytable for macrophages.

In protozoan infections, the predominant immune response appears to be the formation of specific IgG antibodies, which is under the control of T helper cells. In general, they confer only partial protection to reinfections and are not efficient in eliminating existing infections, but only keep the extent of parasitic burden at a low level. They are usually not directed against, or do not affect, the adult, replicating parasite: thus, in malaria, IgG antibodies are produced against merozoites which confer protection against reinfection of the same strain; they are complement independent and apparently neutralize merozoites in a way comparable to virus neutralization; they are specific for glycoproteins on the surface coat of the parasite. This surface coat can undergo variations, thus eluding the action of antibodies (see below). There are no protective antibodies against the gametocyte in erythrocytes or the trophozoite (replicating stage) in liver parenchyma cells. In amebiasis, high titers of circulating antibodies can be demonstrated, yet there is no indication of acquisition of resistance to reinfections (colitis); however, recurrence of amebic liver abscesses after cure are rare. In diffuse cutaneous and visceral leishmaniasis high titers of specific antibodies in addition to generally elevated immunoglobulin levels are detected, but they are not protective. Since in the cutaneous form, the specific antibody titer is low, it is assumed that immunity in leishmania infections is established by cellular mechanisms (see above). In *Tr. brucei* infections, complement-activating antibodies are formed against predominant blood variants; however, new variants escape their actions (see below). Complement-activating and opsonizing IgG antibodies are produced in the course of *Tr. cruzi* infections, which confer in collaboration with cellular mechanisms a certain degree of immunity. Lytic and op-sonizing IgG antibodies are demonstrable in toxoplasmosis; however, they appear to be protective only in the presence of (lymphokine) activated macrophages; in immunologically impaired individuals, this necessary activation of macrophages by sensitized lymphocytes is apparently absent or inefficient.

Metazoal infections. Metazoan infections are characterized by eosinophilia and the production of specific (and unspecific) IgE antibodies, in addition to IgG antibodies, as well as local infiltration of macrophages, basophils, mast cells, and eosinophils at the site of infection. These reactions occur against tissue invasive and penetrating larvae forms of the parasites: schistosomiasis, fascioliasis, paragonimiasis, echinococcosis (hydratid cyst disease), ascariasis (particularly the pulmonary phase), strongyloidiasis, trichinosis, and filariasis. Parasites which neither enter the host tissue, i.e., remain in the intestinal tract, nor induce persistent inflammatory responses do not usually elicit eosinophilia, e.g., enterobiasis, *Trichuris* infections, hookworm infections, and tapeworm *(Taenia)* infections, or only locally at the site of their fixation. In addition to IgE antibodies, IgG (particularly IgG_1) antibodies are formed usually against developmental (molting fluid in filariasis) and metabolic by-products, enzymes (acetylcholinesterase in nematodes), or other secretory products rather than structural components. In addition to specific immune responses, some metazoa activate independent of antibodies the properdin system (see p. 127), which by activation of the late complement components kills the parasites.

IgE Response. High levels of IgE have long been considered a feature of *chronic* metazoan parasitic infections. This potentiated IgE response is T cell dependent as no IgE response are obtained in athymic nude mice. The underlying reasons for the IgE response is unknown, but it has been suggested that antigen persistence in mucous membranes and subcutaneous tissue and disruption of

Table 11.12. Immunologic features of protozoal infections in man

Disease	Vector	Host	Prepatency	Duration of infection	Infected tissue	Cellular activities	Humoral activities	Comments
Malaria (*Plasmodium vivax, ovale, falciparum, malariae*)	anopheline mosquitoe	Human only	24 h	3 years 1 year indef.	Liver parenchymal cells, erythrocytes	CMI present; increase of phagocytic activity; T helper cell activation	IgG against merozoite antigens (partially protective)	Exoerythrocyte stages do not induce antibody formation; hypergammaglobulinemia, autoantibodies, immunosuppresion; immunopathology (nephrosis due to immune complexes and autoantibodies)
Amebiasis (*Entamoeba histolytica*)	Primates, domestic animals		8–35 days	Indefinitely	Intestinal cell wall, portal circulation, liver	CMI present	IgG, IgM, IgE; Arthus reaction	No evidence that Igs are protective
Leishmaniasis Cutaneous L. (*L. tropica*) Oriental Sore	Phlebotomus (sand fly)	Rock hyrax	Days to months	6 Months	Cutis macrophages	Early and strong delayed hypersensitivity	Little antibody response	Cell-mediated protection; development of immediate hypersensitivity coincides with healing
Visceral L. (*L. donovani*) Kala-Azar	"	Hamster, gerbil, dog		Indefinitely	Dermis, macrophages, RES, liver, spleen	No CMI; only after spontaneous recovery or treatment	Polyclonal Ig response; circulating L. antigens	CMI suppressed (defective host response); immune complexes. CMI plays role in resolution of disease
Mucocutaneous L. (*L. braziliensis*) Espundia	"	Sloth hamster, opossum		Indefinitely		CMI present, but inadequate	Elevated Ig levels	Immunopathology (immune complex deposits)
Toxoplasmosis (*T. gondii*)	Mammals, partic. cats, birds		2–4 weeks	Indefinitely	All cells and tissue	DTH develops late; if trophozoite is exposed to antibody and C macrophages kill parasite	IgG, IgM, IgA; nonspecific Ig elevated	Ig not protective; immune complexes in kidney
Trypanosomiasis (*T. cruzi*) Chagas disease	Reduviidae bugs (*Triatomae*)	Mammals (dogs)	2–3 weeks	Indefinitely	RES cells, macrophages, glia cells cardiac muscle cells	No effective CMI	Polyclonal antibody response	Reconvalescent sera confer some protection; experimentally: transfer of protective immunity by spleen cells; immunopathology
(*T. brucei*) Sleeping sickness	Tsetse fly (*glossina*)	Human, domestic oxen, antelope	1–3 weeks	1 year	Blood, lymph circulation, cerebral fluid	Increased phagocytic activity	Polyclonal (IgM) + specific antibodies, antibody-antigen complexes	Systemic Arthus-reaction, immune complex deposits, autoantibodies; immunosuppression; >20 antigenic variants with predictable sequence

such structures by migrating or resident metazoa might be (one of) the reason(s). It has been shown that soluble factors present in cell-free culture supernatants of mesenteric lymph node cells from parasite-infected rats *(Nippostrongylus brasiliensis)* induce the conversion of IgM-bearing cells to IgE-IgM-double-bearing cells when added to normal bone marrow cell cultures. The effect of the factor is specific as it does not increase either IgM-bearing or IgG-bearing cells. There are some indications that this factor is derived from B cells rather than from T cells. However, the differentiation from IgM-IgE-bearing B cells to IgE memory cells and IgE-secreting plasma cells requires the interaction of specifically sensitized T helper cells.

IgE antibodies sensitize selectively basophilic granulocytes and mast cells, both of which possess receptors with high affinity for the Fc portion of IgE immunoglobulins. Binding of IgE-antigen complexes leads to bridging of these receptors, which in turn triggers the release of granules from basophils and mast cells. Furthermore, it has been demonstrated that macrophages are able to adhere via their Fc receptor to IgE antibodies, which react with metazoan antigens, and kill the parasite in a complement-independent reaction (see p. 265, and 275).

Mast Cell and Basophil Activity. Two types of mast cells are distinguished (see pp. 8, 268): connective tissue mast cells and mucosal mast cells.

The activity and activation of *connective tissue* mast cells are thymus independent. Thus, nude mice have normal numbers of typical connective tissue mast cells in their skin and these cells function normally in passive cutaneous anaphylactic (CPA, see p. 261) reactions.

Mucosal mast cells are capable of rapidly increasing in numbers, especially in primary immune responses of the intestine to infections with parasitic nematodes. When animals are reinfected with the same intestinal nematode, the number of mucosal mast cells

increases with a reduced latent period and with heightened magnitude. This effect is not seen in athymic nude mice; however, this response can be restored with subcutaneous thymic grafts from normal syngeneic adults. This mucosal mast cell response can be transferred by hyperimmune sera from nematode infected donors, but not by 56 °C-heat-inactivated hyperimmune sera. It appears, therefore, that the activation, proliferation, and accumulation of mucosal mast cells is induced by IgE antibodies, the formation of which is strictly T cell dependent. Upon activation of mast cells by IgE-antigen complexes which bind with the Fc portion to the IgE specific Fc receptor, the mast cells release their granules, containing, among many substances (see below) involved in the acute inflammatory process, chemotaxins for basophils and eosinophils. Mast cells appear to have several important functions in the inflammatory reaction toward metazoan parasites: damage of parasites by the release of granules containing pharmacologically active components and enzymes; recruitment of local accumulation of effector cells such as eosinophils and lymphocytes; and activation of and cooperation with effector cells (see below). Mast cells are probably required in immunity to some metazoa (e.g., schistosomiasis).

Basophils are normally present in the blood and not in the extravascular tissue space (see pp. 8 and 270). Basophils are recruited to enter the tissue as part of specific immune-inflammatory processes guided by soluble factors including antibodies. Basophil-rich immune-inflammatory reactions are rather restricted to the skin and the gut. In the skin these reactions are called cutaneous basophil hypersensitivity (CBH). In guinea pigs, the accumulation of basophils in cutaneous hypersensitivity reactions is mediated by small amounts of low affinity 7S antibodies, IgG_1. The antibody acts via Fc receptors. The mechanism of this antibody-mediated reaction may initially involve antibody-coated mast cells that release mediators when exposed to antigen. Among the

11.13. Human pathogenic metazoa

Metazoa	Vector	Host	Tissue infected	Life span of adult in man	Prepatency
Trematodes					
Schistosoma hematobium	Snails	Human	Venes of urogenital tract; eggs penetrate wall of bladder		3–6 weeks
S. mansoni	Snails	Rodents, human	Mesenterial venes; eggs penetrate wall of colon or disseminate	10 years or more	5–10 weeks
S. japonicum	Snails	Cattle, domestic animals, man			5–10 weeks
Fasciola hepatica	Fluke snail	Herbivore mammals, occ. man	Bile duct (fibrotic capsule)	Several years	7–8 weeks
Paragonimus	(1st) snail (2nd) shrimp	Canides, felides; accid. man	Lung, also dissemination (fibrotic cyst)	Several years	2–3 months
Cestodes					
Diphyllobothrium latum	Fishes	Dog, cat, pig, bear, man	Intestinal lumen	Several years	3 weeks
Taenia saginata	Cattle	Human	Intestinal lumen	10 years	2–3 months
T. solium	Pig, man	Man	Cysticercosis; striated muscle, lymph nodes, occ. brain, eye	20 years or more	2 months
Echinococcus granulosis	Sheep, pig man	Canides	Liver; lung, brain (hytatide cyst)	Life span of host	2 months
E. multilocularis	Rodents, rhesus m., man	Fox, dog, cat	Liver	Life span of host	35–47 days
Nematodes					
Without vector, oral infection					
Trichuris trichiura			Wall of colon	3–3.5 years	6 weeks
Trichinella spiralis			Striated muscle, encapsulation	Life span of host	6 days
Ascaris lumbricoides			Liver, heart, lung (eosinophil infiltrate)	12–18 months	2–3 months
Toxocarna canis			Larvae migrans visceralis	5 years	5–6 weeks
Without vector, percutaneous infection					
Ancylostoma duodenale			Lung		
Necator americanus			Lung		
Strongyloides stercoralis			Lung	Because of self-infection 30 years or more	15 days
With vector, oral infection					
Dracunculus medinensis	Crab	Human	Lymph; subcutaneous tissue	12 months	12 months
Arthropod-borne					
Wucheria banchrofti	Mosquitoes	Vertebrates except fishes	Lymph nodes and vessels	10–15 years	1–2 years
Loa loa	Horse fly	Human	Subcutaneous connective tissue	5–15 years	2–4 years
Onchocerca volvulus	Mosquitoes		Connective tissue (eye!), fibroid capsules (Onchocercosis)	15 years	15–18 months

mediators are chemotactic factors for intra-vascular basophils.

Upon binding of antigen to the Fc-receptor-bound IgE antibody, basophils release mediators such as histamine, and morphologically demonstrate anaphylactic degranulation (see p. 270) via exocytosis. Basophils may also demonstrate "piecemeal" degranulation: this consists of progressive dissolution of the granules, without fusion of granule-containing vacuoles with each other, or extrusion of granules from cytoplasm.

Eosinophilia. The fact that eosinophils are involved in allergic reactions and metazoan parasitic infections has been documented for a long time. Irrespective of the specific time course of the hypersensitivity (inflammatory) reaction, eosinophils arrive *after* the humoral phase. The activation of eosinophil proliferation in the bone marrow is T cell dependent: allergogenic and certain metazoan antigens, or substances released from cells or tissue in contact with allergens or metazoa, induce T cells to produce an eosinophilic colony-stimulating factor (CSF) which augments the generation of eosinophils. The eosinophils are then attracted to migrate to the site of inflammation by chemotactic factors released from tissue which the parasite invades. IgE-dependent activation of fragments of human lung tissue have been shown to release an array of eosinophilic chemotactic stimuli from mast cells and basophils, including histamine and low molecular weight peptide eosinophil chemotactic factors of anaphylaxis, ECF-A (see pp. 267 and 302). But in addition to those mediators, T lymphocytes are critical to the stimulation by eosinophil chemotactic lymphokines, e.g., eosinophil stimulation promotor (ESP) (see p. 310). The T cell dependency of eosinophilia and tissue eosinophil accumulation during parasite infections has been demonstrated in experimental animal models; thus, eosinophils are present in hypothymic nude mice, but such mice fail to mount a response to infections involving eosinophilia or accumulation in localized sites.

Eosinophils have been found to act in two ways in parasitic inflammatory reactions: (1) antibody-dependent parasitocidal, and (2) mediating tissue repair by neutralizing the products of mast cells and basophil degranulation in immediate hypersensitivity reactions, and by limiting the extent of fibrotic encapsulation (e.g., in *Fasciola hepatica, Paragonimus, Onchocera*, and *Trichinella* infections), wound repair, and granuloma formation during parasitic infections.

Human eosinophils can damage schistosomula (invading larvae of schistosomes) in vitro in the presence of sera from schistosome-infected patients, through an opsonizing, IgG-antibody-dependent, and complement-independent reaction (ADCC): IgG antibodies attach to antigenic determinants on the parasite and then eosinophils adhere via surface Fc receptors for IgG. The attached eosinophils spread out along the surface of the parasite, degranulate, and damage the underlying tegument of larvae; after degranulation, eosinophils are autolytically destroyed. One of the factors damaging to the metazoa was identified as eosinophilic major basic protein. Mast cells are required for the parasitocidal activity of eosinophils, since depletion of mast cells in eosinophil-rich effector cell populations significantly decreases the cytotoxicity. However, when purified mast cells which by themselves show no cytotoxicity are added to purified eosinophils, there is a significant augmentation in antibody-dependent, eosinophil-mediated cytotoxicity compared to the effect of purified eosinophils alone (mast cell-eosinophil cooperation). The mast-cell-mediated augmentation of eosinophil cytotoxicity seems to depend, in the mouse, on IgG_{2a} antibody or its Fc fragment. The mast cell effect can be replaced by supernatants of mast cells that have released mediators in response to IgE or IgG_{2a}. Eosinophil-IgG-mediated cytotoxicity develops in the early phase of the immune response; macrophage-

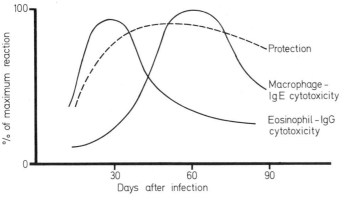

Fig. 11.8. Development of eosinophil-IgG and macrophage-IgE mediated immunity in *S. manson* infections in the rat

IgE-mediated cytotoxicity occurs most effectively in the later phase of the infection (Fig. 11.8).

The prominent protective role of eosinophils in the host response to a variety of helminth, has been amply demonstrated: larvae of *Schistosoma* migrating in immune animals are damaged as they penetrate the skin and the histopathology of the infiltrates around them are predominantly eosinophils. Similarly, when larvae are introduced into the lungs without penetrating the skin, the intensity of local eosinophil infiltration is greater in immune animals (rats) than in those not sensitized previously. Administration of monospecific antieosinophil serum to immune mice prior to reinfection with *S. mansoni* abolishes the protective effect of active antimetazoan immunity. Depletion of other leukocytes by specific antisera did not affect the level of protection. Utilizing the release of ^{51}Cr from prelabeled larvae of *S. mansoni* as a measure of cytotoxicity, complement-independent metazoicidal activity of human leukocytes in the presence of opsonizing IgG antibodies has been demonstrated; the reaction was ablated by antieosinophil serum, and was not dependent on the presence of monocytes. The cytotoxic effect was inhibitable by the addition of immune complexes which block eosinophil Fc receptors and prevent adherence of eosinophils to the parasite. Eosinophil-mediated cytotoxicity has also been demonstrated for epimastigotes of *Tr. cruzi*.

The second function, containment of inflammatory reactions, is deduced from the fact that eosinophils are known to produce and release prostaglandins E_1 and E_2, which inhibit histamine release from mast cells and basophils by increasing the intracellular cyclic AMP level. They also contain in their granules histaminase, arylsulfatase B, phospholipase D, lysophospholipase, enzymes which degradate histamine, SRS-A (slow reacting substances of anaphylaxis, see pp. 267), platelet lytic factor (PLF, which causes release of serotonin from platelets), and lysophospholipids, all substances which are released by cells others than eosinophils in an inflammatory reaction. In addition, eosinophils phagocytose extruded mast cell granules containing heparin and cationic proteases. Part of their postulated repair function may, therefore, be to limit the pathological consequences of chronic inflammation or even the extent of acute inflammations resulting from tissue penetration and damage by parasitic larvae. Thus, at certain stages of schistosomula egg-induced hepatic granuloma formation, eosinophils compose approximately 50% of the cells within the lesion. In *Ascaris lumbricoides* infections, there is a heavy eosinophil cell infiltration in the lung alveoles in which the parasite resides. In nematode infections *(Ancylostomatidae)*, there is a local infiltration of eosinophils, basophils, and mast cells at the site of parasitic fixation in the intestinal mucosa.

Escape from Immune Defense Mechanisms.
In many protozoan and metazoan infections, a specific immune response is clearly
detectable and yet parasites evade these possible attacks of the immune system. Apparently, parasites have developed mechanisms which permit them to escape the
host's protective responses. Demonstrated
or postulated mechanisms are listed in
Table 11.14.

Anatomical Inaccessibility. It appears that
some parasites, particularly *D. latum* and
T. saginata, are inaccessible for immune
mechanisms since they stay in the luminal
space of the intestine. However, they are
fixed to the mucosa at one point. The immune system is principally able to mount an
effective reaction against the parasite as
demonstrated in rats with *Nippostrongylus*;

the parasite is rejected by a locally elicited
immune response within 2 weeks after primary fixation. That some parasites escape
such an attack can only mean that they have
developed mechanisms which protect that
part of their tissue in close contact with the
host mucosa; the nature of these mechanisms is not known.
Other parasites such as *Fasciola hepatica,
Paragonimus, E. granulosus, T. spiralis,* and
O. volvulus are more truly inaccessible although they are in the tissue of the host; they
provoke the formation of fibrotic capsules
around them which protect them from even
most vigorous immune responses (e.g., particularly *Echinococcus*).

Seclusion Inside Host Cells. All human
pathogenic protozoa except *Tr. brucei* are
intracellularly replicating parasites, and

Mechanism	Parasite
Anatomical inaccessibility	Intestinal parasites, encapsulated or encysted parasites (*Echinococcus, F. hepatica, Paragonimus, T. solium, T. spiralis, T. gondii*)
Seclusion inside host cells	*Plasmodium* (trophozoites in liver parenchymal cells), *Leishmania* (macrophages and cells of the RES), *Tr. cruzi* (macrophages, muscle cells), *T. gondii* (virtually all cells)
Antigenic variation	*Plasmodium, Tr. brucei*
Molecular masking	*Schistosoma*
Loss of MHC antigens	*Leishmania*
Immunosuppression	
Disruption of lymphoid tissue	Trypanosomes
Antigen competition	*Plasmodium*, trypanosomes, schistosomes, microfilaria
Mitogenic exhaustion of B cell clones	?
Vigorous antibody response blocking T cell recognition (?)	*Leishmania*
Lymphotoxic factors	*T. spiralis, F. hepatica, Tr. brucei*
Lymphocyte suppressive factors	*Tr. brucei*
Soluble antigens	*Plasmodium, L. donovani*, trypanosomes,
Effector cell blockade	filariae, toxoplasma, and
Feedback inhibition	schistosomes
Suppressor T cell activation (?)	
Clonal abortion by toxic Antigens	

Table 11.14. Mechanisms of evasion of host-protective responses by parasites

they are protected from the activity of antibodies and cellular immune reactions by the host's cell membrane, as long as infected cells do not express parasitic antigens on their surface. Some of the parasites have, additionally, developed mechanisms to avoid the microbicidal activity of macrophages after phagocytosis by or penetration into these cells: *L. donovani* is resistant to the activity of lysosomal enzymes, *T. gondii* inhibits phago-lysosomal fusion, trypomastigotes escape into the extravacuole space (cytoplasm) after phagocytosis.

Antigenic Variation. It has been shown that malarial parasites and *Tr. brucei* protozoa have a repertoire of intrastrain variants which appear sequentially during infections. It appears that the change from one variant to the next is independent of the immune (antibody) response. Since the sequence of variation occurs in a predictable pattern, it is assumed that the antigenic variants are genetically determined. It is not known which mechanism(s) effect(s) the sequential predominance of one variant above the others. The variable surface layer induces in the host the formation of specific antibodies which are toxic for the parasites. This response is T cell dependent, and there are some indications from experimental studies that T helper cells recognize strain specific antigens (carrier) common to all antigenic variants, thus helping B lymphocytes to react in an anamnestic fashion to antigens specific for each successive variant. However efficient the immune response might be, it will be defeated by the extreme plasticity these parasites exhibit: the parasite will be always ahead of the "floundering" immune response.

Molecular Masking. Adult schistosomes are living and reproducing in the blood stream; although an infection confers strong immunity to reinfection (concomitant immunity, see above), the established parasites are unharmed by this immune response. In a series of very elegant experiments, Smithers, Ter-ry, and Hockley could demonstrate that schistosomes a few days after host invasion have coated themselves with host material containing blood group glycolipids and major histocompatibility gene products. It has been thought that the masking of parasite antigens by host-derived material serves as a disguise preventing any effect of the immune response. However, it has recently been shown that schistosomes acquire resistance also in macromolecule-free solutions; the proposed mechanism of antigen masking in order to escape the host's immune response appears, therefore, at least doubtful.

Loss of MHC Antigens. Experimental studies show marked differences of susceptibility between mouse strains to infections with *L. tropica*. BALB/c mice are highly susceptible and develop persistent expanding ulcerated lesions similar to diffuse cutaneous leishmaniasis in man. In contrast, CBA mice develop lesions that resolve within a few weeks like oriental sore in man. Uninfected macrophages from these strains can be used as efficient in vitro blockers of alloreactive cytolytic T cells. When BALB/c macrophages are infected with *L. tropica*, they are no longer efficient blockers of alloreactive killing, but macrophages from CBA mice infected with *L. tropica* remain effective blockers. This suggests that *L. tropica* infections in susceptible BALB/c cause a decrease in the surface expression of MHC coded molecules which may result in defective T cell recognition of parasitized macrophages.

Immunosuppression. Reduced responses to nonparasite antigens have been demonstrated in *Plasmodiae*, *Babesia*, trypanosome, toxoplasma, leishmania, and some metazoan (schistosome, fasciola, *T. spiralis*) infections. The immunosuppression is in general not complete but rather selective and results in partial inhibition of certain immune responses (so as not to threaten the survival of the host). Immunosuppression may have several causes: disruption of lymphoid tissue (trypanosome infection); antigenic competition in infections with high antigen load due to destroyed parasites (e.g., malaria, trypanosomiasis, schistosomiasis, microfilaria) resulting in a blockage of the macrophage-reticulo-endothelial system; parasite-derived mitogens which lead to an exhaustion of B cell clones – thus far, no mitogen has been identified; induction of an early and strong antibody response as in visceral leishmaniasis, which may prevent T cell activation or effectiveness by covering target antigens normally recognized by T cells; lymphocytotoxic factors such as agglutinins produced by *T. spiralis* and trypanosomes, or secretory and excretory products of *fasciola hepatica*, which in addition to being toxic inhibit attachment of adherent cells to flukes in the presence of serum. Similarly, trypanosomes cover themselves with sialoglycoprotein from the host's serum which impedes the attachment of antibodies and antigen recognition by T cells; parasite-derived lymphocyte suppressive factors such as tryptophol, a substance synthesized by *Tr. brucei*, which suppresses thymidine incorporation, and a low molecular weight, heat-stable factor produced by schistosomes, which suppress B as well as T cell proliferation.

Soluble Antigens. Soluble antigenic material is present in the serum after infections with *Plasmodiae*, *L. donovani*, trypanosomes, filariae, toxoplasma, and schistosomes. There are several effects soluble antigens may have on the antiparasite immune response: (1) lymphocyte (effector cell) blockage by antigens; (2) feedback inhibition by antibody (see p. 104), (3) "weak" immunogenic antigens may stimulate suppressor T cells (thus far, there is no evidence for suppressor cells in parasitic infections); and (4) clonal abortion of specific B and T cells. Thus, trypanosomes release from their surface coat exoantigens (filopodia), which in addition to blocking antibodies are toxic for cells which absorb them; if the cells are lymphocytes specifically binding these antigens, a depletion of these specifically reacting

clones might be the result. (5) Formation of antibody-antigen complexes can lead to immunosuppression in several ways: (a) Immune complexes may block antibody formation at the B cell level through interaction with both antigen and Fc receptors of antigen-reactive cells. Cross-linking of antigen receptors (surface Ig) and Fc receptors by immune complexes has been shown to be a direct blocking signal for B cells without participation of T cells or macrophages. (b) Immune complexes may suppress the immune response via activation of Fc-receptor-bearing suppressor T cells (see pp. 41, 50, 341). (c) Immune complexes can lead to effector cell blockage, i.e., inhibition of antibody secretion from terminally differentiated B cells after interaction with small amounts of antigen complexed to antibodies. (d) Immune complexes bound to Fc receptors on B cells can block the immune response nonspecifically, probably by inhibition or "freezing" of the movement of surface molecules necessary for the activation of the cells. (e) Immune complexes induce the release of soluble factors from T cells combining with the Fc portion of antigen-complexed IgG and inhibiting C' fixation.

Acquisition of Immunity

An organism may acquire immunity through a passive process, by transfer of antibodies synthesized in another organism, e.g., maternal antibodies, reconvalescent antisera, immune sera of animals, or transfer of immune cells (adoptive immunity). It also may acquire immunity through an active process, i.e., natural infections, which leads to the formation of its own protective antibodies and sensitized cells, or artificial infection with attenuated or killed microorganism (vaccination). Hence, different forms of acquired immunity are classified according to the following scheme; their differences are summarized in Table 11.15:

	Active immunity	Passive immunity
Origin of the antibodies	Same organism	Other organism
Intensity	High	Moderate to low
Mode of acquisition	1) Disease a) Clinical b) Subclinical 2) Vaccination a) Killed or attenuated vaccines b) Toxoids	Administration of antibodies: 1) Through placenta 2) Via colostrum 3) Serotherapy
Time required for development	5–14 days	Immediately after injection
Duration	Months to years	Days to weeks
Reactivation	Easy via booster doses	Risk of anaphylactic shock
Use	Prophylactic	Prophylactic, therapeutic

Table 11.15. Comparison between active and passive immunity

1. Passively acquired immunity
   a) natural (congenital)
   b) artificial (serotherapy, adoptive immunity)
2. Actively acquired immunity
   a) natural (postinfection)
   b) artificial (vaccination).

Passively Acquired Immunity

Maternal-Fetal Transfer. Passively acquired immunity occurs under normal conditions by passage of maternal antibodies to the fetus (passive congenital immunity). The mechanism of this transfer varies according to the species under study. In man, the placenta, which is of the hemochorial type, permits the transfer of IgG antibodies; these enter the circulation of the fetus and provide protection to the newborn during the first weeks of life. In other species, the passive transfer of immunoglobulins occurs only after parturition, through the colostrum of the milk, which contains appreciable quantities of IgG, IgA, and IgM. In this case, immunoglobulins are taken up at the level of the in-

testinal mucosa, which at this time is not yet fully developed. In primates, the milk possesses a certain amount of IgG and IgA, but the newborn resorbs hardly any; thus in primates, the principal manner of transfer is transplacental. Nevertheless, the immunoglobulin present in the colostrum and in the milk can be important in the local protection of the gastrointestinal mucosa. The principal routes of maternal-fetal transfer in different species are listed in Table 11.16.

Table 11.16. Alternative paths of maternal-fetal transfer of immunoglobulins

Species	Yolk sac	Placenta	Colostrum
Birds	+		
Rodents	+	−	+
Swine	−	±	+
Cattle	−	±	+
Sheep	−	−	+
Primates	−	+	−

Regardless of the path of maternal-fetal transfer, the immunoglobulin levels in the

Fig. 11.9. Variation of the serum levels of IgG after birth. The dotted line parallel to the abscissa indicates the lower limit of normal gamma globulin. There is a physiologic hypogammaglobulinemia between the first and fifth months

newborn diminish considerably in the first weeks of extrauterine life (Fig. 11.9). Between the first and the tenth week, a slow but continuous increase begins in the immunoglobulin level, now due to the individuals own immune system, establishing normal adult levels (600–1,600 mg/ml pf plasma) within 1–4 years of age.

The IgG and IgA immunoglobulin concentrations gradually approach normal levels whereas IgM quickly attains such values, especially in the event of a neonatal infection. The initial decline of the immunoglobulin concentration (Fig. 11.9) is due to the degradation of the maternal immunoglobulins, and the ascent reflects the rate of immunoglobulin synthesis in the newborn. The greater or lesser rapidity with which this portion of the curve reaches normal values reflects the state of development of the immune system and the number and nature of antigenic stimuli experienced.

Ontogenic Development of Immunologic Capacity. Generally speaking, the reactive capacity of the immune system, measured by the production of circulating antibodies, is less in the fetus and in the newborn than in the adult. The majority of fowl, for example, only reach a state of immunologic maturity 5 weeks after hatching. Similar results have been obtained for the majority of mammals. This is why newborns are practically

without isoagglutinins for the AB0 system and also do not respond to certain antigens such as antityphus vaccine. Influenced by these observations, some pediatricians think vaccination to be indicated only after the sixth month or even later. In fact, if certain vaccines, for example that against poliomyelitis with attenuated virus, are applied within the first 10 weeks, 95% of those vaccinated produce antibodies for type two, 75% for type three, and only 25% for type one. However, when this vaccine is given to infants over 1 year of age, it induces antibodies for the three types of poliovirus in nearly 100% of those vaccinated. For other vaccines such as against whooping cough, tetanus, and diphtheria, this does not occur; infants vaccinated even in the first weeks of life can be effectively protected.

Immunotherapy. Passive artificial immunity is in general achieved through injection of hyperimmune serum, particularly of antitoxin sera (against snake venom, diphtheria toxin, tetanus toxin, and others, see below), that is either produced in animals (e.g., horse) or obtained from hyperimmunized human (either postinfection or after vaccination, e.g., rabies).

Although active vaccination is long term, the protection conferred by serum is immediate but of short duration because the foreign immunoglobulins are quickly eliminated from the organism (see Fig. 10.13, p. 286).

In man, the metabolic elimination of allogeneic immunoglobulin corresponds to a half-life of 20–30 days[3] – which means that in this period of time the concentration of antibodies is reduced by one-half. The allogeneic immunoglobulins, because of their gradual elimination, are capable of conferring passive immunity for relatively long periods, affording better prophylactic and therapeutic prospects than xenogeneic immunoglobulins; evidence for that are the particularly favorable results observed in the treatment of certain virus diseases (e.g., measles, hepatitis, rabies) and in the prophylaxis of newborn hemolytic disease.

Xenogeneic and Allogeneic Serotherapy. Because of the availability of chemotherapeutic agents and antibiotics for the treatment of bacterial infections, serotherapy today is restricted to treatment of toxic infections, accidents with venomous animals, and to treatment of virus infections.

Two classes of products are utilized for passive immunization: (a) hyperimmune, xenogeneic sera, generally obtained from horses, and (b) human gamma globulin concentrates from normal donors (measles, infectious hepatitis, hepatitis B, vaccinia, varicella) or hyperimmunized donors (rabies, tetanus) (Table 11.17).

The methods for purification of horse antitoxins and the fractionation technique with cold ethanol (Cohn's fractionation) used for obtaining human gamma globulin in concentrates were described in Chap. 7 (p. 78). The antitoxins are measured in international units (IU), and the human gamma globulin concentrates generally are adjusted to a protein concentration of not more than 15%.

Special mention should be made of the prophylaxis of fetal erythroblastosis by postpartum administration of anti-D gamma globulin. Rh^+ red cells of the fetus in the Rh^- mother do not stimulated an immune response in the first pregnancy because of the insufficient quantity of fetal blood that passes into the maternal circulation through the intact placenta. At the time of parturition, however, transplacental hemorrhage can deliver the necessary immunogenic stimulus leading to the occurrence of fetal erythroblastosis in subsequent pregnancies. The injection within 72 h postpartum of only 300 µg of anti-D is effective in preventing erythroblastosis through two nonexclusive mechanisms: (1) the elimination of opsonized fetal erythrocytes; and (2) repression of the formation of maternal anti-D antibodies through passively inoculated anti-D antibodies that prevent the binding of the antigen to the receptors of the corresponding maternal lymphocytes.

In a well-controlled study in the United States with two groups of approximately 600 women treated or not treated with anti-D, the formation of antibodies was observed in 76 individuals in the control group and in only one in the treated group – indicating a protection index of 99.8%. Failures have been recorded, however, and they can be attributed either to massive transplacental hemorrhage or to intense secondary stimuli in repeated pregnancies.

Serotherapy Accidents. The administration of horse serum can cause serum sickness and, in rare cases, anaphylactic shock. To avoid the latter, which can be extremely severe, especially in individuals who have previously been injected with serum or who have a history of allergies, it is advisable first to perform a sensitivity test. This is done by intradermal injection of 0.05 ml of serum at a dilution of 1:10. If there is a positive reaction (development of an urticarial papule within 15 min), it is expedient to adopt the following precautions: (1) Injection of an antihistamine ½ h before injection of the serum, (2) injection of fractionalized doses of serum subcutaneously, starting with 0.1 ml and increasing progressively, with

---

3 The half-life of gamma globulin (IgG), up to a certain point, is proportional to the size of the animal: 15–20 days for sheep, 5–7 days for rabbits and guinea pigs, and 3–4 days for mice

Table 11.17. Serotherapeutic materials used in human diseases

Disease	Product	Dosage[a]	Comment
Toxic infections			
Botulism	ABE polyvalent anti-toxin from horse	1 vial iv, 1 vial im	Repeat if symptoms persist
Diphtheria	Antitoxin from horse	Prevention: 1,000 IU Treatment: 30,000–60,000 IU	
Tetanus	Immune globulin from human	Prevention: 1,000 IU Treatment: 3,000–6,000 IU	Recommended only for exposed individuals who have fewer than two doses of toxoid at any time in the past
Viral infections			
Hepatitis B	Immune globulin from human	0.06 ml/kg	As soon as possible after exposure up to 7 days
Measles	Immune globulin from human	0.25 mg/kg	As soon as possible after exposure
Rabies	Immune globulin from human	20–40 IU/kg	Give until 72 h after exposure
Vaccinia	Immune globulin from human	Prevention: 0.3 ml/kg Treatment: 0.6 ml/kg	
Varicella	Immune globulin from human	3–5 ml	Within 72 h of exposure
Poisonings			
Black widow spider bite	Antivenin from horse	1 vial im or iv	
Snakebite	Coral snake or crotalide antivenin from horse	3–5 vials iv	
Others			
Fetal erythroblastosis	Anti-D gamma globulin from human	300 μg antibody	Give within 72 h of exposure

[a] Passive immunotherapy or immunoprophylaxis should always be administered as soon as possible after exposure; antisera are always given intramuscularly (im) unless otherwise stated. iv, intraveneously

15 minutes intervals between successive doses, (3) conceivably, intravenous injection of the serum. In any case, it is always safe to have on hand a solution of 1:1,000 of epinephrine to inject (0.5 ml intramuscularly) in the event of peripheral collapse.

As with sera, gamma globulin preparations should be injected intramuscularly and only exceptionally intravenously. In the latter case, it is indispensable to use preparations that do not contain aggregates, for these produce anaphylactoid reactions resulting from the formation of kinins and of anaphylatoxins due to activation of the complement system.

Adoptive Transfer. Adoptive immunity is that which the organism acquires through the transfer of lymphocytes from a sensitized individual to a normal individual. Attempts have been made to transmit cell-mediated immunity, e.g., to vaccinia virus in immunologically incompetent hosts; to *Coccidioides immitis* in patients with disseminated coccidioidomycosis; and to *M.leprae* in lepromatous leprosy. Whole blood, leukocyte-rich buffy coat, and leukocyte-derived transfer factor have been used. The value of the therapy is uncertain, and these procedures are still rather experimental.

Actively Acquired Immunity

The first known method for active artificial immunization (vaccination) was immunization against smallpox, discovered by Edward Jenner in 1796. Jenner having noted the popular observation that dairymaids became immune to smallpox after being infected with the cowpox virus (vaccinia), concluded that a cross-immunization had occurred, and decided to inoculate the vacci-

nial pustule from a milkmaid (Sara Nelmas) into the skin on the arm of an English youth, James Philipp. The latter acquired a localized pustule like that seen today when the vaccine "takes," and upon being inoculated 6 weeks later with the smallpox virus, was found to be immune: the "humanized" cowpox virus was effective in imparting immunity to smallpox.

Experimenting further, Jenner in 1798 inoculated into a youth named Summers material taken directly from the vaccinia pustule of a cow. The pustule resulting from this inoculation material was passed by vaccination to a second child and so on, until the process had been repeated for a fifth time: the cowpox virus could be artificially humanized by serial inoculations (passages) into human skin.

Type	Live vaccine	Killed vaccine
Viral	Smallpox Rubella Measles Rabies (veterinary use)	Poliomyelitis Influenza Rabies Foot-and-mouth disease (veterinary use)
	Yellow fever Mumps Newcastle's disease (veterinary use)	Typhus
Bacterial	Tuberculosis (BCG) Brucella (veterinary use)	Cholera Typhoid Whooping cough
Bacterial toxoids	Diphtheria Tetanus *Cl. welchii* (veterinary use)	
Helminths	Cattle lung worm Sheep lungworm Dog hookworm ⎬ veterinary use Bovine babesia Schistosoma bovis	

Table 11.18. Types of vaccines currently in general use or only used occupationally, or in experimental stage

Occupational use or experimental:
Adenovirus (attenuated oral virus), arborvirus (equine encephalitis, occupational use), cytomegalovirus (live attenuated vaccine), hepatitis B (experimental), herpes virus hominis (experimental), influenza (live attenuated, orally administered, experimental); anthrax (protein antigen extracted from culture filtrates, occupational use), cholera (purified haet- and formalin-inactivated toxin), streptococci (dental caries, experimental), gonococci (experimental), typhoid (live attenuated oral); malaria (falciparum merozoites, experimental)

These experiments resulted in the general use of the Jennerian vaccination with humanized (attenuated) vaccinial viruses. The procedure rapidly spread from country to country, with the vaccinia lymph passed from arm to arm. Soon it was realized, however, that the humanized vaccinia virus tended to weaken, losing its immunizing effectiveness; for this reason, the direct animal vaccine later came into use.

Eighty-five years later, Pasteur discovered vaccination with artificially attenuated germs (fowl cholera, hematic anthrax, rabies). In deference to Jenner and his fundamental discovery, he proposed that the name vaccine (Lat. *vacca*, cow) be given to the suspensions of attenuated germs utilized to produce active immunization.

Later, when it was verified that in certain cases, suspensions of dead germ or products derived from bacterial toxins (anatoxins or toxoids) are both capable of conferring immunity, the word vaccination was used as a synonym for active, artificial immunization.

Vaccines. The vaccines available today and used in human medical and veterinary practice are summarized in Table 11.18. A scheme for active immunization is found in Table 11.19, and vaccines used in special cases (occupation, travel, accidents, epidemics) are summarized in Table 11.20. For obvious reasons, the use of live vaccines in man has been restricted as much as possible; with the exception of the tuberculosis vaccine (BCG) they are used only in the prevention of certain virus diseases. In veterinary practice, however, live vaccines are used in the prophylaxis of bacterial infections, virus infections, and parasitic infections. Attenuation of microorganisms for the use of vaccines can be achieved by passages and selec-

Table 11.19. Scheme of active immunization

Vaccine	Age	First immunization		Revaccination or booster; comments
		Route[a] Doses	Interval	
BCG	Until 3 months id	1×0.05 mg	—	Revaccination in absence of allergy
	After 3 months id	1×0.1 mg	—	
DTP	2 months to 5 years	im 3×0.5–1.0 ml	1–2 months	1 and 5 years after the 1st dose
DT	5–7 years	im 2×0.5–1.0 ml	1–2 months	Annually until age of 7; thereafter only tetanus (T)
Measles[b]	6 months to 4 years	sc 1×0.5 ml	—	May prevent natural disease if given less than 48 h after exposure
Mumps[b]	After 1 year	sc 1 dose	—	Reimmunization if given before 1 year of age
Rubella[b]	After 1 year (usually girls at age 10–12)	sc 1 dose	—	Contraindicated during pregnancy; women must prevent pregnancy for 3 months after immunization
Sabin[c] (trivalent)	3 months and after	oral 3×1 drop	2 and 6 months	5 years after the first dose
Smallpox[d]	2 years	id 1 drop	—	Revaccination after 5 years
Tetanus	Only after 7 years	im 2×0.5–1.0 ml	1–2 months	In the event of exposure

[a] id, intradermally; im, intramuscularly; sc, subcutaneously
[b] available as combination vaccine (MMR)
[c] Can be combined with first and second dose of DTP
[d] No vaccination if child or contacts have eczema or (any) skin disease

Table 11.20. Additional vaccines against infectious microorganisms

Disease	Vaccine	Route of administration[a]	First immunization	Duration of effect	Comments
Cholera	Killed bacteria	sc, im	2 doses 1 week or more apart	6 months	Only partially protective
Influenza	Killed whole or split virus A and/or B (chick embryo)	im	1 dose	1 year	Vaccination in November; composition of the vaccine varies depending upon epidemiologic circumstances
Meningo-coccus	Meningococcal polysaccharide group A or C	sc	1 dose	Permanent	Recommended in epidemic situations
Plague	Killed bacteria	im	3 doses 4 weeks or more apart	6 months	Only occupational exposure and residents of endemic areas
Pneumo-coccus	Pneumococcal polysaccharide, polyvalent	sc, im	1 dose	At least 3 years	Recommended for patients with cardiorespiratory diseases and sickle cell disease
Rabies	Killed virus (duck embryo)	sc	Preexposure: 2 doses 1 month apart; 3rd dose 6–7 months later Postexposure: always give human rabies immune globulins. 23 doses: 2 doses for the first 7 days, then 7 daily doses, and boosters on days 24 and 34	2 years	
	(Human diploid)[b]	im (m. deltoides)	Preexposure: 3–4 doses Postexposure: immune globulin; 6 doses: days 0, 3, 7, 14, 28, and 90		
Typhoid	Killed bacteria	sc	2 doses 4 weeks or more apart	3 years	Recommended only for exposure from travel, epidemic or carrier
Typhus	Killed virus	sc	2 doses 4 weeks or more apart	6–12 months	Recommended only for occupational exposure
Yellow fever	Live virus (chick embryo)	sc	1 dose	10 years	Recommended for residence in or travel to endemic areas

[a] sc, subcutaneous; im, intramuscular
[b] In some countries not (yet) in general use

tion of less pathogenic variants (viruses), and by irradiation (protozoa and metazoa).

References

Allison AC (1974) On the role of mononuclear phagocytes in immunity against viruses. Prog Med Virol 18:15

Cline MJ (1975) The white cell. Harvard University Press, Cambridge/Mass.

Cohen S, Sadun EH (eds) (1976) Immunology of parasitic infections. Blackwell, Oxford

Dixon FJ (ed) (1979) Viral immunopathology. Springer Sem Immunopath 2:233

Dönges J (1980) Parasitologie. Thieme, Stuttgart

Fudenberg HH, Stites DP, Caldwell JI., Wells JV (1980) Basic and clinical immunology, 3 rd ed. Lange Medical Publications, Los Altos/Calif.

Gadebusch HH (ed) (1979) Phagocytosis and cellular immunity. CRC Press, Boca Raton, Fla.

Goodwin LG (1974) Pathology of african trypanosomiasis. In: Trypanosomiasis and leishmaniasis. Ciba Foundation Symposium, Elsevier-North Holland, Amsterdam

Gupta S, Good RA (eds) (1979) Cellular, molecular, and clinical aspects of allergic disorders. Plenum, New York

Jawetz E, Melnick JL, Adelberg EA (1978) Review of medical microbiology, 13 th ed. Lange Medical Publications, Los Altos/Calif.

Klebanoff SJ, Clark RA (1978) The neutrophil. Function and clinical disorders. North-Holland, Amsterdam

Kraus R (ed) (1980) Immunopathology of parasitic diseases. Springer Sem Immunopath 2:355

Mims CA (1977) The pathogenesis of infectious disease. Academic, New York

Mitchell GF (1979) Responses to infections with metazoan and protozoan parasites in mice. Adv Immunol 28:451

Möller G (ed) (1974) The immune response to infectious diseases. Transplant Rev 19

Najjar VA, Schmidt JJ (1980) The chemistry and biology of tuftsin. Lymphokine Rep 1:157

Nelson DS (ed) (1976) Immunobiology of the macrophage. Academic, New York

Notkins AL (1974) Viral infections: Mechanisms of immunologic defense and injury. Hosp Pract 9:65

Rocklin RE, Bendtzen K, Greineder D (1980) Mediators of immunity: Lymphokines and monokines. Adv Immunol 29:56

Steward II WE (1979) Interferon. Springer, Wien New York

Stossel TP (1974) Phagocytosis. N Engl J Med 290: 717, 774, 833

Theofilopoulos AN, Dixon FJ (1979) The biology and detection of immune complexes. Adv Immunol 28:89

Zinkernagel RM, Doherty PC (1979) MHC restricted cytotoxic T cells: Studies on the biological role of polymorphic transplantation antigens determining T cell restriction-specificity, function, and responsiveness. Adv Immunol 27:52

Chapter 12   Immunodeficiencies

Wilmar Dias da Silva and Dietrich Götze

Contents

Control of infectious diseases by immunotherapy and chemotherapy has made possible the survival of individuals genetically predisposed to a series of diseases including immunodeficiencies that formerly resulted in death before the individual reached reproductive age. As a result, today, rare genes are expressed, which formerly were the exception. Thus, immunodeficiencies may cease to be rare diseases in the not too distant future.

The immunodeficiencies, conceptualized as aberrations in immunologic functions, might be considered as experiments carried out by nature, which immunologists have (also) studied in order to elucidate important aspects of the immune response.

As described in previous chapters, the immune response is made up of several subsystems: B lymphocytes and their immunoglobulin-secreting descendants, the plasma cells, and their products in the serum: IgM, IgG, IgA, IgE, and IgD; T lymphocytes, which help or suppress the function of B or other T lymphocytes, release lymphokines, and destroy specifically target cells upon stimulation; macrophages and polymorphonuclear cells, which are very effectively involved in the defense against infections and in enhancing the activity of lymphocytes (see Chap. 11). Deficiency of any part of the defense system will result in disturbance of the whole system.

Evaluation of the Immune System Functions

The first stage in the identification of immunodeficiencies is to evaluate the functional state of each of the components of the immune system: immunoglobulins, B and T lymphocytes, polymorphonuclear cells and macrophages, and the complement system.

Immunoglobulins and Antibodies

The immunoglobulin level is evaluated by serum electrophoresis and immunoelectrophoresis of the total serum; the concentration of immunoglobulin classes is assessed by the Mancini test (IgG, IgM, IgA, and IgD) or radioimmune assay (IgE) (see p. 275). Furthermore, the following parameters are usually determined: (1) the titer of IgM isoagglutinins and heteroagglutinins to rabbit and sheep erythrocytes as well as against *B. pertussis;* (2) the titer of IgG antibodies after immunization with diphtheria toxoid using the Schick reaction (see p. 312) or the quantification of diphtheria antitoxin in guinea pigs; (3) neutralizing antibody titer for measles by hemagglutination inhibition, and (4) the quantification of complement-fixing antibodies against mumps, and other previous infections or immunizations.

Under normal conditions, the immunoglobulin levels remain relatively constant due to an equilibrium between synthesis, distribution in the vascular and tissue compartment, and degradation. The synthesis of immunoglobulins has preference over that of other proteins in relation to the utilization of the essential amino acids available; more over, as mentioned already, the synthesis of immunoglobulins is normal even in cases of extreme malnutrition. It has been calculated that each IgG-producing plasma cell synthesizes 2,000 molecules of immunoglobulin per second, which corresponds to 1.5–2.5 g per day in an individual weighing 70 kg (154 lb). With these values, it was possible to determine the number of functioning IgG-producing plasma cells which, under normal conditions, is of the order of 5.5×10^{10}. For IgM and IgA, the median synthesis values are of the order of 0.4 g and 3.0 g per day, respectively, in the adult.

The distribution of immunoglobulins in the organism is not homogeneous. IgG is equally distributed in the intravascular and interstitial spaces and in such a way that variations in serum levels are reflected in the interstitial spaces. A similar distribution is observed for IgA, although it should be noted that IgA is most abundant in the secretions. IgM is found almost exclusively in the intravascular spaces, whereas IgE is de-

tectable in the blood only in cases of increased synthesis (allergic conditions and IgE myeloma).

The catabolic elimination of the immunoglobulins that are not combined with antigens occurs principally in the digestive tract, the liver, and the lungs. In man, the half-life of the immunoglobulins is 26 days for IgG, 6 days for IgA, 5.1 days for IgM, 2.8 days for IgD, and about 2 days for IgE. When the immunoglobulins are combined with antigens in the form of immune complexes, the elimination is rapid and occurs through phagocytosis by macrophages.

To evaluate the capacity for the formation of antibodies in vivo, the commonly employed antigen is diphtheria toxoid, and the intensity of the humoral response is verified by the Schick test.

B Lymphocytes

Under normal conditions, about 10%–30% of the lymphocytes in the peripheral blood are B lymphocytes expressing surface immunoglobulins. Their fraction among lymph node lymphocytes is about 20%, in tonsils about 40%, and in the spleen about 35%. Pre-B cells in the bone marrow have no surface immunoglobulins (Ig) but cytoplasmic IgM which can be assayed by fluoresceinated anti-immunoglobulins. Mature B cells possess, in addition to surface IgM, receptors for C 3 b and the Fc portion of IgG, and surface IgD. Antigen-stimulated B cells, mostly memory cells, express instead of IgD IgA or IgA together with IgM (see Chap. 1, pp. 11–12).

B cell function can be assayed in vitro by pokeweed mitogen stimulation, which induces normal B lymphocytes to proliferate (thymidine uptake) and to differentiate into mature antibody-secreting plasma cells of all classes. For this response to occur, B cells have to be co-cultured with helper T cells which are purified from healthy donors. Ig production is assessed at the end of the culture period by radioimmune assay of the culture supernatant fluid, or by the determination of uptake of labeled amino acid precursors, or by the demonstration of cytoplasmic Ig with fluoresceinated antisera.

T Lymphocytes

Human T cell function is evaluated by (1) enumeration of circulating T cells and T cell subpopulations, and (2) in vivo and in vitro testing of T cell functions.

The percentage and absolute numbers of T cells in the peripheral blood can be assessed by their ability to form rosettes with neuraminidase-treated sheep red blood cells (SRBC). Normally, about 75% of the circulating lymphocytes are T cells, in absolute numbers: 1,600–4,300 per mm³ until 18 months of age, and 600–3,000 per mm³ thereafter. Subpopulation of T cells can be distinguished by appropriately absorbed specific anti-T cell sera; about 50%–60% of peripheral blood T cells possess an antigenic marker, TH1, detected by such antisera. These T cells react in the allogeneic mixed lymphocyte culture (see p. 240), produce lymphocyte mitogenic factors, possess helper activity for B cells, and act as allogenic killer cells (see pp. 39, 51). TH1⁻ lymphocytes do not participate in these reactions but proliferate in response to soluble antigens. Both T cell populations proliferate in response to phythemagglutinin (PHA) and concanavallin A (ConA). In addition, circulating T lymphocytes differ in terms of their surface receptors for immunoglobulin molecules (see p. 50): Tγ cells with a receptor for IgG-Fc, and Tμ cells with receptor for IgM-Fc. Rosetting with oxerythrocytes bearing either rabbit IgG or IgM on their surface shows that about 65% of the peripheral blood T cells are Tμ, and 10%–15% are Tγ cells. The functional capacity of Tμ and Tγ can be evaluated in terms of their capacity to help or suppress Ig production in response to pokeweed mitogen (see above); in this test, Tμ are helper cells, whereas Tγ are suppressor cells. The suppressive effect can be eliminated by irradiation (1,000–2,000 r) of the purified T cell suspension prior to coculturing. There are some indications that Tγ can transform into Tμ cells after incubation at 37 °C.

The functional tests for T cells comprise (a) delayed type hypersensitivity skin tests, (b) proliferation assays, (c) demonstration of release of soluble factors (lymphokines, see p. 310, 313), and (d) assessment of killer, helper, and suppressor activity.

The following skin tests are usually applied: mumps, trichophytin, PPD, Candida, and streptokinase-streptodornase. Patients with no positive skin test to recall antigens are stimulated with 2-4-dinitrochlorbenzene or keyhol limpet hemocyanin.

Proliferation assays employ either unspecific mitogens such as PHA, ConA, and PWM, or antigens. Commonly used anti-

Table 12.1. B and T lymphocyte specific characteristics

Characteristics	T cells	B cells	K cells	Method of detection
SRBC receptor (E rosettes)	+	−	−	Binding of sheep red blood cells
HT1	+	−	−	Cytotoxicity, fluorescence
Receptor for rabbit IgM	+ (Tμ)	−	−	Rosette formation with ox erythrocytes
Receptor for rabbit IgG	+ (Tγ)	−	+	coated with rabbit IgM or IgG, respectively
Receptor for Ig-Fc	−	+	+	Aggregated Ig; immunofluoresence
Receptor for C3b (EAC rosettes)	−	+	?	Binding of complement and IgM-coated sheep or ox red blood C.
Surface Ig	−	+	−	Immunofluorescence
Proliferation to PHA	+	−	?	Thymidine up-take
Proliferation to ConA	+	−	?	
Proliferation to PWM	+	+	?	
Radiosensitivity	Tμ−, Tγ+	+	?	PWM induced plasma cell maturation

gens are: PPD, Candida, tetanus, diphtheria. Cells of patients who had no prior encounter with these antigens do not proliferate. In stimulation experiments with allogeneic cells (MLR, see p. 240), B cell lines
or T cell depleted normal cells, irradiated or
mitomycin treated, should be used as stimu-
lators to avoid the release of blastogenic
factors.

The production of lymphokines (MIF, interferons, lymphotoxins, see p. 310) can be
by B and T cells; therefore, purified cell populations have to be used in determining the
capacity of T or B lymphocytes to release
these substances.

In order to assess helper and suppressor activity of T cells, the pokeweed mitogen-in-
duced maturation of B cells into Ig-secreting
plasma cells is used (see above). Normal peripheral B cells and monocytes are rigorously depleted of T cells and cocultivated
with T cells of patients. Two cultures are run
simultaneously, one with irradiated (1,000–
2,000 r) T cells (T suppressor cells are
radiosensitive), and the other with nonirradiated T cells. The ability to generate
cytotoxic T cells is best studied after in vitro
allogeneic stimulation as described in
Chaps. 2 (p. 42) and 6 (p. 142).

Phagocytes

Polymorphonuclear and mononuclear cell
functions in a defense reaction can be, for
practical purposes, separated into distinct
operations: chemotactic (directed) and random movement, adherence to microbes, ingestion of microbes, degranulation of lysosomes into phagosomes or exterior, and killing of microbes (Fig. 12.1).

Motility. Random motility can be tested for
by the capillary tube migration test. Purified
neutrophils (5×10^6/ml in 0.1% albumin solution) are placed in siliconized microhe-
matocrit tubes; the tubes are heat sealed at
one end and centrifuged at 1,500 rpm for
10 min. The tubes are then severed at the top
of the leukocyte pellet and the truncated
capillary tube is placed horizontally in a Pe-

Fig. 12.1. Functional steps of phagocytosis in neutrophils: *1,* chemotaxis; *2,* opsonization; *3,* ingestion; *4,*
phagosome; *5,* degranulation (phagolysosome formation); *6,* bacteriolysis. *G,* granules containing lytic enzymes

tri dish containing a suitable medium at
37 °C. During this incubation, the cells migrate out of the tube in a fan-shaped manner
(see Fig. 10.16, p. 291).

Chemotactic movement is tested by the use
of Boyden's chambers (see Fig. 5.8). Cells to
be tested are placed in the upper chamber
and are separated from the lower chamber
containing a chemotactic substance by a
millipore filter (pore size usually 3 µm).
Neutrophils can enter the filter membrane
but are trapped in transit through the membrane. After several hours of incubation at
37 °C, the filter is removed and stained, and
the underside is microscopically examined
for the presence of neutrophils.

Another technique, migration under
agarose, permits the determination of random and chemotactic movement at the same
time. Wells are cut in an agarose medium.
The center well is filled with a suspension of
purified cells while two peripheral wells are
filled with medium and chemotactic materi-

al, respectively. The cells respond to the chemotaxin and migrate in a tear-drop fashion toward that well. By measuring the distance of migration from the leading edge to the center well, one can quantitate the intensity of the chemotactic stimulus. The random migration is measured by the degree of migration toward the control well.

Adherence. Neutrophil and monocytes adherence is evaluated by their ability to spread on certain surfaces (glass, plastic).

Opsonization. Opsonization is measured in terms of increased phagocytosis of microorganisms coated with antibodies and complement in comparison to noncoated microorganisms.

Ingestion. Methods for quantitation of ingested material include direct counting of ingested microbes by light microscope, estimation of cell-bound radioactivity after ingestion of labeled microbes, and measurement of stained particles after ingestion.

In the first procedure, cells are mixed with appropriate bacteria; after a suitable incubation time (usually 30–60 min), the cells are fixed. Internalized bacteria are directly counted with the light microscope from stained smears.

The second procedure uses bacteria which have been grown on ^{14}C-amino acids or ^{3}H-thymidine. The opsonized, labeled bacteria are incubated with cells for varying periods of time and the reaction is terminated by the addition of cold buffer containing an inhibitor of glycolysis (NaF). Free bacteria are removed from ingested bacteria by repeated washings. The cell-associated radioactivity is then measured.

The third method utilizes paraffin oil emulsions containing a dye, oil red O. Following incubation of the neutrophils with the test emulsion and removal of noningested paraffin, the amount of cell-associated dye is quantitated spectrophotometrically.

Degranulation. Degranulation is tested by "frustrated phagocytosis": heat-aggregated γ-globulin or immune complexes are fixed to the plastic surface of a Petri dish so that they cannot be ingested. Neutrophils are placed in Petri dishes with and without attached γ-globulin. They are stimulated and discharge their intralysosomal content, particularly β-glucuronidase and acid phosphatase, into the suspending medium. Nonspecific cell death or cytolysis can be estimated by measuring the discharge of lactate dehydrogenase, a cytoplasmic (nongranule) enzyme into the medium.

Intracellular Killing. Intracellular killing is assessed by two methods: the nitroblue tetrazolium dye reduction test (NBT) and the intraleukocytic killing test.

Nitroblue tetrazolium is a clear, yellow, water-soluble compound that forms formazan, a deep blue dye, on reduction. Neutrophils can reduce the dye following ingestion of latex or other particles subsequent to the respiratory burst. The reduced dye can be easily measured spectrophotometrically at 515 nm after extraction from neutrophils with the organic solvent pyridine. For the mechanism of dye reduction, see p. 304.

In the intraleukocytic killing test, bacteria (about 5 per neutrophil in the final test) and opsonins are incubated with neutrophils for 1, 2, or 3 h at 37 °C. After incubation, extracellular bacteria are killed by the addition of antibiotics. Intracellular bacteria are liberated by lysis of neutrophils by sterile water, and the number of viable bacteria is estimated from the number of bacterial colonies after plating. Additional tests for the evaluation of the status of leukocytes are listed in Table 12.2.

Classification of Immunodeficiencies

The defense system consists of several distinct functional complexes, the cooperation of which confers protection against the constant assault by viral, bacterial, fungal, protozoal, and noninfectious agents (see Chap. 11). Dysfunction of any of these systems, i.e., T lymphocytes, B lymphocytes,

Table 12.2. Additional tests for the evaluation of the white blood cell status

Tests	Comments
Special stainings	
Myeloperoxidase	*Negative:* neutrophils with toxic granulation during severe infections
	Positive: neutrophils and eosinophils
Acid phosphatase	*Negative:* normal plasma cells; *positive:* plasmocytoma cells
PAS reaction (periodic acid Schiff reaction)	*Negative:* myeloblasts; *positive:* lympho- and monoblasts
Esterase reaction with α-naphthyl-acetate	*Positive:* monocytes
Functional tests	
Rebuck skin window test	Chemotaxis in vivo
H_2O_2 generation	Evaluation of different ingestive and bactericidal functions
O_2-consumption	during phagocytosis
Glucose-1-^{14}C-oxidation	
Format-^{14}C-oxidation	
Superoxide production	
Iodination of phagocytosed particles	
Leukocyte survival time with DF ^{32}P or ^{51}Cr	
Adrenaline test	Evaluation of marginated pool
Endotoxin-, etiocholanolon- and prednisolone test	Evaluation of granulocyte pool in the bone marrow
Serum lysozyme (muramidase)	Leukocyte turnover
Anti-neutrophil antibodies	
Radiological examination	Thymus aplasia, thymom, a.o.

phagocytes, and complement, will result in an overall deficiency, usually expressed in enhanced susceptibility to infections. The known deficiencies can be classified according to the system(s) involved:

1. B cell deficiencies
   Hypo- or agammaglobulinemias
   Transient hypoglobulinemia in infants
   Congenital Bruton-type (X chromosome) agammaglobulinemia
   Acquired primary and secondary hypogammaglobulinemias
   Selective, variable hypogammaglobulinemias
   Hypergammaglobulinemias, disorders of Ig-secreting cells
   Monoclonal gammopathies
   Polyclonal gammopathies
2. T cell deficiencies
   DiGeorge's syndrome
   Chronic cutaneous candidiasis
   Hodgkin's disease

3. Combined T, B cell deficiencies
   Severe combined immunodeficiencies (SCID)
   Lymphoid stem cell defect (Swiss type)
   Adenosine-deaminase deficiency
   Purine nucleoside phosphorylase deficiency
   Transcobalamin II deficiency
   Nezelof's syndrome
   Ataxia telandiectasia
   Wiskott-Aldrich syndrome
4. B and T lymphocyte proliferative disorders
   Lymphomas
   Cutaneous T cell lymphomas
   Leukemias
5. Phagocytic dysfunctions
   Neutropenias
   Chemotactic deficiencies
   Ingestion deficiency
   Bactericidal deficiencies
6. Complement deficiencies.

B Cell Deficiencies

Hypo- and Agammaglobulinemias

Transient hypogammaglobulinemia in infants. A full-term neonate possesses approximately 1 g IgG per 100 ml of maternal origin, whereas IgM and IgA are practically absent. In the first weeks of life, the IgG level falls progressively, reaching concentrations of 250 mg per ml at the third month of age. By this time, the infant begins to synthesize its own immunoglobulin, first IgG and IgM, then a little later IgA; by the fourth month, a progressive elevation of immunoglobulin levels to approximately 560 mg per ml has occurred. The period of depression of serum immunoglobulin levels in the third month coincides with the elimination of maternal IgG and generally signals the onset of synthesis of the infant's own immunoglobulins. In certain cases, however, this synthesis of immunoglobulins is retarded; during such a phase, the infant exhibits increased susceptibility to infections such as pneumonia, otitis media, and pyoderma. This abnormal condition is called transient hypogammaglobulinemia. This period is characterized immunoelectrophoretically by a shortening of the IgG anionic arc. The restoration of normal serum levels of immunoglobulins generally occurs between the third and the 30th month of life.

Fudenberg proposed an interpretation for transient hypogammaglobulinemia in infants of both sexes that is distinct from congenital autosomal agammaglobulinemia which is discussed later. Transient hypogammaglobulinemia may represent the isoimmunization of the mother against fetal IgG carrying different Gm allotypes that give rise to the formation of antigen-antibody complexes that can be eliminated rapidly by the mononuclear phagocytic system.

Congenital and Hereditary and Acquired Agammaglobulinemias. The term agammaglobulinemia is restricted to cases in which the total serum level of immunoglob-

ulins is less than 100 mg per 100 ml; above this level the expression hypogammaglobulinemia is used. Agammaglobulinemias customarily are separated into two groups: congenital and acquired. The former appear in the first two months of life, whereas the latter appear later in puberty or adulthood. At times it is difficult to decide whether an agammaglobulinemia manifesting itself at puberty is in fact an acquired form, or whether it represents the delayed appearance of a hereditary disease.

Congenital Hypogammaglobulinemia Bruton-Type. This type of X-linked, infantile hypogammaglobulinemia is due to a regulatory gene defect that affects pre-B cell differentiation (see Fig. 12.4). In general, patients lack B cells, although normal numbers of pre-B cells (approximately 0.6% of nucleated bone marrow cells) are observed in bone marrow samples. The cellular immunity appears to be normal. The number of circulating lymphocytes is usually normal, but the thymus-dependent areas of the lymphoid organs are poorly delimited, and there are hardly any follicles or plasma cells. There is a scarcity or absence of pharyngeal lymphoid tissue. The latter phenomenon can be shown radiographically by the increased size of the nasopharyngeal space (Newhauser's space). The thymus is generally normal; however, there can be a scarcity of Hassal's bodies. Successive and recurring gram-positive infections occur insidiously from the sixth month onward in distinct locations (e.g., otitis media, pyoderma, and pneumonia). It is believed that the resistance in these patients to gram-negative bacterial infections and to viruses is due to the properdin system and the cellular immunity, which appear to be unaffected. The frequency of autoimmune diseases and malignant tumors of the lymphoid tissue in such patients is relatively high. This form of immunodeficiency exhibits a pattern of anomalies of the immune system similar to those observed in the experimental model resulting from bursectomy in the chicken.

Acquired Primary Hypogammaglobulinemias. These hypogammaglobulinemias appear after a period of normal functioning of the immune system. The age at which the disease appears varies between 30 and 50 years, and generally precedes by some years the appearance of malignant tumors of the lymphoid tissue. Those afflicted exhibit low levels of IgG, IgM, and IgA; they respond poorly to antigenic stimulation, although they are capable of producing delayed hypersensitivity reactions and rejection of allografts. The number of circulating lymphocytes is normal, these cells being capable of producing a normal blastogenic response to stimulation by phythemagglutinin. The peripheral lymphoid organs are practically devoid of plasma cells, the number of lymphoid follicles being sharply reduced. In some cases, lymphoid hyperplasia occurs, especially in the small intestine; the resultant picture is that of intestinal malabsorption and loss of proteins. There is a correlation in about 10% of all cases between this immunodeficiency and tumors of the thymus; in those cases, an excessive activity of T suppressor cells have been found, and Tγ cells are increased.

Acquired Secondary Hypogammaglobulinemias. This group includes all forms of hypogammaglobulinemias associated with processes that do not directly affect the lymphoid organs.

Selective, Variable Hypogammaglobulinemias

These are selective deficiencies of one or more classes of immunoglobulins that are always accompanied by a deficient response to certain antigens. These disorders are attributed either to the absence of synthesis of a particular class of immunoglobulins or to the production of functionally abnormal immunoglobulins. From the innumerable combinations of immunoglobulin deficiencies possible, only a few types have been studied extensively. Almost all patients exhibit recurring infections – principally in

cases of IgG deficiency. Cellular immunity remains normal.

Selective IgM Deficiency is characterized by a selective lack of IgM in the serum. In some cases, B cells with IgM on their surface are present in normal numbers; apparently, IgM cannot be secreted probably because of a defect in the secretory peptide (see p. 100). In other cases, suppressor T cell activity specific for the IgM class has been demonstrated. Clinical observation reveals sudden episodes of septicemia caused in general by gram-negative bacteria. This disease illustrates the biologic role of IgM as an immunoglobulin with intravascular protective activity.

Selective IgG Deficiency involves imbalances in the production of IgG subclasses, and has been defined as inherited structural gene defects by using allotype markers specific for each subclass. In a few patients, B cells are able to synthesize IgG upon stimulation by a T-cell-derived mitogenic factor but can not secrete it. The secretory defect of these cells has been associated with a failure in glycolyzation of newly synthesized IgG; this process normally occurs just before secretion of IgG. Clinically, such patients exhibit repeated pyogenic infections, the occurrence of which is extremely similar to those in patients with Bruton-type agammaglobulinemia.

Selective IgA Deficiency is the most common immunodeficiency disorder, and occurs in two forms: in one, there is a deficiency in serum as well as secreted in IgA, and in the other, there is only a deficiency in secreted IgA. The first form is autosomal dominantly or recessively inherited, but sometimes occurs sporadically. In a few patients it is observed together with one of the following disorders: ataxia-telangiectasia, malabsorption syndrome, and recurrent respiratory infections; an increased incidence of autoimmune diseases has also been observed.
In patients with serum and secrete-IgA deficiency, B cells are normal and express IgA on their surface; however, the differentiation

of the B$^{\alpha}$ cells to plasma cells is defective. In some patients, an increase of suppressor T cells specific for IgA has been demonstrated. In other patients, a deficiency in the helper function of T cells specific for IgA-B cells has been suggested.

Patients who lack IgA in their secretions, but who have normal IgA serum levels, have a deficiency in the formation of the secretory piece in the intestinal mucosal cells; the number of IgA-B cells in the blood is often elevated. Clinically, infections of the respiratory tract, otitis media, and recurrent pneumonias are observed.

Selective IgG and IgA Deficiency is often accompanied by elevated (normal) IgM levels (100–150 mg/ml). In some cases, the deficiency is X-linked inherited, but apparently the deficiency can also be acquired in later life, and then affects both sexes. It is assumed that the underlying mechanism, at least in the inherited form, is a regulatory gene defect resulting in the inability of mature B cells to switch from IgM to IgG and IgA production, maybe primarily to IgG production (see p. 49, 99 and 160). Clinically, recurrent pyogenic infections of the lungs occur. Transient neutropenia is common during severe septicemic infections. In addition to infections, these patients also exhibit autoimmune diseases (thrombocytopenia, neutropenia , hemolytic anemia). Histologic examination of the spleen and lymph nodes indicates an increase in IgM-producing plasma cells characterized histochemically by intense staining with periodic acid (Schiff's reaction) due to the high level of IgM carbohydrates.

Selective IgA and IgM Deficiency is characterized by a simultaneous IgM and IgA deficiency, along with normal concentrations of IgG. The ratio of male to female among affected patients is 4:1. In some patients, the produced IgG appears to be inert, i.e., functionally defective. Patients exhibit recurrent bacterial infections, and have a reduced capacity to respond adequately to a large number of antigens.

Secondary Immunologic Deficiencies are defects in the immunologic activity associated with other pathologic entities. They may derive from exaggerated catabolism of immunoglobulins, e.g., in the nephrotic syndrome, or in enteropathies with protein loss, or from dysfunction of the bone marrow due to toxic factors (e.g., renal insufficiency, drugs), or they may be due to reticuloendothelial neoplasias such as reticulosarcoma, Hodgkin's disease, lymphosarcoma, chronic lymphocytic leukemia, and thymoma.

Hypergammaglobulinemias,
Disorders of Ig-Secreting Cells

Monoclonal Gammopathies. These result from the abnormal proliferation of a particular clone of plasma cells, with production of elevated quantities of immunoglobulins of one class, one type, and one specificity. Included among these are multiple myeloma (plasmocytoma), Waldenström's macroglobulinemia, heavy chain diseases, and light cain diseases.

Monoclonal gammopathies can involve any class of immunoglobulin. They consist of a paraprotein generally called the "M" (myeloma) component. In certain cases, light chains (λ or κ) are encountered free in the serum and in the urine (Bence Jones protein).

Multiple myeloma is characterized by malignant proliferation of plasma cells in delineated regions of the bone marrow. The M component can be demonstrated electrophoretically. The component can belong to any class of immunoglobulins: in about 16% of cases, Bence-Jones protein can be demonstrated in the urine. Functional hypogammaglobulinemia (relative!) and deficiencies of other immunoglobulins are almost always present, making the patient singularly susceptible to infections, pneumococcal pneumonia in particular.

In parts a, b, and c of Fig. 12.2, the electrophoretic diagrams of a normal individual, of a patient with hypogammaglobulinemia,

	Relative %	g/100 ml
Total amont		7.1
PreA	0.0	0.0
Albumin	66.5	4.72
Alpha₁	3.0	0.21
Alpha₂	10.0	0.71
Beta	7.5	0.53
Gamma	13.0	0.93

a

	Relative %	g/100 ml
Total amont		4.8
PreA	0	0.0
Albumin	74.5	3.58
Alpha₁	4.0	0.19
Alpha₂	9.0	0.43
Beta	7.5	0.36
Gamma	5.0	0.24

b

	Relative %	g/100 ml
Total amont		7.3
PreA	1.0	0.07
Albumin	54.0	3.94
Alpha₁	2.0	0.15
Alpha₂	4.0	0.30
Beta	11.0	0.80
Gamma	28.0	2.04

c

	Relative %	g/100 ml
Total amont		12.6
PreA	1.0	0.13
Albumin	29.0	3.65
Alpha₁	3.0	0.38
Alpha₂	4.0	0.50
Beta	7.0	0.88
Gamma	56.0	7.06

d

	Relative %	g/100 ml
Total amont		9.1
PreA	0	0.0
Albumin	48.0	4.37
Alpha₁	2.0	0.18
Alpha₂	4.0	0.36
Beta	36.0	3.28
Gamma	10.0	0.91

e

	Relative %	g/100 ml
Total amont		9.2
PreA		
Albumin	26.6	2.45
Alpha₁	6.0	0.55
Alpha₂	7.9	0.73
Beta	7.2	0.66
Gamma	52.3	4.81

f

Fig. 12.2 a–f. Electrophoretic profiles of human sera: **a** normal; **b** hypogammaglobulinemia; **c** polyclonal hypergammaglobulinemia. Monoclonal hypergammaglobulinemias: **d** IgG myeloma; **e** IgA myeloma; **f** IgM myeloma. (Courtesy of Dr. Rubens G. Ferri)

and of one with polyclonal hypergammaglobulinemia, respectively, are shown; parts d, e, and f correspond to profiles of IgG, IgA, and IgM, respectively (Waldenström's macroglobulinemia) myelomas.

Figure 12.3 shows electrophoretic diagrams of normal serum and of IgA (a), IgG (c), IgD (e), and IgM (f) myeloma sera as well as that of urine containing the Bence Jones protein (g). IgG and IgA myelomas are relatively more frequent, especially the former, whereas those of IgD and IgE are exceptional.

The myeloma proteins possess structural and antigenic properties similar to those of corresponding normal immunoglobulins.

Fig. 12.3 a–g. Immunoelectrophoretic diagrams of human sera: **a** IgA myeloma; **b** normal IgA; **c** IgG myeloma; **d** normal serum; **e** IgD myeloma; **f** IgM myeloma; **g** Bence Jones-protein (urine). (Courtesy of Dr. Rubens G. Ferri)

Antibody-type activity, such as that of cold agglutinin, antiglobulin, antistreptolysin, and others, has been demonstrated for myeloma proteins. Exceptions include the paraproteins encountered in heavy chain disease and Deutsch's paraproteins.

Waldenström's Macroglobulinemia is a proliferative disorder of IgM-producing cells. Serum levels of IgM are significantly elevated (β_2-globulins); due to the high molecular weight of this immunoglobulin, a great increase in the viscosity of the serum of these patients occurs. Antibody activity has been detected in these monoclonal IgM-immunoglobulins (e.g., antierythrocyte and anti-IgG activity), responsible for hemolytic anemia and for glomerular lesions that usually appear in association with this disease. Figure 12.2 f and 12.3 f show the electrophoretic and immunoelectrophoretic diagrams of the serum of a patient with Waldenström's macroglobulinemia.

Monoclonal Gammopathies with Abnormally Structured Immunoglobulins. Gammopathies associated with abnormally structured immunoglobulins appear under certain pathologic conditions of immunocompetent cells, as in heavy chain disease, light chain disease, and Deutsch's paraproteinemia.

Heavy Chain Disease (γ-chain or Franklin's disease) involves a lymphoma that preferentially affects the cervical, axillary, mediastinal, and abdominal lymph nodes. Among the cases described, the male-female ratio is 3:2, with greatest prevalence around 50 years of age.

There is an abnormal production of a paraprotein with a molecular weight of 55,000 daltons, containing IgG antigenic determinants. Basically, this involves a deletion in the Fc fragment of the heavy chain so that no disulfide bridges can be formed between the light and the heavy chains. It is not known whether these proteins represent intact products of genes with deletion of the codifying nucleotides of the N-terminal region, or whether they are products of post-synthetic degradation of a heavy chain polypeptide. In some of the proteins in which the amino acid sequence has been determined, the N-terminal sequences were normal, extending from the V region to the greater part of the C_H-1 region and always terminating at position 216. These observations suggest that the proteins represent the product of aberrant synthesis and not that of a degradation process. The majority of patients do not exhibit positive reactions to a test for Bence-Jones proteins. The heavy chain excreted in the urine possesses high carbohydrate levels.

Alpha Chain Disease (Mediterranean Lymphoma) is characterized by an infiltrative lymphoma involving the small intestine and the mesenteric lymphoid nodules. It occurs preferentially in young individuals, and there appears to be a close relationship between the incidence of this disease and endemic intestinal parasitosis. Also in this case, the disturbance is in the Fc fragment, however, in the heavy chain of IgA.

Mu Chain Disease. Thus far, only one case has been described. In that case, light chains appeared in the urine along with the heavy chains, although they were not combined.

Deutsch's Paraproteinemia is characterized by the appearance of paraproteins containing IgG_1 antigenic determinants with a deletion in the region of the heavy chains in which the Gm factor is localized. Since normal IgG molecules of the same patient possess the same genetic marker, Deutsch's protein must be a product of abnormal synthesis by a specific cellular clone.

Light Chain Abnormalities have been described in a few immunodeficient patients who completely fail to produce antibodies with kappa light chains. Circulating B lymphocytes, which were examined for light chain expression and surface immunoglobu-

lins, were exclusively lambda chain in type. Since the kappa chain family contains its own set of variable region genes, it is worth noting that kappa-chain deficient patients have an important gap in their antibody repertoire. Another patient, whose serum Ig and plasma cells were virtually all of the lambda chain type, had a normal κ/λ ratio for surface bound Ig on circulating B lymphocytes and cytoplasmic Ig in PWM-induced plasmablasts, thus suggesting that the deficiency of chain production resulted from an abnormality of terminal differentiation.

Polyclonal Gammopathies are hypergammaglobulinemias with increase in the levels of more than one immunoglobulin class. Electrophoresis of the sera of these patients shows a diffuse increase of the gamma globulin fraction and a reduction of the albumin fraction. These conditions always appear to be associated with alterations in the connective tissue such as systemic lupus erythematosus and rheumatoid arthritis, hepatopathies, chronic infections, and sarcoidosis. There can be an increase of three immunoglobulin classes (triclonal gammopathies) or of just two (diclonal gammopathies), but in any case the components of the paraproteins are homogeneous. By using idiotypic antibodies, it is possible to verify that many of the diclonal components possess identical V regions bound to different heavy chains. However, not all diclonal paraproteins exhibit the same idiotype. The paraprotein can be of the κ or λ type, even when the V regions of the heavy chains are identical, in which case the light chains would be of different allotypes.

T Cell Deficiencies

Thymus-dependent immunologic deficiencies are those that affect the thymus-dependent immune system. In general, these patient exhibits lymphopenia of variable intensity, are incapable of developing delayed-type hypersensitivity, and their lymphocytes do not undergo blast transformation when incubated with phytohemagglutinin or other plant mitogens. However, the patient possesses normal serum levels of immunoglobulins. The most important forms that have been described are DiGeorge's syndrome, Nezelof's syndrome, and the immunologic deficiency associated with Hodgkin's disease.

DiGeorge's Syndrome

DiGeorge's syndrome is a diseae characterized by simultaneous agenesis of the thymus and parathyroids and consequent defects in the development of the III and IV pharyngeal bursas. In addition to the deficiencies in cellular immunity described previously, the patient exhibits symptoms of hypoparathyroidism such as tetany and hypocalcemia. The patient generally succumbs to viral or mycotic infections. Histologic examination of the peripheral lymphoid organs reveals depression of lymphocyte levels in thymus-dependent areas; the lymphoid follicles are normal and rich in plasma cells.

Mucocutaneous Candidiasis

This disorder is associated with a selective defect in cell-mediated immunity to candida in form of an absent delayed type hypersensitivity skin test response. Antibody-mediated immunity is intact, resulting in a normal antibody response to candida. The numbers of T cells in the peripheral blood are usually normal; they respond to PHA, to allogeneic cells, and to antigens others than candida. In some patients, increased numbers of suppressor T cells have been found. A familial occurrence has been reported, suggesting an autosomal-recessive inheritance. The clinical picture is characterized by persistent candida infections of skin and mucosa (respiratory and gastrointestinal tracts) and by a series of endocrine disturbances.

Hodgkin's Disease

Hodgkin's disease, a pathologic condition occurring exclusively in human, exhibits two pathognomic characteristics: it is granulomatous, and it shows accentuated cellular pleomorphism. Hodgkin's disease has some characteristics of an infectious disease, probably due to a virus, which leads to an ineffective proliferation of T cells with depletion of T cells in time combined with neoplastic monoclonal proliferation of B lymphocytes or B cell precursors (Reed-Sternberg's giant cells in granulomas). The course of the disease depends to a great extent upon the competency of the immune system, which is, in turn, threatened by the disease itself. Patients with Hodgkin's disease who are over 60 years of age tend to have disseminated lymphocyte-depleted tumors, and a relatively poor clinical prognosis. Grafts of fetal thymus tissue into such patients have been followed by a degree of immunological reconstitution. Serum immunoglobulin levels are normal or even somewhat elevated, but cellular immunity is depressed. The patients, though capable of resisting bacterial infections, are highly susceptible to viral and mycotic infections.

Combined T, B Cell Deficiencies

Combined immunodeficiency diseases are due to various causes and are of variable severity. Defective T and B cell immunity may be complete (as in severe combined immunodeficiency, SCID), or partial. The onset of symptoms in patients with combined immunodeficiency diseases, symptoms usually appear early in infancy.

Severe Combined Immunodeficiency Syndromes (SCID)

These are defined as all diseases resulting from marked and long-lasting functional impairment of both the T and B cell systems. Accordingly, the clinical symptoms and signs involve many organs and invariably lead to death. An almost constant feature is thymic dysplasia.

Immunologically, patients are lymphopenic, and B and T cells are severely diminished in absolute numbers. The severe depression of immunoglobulin synthesis becomes manifest after the age of 3 months, when maternal IgG has been exhausted; IgM deficiency might be detected earlier. All cell-mediated immune functions are absent. The architecture of the lymphatic tissue is severely disrupted. Lymph nodes are very small, and they lack germinal centers and plasma cells. The intestinal mucosa shows severe atrophy of the lymphatic system. If the thymus can be found, its architecture can barely be recognized. There are very few lymphocytes, the predominant cells being large, clear reticulum cells, and complete absence or severe diminution of Hassall's corpuscles is a constant finding. The syndrome is caused by several distinct clinical entities with different pathogenesis.

Lymphoid Stem Cell Defect. The SCID syndrome caused by a failure of maturation of bone marrow stem cells into lymphoid precursor cells was the first SCID syndrome described by Swiss authors; it was, therefore, called "Swiss-type" deficiency. The majority of these cases are hereditary; two modes of inheritance have been demonstrated: in some families the disease follows a sex-linked pattern, but in others, it is transmitted as an autosomal recessive trait. It has been claimed that this form is associated with the HLA-A1 or HLA-B7 types, but this is not accepted unanimously.

Adenosine-Deaminase Deficiency. In 1972, it was found that some SCID patients lacked the enzyme adenosine-deaminase (ADA). Meanwhile, it is recognized that ½ to $^1/_3$ of SCID patients with autosomal recessive transmission are ADA deficient; ADA deficiency without immunodeficiency has never been observed. ADA is an enzyme of the purine salvage pathway which catalyzes the deamination of both adenosine and deoxyadenosine to yield inosine and

deoxyinosine, respectively. The structural gene for ADA is located on chromosome 20 in man. This low molecular weight (32,000 daltons) ADA enzyme is found free in erythrocytes, thymus cells, and spleen and lymph node cells. ADA deficiency apparently results in an accumulation of deoxyadenosine and deoxyATP; deoxyATP is a potent inhibitor of the ribonucleotide reductase activity responsible for the generation of the 2'-de-oxyribonucleotides and thus for the production of the substrate for DNA synthesis.

Purine Nucleoside Phosphorylase (PNP) Deficiency. PNP is also an enzyme in the purine salvage pathway and catalyzes reversibly the phosphorolysis of guanosine, inosine, deoxyguanosine, and deoxyinosine. The human enzyme is a trimer consisting of subunits with molecular weights of 30,000. The PNP locus has been mapped to chromosome 14; the deficiency is inherited as an autosomal recessive disorder. Patients have severe T cell dysfunction but less impaired humoral immunity. The effect of PNP deficiency is similar to that of ADA deficiency only that in this case, deoxyGTP is the toxic product inhibiting ribonucleotide reductase activity and resulting in depletion of the cells for one of the necessary substrates for DNA synthesis. PNP activity – like ADA activity – is predominantly found in peripheral T cells and thymus, which might be an explanation for the T cell specific effect of PNP deficiency.

Transcobalamin II Deficiency. Transcobalamin II is the binding protein necessary for transporting vitamin B_{12} into cells. Patients deficient in this protein develop agammaglobulinemia, macrocytic anemia, leukopenia, thrombocytopenia, and severe malabsorption due to atrophy of the small intestinal mucosa. This deficiency appears to result in a block in clonal expansion and maturation of lymphocytes, but not in differentiation of antigen specific memory cells.

The lack of cobalamin impedes the production of tetrahydrofolate from N^5-methyltetrahydrofolate which is necessary for the synthesis of thymidylate and TTP, a substrate required for DNA synthesis.

Nezelof's Syndrome. This is characterized by impaired cell-mediated immune responses due to thymic dysplasia (embryonal thymus) and variable (up to normal) circulating antibodies. However, the antibody response to specific antigens is usually absent. It is not associated with endocrine dysfunctions, thus distinguishing it from DiGeorge's syndrome. The disease is transmitted as an autosomal recessive trait.

Reticular Dysgenesia. This is a particularly malignant congenital deficiency of all blood leukocytes. Presumably, it is caused by a lack of differentiation of the primitive he-

matopoietic stem cell into a common precursor cell.

Wiskott-Aldrich Syndrome

The Wiskott-Aldrich syndrome is characterized by thrombocytopenia, eczema, recurrent bacterial infections, and is transmitted in an X-linked pattern. Immunologically, it is characterized by normal IgG, decreased IgM, increased IgA and IgE levels, normal numbers of B cells, but an inability to respond to polysaccharide and lipopolysaccharide antigens. T cell-mediated immune responses are initially intact, but become severe with advancing age. The patients, in general, do not survive their first decade, succumbing to infections accompanied by hemorrhagic processes.

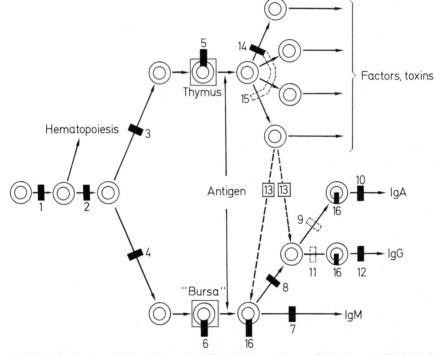

Fig. 12.4. Localization of defects along the differentiation pathways of lymphocytes. The black bars indicate positions of maturation or differentiation arrest; dashed boxes indicate conceivable block; open boxes on dashed lines regulatory (here, inhibitory) interactions. *1*, reticular dysgenesia; *2* (or *3* and *4*), severe combined immunodeficiencies, SCID; *5*, thymus dysplasia; *6*, X-linked hypogammaglobulinemia; *7*, selective IgM deficiency, Wiskott-Aldrich syndrome; *8*, selective IgG and IgA deficiency with elevated IgM (X-linked); *7* and *9*, selective IgA and IgM deficiency; *10* (and *9*), selective IgA deficiency; *12* (and *11*), selective IgG deficiency; *13*, acquired primary hypogammaglobulinemia (suppressor T cells?); *14*, mucocutaneous candidiasis (clonal T cell abortion?); *15*, Hodgkin's disease associated immunodeficiency (ineffective T cells?); *16*, gammopathies with abnormally structured immunoglobulins (deletion, translation defect?)

Ataxia Telangiectasia

This syndrome is transmitted in an autosomal recessive pattern. Patients exhibit progressive degeneration of the cerebellum with ataxia, multiple telangiectasia of the skin and conjunctiva, and susceptibility to infections. The most common immunologic abnormality is a simultaneous deficiency of IgA and IgE in the serum and in the secretions in approximately 60% of patients. Cellular immunity is depressed in many cases and becomes more severe with advancing age.

A synopsis of the localizations of defects in the lymphocyte differentiation pathways from the primitive stem cell to the finally differentiated plasma cells and T effector cells is given in Fig. 12.4.

B and T Lymphocyte Proliferative Disorders

Lymphomas

Lymphomas are disorders of hemopoiesis associated with defects in the regulation, maturation, and/or differentiation mechanisms of lymphocyte lineages resulting in an uncontrolled growth which eventually leads to immunologic deficiencies due to loss of functionally active cells. Non-Hodgkin lymphomas are tumors of lymphatic origin, which are characterized by infiltrative growth of abnormal lymphoblast cells, usually clonally derived from B, or B/T precursor cells, less frequently from T cells.

The classification of non-Hodgkin lymphomas follows morphological (Rappaport) or functional (Lukes and Collins), or functional and malignancy (Lennert) criteria: The classification proposed by Lukes and Collins, and that proposed by Lennert (also called "Kiel" classification) are similar and are given in Table 12.3 together with Rappaport's classification which has found wide acceptance because of its practical clinical usefulness and the separation of the prognostically more favorable nodular lymphomas from diffuse lymphomas. Fig-

ure 12.5 depicts a differentiation and maturation scheme identifying the stages from which lymphomas may originate, and on which the Kiel classification is based.

All forms may be histologically divided into those with nodular and those with diffuse architecture. Nodular lymphomas arise from follicular center cells and have been proven to be B cell derived malignancies with usually a high density of Ig molecules bound to the membrane of the neoplastic cells. These cells bear also C3 receptors as the predominant cell of the lymphoid follicle does.

Burkitt's Lymphoma. Two forms of Burkitt's lymphoma are distinguished. *African Burkitt's lymphoma* is endemic in some areas in Africa and New Guinea and affects predominantly small children; it is expressed as a tumor localized in the yaw and/or orbita bone as well as in the abdomen (lymph nodes, ovaries, kidney, and adrenal gland). The affected cells contain EB virus DNA or EB virus specific nuclear antigen. *European* and *American Burkitt's lymphoma* is identical to the African form in its cytology. Cervical and abdominal lymph nodes are predominantly affected, and no EB virus can be identified. In both instances, B lymphocytes are the infected cells.

Most cases of diffuse poorly differentiated lymphocytic lymphomas in adults are malignancies of B cell origin (presence of cleaved cells). In approximately 10% of cases, the neoplastic cells have T surface characteristics, and a similar proportion of cases has not detectable surface markers (0 cells).

Childhood Lymphoblastic Lymphoma is a subgroup of childhood lymphomas of the diffuse poorly differentiated lymphocytic lymphomas that has been defined by immunologic studies. The proliferating cells may have a convoluted appearance, and in most cases, the neoplastic cells bear T lymphocytic markers [complement receptors, human T lymphocyte antigen (HuTLA), presence

Table 12.3. Classification of non-Hodgkin lymphomas according to Lukes and Collins, Lennert ("Kiel" classification), and Rappaport

Lukes and Collins	Lennert (Kiel classification)
Low malignancy	
B cell-small lymphocyte, CLL	Lymphocytic lymphomas (L), e.g. CLL, Hairy cell L
B cell plasmocytoide lymphocytic	Lymphoplasmocytic L
B cell-small cleaved follicular center cell (FCC)	Centrocytic L
B cell cleaved FCC (small and large)	Centrocytic-blastic L
High malignancy	
B cell-large cleaved FCC	Centroblastic L
B cell-small non-cleaved FCC	Lymphoblastic L
Burkitt's type	Burkitt's type
Non-Burkitt's type	Non-Burkitt's type
T cell convoluted lymphocytic	convoluted or acid phosphatase type, others
0 cell-undefined, unclassifiable	
B cell immunoblastic sarcoma	Immunoblastic L
T cell immunoblastic sarcoma	

Rappaport's classification on the basis of morphology

Nodular pattern	Diffuse pattern
NLWD Lymphocytic well differentiated	DLWD Lymphocytic well differentiated
NLPD Lymphocytic poorly differentiated	DLPD Lymphocytic poorly differentiated
NH Histiocytic	DH Histiocytic
NM Mixed histiocytic-lymphocytic	DU Undifferentiated (non-Burkitt)

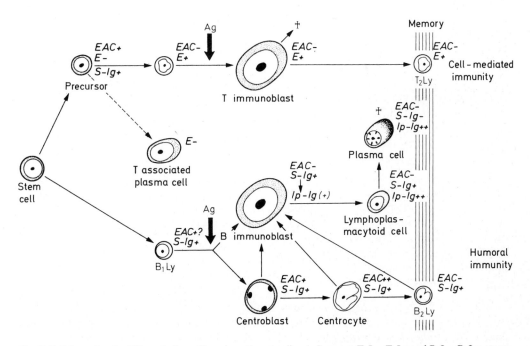

Fig. 12.5. Scheme for the differentiation of lymphocytes according to Lennert: T_1Ly, T_2Ly and B_1Ly, B_2Ly, stages of differentiation of T and B cells, respectively; E, receptor for sheep red blood cells; EAC, eyrthrocyte-antibody-complement-(C 3) receptor; $S–Ig$, surface membrane bound Ig; $Ip–Ig$, intraplasmatic immunoglobulin. (Reproduced with kind permission from Lennert K, 1977, Klassifikation der Non-Hodgkin-lymphome im Kindesalter. Klin. Pädiat. 189:7)

of acid phosphatase], and it is very likely that they are of thymus cell origin. In many of these patients, acute lymphoblastic leukemia develops rapidly, and it is probable that these two diseases are closely related.

Diffuse large cell lymphomas (reticulum cell sarcomas, histiocytic lymphomas) represent a heterogeneous group of lymphomas: some of them are of monocytic origin (lysozyme synthesis); more than half originate from B cell clones; less than 10% are T cell derived; and in more than 30% of the cases, the neoplastic cells are devoid of the usual membrane markers of B or T lymphocytes.

Cutaneous T Cell Lymphomas

Mycosis fungoides is a chronic disease of the lymphoreticular system. Clinically, it is confined to the skin for a long period of time with the development of scaly, eczematous, or erythematous patches, followed by infiltrated lichenified plaques, and progressing to ulcers and tumors of lymph nodes and internal organs. The proliferating cells in cutaneous lesions have surface marker characteristics of thymus-derived lymphocytes and are morphologically similar to PHA-stimulated normal lymphoblasts.

The disease occurs more commonly in males than in females, and is less common in blacks than in whites. The disease usually appears in the fifth decade of life. In advanced stages, patients show decreased numbers of B and T cells, but increased numbers of null cells in the circulation. Skin testing reveals an impaired cell-mediated immunity; the lymphoproliferative response in vitro is also impaired. Serum levels of IgA and IgE are increased, and a high level of leukocyte-inhibition factor (MIF) as well as thymic factor has been observed in the serum.

Sézary Syndrome (SS) is characterized by generalized exfoliative erythrodermia, intensive pruritus, and the presence of atypical cells (Sézary cells) in the peripheral blood as well as the cellular infiltrate of the skin. The observed blood leukocytosis is due to an increase of lymphocytes; atypical lymphocytes account for about 10% or more of peripheral blood cells.

These abnormal cells are lymphocytes of thymus-derived origin. It is believed that the Sézary syndrome and mycosis fungoides are identical diseases with proliferation of T lymphocytes, one with a leukemic presentation (SS), and the other without it.

Leukemias

According to the clinical course, two major groups of leukemias can be distinguished, with subgroups according to the cell types involved: acute and chronic leukemias (Table 12.4).

Akute Leukemias, particularly acute lymphoblastic leukemias and acute myeloblastic

Table 12.4. Forms of leukemias (L); in parenthesis classification of the French-American-British (FAB) co-operative group

---

I. Acute leukemias
  Acute lymphoblastic leukemias, ALL (L_1-L_3)[a]
    B cell type approx. 4%
    T cell type approx. 26%
    0 cell type approx. 70%
  Acute myelocytic leukemias, AML
    Granulocytic
      (myeloblastic without and with maturation, M_1 and M_2; hypergranular promyelocytic, M_3) L
    Myelomonocytic L (M_4)
    Monocytic L (M_5)
    Erythroleukemia (M_6)
    Eosinophil L
    Basophil L
    Mast cell L
    Plasma cell L
    Megakaryocytic L
II. Chronic leukemias
  Chronic lymphatic leukemia (CLL)
  Chronic myeloid leukemia (CML)
  Chronic myelomonocytic leukemia (CMML)

---

[a] L_1-L_3 does not correspond to B, T, or 0 cell type leukemia; L_1-L_3 denote morphological characteristics: L_1, small cell type; L_2, large, heterogeneous type; L_3, large, homogeneous type

leukemias occur predominantly in children, with the highest incidence between 3 and 5 years of age. Boys are more often afflicted than girls. Chronic lymphocytic leukemia is typically a disease of the elderly; chronic myeloid leukemia is commonly observed between the third and fifth decades.

In many animal leukemias, lymphomas, and sarcomas, RNA-containing oncornaviruses with reverse transcriptase and high-molecular weight RNA have been found. In analogy, it is assumed that similar viruses play an important etiologic role in human leukemias, although direct evidence for this contention has not been unambiguously presented thus far – except for the herpeslike Epstein-Barr virus in Burkitt's lymphoma (see above) and lymphoepithelial nasopharyngeal carcinoma. However, reverse transcriptase and high-molecular weight RNA have been identified in human leukemic cells which are not present in normal cells. Genetic and environmental factors are apparently the triggers which permit the phenotypic expression of uncontrolled proliferation. Thus, a number of genetic disorders characterized by constitutional chromosomal instability and/or immunodeficiency (Fanconi's anemia, Bloom's syndrome, Chediak-Higashi syndrome) or aneuploidy (Down's syndrome) are associated with a high incidence of acute (mainly myeloid) leukemia; exposure to radiation (therapeutic; in Japan after World War II) increases particularly acute leukemias and chronic myeloid leukemia; exposure to chemicals (benzene, alkylating agents) increases the risk of acute leukemias.

Chromosomal and biochemical findings strongly suggest that leukemias are of monoclonal origin. Normal leukocytes are formed in leukemic patients; but their generation is more and more decreased, which is not only due to "lack of space," but also to a regulatory phenomenon. The leukemic lymphocytes show an increased spontaneous proliferative response, which is inhibitable by PHA, a disturbed lymphotoxin formation, and they are immunologically inactive. Leukemic granulocytes and monocytes show impaired migration, phagocytosis, and bacterial killing.

Clinical symptoms are pallor, fatigue, recurrent fever with severe or without apparent infections (gram-negative bacteria, fungi, *Pneumocystis carinii*), hepatosplenomegaly, hemorrhage, ostealgia, and arthralgia. Each organ can be infiltrated and this causes additional "organ-specific" symptoms.

Cells from which lymphoblastic leukemias arise are thought to be precursor cells of T and B lymphocytes. Accordingly, acute lymphoblastic leukemias can be subdivided in respect to their membrane markers (Fig. 12.6). This classification has proven invaluable for diagnosis of preleukemic stages, early recognition of relapses, and prognosis (B cell type ALL has the poorest, 0 cell type – pluripotent stem cell ALL – the best prognosis). B cell type acute leukemias may be in most instances lymphomas (see below) with leukemic presentation. 0 cells type ALL possess in the majority markers similar to thymocytes or T cells rather than B cells. It appears, therefore, that acute lymphoblastic ALLs are primarily T cell disorders, whereas acute B cell disorders manifest themselves rather in the form of lymphomas (see below).

It is generally believed that acute myeloid leukemias (M_1–M_6) have a common precursor cell, namely a cell committed to myeloid differentiation. Among the acute myelytic leukemias (AML) those with predominant granulocytic differentiation character (M_1–M_3) are more frequent than myelomonocytic and monocytic leukemias (M_4 and M_5, leukemias of the monocyte-macrophage system with elevated serum muramidase activity), or erythroleukemia; eosinophil, basophil, and mast cell leukemias are rare.

Chronic lymphatic leukemias can be divided, again, by surface markers into those with (a) B cell characteristics of a single clone (the vast majority of CLL), (b) T cell characteristics, and (c) some B cell (surface bound Ig, SmIg) and some T cell (E rosetting, reaction with anti-T serum) characteristics.

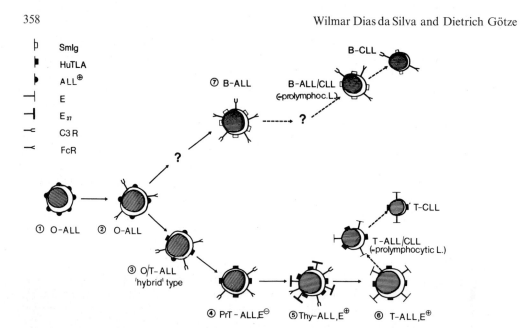

Fig. 12.6. Scheme for the differentiation pathway of early, immature lymphoid cells, based on the phenotypes of various numbered ALL-subtypes; *1*, O-All (All$^+$); *2*, O-ALL (ALL$^+$, Fc-R$^+$, C 3-R$^+$, acP$^+$); *3*, O/T-ALL (ALL$^+$, HuTLA$^+$, Fc-R$^+$, C 3-R$^+$); *4*, Precursor-T-ALL (HuTLA$^+$, Fc-R$^+$, C 3-R$^+$, acP$^+$); *5*, Thy-ALL, E$^+$ (HuTLA$^+$, E-R$^+$, Fc-R$^+$, C 3-R$^+$, acP$^+$); *6*, T-ALL, E$^+$ (HuTLA$^+$, acP$^+$); *7*, B-ALL (SmIg$^+$, Fc-R$^+$, C 3-R$^+$). SmIg, surface immunoglobulin; HuTLA, human T lymphocyte antigen; ALL$^+$, anti-O-ALL serum, specific for common ALL of non-T, non-B-type; E, receptor for sheep erythrocytes at 0 °C; E$_{37}$, receptor for sheep erythrocytes at 37 °C; C 3-R, C 3-receptor; Fc-R, Fc-receptor; acP, acid phosphatase. (Reproduced with kind permission from Thierfelder et al., 1977)

As a general rule, CLL represent B cell-derived monoclonal proliferations with expression of IgM. In rare cases, IgG or IgA are produced. In patients in whom several Ig classes are found, all have the same light chains, idiotype specificity, and antibody activity.

In most patients with CLL, the cells do not secrete monoclonal protein, but show a uniform and faint fluorescence pattern with SmIg density much lower than on normal lymphocytes, suggesting that their development is apparently "frozen" with a block in maturation along the pathway of differentiation of the B cell lineage.

In patients with CLL and a serum monoclonal Ig, the very same Ig chain with identical idiotypic determinants are found on the leukemic cell and serum monoclonal Ig. These findings indicate that such cases represent a B cell proliferation with some degree of persistent maturation of the neoplastic clone into plasma cells, a situation intermediate between that of common CLL (without serum monoclonal Ig) with a complete block in the maturation process and Waldenström's macroglobulinemia (see above, p. 349) with interrupted maturation of the proliferating clone up to the IgM secreting cell.

The proliferating lymphocytes of B-derived CLL are different in some respect for their markers from normal B cells: they possess a complement receptor for C 3d, but lack the receptor for C 3b; and they have a receptor for *Helix pomatia A* hemagglutinin, which is usually found on T lymphocytes in normal individuals.

Chronic myeloid leukemia (CML) is characterized by an increase of stem cells and myeloblasts which results in an increased production of granulocytic cells, the lifespan of which is additionally prolonged in the peripheral blood. These two mechanisms cause an excessive enlargement of the pool of myelopoietic cells (leukocyte numbers in the peripheral blood reach 100,000 per mm^3 and more). More than 90% of the cases of CML show an *acquired* chromosomal abnormality, the Philadelphia (Ph^1—) chromosome.

Chronic myelomonocytic leukemia (CMML) occurs only in adults with a predominant increase of promonocytes and monocytes. It is not clear whether or not this form represents a leukemia; it may be only an extreme and benign proliferation of monocytes.

Phagocyte Deficiency Diseases

Susceptibility to infections in phagocytic dysfunction syndromes may range from absence of clinical symptoms to mild recurrent skin infections to severe overwhelming, fatal systemic infections. Characteristically, patients are susceptible to bacterial infections and have little difficulty with viral or protozoal infectious processes.

Neutropenias

Infantile genetic agranulocytosis was described by Kostmann as an autosomal recessive disorder. It is assumed that it is caused by a defect interaction of stroma cells and granulocyte precursor cells resulting in a reduced production of granulocytes. The few granulocytes detectable are functionally normal. The disease appears within the first year of life with chronic and recurrent bacterial infections, usually leading to death. There is a marked neutropenia in the blood, occasionally accompanied by eosinophilia and monocytosis. In the bone marrow, cells after the stage of promyelocyte/myelocyte are completely absent.

Familial severe neutropenia is an autosomal dominant disorder of unknown pathogenesis. Bacterial infections occur early after birth. Patients show neutropenia accompanied by monocytosis; the bone marrow shows a deficiency in granulocytes beyond the myelocyte stage.

Cyclic neutropenia is autosomal-dominantly inherited. The pathogenic mechanism causing the cyclic variation of the number of monocytes and reticulocytes is unknown, but presumably involves a regulatory (feedback) defect. The function of granulocytes is normal. The neutropenic phases appear in intervals of 14–45 days and last 4–10 days. During this time, patients show fever, mucosal ulcerations, peridontitis, and skin infections.

Immunoneutropenias comprise at least two disease entities: (a) a transitory form caused by maternal antibodies transferred transplancentally against paternal neutrophil antigens present in the newborn; and (b) a form caused by autoantibodies to granulocyte antigens (NA 1, NA 2, NB 1, NCVaz; see p. 254).

Chemotactic Deficiencies

Chediak-Higashi syndrome (CHS) is an autosomal recessive disease. Patients show oculo-cutaneous albinism and recurrent pyogenic infections. The syndrome is characterized by giant granules in all granule-possessing cells which are abnormal primary lysosomes. It is assumed that the enlarged size of the granules causes reduction in mobility and plasticity, and slowed migration. Phagocytosis is not disturbed; however, degranulation (phagolysosome formation) is defective, which results in reduced intracellular killing of bacteria. The defective phagolysosome formation is thought to be caused by absence of induction of microtubulin formation (assembly). Cyclic GMP and cholinergic agents (carbachol and bethanechol) elevate intracellular cyclic GMP and enhance microtubule assembly; and, indeed, the function of leukocytes from CHS patients (degranulation and bactericidal activity) is partially corrected when they are incubated in vitro with cyclic GMP or cholinergic agents. Intraleukocytic concentrations of cyclic AMP are markedly elevated in CHS leukocytes; cyclic AMP has been shown to suppress neutrophil degranulation and mobility. Reduction of intracellular cyclic AMP to normal levels by treatment with high doses of ascorbic acid results in normal chemotaxis, degranulation, and bactericidal activity.

Job's syndrome: There are a number of single case reports about severed chemotactic activity of neutrophils as the only pathologic parameter detectable, accompanied by recurrent staphylococcal infections of the dermis (pyogenic abscesses) and respiratory tract (pneumonia). Some of these patients exhibit an extremely high serum IgE level (19,000–24,000 ng per ml; normal value about 330 ng per ml). In most patients, humoral and cell-mediated responses were normal, as were phagocytosis and bactericidal activity. In some, however, there is also a reduced bactericidal activity. It might be assumed that the high IgE level is caused by the persistent presence of bacterial antigenic material in skin and mucosa (see p. 325). Defective chemotactic activity has also been observed in a number of patients with epidermal disorders such as ichthyosis, eczema, and dermatitis.

Lazy leukocyte syndrome is characterized by neutropenia associated with impaired random as well as chemotactic locomotion of neutrophils. Patients show recurrent infections. All other phagocytic parameters are normal, but some patients show an elevated IgE level.

Actin polymerization deficiency is characterized by recurrent staphylococcal infections of newborns without development of pus. Infiltrations consist only of monocytes and histiocytes. The migration of neutrophils is extremely impaired, but also ingestion is retarded. It is thought, thought not proven, that the cause is a defect in actin polymerization.

Table 12.5. Disorders of neutrophil chemotaxis

Lazy leukocyte syndrome
Wiskott-Aldrich syndrome
Chediak-Higashi syndrome
Job's syndrome
Actin dysfrome
Hyperimmunoglobulin E
Hyperimmunoglobulin A
Mucocutaneous candidiasis
Cellular immune defects
Toxic neutrophils
Measles
Hodgkin's disease
Cirrhosis
Diabetes mellitus
Rheumatoid arthritis
Malignancy
Protein-calorie malnutrition

Ingestion Deficiency

Tuftsin deficiency (see p. 303) is an autosomal recessive disorder. Patients exhibit a generally increased susceptibility to infections of the respiratory tract and skin. Tuftsin is a tetrapeptide cleaved from a gamma globulin (Leukokinin; C 2 domaine, position 289–292) by the combined action of two proteolytic enzymes, one present in the spleen cleaving the carboxy-terminal part between residue 292 and 293, and the other one localized in the membrane of neutrophils (leukokininase) liberating the tetrapeptide by cleavage between position 288 and 289. The free tetrapeptide stimulates neutrophils to increased phagocytosis. The defect is probably caused by the absence of the splenic enzyme.

Bactericidal Deficiency

Chronic granulomatous disease (CGD) of childhood is characterized by a defect of granulocytic bactericidal activity of catalase-positive bacteria. The critical defect appears to be the inability of granulocytes to generate H_2O_2 (NADPH-oxidase deficiency). The increased O_2-consumption and activation of the hexose-phosphate shunt (see pp. 304–306) after phagocytosis is absent. The granulocytes are unable, therefore, to kill catalase-positive bacteria (catalase reaction: $2\,H_2O_2 \rightarrow 2\,H_2O + O_2$; these bacteria destroy H_2O_2 which they produce by themselves; catalase-negative bacteria – pneumococcus, β-hemolytic streptococcus – are killed by their own H_2O_2). The bacteria remain intracellularly, and are protected against the action of not only antibodies but also that of antibiotics. Inside granulocytes, they spread all over the organism and cause granulomas. The clinical picture is characterized by recurrent infections (particularly pneumonia), lymphadenitis, formation of abscesses, and hepatosplenomegaly. Also typical are granulomatous, eczematoid, or lupus-like skin lesions, liver abscesses, and osteomyelitis. Histologic examination reveals typical granulomas in lymph nodes, lungs, liver, spleen, and skin with giant cell formation, central necrosis, and lymphohistiocytic inflammation.

The inheritance is X-linked recessively in patients in whom the disease is caused by a deficiency of the NADPH-oxidase; some cases have been described, however, for which an autosomal-recessive pattern is more likely; in these cases, glutathion-peroxidase deficiency in addition to oxidase deficiency has been demonstrated. Furthermore, the sex-linked dominantly inherited glucose-6-phosphate dehydrogenase deficiency results in the same clinical disease if the deficiency occurs not only in erythrocytes but also in leukocytes.

Some patients with X-chromosomal recessive CGD show an association to the rare McLeod phenotype of the Kell blood group ($= K_o$). The absence of K_x on leukocytes reduces their bactericidal activity.

Immunologically, humoral as well as cell-mediated immune responses are normal. The phagocytic functions of neutrophils are all normal, i.e., chemotactic migration, ingestion, degranulation, except bacterial killing (Fig. 12.7). The NBT test is always negative.

Lipochrome histiocytosis has a course similar to CGD including negative NBT, but without granuloma formation; there is a li-

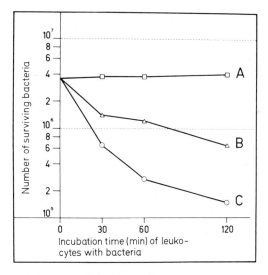

Fig. 12.7. Intracellular killing of *Staphylococcus aureus* in leukocytes of CGD patients *A*; conductors *B*; and normal, healthy individuals *C* as assessed by the intraleukocytic killing test (see p. 343). (Reproduced with kind permission from Hitzig WH, Weber Ch 1980)

pochrome pigmentation of histiocytes, which is pathognomonic. Lipochrome histiocytosis is autosomal-recessively transmitted.

Myeloperoxidase (MPO) deficiency in neutrophils and monocytes is autosomal-recessively inherited. Generally it does not *cause disease;* however, disseminated candidiasis and acne vulgaris have been described.

Complement Deficiencies

Deficiencies for each complement component of the classical pathway were described

Table 12.6.
Disorders of neutrophil bactericidal function

Chronic granulomatous disease (CGD)
Glucose-6-phosphate dehydrogenase deficiency
Myeloperoxidase deficiency
Chediak-Higashi syndrome
Acute leukemia
Down's syndrome
Leukocyte alkaline phosphatase deficiency
Felty's syndrome

Table 12.7. Survey of complement component deficiencies

Deficient component	Clinical symptoms	Inheritance	Laboratory findings[a]
C1q	Usually found in combination with severe combined immuno-deficiencies (SCID) like Swiss- or Bruton-type (see p. 351)	Depending on basic disease	Lack of C1q
C1r	Infections of the respiratory tract, chronic glomerulonephritis, LE-like skin lesions	Autosomal, recessive	Lack of C1r, decrease of C1s, increase of C4, C1-inhibitor; decreased bacteriocidic activity
C1s	LE-like systemic symptoms; persistent antigen-antibody complexes	Autosomal, dominant	Lack of C1s; increase of C4 and C2
C1-inhibitor	Also called Hereditary angioneurotic syndrom. Two forms exists: (a) lack of inhibitor, and (b) functionally inactive inhibitor. Symptoms are edemas of extremeties, face, and respiratory tract (glottis, bronchi) and abdominal pain attacks. C1-inhibitor also physiologically blocks factor XII (Hagemann) of the clotting system; the lack of it causes kinin liberation and, via plasmin activation, fibrinolysis. Degraded fibrin activates the complement system, and since C1s is not inactivated, a continuous consumption of C4 and C2 reduces their serum level	Autosomal, dominant	(a) Lack of C1-inhibitor, (b) increased C1-inhibitor (inactive) with abnormal electrophoretic mobility; decrease in C4 and C2, increase in C1s
C4	Most carriers are healthy; few cases have been reported to have shown a LE-like picture without LE-cells, and Ig- and C3-deposits in the skin. In some patients, the IgM to IgG switch does not occur after immunization	Autosomal, recessive; association with HLA	Lack of C4; defect in chemotaxis
C2	Usually, no symptoms; occasionally, autoimmune-like syndroms (lupus erythematodes, dermatomyositis, glomerulonephritis)	Autosomal, recessive; association with HLA	Lack of C2
C3	Recurrent, severe bacterial infections without (expected) leukocytosis	Autosomal, recessive	Lack of C3; deficient chemotactic activity, opsonisation, and bacteriocidic activity
C3-inactivator	Increased susceptibility to infections. C3 catabolism is increased, this causes a high level of C3a (anaphylatoxin) and C3b. C3b activites properdin which, in turn, leads to high catabolism of factor B. Increased C3a activates histamin-release	Autosomal, recessive	Lack of C3b-inactivator; deficient chemotactic activity, opsonisation, particle ingestion, and bacteriocidic activity; histamine in urine
C5	Two forms are known: (a) lack of C5, and (b) dysfunction of C5. (a) Frequent and recurrent bacterial infections, and visceral LE-like symptoms. (b) Eczema, diarrhea, increased susceptibility to bacterial (staphylococcal) infections	(a) Autosomal, recessive; (b) unclear	(a) Lack of C5; decreased chemotactic activity. (b) Defect in properdin pathway?; reduced opsonizing activity; lack of C6; reduced bacteriocidic activity

	Symptoms	Inheritance	
C6	Usually healthy; occasionally Raynaud-like symptoms; increased susceptibility to gram-negative (meningococcal, gonococcal) infections		
C7	Usually healthy; in some cases Raynaud-like symptoms with sclerodactyly and teleangiectasy	Autosomal, recessive	Lack of C7; increased levels of C8 and C9. Reduced chemotactic activity, opsonisation, and bacteriocidic activity
C8	Usually healthy; occasionally increased susceptibility to infections with N. meningococcus and N. gonorrhoea; LE-like symptoms	Autosomal, recessive	Lack of C8; reduced bacteriocidic activity
C9	Healthy	Autosomal, recessive	Lack of C9

[a] All deficiencies show a significant reduction of the total hemolytic activity (CH_{50}) (see p. 113)

by 1980. All these deficiencies are rare, the most common being a C1-inhibitor deficiency, and a lack of C2 expression. All deficiencies are inherited; C4 and C2 deficiencies are associated with HLA genotypes (see p. 147). In many patients, complement deficiencies exist without signs of disease. When symptoms do appear, they usually develop within weeks after birth until early childhood and consist of an increased susceptibility to infections (skin, respiratory tract, joints, kidney), and sometimes they are similar to autoimmune diseases (lupus erythematosus-like but without LE cells, anti-nuclear antibodies, and Ig- and C3-deposits in the skin). In all patients, laboratory tests reveal a significantly reduced total hemolytic activity of the serum (CH_{50}), lack of the respective single complement component, and, depending upon which component is deficient, decreased chemotactic activity of polymorphonuclear cells (C4, C3b-inactivator, C5, C7), reduced opsonization (C3, C5, C7), and reduced phagocytosis (C1r, C3, C3b-inactivator, C6, C7, C8). The deficiencies are summarized in Table 12.7.

References

Agnello V (1978) Complement deficiency states. Medicine 57:1

Chandra RK, Cooper MD, Hitzig WH, Rosen FS, Seligman M, Scoothill JF, Terry RJ (1979) Immunodeficiency: Report of a WHO scientific group. Clin Immunol Immunopathol 13:296

Clinical Oncology (1978) A manual for students and doctors. Edited under the auspices of the International Union Against Cancer (2nd edition). Springer-Verlag, Heidelberg New York

Cooper MD, Seligman M (1977) B and T lymphocytes in immunodeficiency and lymphoproliferative diseases. In: Loor F, Roelants GE (eds) B and T cells in immune recognition. Wiley, p 347

Cooper MD, Lawton AR, Miescher PA, Müller-Eberhard (eds) (1979) Immunodeficiency. Springer, New York

Gallin JI, Quie PG (eds) (1978) Leukocyte chemotaxis. Raven

Güttler F, Seakins JWT, Harkness RA (eds) (1979) In-
born errors of immunity and phagocytosis. MTP
Press, Falcon House, London

Hitzig WH, Weber CH (1980) Die progressive septische
Granulomatose. Adv Int Med Ped 44:37

Kobayashi N (ed) (1978) Immunodeficiency. University Park Press, Baltimore

Mendes NF (1973) Technical aspects of the rosette tests
used to detect human complement receptor (B) and
sheep erythrocyte-binding(T) lymphocytes. J Immunol 111:860

Thierfelder S, Rodt H, Thiel E (eds) (1977) Immunological diagnosis of leukemias and lymphomas.
Springer-Verlag, Heidelberg New York

Chapter 13　Autoimmunity

WILMAR DIAS DA SILVA and DIETRICH GÖTZE

Contents

Autorecognition

Paul Ehrlich introduced the term "horror autotoxicus" to circumscribe the observation that an organism would not react under normal conditions against its own constituents (containment of auto-reactivity, self-tolerance). A mechanism by which self-tolerance might be established was proposed by Burnet and became known as clonal abortion (deletion) theory: during fetal life, lymphocytes for self-determinants are eliminated (forbidden clones). First indications that this theory might not be an explanation for self-tolerance were obtained by Witebsky and Rose in 1956. These authors could demonstrate that rabbits were able to produce antibodies specific for their own thyroglobulin when immunized with thyroglobulin in complete Freund's ad-

juvant. Subsequent studies revealed that normal individuals possessed B lymphocytes able to bind specifically thyroglobulin. Elimination of these B cells by binding of highly labeled thyroglobulin (suicide) prevents the formation of antibodies and the development of an autoimmune thyroiditis. Since then numerous experiments have provided ample evidence that auto-antibodies against a large number of self-antigens are found naturally in the serum of normal, healthy individuals, and that auto-antibodies against virtually all self-constituents can be elicited when appropriately immunized or stimulated; thus, polyclonal B cell mitogens such as lipopolysaccharide can indiscriminately activate potentially auto-reactive cells in vivo, causing the production of measurable concentrations of serum auto-antibodies. This LPS-induced autoimmune state tends to be self-limiting, and the auto-antibodies disappear within a short time after the last LPS administration.

Furthermore, auto-antibodies can be demonstrated in many pathologic events, e.g., infectious diseases, which are usually only transiently present and not harmful to the individual (Table 13.1). Moreover, Cohn and Weckerle could furnish evidence that cell-mediated auto-reactivity is also present under normal conditions: They incubated lymphoid cells for 5 days on syngeneic fibroblast monolayer cultures, after which time specifically sensitized T lymphocytes were able to lyse syngeneic target cells, and to induce a graft versus host-like reaction of splenomegaly or lymph node enlargement after in vivo transfer into syngeneic hosts. Adsorption experiments on syngeneic fibroblasts, followed by transfer onto syngeneic

Table 13.1. Examples of autoantibodies in nonimmunized normal individuals and nonautoimmune diseases

Normal	Disease
Cold agglutinins, e.g. anti-I and anti-i (see p. 229) Pan-agglutinins, react with neuraminidase-treated RBC, lymphocytes, spermatozoa	Antibodies to: Nuclei, kidney, heart, gastric tissue, thyroglobulin, tumor tissue, cardiolipin, complement (immuneconglutinins, anti-C3, C4)
Antibodies to lung tissue, elastin, nuclear components, immunoglobulins (particularly their degradation products), myelin	Skin, tumor tissue (particular colon tumor), liver surface lipoprotein, insulin

or allogeneic sensitizing monolayers, have demonstrated that T cells endowed with specific recognition structures for self-antigens exist in the spleen prior to in vitro sensitization. The induction of autoreactive T lymphocytes could be blocked by the addition of syngeneic, but not allogeneic, serum; this inhibition is caused by soluble antigens.

Thus, auto-reactive B and T lymphocytes constitute a normal fraction of the immunologically reactive cell pool, and auto-antibodies are permanently present under normal conditions, though at low concentrations. Tolerance and (concomitant) immunity are both a continuously acquired property of the immune system, kept in an equilibrium by regulatory interactions of the immune cells, actually based on continuous self-recognition (see Chap. 6, p. 155; and Chap. 9, p. 248). Disturbances of these regulatory interactions result in autoimmunity (or allergy, or anergy). The mechanisms by which tolerance is established and maintained are thought to be (1) clonal inactivation of maturing lymphocytes by the continuous presence of small amounts of auto-antigens (e.g., thyroglobulin, peptide hormones, plasma membrane glycolipids – HLA, H-2 –, and others); (2) antibody-mediated inhibition; and (3) T cell regulation (see also Chap. 9, pp. 245–249).

Clonal inactivation: In 1975, Nossal extending Burnet's deletion theory, proposed that at some stage during their differentiation from stem cells to mature antibody-forming cells, B lymphocytes go through a phase during which contact with antigen induces tolerance only and not immunity. Indeed, it could be demonstrated that primary B cells which start to express surface IgM are highly susceptible to induction of tolerance, and that tolerance is very rapidly induced in these cells. The underlying mechanism(s) for the preferential development of tolerance rather than stimulation to antibody-secreting cells is not known, but it might be related to the observation that immature B cells are unable to regenerate receptors once removed (e.g., by capping, see p. 150). It has been suggested that this form of tolerance induction is only possible as long as there is a deficiency of high avidity cells as in the newborn in comparison to adults. Additional mechanism(s) appear to be required, therefore, to explain self-tolerance.

Since B lymphocytes have a rather short lifespan, and there is a continuous generation of new B cells, functional inactivation has to occur over and over again whenever new lymphocytes mature that possess receptors for self-determinants. It is, therefore, conceivable that even under normal conditions, but particularly under pathologic conditions, some B cells with anti-self specificity reach the mature stage without having been inactivated (they escaped).

The same mechanism(s) may operate for tolerance induction of T lymphocytes (see p. 247, low zone tolerance).

Antibody-mediated inhibition: It has been demonstrated that antibodies can contribute to an unresponsive state by competing with lymphocyte receptors for available antigens. Furthermore, anti-idiotypic antibodies may contain the anti-self-reactivity of lymphocytes (see pp. 104–108). In addition, immune complexes can act as blocking factors (see p. 330, and immunologic enhancement p. 245). The effect of immune complexes might be due to (a) a free combining site of the complexed antibody binding to cell-bound antigen and thus masking it so that it can not be recognized by potential effector cells, and/or (b) free antigenic determinants which may interact with surface receptors and induce lymphocyte inactivation (see above).

T cell regulation: It is now recognized that the activity of effector cells (B/plasma cells, cytotoxic T cells) is regulated by at least two types of T lymphocytes: T helper cells and T suppressor cells (see Chap. 2, p. 51; Chap. 4, pp. 106–108; Chap. 6, p. 162; and Chap. 9, p. 248). Containment of autoreactivity might be achieved by two means: activation of suppressor T cells or inactivation (or nonactivation) of helper T cells. These effects might result from antigen-inactivation of T helper cells as outlined

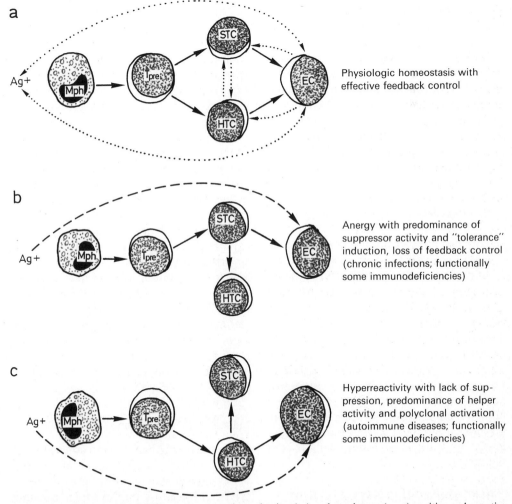

Fig. 13.1 a–c. Homeostasis of the immune system by activating (→) and regulatory (----→) positive and negative feedback interactions of antigen (Ag), macrophages (mph), suppressor T cells (STC), helper T cells (HTC), and effector cells (EC; cytotoxic T cells or B/plasma cells and their products, antibodies). **a** System in equilibrium, physiologic condition; **b** Predominance of suppressor T cell activity with loss of stimulating helper activity resulting in antigen specific or general anergy; **c** Predominance of helper T cell activity with loss of suppressor activity resulting in antigen-specific or general hyperreactivity

above for B cells, or antigen-activation of suppressor T cells, or anti-idiotypic interactions as described in Chap. 4 (pp. 104–108), and thus, does not only include the two mechanisms described above, but also fits more the actual findings. Since B lymphocytes will react against most antigens only if helped by T lymphocytes, the inactivation of T helper cells (by antigen, by suppressor cells) would be a sufficient requirement to establish tolerance in the intact organism.

Both types of unresponsiveness, i.e., due to inactivated T helper cells and to activated suppressor cells, are transferable into "B animals" (depleted of T cells); however, responsiveness can be restored by mature T cells in case of inactivated T helper cells only. Which type of tolerance prevails for a given antigen depends upon the nature and dose of the antigen and the immunologic experience of the organism, as well as the genetic make-up of the individual with respect to the alleles of its MHC (see Chap. 6, pp. 164–167).

Autoimmunity

As outlined above, autoimmunity or better still auto-recognition, appears to be a normal feature of the immune system's reactivity, i.e., is a physiologic event far removed from the immunopathology of autoimmune diseases, and an important device for the maintenance of a state of equilibrium of the immune system (see Chap. 6, pp. 156–163). Talal has suggested, therefore, the distinction of three stages in the response to self: auto-recognition, autoimmunity, and autoimmune diseases, in order to indicate the range of reactivity from normal (regulated) to pathologic (deregulated) conditions.

Auto-recognition of membrane idiotypic receptors and MHC molecules appears to be a fundamental principle facilitating regulatory interactions between cells constituting the immune system in order to adjust their response to signals from within as well as

outside. In addition, the continuous interaction of receptors with soluble self-antigens which are always present in low concentrations, is necessary in order to maintain a state of tolerance.

This state of auto-recognition as described has been interpreted by Grabar not only as a necessary means of immune system regulation, but as the essence of the immune system's physiologic function (theory of immunoglobulins as "transporters"): namely, handling and eliminating metabolic and catabolic substances regardless of their origin, self or nonself.

Autoimmunity is then characterized by enhanced auto-reactions concomitant to nonself reactions due to temporary disturbances (e.g., infections and injuries), in which the immunologic network is fundamentally intact.

Autoimmune diseases are severe derangements of the immunologic network (or a part of it) that are non-reversible from within the systems and lead to pathologic conditions. Autoimmune states might be the result of intrinsic defects of the immune system (e.g., experimental systemic lupus erythematosus (SLE) in NZB mice, see below), or the result of either an induced, inadequate immune response (active chronic hepatitis) or an antigen-specific deficient recognition (e.g., probably most autoimmune diseases associated with certain HLA types, see Chap. 6, Table 6.21, p. 165, and below) of an otherwise normally functioning immune system.

Induction of Autoimmunity

Three major mechanisms are considered to bring about the development of autoimmune disease states: (1) Antigen seclusion, (2) T cell bypass, and (3) disordered immunologic regulation.

Antigen seclusion: Antigens confined inside cells, or located at anatomical sites not in contact with the circulation are thought not to participate in the induction of tolerance of lymphocytes. Whenever those self-components come into contact with lymphocytes, for example after tissue damage due to infections or injuries, a normal immune response will follow. Such a mechanism may underly the reactivity toward the basic protein of myelin, organ-specific microsomal antigens of the thyroid gland, the testicles, and gastric parietal cells, nuclear antigens, and the crystalline lens.

T cell bypass: As was pointed out above, tolerance appears to be maintained by the inactivation (nonactivation) of T helper cells (and/or activation of suppressor T cells) due to the continuous presence of small amounts of antigen; this resembles low zone tolerance (see p. 247–249), which affects primarily T lymphocytes but not B lymphocytes. However, since B lymphocytes need the help of T cells for activation to differentiate into antibody-secreting cells, the overall effect on the organism is tolerance. Any mechanism, therefore, which can circumvent the T cell participation-requirement (mitogens, adjuvants), or cause T helper cell activation (providing helper determinants = carrier) may lead to the activation of (non-tolerant)

B cells. Such mechanisms are: Drugs that bind to body constituents, partially degraded autoantigens, bacterial, viral, and parasitic infections, and graft-versus-host reaction (Table 13.2).

Many drugs are known today to cause autoimmune thrombocytopenia, Coombs'-positive hemolytic anemia, leukopenia, and/or immune complex syndromes. The underlying mechanisms are thought to be due to binding of the drug to proteins and/or cell surfaces (platelets, erythrocytes, leukocytes, tissue cells) so that T helper cells are activated which, in turn, activate B cells specific for the drug, but sometimes also drug-associated (self) components. Antigen-(drug)-antibody complexes activate complement which results in inflammatory reactions and cell-lysis.

Partially degraded self-components may expose antigenic determinants to which the immune system is not tolerant, and thus may elicit a regular immune response.

Many microorganisms possess or release substances such as lipopolysaccharide, tuberculin, *B. pertussis* components, *T. brucei* components, that act as polyclonal B cell (and T cell) mitogen, and are experimentally used as adjuvants. That such substances in-

Table 13.2. Mechanisms to bypass T cells in B lymphocyte activation

Mechanism	Mode of action
Drugs	provide helper determinant(=carrier) to T cells, e.g. α-methyldopa (anti-e of Rh), procainamide and hydralazine (anti-nuclear), hydantoin (anti-MHC), nitrofurantoin
Partially degraded autoantigens	Presentation of antigenic determinants to which no tolerance exists, e.g. thyreoglobulin, collagen, immunoglobulins
Bacterial infections	Polyclonal B (and T) cell activation, adjuvant effect (e.g., lipopolysaccharide, PPD, *B. pertussis*); presentation of determinants cross-reacting with self (e.g., polysaccharide antigens of E. coli 0:14 with colon antigen, basement membrane antigens (?), and group A hemolytic streptococcus antigen with cardiac muscle)
Viral infections	Viral antigens form complexes with self-antigens (MHC); polyclonal B cell stimulation (e.g. EB-virus) among them autoantibodies
Graft-versus-Host reaction	Donor T helper cells stimulated by host antigens induce proliferation of host B cells (allogenic effect)
Multiple specificities of antibodies	According to Richards et al. an antibody combining site may be able to react with several structurally completely unrelated determinants; by accident, an antibody specifically produced against an infectious agent may turn out to also react with a self-antigen (RF?)

deed induce autoimmune diseases is amply demonstrated by the fact that Freund's adjuvant (see p. 66) is widely used to induce experimental autoimmune diseases; furthermore, it has been shown that after stimulation of B cells with mitogens, large numbers of cells are found forming antibodies against autologous red cells. Well known are antibodies to cardiolipin (Wassermann) and cold auto-antibodies to erythrocytes in syphilis, auto-antibodies to the lung in tuberculosis, antibodies against thyroglobulin, immunoglobulins (rheumatoid factor, RF), cardiolipin, and nuclear components in lepromatous leprosy, cold agglutinins in *Mycoplasma* pneumonia infections, and auto-antibodies in parasitic infections.

Another effect of microorganisms is that they provide helper determinants. Thus, in rheumatic fever, streptococcal determinants cross-react with cardiac tissue antigens. Type 12 streptococcus infections are usually accompanied by glomerulonephritis, probably because they possess antigens resembling those encountered in renal glomeruli, and the antibodies produced against these antigens react with glomerular basement membrane.

In other instances, bacterial glycolipids may become inserted into host cell membranes and in this way activate T helper cells for auto-antigen specific B cells. Similarly, many viruses express viral antigens in the membrane of the infected host cell, and these antigens are recognized by immune cells; interaction of virus-infected host cells with immune cells causes destruction of the former, liberating intracellular components which might be immunogenic (e.g., active chronic hepatitis).

Lymphocytes infected by viruses might be induced to proliferate and differentiate to a certain functional stage; since this would be, in general, a polyclonal activation, severe disturbances of the immune regulation might be expected (e.g. systemic lupus erythematosus; usually not severe: infectious mononucleosis).

The production of antibodies of recipient origin (demonstrated by allotype markers)

against erythrocytes, basement membranes, and cytotoxic antibodies could be demonstrated during graft-versus-host reactions.

The concept of T cell bypass as an important mechanism for the initiation of an autoimmune disease implies that most autoimmune diseases are, indeed, caused by antibody activities. As a matter of fact, this has been demonstrated to be true in many instances.

T cell dysregulation: The immune response is controlled by the activity of T lymphocytes. Defects in these controlling elements are, therefore, expected to cause aberrant immune reactions (Table 13.3). An increase in the activity of suppressor T cells may lead to the complete absence of any detectable *specific* immune response (anergy); the concurrent presence of a polyclonal B cell mitogen leads to an elevation of (unspecific) antibodies, including auto-antibodies. Deficiency in suppressor T cell activity may cause the opposite effect: a general "unleashing" of B lymphocytes due to the overwhelming ac-

Table 13.3. T cell dysregulations

Decreased T suppressor cell activity:[a]
Experimental allergic encephalomyelitis (?)
Multiple sclerosis (?)
Systemic lupus erythematosus
Rheumatoid arthritis (?)
Sjögren's syndrome
Experimental autoimmune thyroiditis
Autoimmune active chronic hepatitis
Pemphigus vulgaris
Progressive systemic sclerosis (scleroderma)
Increased T suppressor cell activity:
Lepromatous leprosy
Fulminant tuberculosis
Candidiasis (some)
Histoplasmosis
Measles
Myxo- und Paramyxo-viruses
Infectious mononucleosis
Mucocutaneous leishmaniasis
Acquired hypogammaglobulinemia (some)
Selective IgA deficiency (some)
Hodgkin's disease
Acute lymphatic leukemia

[a] An increase in T helper cell activity equals a deficiency in T suppressor cells

tivity of T helper cells, (e.g., experimental SLE, see below). Other mechanisms may involve (a) unresponsiveness of effector cells to controlling signals of regulator cells, or (b) inefficiency of effector functions with uncoupling of feedback control mechanisms. Disturbances of these latter kinds are observed in many lymphoproliferative disorders, and some infections (e.g., chronic lymphatic leukemia, lymphosarcoma, infectious mononucleosis).

Factors Influencing Autoimmunity

Factors influencing the development of autoimmune diseases are of environmental (drugs, food, dust; infections) and organism-inherent (genetic, immunodeficiency, hormonal, thymic, and age) origin.

Many drugs induce autoimmune reactions which are often asymptomatic, and/or disappear after discontinuation of exposure. Food, dust, and other agents may cause autoimmune symptoms, usually of the immediate hypersensitivity (see pp. 257–281) type I rather than of other types.

Many infections by viruses, bacteria, fungi, and parasites cause temporary autoimmune symptoms, particularly rheumatoid factor and anti-nuclear antibodies (Table 13.4). Some acute virus infections (e.g. infectious mononucleosis) and parasite infections (e.g., African trypanosomiasis) are characterized by polyclonal B cell activation. In general, these symptoms are reversible after eradication of the infectious agent. However, tissue damage caused as a result of excessive immune reactions is not always reversible. The resulting immunopathology in such cases is so similar to many "spontaneous" autoimmune diseases that an infectious cause is strongly suggested for them (Table 13.5). The infectious agents in such cases not only elude our detection so far, but they also de y elimination by the affected organism (persistent infections, slow-virus infections). In other words, many of the so-called autoimmune diseases will probably turn out to be infectious diseases, with which the infected organism cannot cope with appropriately because of some selective immunodeficiencies (see below).

Table 13.4. Examples of autoimmune symptoms associated with infections

Rheumatoid factor	Arthritis	Anti-nuclear antibodies	Coombs' positive hemolytic anemia	Immune complex nephritis	Polyclonal gammopathy
Subacute bacterial endocarditis	Gonorrhea	Leprosy	Syphilis	Streptococcus	Syphilis
Syphilis	Tuberculosis	Tuberculosis	Mycoplasma pneumoniae	S. typhi	Rubella
Lepromatous leprosy	Serum hepatitis	Cytomegalovirus	Hepatitis	Serum hepatitis	Leishmaniasis
Tuberculosis	Yersinia infection	Infectious mononucleosis	Influenza	Infectious mononucleosis	Trypanosomiasis (T. brucei, T. cruzi)
Hepatitis B			Cytomegalovirus	Coxsackie virus	
Influenza A			Infectious mononucleosis	Varicella	
Cytomegalovirus				Measles	
Rubella				Malaria	
Herpes zoster				Toxoplasmosis (congenital)	
Infectious mononucleosis				Schistosomiasis	
Malaria				Filariasis	
Kala-Azar					
Schistosomiasis					

Table 13.5. Infectious agents suspected as inducers of autoimmune diseases

Autoimmune disease	Suspected infectious agent
Rheumatoid arthritis	EB-virus related agent
Insulin-dependent diabetes mellitus	Coxsackie B virus
Multiple sclerosis	Defective measles virus
Sclerosing panencephalitis	
Systemic lupus erythematosus (in NZB mice, in dogs)	C-type RNA virus
Equine infectious anemia	
Sjögren's syndrome	A-type virus (?)
Rheumatic fever	Group A streptococcus
Ankylosing spondylitis	Chronic infections of the bowl and genitourinary tract
Reiter's disease	Shigellae
Ulcerative colitis	Rheovirus-like agent
Crohn's disease	
IgG(warm) antibody-mediated hemolytic anemia	Mycoplasma pneumoniae
Guillain-Barré-Strohl syndrome	Viruses, e.g., influenza, cytomegalo, varicella-zoster, measles, mumps, rubella, vaccinia

Genetic factors play an important role as demonstrated by the fact that almost all autoimmune diseases show a preferential association to certain HLA alleles (see Table 6, p.165). The underlying mechanisms of these associations are discussed at the end of Chap.6 (pp.166–167). In view of the suspicion that many of the autoimmune diseases may have been initiated by infections, the immune response theory of these associations is most likely correct, i.e., a certain allele predisposes to low responsiveness which leads to a persistent infection followed by aberrant or inadequate immune responses which are not effective in eliminating the causative agent but, to the contrary, now cause the pathology; the process of inadequate immune reactions may eventually become dissociated from the infections and perpetuate themselves.

Many immunodeficiencies are genetically determined and are associated with autoimmune reactions (Table 13.6). It should be kept in mind that an existing immunodeficiency leads to the net effect that an infectious agent cannot be eliminated, thus resembling the picture of a persistent or "slow-microbe" infection, which of course will result eventually in immunopathologic lesions identical to those of "autoimmune diseases" (e.g. CGD, p.360).

Hormonal factors, particularly sex hormones, have a critical influence on the expression, severity, and time course of many autoimmune diseases. Thus, systemic lupus erythematosus, Hashimoto's thyroiditis, Graves' disease, Addison's disease, and scleroderma show a high prevalence for females, and usually during pregnancies, the disease exacerbates. Systemic lupus erythematosus in female NZB mice appears much earlier and more severely than in males; prepubertal castration of males causes the "female-type" disease, and prepubertal castration of females with subsequent administration of androgens reverts the disease to the "male-type."

For all these influences to occur a functioning thymus is needed. Severe autoimmune diseases are not seen in nude (athymic) mice. For many autoimmune diseases, there is an age-related peak incidence; however, autoimmune diseases in general are not clearly related to older age groups.

Table 13.6. Immunodeficiencies associated with autoimmune symptoms

Immunodeficiency	Autoimmune symptoms
Hypogammaglobulinemia:	
Congenital	Rheumatoid arthritis, dermatomyositis, scleroderma, Felty's syndrome, hemolytic anemia
Acquired	Hemolytic anemia, pernicious anemia
Selective IgA deficiency	Systemic lupus erythematosus, rheumatoid arthritis, dermatomyositis, pernicious anemia, thyreoditis, celiac disease (autoantibodies to double stranded DNA, to basement membrane), Addison's disease, thrombocytopenic purpura, regional enteritis
Dysgammaglobulinemias (selective IgG, selective IgM deficiency)	Hemolytic anemia, systemic lupus erythematosus, thrombocytic purpura
Chronic mucocutaneous candidiasis	Endocrinopathies (Addison's disease), pernicious anemia
Wiskott-Aldrich syndrome	Hemolytic anemia (Coombs' positive)
Ataxia telangiectasia	Autoantibodies against thyroglobulin, immunoglobulins, parietal cells, smooth muscle, nuclear material, basement membrane
Chronic granulomatous disease (female carriers)	Discoid and systemic lupus erythematosus with autoantibodies to DNA
Complement deficiencies (C1r, C1s, C2, C4, C5, C1-inhibititor)	Systemic lupus erythematosus

Autoimmune Diseases

Tissue Lesions in Autoimmune Diseases

Tissue lesions in autoimmune diseases can be produced by humoral, by cellular, or by a combined mechanism. In the former instance, antibody-antigen complexes are deposited in the tissue, particularly if the antibody is of the IgG type, complement is activated, and these effects result in inflammatory reactions, particularly of blood vessels (vasculitis, see Chap. 10, type III hypersensitivity), and lysis of cells in cases where the antigen is cell-bound (Type II hypersensitivity). Cell-mediated lesions are caused by the direct action of cytotoxic T cells as well as by antibody-dependent, cell-mediated cytotoxicity of killer cells and macrophages (see pp. 287–294; Chap. 10, type IV hypersensitivity) (Fig. 13.2).

Some Autoimmune Diseases

The presence of auto-antibodies or even their distribution in the tissues does not necessarily imply that the cause of the lesions and of the clinical symptoms of the disease is necessarily the autoimmune process itself.

For a given disease to be considered autoimmune, the following criteria must be fulfilled: (1) For at least some stages of the evolutionary process of the disease in question, the existence of an immune response must be demonstrated, as indicated by the presence of autoantibodies or of sensitized cells, with specificity for auto-antigens localized in the injured tissue. (2) The sensitizing agent should be identified or characterized. (3) The disease should be reproducible by the injection of purified or partially purified auto-antigens into laboratory animals. (4) The pathologic events in experimental animals should correspond to those in man. (5) It should be possible to transfer the disease produced in laboratory animals to syngeneic animals by serum or lymphocytes.

There are several possible ways of classifying autoimmune diseases; since we do not understand the underlying mechanism for all these diseases (which would probably lead to a more logical classification), the classification as organ-specific or systemic appears to have some etiologic significance. The organ-specific autoimmune diseases are possibly related to the liberation of endogenous tissue constituents or modified auto-antigens. On the other hand, the systemic

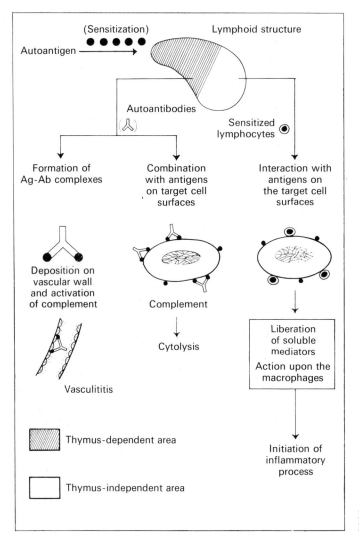

Fig. 13.2. Mechanism of tissue lesions in autoimmune processes

autoimmune diseases are probably due to alterations in the recognition mechanism of the central immune system (Table 13.7).

Autoimmune Diseases of the Central Nervous System

The diseases that affect the central nervous system and in which the autoimmune phenomena probably play an important part are: (1) experimental allergic encephalomyelitis (EAE), (2) multiple sclerosis, (3) acute disseminated encephalomyelitis, (4) acute postinfectious encephalomyelitis, and (5) postrabies vaccinal encephalomyelitis.

Experimental allergic encephalomyelitis (EAE) was first described by Rivers and his colleagues in 1933. The disease was elicited by repeated injections of brain extracts into monkeys; after 6–12 months, a demyelinating disease caused the death of some of the animals. Later, it could be demonstrated that brain extracts in complete Freund's adjuvant produced the disease with much greater regularity and in a far shorter period of time (10–30 days after the injection). The disease can also be produced in other species such as guinea-pigs, rabbits, mice, rats, and birds. In rats, the disease has been evaluated exhaustively using inbred strains: some

Table 13.7. Classification of the autoimmune diseases

Autoimmune diseases	Characteristics
Organ-specific	a) The antibodies usually are specific for one or more antigens of a particular organ b) The antigens are usually "segregated," c) The lesions can be reproduced experimentelly by injecting the antigen in complete Freund's adjuvant Examples: encephalomyelitis, thyroiditis, orchitis, epididymitis, glomerulonephritis, and autoimmune nephroses
Systemic	a) Antibodies exist for antigens of various tissues or organs; antigens react with antibodies obtained from either the same or different species b) The antigens are not "segregated"; under normal conditions the immune system is tolerant to them c) The diseases appear spontaneously in animals of the appropriate genotype (e.g., in NZB mice) Examples: lupus erythematosus, rheumatoid arthritis, some forms of acquired hemolytic anemia
Combination of both forms: organ-specific and systemic	a) Diseases that generally involve antibodies for various tissues, even though the inflammatory lesions are restricted to a small number of organs Examples: Sjögren's syndrome, ulcerative colitis, lupoid hepatitis, primary biliary cirrhosis, and some forms of acquired hemolytic anemia

strains are more susceptible to the development of the disease than others, and this susceptibility is genetically associated with certain alleles of the major histocompatibility complex. Similar results have been obtained in mice, in which susceptibility was found to be associated with the H-2^s haplotype, more precisely with the I-A^s allele.

The clinical symptoms vary from species to species but usually include paraparesis with urinary incontinence progressing to tetraplegia or death; weight loss is common.

The antigen responsible for the pathologic reactions in EAE has been identified as myelin basic protein, which is found in the myelin sheath in the white matter (it is not found in the newborns; EAE is, therefore, not induced in very young animals). Myelin basic protein has been completely characterized as a heat-stable, acid-resistant protein with a molecular weight of about 18,000 dalton with 170 residues. Residues 116–122 contain the only tryptophan in the molecule, and this part of the molecule represents the major encephalitogenic region for the guinea-pig.

66 67 68 69 70 71 72 73 74 75
Thr–Thr–His–**Tyr–Gly**–Ser–Leu–Pro–**Gln–Lys**

113 114 115 116 117 118 119 120 121 122
Arg–Phe–Ser–**Trp–Gly**–Ala–Glu–Gly–**Gln–Lys**

Residues 66–75 appear to be the major encephalitogenic determinant for the rabbit and the rat (the similarity of the important positions are indicated).

Histopathologically, there are two fundamental alterations: inflammatory infiltrations and demyelination. Other alterations such as vasculitis, necrosis of the nervous tissue, and hemorrhage are less frequent and appear only in the most severe cases. At first, the lesions are characterized by perivenular infiltrations of macrophages and lymphocytes, with small lymphocytes predominant. The infiltrations appear first in the white matter, from which they can spread to the meninges and choroid plexus. Within 48–72 h, macrophages become predominant; myelin destruction is accomplished by macrophages. The histopathologic aspect of EAE closely resembles that encountered in postrabies vaccinal and acute postinfectious encephaloyelitis (Fig. 13.3).

Electron microscopic studies of the lesions have revealed interesting pecularities with respect to the disposition of the cells of the inflammatory infiltrates. For example, it has been observed that in the areas where demyelination has occurred, the macrophages generally envelop the axis cylinders (Fig. 13.4) with their pseudopodia, which suggests that these cells are directly impli-

Fig. 13.3. Autoimmune encephalomyelitis. Perivenular inflammatory infiltrate of mononuclear cells. Bovine brain vaccinated with antirabies vaccine. (Courtesy of Prof. José M. Lamas da Silva, Departemento de Patologia, Escola de Veterinária, Universidade Federal de Minas Gerais)

Fig. 13.4. Ultrastructure of autoimmune encephalitis. The cytoplasm of a mononuclear cell is enveloping the axons A, A_1, and A_2, which are demyelinated. Rubis JJ, Luse SA (1964) Am J Path 44:299

cated in myelinolysis. These are focal areas that correspond in general to the zones of inflammatory infiltrations. In addition to the destructive processes, areas of remyelination also exist, which could explain the remission of paralysis in some patients.

EAE is a T cell-dependent and cell-mediated disease, and antibodies are not of major importance for its development. Thus, the disease will not develop in thymectomized animals, but can be induced in bursectomized chicken. Furthermore, the disease can be passively transmitted with cells, but not with serum. Delayed-type hypersensitivity to basic protein can always be demonstrated by skin testing, and peripheral blood lymphocytes from EAE animals show a prolifer-

ative response to basic protein in vitro. Cells from EAE animals can destroy cultured myelinated nerve cells.

Animals can be protected from EAE by administration of basic protein in incomplete Freund's adjuvant, most probably because of the induction of suppressor T cell activity.

Multiple sclerosis (MS) is a demyelinating disease of the CNS in man; epidemiologic studies indicate that it occurs more commonly in regions with temperate or harsh climates and is rare in regions with warm climates. An environmental factor is, therefore, assumed to be important in the development of this disease. Immunogenetically, the HLA-D2/DR2 type is overrepresented in MS patients.

Histopathologically the disease shows a picture similar to EAE, and is characterized by plaques which consist of discrete regions in the white matter within which myelin and oligodendrocytes (the cells synthesizing myelin) are lost. During the acute inflammatory stage, large numbers of lymphocytes and macrophages are seen around the venules within plaques.

The etiology of the disease is still unknown, but it is suspected to be caused by immune reactions to cells infected with defective measles virus; alternatively, it might be an autoallergy. The target antigen does not appear to be the basic protein of myelin.

In the majority of MS patients, T cells in the peripheral blood are significantly reduced – however, this might be due to recruitment of T cells into the CNS. Con-A activated nonspecific T cell suppressor function is depressed in MS patients; it also has been shown that T cells (suppressor T cells) are markedly reduced in their number during active stages of the disease.

Acute disseminated encephalomyelitis appears as a sequel to infections such as measles, smallpox, chicken pox, and mumps, and is relatively similar to EAE. The lesions are found more frequently in the optic nerve, brain stem (in particular in bridges with ocular muscle nuclei), in the cerebellum and cerebellar peduncle, the pyramidal tracts, the base of the fourth ventricle, and in the posterior column of the spinal cord. It appears that the virus or viral components responsible for these lesions modify the structure of certain components of the neural tissue, possibly by the action of neuraminidase, or by the incorporation of liberated antigenic constituents of the host from the blood.

Another form of acute disseminated encephalomyelitis can occur after treatment with antirabies vaccine prepared with attenuated virus (see Fig. 13.3). In this case, the autoimmune response is unleashed by the presence of neural tissue components in the vaccine, the entire process presumably being almost analogous to that of experimental allergic encephalomyelitis.

Myasthenia gravis is characterized by weakness due to a defect in neuromuscular transmission. The disease is more frequent in women than in man; familial cases are know; the HLA-B8 type is overrepresented in patients with myasthenia gravis. The weakness symptom is abrogated by anti-cholinergic drugs, are which a sign frequently employed as a diagnostic test. The underlying defect appears to be a depletion of acetylcholine-receptors, or a block of the receptors, in the subsynaptic region of myoneural junctions. In more than 90% of patients, antibodies to acetylcholine receptors can be demonstrated. This antibody is responsible for the disease since myasthenia gravis symptoms can be induced to occur in mice to which the antibody has been transferred.

In 60%–70% of patients, there are alterations of the thymus that vary from simple hyperlastic to thymoma (about 10%), occasionally malignant. In the hyperplasia form, numerous lymphoid follicles differentiate in the medullary zone with germinal centers rich in plasma cells. The cortex, although there are no fundamental changes, shrinks little by little to a fine layer. The medulla is proportionally enriched in lymphoid follicles with many B lymphocytes. This (and the findings of an increased incidence among myasthenia gravis patients of diseases with known or presumed autoimmune character such as thyroiditis, pernicious anemia, pemphigus, rheumatoid arthritis, systemic lupus erythematosus, insulin-dependent diabetes mellitus, and adrenalitis) have suggested an autoimmune pathogenesis of the disease.

Many myasthenics have antibodies against nuclear material, parietal cells, thyroid, and gammaglobulin (RF) in their sera. Moreover, with immunofluorescence methods, auto-antibodies can be detected which react specifically with the A and/or I band of myofibrils of normal individuals. These auto-antibodies react also with epithelial cells of the thymus, probably because of the presence of constituents common to the two types of cells; these antibodies can also be absorbed by thymus epithelial cells. These antibodies are not related to the disease, and are found in those patients in whom thymus alterations are observed.

Cellular immunity appears to be slightly abnormal, and in many patients, thymectomy apparently improves the prognosis. Although the etiology is not known, it is speculated that a viral infection (oncogenic virus?) of the thymus might be the cause.

Autoimmune Diseases of Endocrine Glands

The endocrine system is characterized by two important features: its activity is mediated by hormones via receptors, and the activity is regulates via feedback control. Therefore, immune reactions may play an important role at different levels: affecting the endocrine gland (e.g. Hashimoto's thyroiditis, Addison's disease, and insulin-dependent diabetes mellitus), intercepting circulating hormones (e.g., hypothyroidism, diabetes due to antibodies against insulin), and/or interfering with the receptor of the (hormone) target cell and thus disturbing the regulation (e.g., Graves' disease and insulin-resistant diabetes mellitus).

Experimental autoimmune thyroiditis. Witebsky and Rose demonstrated first that injection of thyroid lobe extracts in Freund's adjuvant into rabbits produced thyroiditis; since then, this model and other animal models (guinea-pig, dog, rat, mouse, chicken, and monkey) have been used to study this disease. Thyroiditis induced with thyroid extract in Freund's adjuvant is characterized by lymphocytic infiltrations of the thyroid gland and circulating antibodies to thyroglobulin. Although this disease is in some aspects similar to Hashimoto's thyroiditis in man (see below), it differs in that no germinal centers are found in the thyroid gland, and in that the antibodies produced are almost only anti-thyroglobulins. More similar to Hashimoto's thyroiditis are the thyroid disorders which occur spontaneously in the obese chicken strain and in buf-

falo (BUF) rats. It appears from studies in these animals that the production of antibodies is necessary for the development of the disease, but that T cells play an important part in controlling this development: thymectomy increases the incidence of the disease, whereas bursectomy inhibits the production of antibodies and decreases the incidence of the disorder. From these and other studies, it is assumed that a decrease in functionally active suppressor T cells (the same effect would be achieved by hyperreactive helper T cells!) may be the cause of the occurrence of the disease.

Hashimoto's thyroiditis or chronic lymphocytic thyroiditis represents a form of goiter occuring more frequently in women than in men, and is always associated with hypothyroidism.

Histopathologically, the first observed alterations appear as centers of perivascular inflammatory infiltrations, rich in lymphocytes and macrophages, and irregularly distributed but predominating in the capsule. As the process advances, the infiltrates spread out in the parenchyma between the thyroid vesicles. As revealed by electronmicroscopy, the mononuclear cells can penetrate the cells of the epithelium; in these areas, one encounters ruptures of the follicles and spreading of the colloid into the interstitial tissue (Fig. 13.5).

A variety of antibodies to different components of thyroid tissue has been found in the circulation of patients (Table 13.8). The role of these antibodies in relation to the disease is uncertain; the disease is not transferable to monkeys by serum of Hashimoto patients, and there is no correlation between the levels of circulating auto-antibodies and the intensity of lesions. On the other hand, cutaneous delayed-type hypersensitivity turns positive at the same time that lesions appear, whether or not circulating antibodies are detectable in the serum. From the histologic point of view the degenerative alterations occur only in thyroid follicles that are in contact with mononuclear cell infiltrates, the intensity of the alterations being

Fig. 13.5 a–c. Hashimoto's Thyroiditis. **a** Intense infiltration of lymphocytes in the glandular parenchyma with formation of lymphoid follicles exhibiting germinal centers. **b** Detail showing lymphocytic infiltration among the glandular follicles, with destruction of the same. **c** Lymphoid follicle in the interior of the glandular parenchyma, with distinct germinal center. (Courtesy of Prof. Fausto E. Lima Pereira, Departemente de Anatomia Patologica, Faculdade de Medicina, Universidade Federal de Espirito Santo)

proportional to the quantity of the infiltrate. More importantly, autoimmune thyroiditis can be transferred to normal guinea-pigs using suspensions of lymphoid cells of diseased animals. Furthermore, lymphocytes from patients show a proliferative response to thyroid antigens in vitro, and their lymphocytes are cytotoxic to thyroid cells in culture. Moreover, antibody-dependent cell-mediated cytotoxicity might be involved in the pathologic process: thus, cytotoxicity has been demonstrated using patients' lymphocytes and normal serum (i.e., activated "armed" K cells).

Table 13.8. Antibodies found in Hashimoto's thyroiditis

Antigen	Nature	Antibody	Detection[a]
Thyroglobulin (TG)	Glycoprotein, m.w. of 660,000, organ-specific	IgG, complement fixing	AG, CF, RIA
Microsomes	Membrane lipoprotein, organ-specific	IgG, complement fixing	CF, FAT, RIA
Antigen$_2$. colloid	Colloid protein, organ-specific	IgG, noncomplement fixing	FAT
Surface membrane	Organ-specific	IgM, IgG	FAT
TSH receptor	Glycoprotein, 200,00 mol. w.	IgG	RIA

[a] AG, agglutination of TG-coated latex particle; CF, complement fixation; FAT, fluorescence antibody technique; RIA, radioimmune assay

Graves' disease is a disorder characterized by hyperthyroidism, infiltrative ophthalmopathy, and pretibial myxedema. The thyroid hyperfunction is the result of stimulation of the thyroid gland by an auto-antibody with specificity for the TSH (thyroid stimulating hormone) receptor (long-acting thyroid stimulator, LATS). As a result, nearly all patients have elevated serum T_3 and T_4 concentrations, and show an increased thyroidal uptake of radioiodine.

An association of the disease occurrence with the HLA-D 3 type (and HLA-B 8 which is linkage disequilibrium with HLA-D 3) has been found.

Some circumstantial evidence suggests that Graves' disease is an autoimmune disorder: there is an incidence of thymic hyperplasia, lymphadenopathy, splenomegaly, peripheral lymphocytosis, and diffuse lymphocytic infiltrates in the thyroid gland. However, nothing is known about the etiology and pathogenesis.

Addison's disease is, in the majority of patients, caused by adrenal tuberculosis; the remaining cases result from amyloid degeneration, from Waterhouse-Friderichsen syndrome or its sequelae, or from prolonged administration of corticosteroids. In rare cases, Addison's disease is idiopathic; this form is more common in females than in males, and appears to be associated with an increased incidence of HLA-B 8.

The underlying pathogenic mechanism appears to be an autoimmune reaction to adrenal tissue. This is suggested by (a) its association with other autoimmune diseases (e.g., Hashimoto's thyroiditis); (b) its histology, characterized by atrophy and diffuse lymphocytic infiltration, particularly in the cortex, the structure of which is completely disrupted whereas the medulla is often preserved; (c) the presence of anti-adrenal antibodies, the antigen to which they are produced being unknown; (d) evidence for the presence of cell-mediated immunity, since patients show delayed-type hypersensitivity skin reactions to adrenal extracts; and (e) the production of experimental autoimmune adrenalitis after injection of adrenal gland extracts in Freund's adjuvant into rabbits or guinea-pigs. In these animals, the disease cannot be transferred by serum, but by cells.

Autoimmune pancreatitis: Diabetes mellitus is a symptom (sweet urine) and comprises a variety of different etiologic and pathogenic disease entities. Of the different forms of diabetes mellitus, a classification into insulin-dependent and insulin-independent has been suggested in recent years, providing a better understanding of the pathophysiology and genetics of diabetes than a classification based on the age of onset. Of these two groups, the insulin-dependent forms are those in which autoimmune phenomena play an important role.

Insulin-dependent diabetes mellitus is characterized by an early (usually less than 30 years of age) and rapid onset, a male predominance, severely reduced islet mass with inflammatory reactions in the islets, an association with HLA-D 3/D 4 types and other endocrinopathies (e.g. autoimmune adrenal or autoimmune thyroid diseases), and immunologic symptoms (cell-mediated immunity and auto-antibodies to endocrine pancreas, but also a high prevalence of auto-antibodies to nonpancreatic antigens).

Histologically, the islets are infiltrated by lymphocytes and large mononuclear cells (insulitis) with a reduction in the number of islets and gross atrophy of those which remain.

Insulitis can be induced in experimental animals by injection of endocrine pancreas homogenates; it is also seen in animals infected with encephalomyocarditis virus, suggesting a possible etiology of insulin-dependent diabetes in man (see Table 13.5).

Two types of auto-antibodies are found in the serum of patients: early after onset of the disease, an auto-antibody with specificity for cytoplasmic or microsomal membrane fractions can be detected with the fluorescence antibody technique; this antibody is usually of IgG type and fixes complement; it is organ-specific, but not species-specific. A second antibody is found reacting specifically with the surface membrane of islet cells, usually of the IgM or IgG type. It is not clear, whether or not these antibodies are important for the generation of the disease. The fact that a diabetic syndrome can be provoked in nude mice after transfer of lymphocytes from insulin-dependent diabetes mellitus patients strongly suggests that the disease is mediated by cellular immune mechanisms. It can be shown that lymphocytes of patients possess a specific cytotoxic activity to cultured insuloma cells; this cytotoxicity could be enhanced by addition of serum from diabetes mellitus patients, perhaps indicating that T cell-mediated as well as antibody-dependent cell-mediated reactions are important.

Acanthosis nigricans is a rare disease of the skin with a wart-like hyperplasia of the stratum spinosum of the epithelium with pigment deposits. In some of these patients, a severe impairment of insulin binding to lymphocyte receptors has been diagnosed. This impairment is caused by anti-receptor antibodies competing with insulin. In those patients, an increase in serum gammaglobulin, leukopenia, the presence of anti-nuclear antibodies and arthralgia has been observed.

Hematologic Autoimmune Diseases

Autoimmune hemolytic anemia: The hemolytic anemias comprise a group of diseases in which the life of the red blood cells is abnormally short, even though all the conditions for erythropoiesis are normal.

In the congenital forms (congenital hemolytic anemia), cellular fragility is due to defects in the erythrocytes themselves and is genetically controlled. In the acquired forms, however, the defect appears to have no familial distribution, nor does it relate to the structure of the erythrocyte. These differences can be demonstrated through cross-transfusion, by studying the survival of erythrocytes transferred to normal persons or

to persons with acquired hemolytic anemia. Red blood cells of patients with congenital hemolytic anemia are short-lived even when transferred to normal individuals. On the other hand, the red blood cells obtained from patients with acquired hemolytic anemia reveal normal longevity when transferred to normal individuals. For these reasons, the congenital forms are called "intraerythrocytic" or "intracorpuscular", and the acquired forms "extraerythrocytic" or "extracorpuscular".

In 50%–60% of all cases, the acquired hemolytic anemias are not associated with any particular disease, and are termed idiopathic. In the remaining cases, they appear to be associated with other processes such as neoplasias of the lymphoreticular tissue, diseases of the "collagen", and with viral or chronic inflammatory diseases; they are then referred to as "symptomatic".

It was long suspected that the acquired hemolytic anemias were autoimmune in origin, especially after the demonstration by Donath and Landsteiner of the presence of autohemolysins in the sera of patients with paroxysmal nocturnal hemoglobulinemia. With the development of the antiglobulin test by Coombs, it could be shown that in the majority of acquired hemolytic anemias, the destruction of the red blood cells was always associated with the presence of autoantibodies on their surfaces.

Antierythrocytic auto-antibodies were classified in two groups: those that were active at body temperature (36°–37 °C), called "warm antibodies," and those that reacted optimally only at low temperatures (4°–10 °C), called "cold antibodies."

Antigens: In more than one-third of autoimmune anemia cases, the antigens correspond to the Rh system, and within this group the "e" antigen appears with the greatest frequency (98% of Rh positive individuals). In addition to these Rh system antigens that stimulate the formation of warm antibodies, other antigens have been described that stimulate the appearance of cold antibodies. The latter are designated by the letter "I."

The erythrocytes that react with the cold antibodies are designated "I-positive" whereas the nonreacting red blood cells are designated "I-negative" or simply "i." The I antigens are genetically controlled and are absent in neonates, whose erythrocytes react only with anti-i antisera; they appear only between 18 months and 2 years of age, at which time the I-positive or i character becomes definitely established.

Antibodies: In addition to the warm and cold antibodies mentioned previously, a third type of autohemolysin is encountered in paroxysmal nocturnal hemoglobinuria, known as the "Donath-Landsteiner antibody," or D–L antibody.

Warm auto-antibodies are immunoglobulins with 7S sedimentation coefficients; the majority are incomplete and do not activate complement. Their presence on the erythrocyte membrane can be disclosed either by the Coombs test (most commonly, see Fig. 13.6a) or by the direct agglutination test using erythrocytes treated with trypsin.

The cold auto-antibodies belong to the IgM immunoglobulin class (sedimentation coefficient, 19S). They function as complete antibodies, i.e., they can be revealed by methods for direct agglutination of normal red blood cells; they bind complement and easily lyse erythrocytes treated with trypsin or erythrocytes from patients with paroxysmal nocturnal hemoglobinuria. Cold antibodies aggregate on erythrocyte membranes at lower temperatures and dissociate when the temperature is raised to 37 °C. Nevertheless, Coombs' test is positive even when care

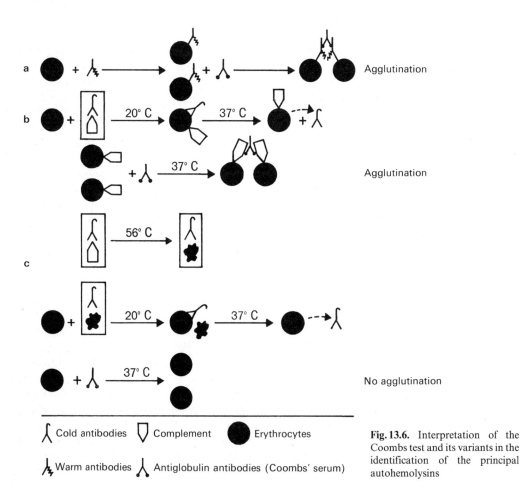

Fig. 13.6. Interpretation of the Coombs test and its variants in the identification of the principal autohemolysins

is taken that the blood is not cooled lower than 37 °C, whereby cold agglutinins become disaggregated and are bound to the erythrocyte membranes (Fig. 13.6).

When the indirect Coombs test is performed (Fig. 13.6), one must take care to warm the serum to be tested to 56 °C to inactivate the complement. The addition of anti-gammaglobulin serum to the mixture does not produce agglutination of the red blood cells. This indicates that the agglutination of the red blood cells by the Coombs serum at 37 °C is not due to cold antibody reaction, but rather to components of complement bound to the red blood cell in the event that there is an erythrocyte–cold antigen reaction. These data suggest that complement, in addition to serving as a "bridge" in the antibody–antiglobulin and erythrocyte reaction, also fosters the binding of the cold antibodies to the erythrocyte membrane.

The D–L antibodies are hemolysins encountered in the sera of patients with paroxysmal nocturnal hemoglobinuria; they possess a sedimentation coefficient of the order of 7 S, and require lower temperatures than do cold antibodies to affix to erythrocyte membranes. They do not require complement (C) to attach to the erythrocytes, but lytic properties are acquired only when the temperature reaches 18°–20 °C – thus the name "diphasic cold antibodies."

Hemolysis mechanisms: The destruction of red blood cells in the different forms of "autoimmune" anemias can occur in two ways: In the first mechanism, the erythrocytes carrying acquired autoantibodies adhering to their surfaces reveal spherocytosis and are retained in the macrophage system, principally in the spleen, where they are ultimately destroyed. In the second mechanism, most commonly observed in paroxysmal nocturnal hemoglobinuria and in the forms of anemia due to cold antibodies, hemolysis of erythrocytes results from the activity of complement. In this case, the autohemolysins attach to the red blood cells and fix complement when in transit through the peripheral vessels of the regions most subject

to low temperature (face, ears, nose, and hands), with hemolysis occurring when the erythrocytes reach warmer regions.

There are three experimental models of autoimmune anemias: (1) homologous disease, produced by introduction of immunocompetent cells into a recipient animal that cannot eliminate them; (2) spontaneous autoimmune anemia observed in NZB mice; and (3) spontaneous autoimmune hemolytic anemia of the dog, with or without disseminated LE syndrome.

Homologous disease (Secondary or Graft-vs-Host Disease): Homologous disease occurs as a consequence of the proliferation of allogeneic immunocompetent cells in a recipient animal incapable of rejecting them, either because it has been rendered immunoincompetent (irradiation, ALS treatment) or because it is tolerant to the transfused cells, or because it is an F_1 hybrid, that has received transplanted immunocompetent cells from one of its parents. These transplanted cells proliferate and react immunologically with tissue components of the host. Among other alterations, destruction of the red blood cells, leukopenia, and sometimes thrombocytopenia are observed. The antibodies eluted from the red blood cells of the F_1 hybrid with homologous disease agglutinate the red blood cells from that parent that did not furnish the immunocompetent cells. The antigens responsible for the establishment of homologous disease belong to the group of histocompatibility antigens and the ABO blood group antigens.

Spontaneous autoimmune anemia of the NZB mouse: This strain of mice was originally selected for cancer research. In the meantime, it was ascertained that from the third month of life these animals exhibited an autoimmune hemolytic anemia characterized by a positive Coombs test, reticulocytosis, jaundice, glomerulonephritis, and hepatosplenomegaly. Contemporaneously with the appearance of the hemolytic-antibodies – unusually warm antibodies – histologic alterations develop in the thymus, characterized by proliferation of lymph cells, with occasional formation of lymphoid follicles. The autoimmune nature of this syndrome was confirmed by transferring lymphocytes during the active phase of the disease to young mice of the same strain.

The renal alterations resemble those encountered in human lupus erythematosus. This form of autoimmune hemolytic anemia constitutes an example of the emergence of "forbidden clones" genetically conditioned for the formation of auto-antibodies directed against the animal's own erythrocyte cell membrane components.

Spontaneous autoimmune hemolytic anemia of the dog: This form of autoimmune anemia appears either alone or accompanied by symptomatology similar to that observed in lupus erythematosus. In the first case, anemia, jaundice, generalized lymphadenopathy, and splenomegaly are observed. The anemia observed is of the macrocytic type, with low hemoglobin levels (about 2.5 g/ 100 ml). Reticulocytosis, hyperplasia of the bone marrow, and thrombocytopenia are also observed in the majority of cases. The Coombs test is always positive; the antibodies can be eluted from erythrocytes, and they react with red blood cells of normal animals. In the symptomatic form, one encounters, in addition to the alterations just described, diffuse glomerulonephritis characterized by thickening and hyalinization of the basement membrane of Bowman's capsule, as well as by sclerosis of the afferent glomerular arterioles. In the majority of cases, one also encounters rheumatoid factor and LE-cells.

Thrombocytopenias: Thrombocytopenic purpura occurs as a primary disease, or as a secondary disease associated with other diseases such as lupus erythematosus or leukemia. In addition to hemorrhagic phenomena, there are alterations in the structure of platelets in the blood and of the megakaryocytes in the bone marrow. The acute forms are usually encountered in children under 8 years of age, of both sexes, whereas the

chronic forms occur more often in adults – mostly in women – and persist for months or even years.

A factor exists in the serum of those afflicted with thrombocytopenic purpura that can produce thrombocytopenia when injected into normal individuals. The nature of this factor has not yet been adequately determined; however, it does exhibit characteristics of an antibody: It is adsorbed by platelets, is species-specific, and is a 7 S globulin. During purpuric crises, an increase is observed in the level of β-glycerol-phosphatase (an enzyme found in the platelets), always coinciding with thrombocytopenia, which suggests intense platelet destruction. Since it is much easier to determine glycerol-phosphatase levels than those of anti-platelet factor, testing for the former is preferred in differential diagnostics. The destruction of the platelets appears to occur either by direct action of the antiplatelet factor, agglutinating and lysing them, or by opsonizing them to facilitate their destruction by the macrophages of the reticuloendothelial system, principally those of the spleen.

The use of drugs such as sulfonamides, chlorothiazides, chlorpropamide, meprobamate, phenylbutazone, quinidine, and the sedative Sedormid can produce thrombocytopenia.

It is presumed that the drug, functioning as a foreign hapten, combines with certain components of the platelet membranes to form autoimmunogenic complexes. These complexes generate antibodies that react with the membrane-drug complex of the platelets.

Autoimmune leukopenias: Some forms of leukopenias appear to be associated with the presence of autoantibodies. Data indicating that these auto-leukoagglutinins are related to destruction of the leukocytes are summarized as follows: (1) auto-agglutinins exist in many cases of neutropenias; (2) when the neutropenia recedes either naturally or upon treatment, the auto-antibodies also disappear; and (3) in some cases of neutropenia, there is no history of transfusions, thus eliminating the possibility of formation of alloantibodies.

Autoimmune Diseases
of the Gastrointestinal Tract and Liver

Gastric atrophy and pernicious anemia: Gastric atrophy is the endstage inflammatory process which begins as superficial gastritis, progresses to atrophic gastritis, and ends in atrophy. Histologically, these three phases are characterized by: first, lymphocytic, plasmocytic, and monocytic infiltrates of the superficial epithelium and lamina propria of the gastric mucosa; in the more advanced phase, mononuclear infiltrates extend more deeply and surround the tubular acini of gastric glands with partial loss of parietal and chief cells; the atrophic phase is characterized by complete loss of gastric glands.

Two types of antibodies are found: one reacting with the Vitamin B_{12}-binding glycoprotein, intrinsic factor, and the other with a lipoprotein antigen present on the microvilli of gastric parietal cells. Anti-intrinsic factor antibodies react either with the Vitamin-B_{12} binding site and compete with the binding of Vitamin B_{12}, or with a determinant away from the binding site. Usually, both antibodies are present; in the serum, they are IgG antibodies, in the stomach often IgA. These antibodies interfere with the uptake of Vitamin B_{12}.

The antiparietal antibody detects an organ-specific, but not species-specific antigen, and it may not be detected in the serum, only in the gastric juice. A high degree of correlation exists between the presence of this antibody and the extent of gastritis and gastric mucosal atrophy.

The histopathologic alterations are assumed to be the result, at least in part, of cell-mediated immunity to gastric mucosa cells. Lymphocytes of patients show an enhanced proliferative response and release leukocyte-migration inhibition factor upon stimulation with gastric mucosa homogenates.

The etiology is not known; a strong familial association exists. There is an association in a few cases between pernicious anemia and thyrotoxicosis; thyroid microsomal and thyroglobulin antibodies are also found in some patients with pernicious anemia.

Ulcerative colitis and Crohn's disease are two inflammatory diseases affecting the mucosa of rectum and colon (ulcerative colitis), and terminal ileum (Crohn's disease); they might be two expressions of a single disease. The diseases are slightly more common in females than in males. The cause is not known, although in recent years some indications have suggested a viral etiology: electron microscopic studies revealed some evidence for virus-like particles, and intestinal lesions have been demonstrated to occur after transfer of mucosa homogenate from patients' colon into laboratory animals.

Antibodies with specificity for colonic mucosal epithelial cell antigen, which is present in sterile, fetal colonic mucosa, and with specificity for polysaccharide antigens of E.coli 0:14 cross-reacting with colon antigen, have been found in patients with ulcerative colitis. These antibodies are of the IgG class, and are not cytotoxic for colon epithelial cells; moreover, neither the presence nor the titer correlates with extent or severity of the disease.

Some indications for cell-mediated immunity have been found: lymphocytes to patients are specifically cytotoxic to allogenic colonnic epithelial cells; this cytotoxicity is inhibited by preincubation with E.coli lipopolysaccharide, is complement-independent, and is mediated by K cells.

Chronic active hepatitis is characterized by periportal inflammation and liver cell injury. As etiologic agents have been identified: hepatitis B virus, drugs, and alcohol.

Two groups of patients can be distinguished: one is HB_sAg negative and presents autoimmune-like symptoms; in these cases, the etiology is not always clear. Women are more frequently affected than men, and there is an overrepresentation of the HLA-B8 type. In addition, these patients usually have high-titer of antibodies to hepatocyte-actin and smooth muscle. The other group consists of HB$_s$Ag-positive patients with males predominant, and an overrepresentation of the HLA-B 35 type.

An antibody to hepatocyte-specific antigen, liver-surface protein (LSP), can be detected in the serum of all patients with acute hepatitis. This antibody usually disappears in patients recovering from this disease, but remains in those who develop chronic active hepatitis (the reason for this is not known). It has been shown that when injected into rabbits, LPS induces chronic aggressive hepatitis, and that the killing of liver cells in culture by lymphocytes of patients can be prevented by adding LSP to the culture.

The pathogenic mechanism leading to chronic disease is assumed to involve virus antigens on the surface of hepatocytes that stimulate T helper cells which, in turn, induce B cells to produce antibodies; this antibody response includes the formation of anti-LSP. The infected cells are killed either by complement-dependent antibody lysis, or by antibody-mediated cell lysis (which has been demonstrated to occur in vitro by K cells). In cases where the infection is controlled, stimulation of T helper cells and antibody production ceases. In persistent virus infections (HB$_s$Ag$^+$), the antibody production continues; in "autoimmune" hepatitis it is assumed that the anti-LSP antibody formation has become autonomous, most probably as a result of deficient suppressor T-cell function (for which there are some hints from in vitro studies).

Autoimmune Diseases of the Kidney

Glomerulonephritis: Two immunologic mechanisms may be distinguished in the production of experimental glomerulonephritis: (a) Antibody-antigen complex deposition in the glomeruli with activation of inflammatory processes due to complement and subsequent polymorphonuclear and mononuclear cell activation (see Chap. 10, p. 287), and (b) nephrotoxic glomerulonephritis (Masugi's nephritis,

glomerular basement membrane antibody glomerulonephritis) induced by antibodies specific for xenogeneic or allogeneic (autoimmune) basement membrane antigen.

Anti-glomerular basement membrane antibody-induced glomerulonephritis: Antikidney or nephrotoxic sera (NS) are produced by injecting kidney extract, emulsified in complete Freund's adjuvant, into animals of different species. Usually, rat kidney extracts have been used to immunize rabbits or, occasionally, ducks.

Intravenous injection of NS into the appropriate species induces a biphasic glomerulonephritis. Application of large amounts of antibasement antibody produces an immediate injury with proteinuria. A second phase appears 8–12 days later, when the host has mounted an immune response to the foreign antibody (see also below).

In the first hours after injection, the capillaries in the affected glomeruli dilate and are invaded by an infiltrate rich in neutrophils. Subsequently, the endothelial cells swell, proliferate, and reduce the capillary lumen, terminating in tubular hemorrhages (Fig. 13.7). The electron microscope reveals that the basal lamina becomes thickened on the capillary side from the deposition of dense material composed of xenogeneic antikidney antibodies and of complement components, among them C 3 and C 4. Continuous deposition of antibodies and complement components can result in the complete obliteration of the capillary (Fig. 13.8). In immunofluorescence staining of kidney sections, a linear configuration appears. When the lesions are focal, they tend to disappear; however, when they are diffuse, the animals either die in the first few days, or the lesions evolve to a chronic state, persisting for months or even years. In this case, the histopathologic picture closely resembles human glomerulonephritis.

The nephritogenic antigen is localized in the glomerular basement membrane, and appears to be a glycoprotein. A similar antigen is encountered in the lung, probably associ-

Fig. 13.7. Electron microscopic appearance of a capillary of the glomerulus of a rat killed 2.5 h after injection of nephrotoxic serum. A polymorphonuclear leukocyte is shown in intimate contact with the basement membrane of the capillary. *BM*, basement membrane; *En*, endothelial cell; *Ep*, epithelial cell; *PMN*, polymorphonuclear leukocyte

ated with the wall of the alveolar capillaries (see below, Goodpasture's syndrome).

The nephrotoxic sera contain IgG and IgM antibodies; in addition to the anti-basement membrane antibodies two other factors may be responsible for the occurrence of the glomerular lesions: complement components and polymorphonuclear cells. The injection of NS into rats decomplementized by prior administration of human IgG aggregates, antigen-antibody complexes, cobra venom, zymosan, a.o., only produces lesions of slight intensity. The same reaction occurs if the animal has been rendered leukopenic by previous administration of nitrogen mustard or similar agents. It appears,

therefore, that lesions are formed only after the antibody-antigen complex on the basement membrane has activated the complement system, with the production of anaphylatoxins and chemotactic factors, followed by the accumulation of neutrophils. Electron microscopic studies show that, in many areas, the polymorphonuclear cells displace the cytoplasm of the endothelial cells and enter into contact with the basement membrane (Figs. 13.7 and 13.8).

The necessity of complement activation for the pathogenesis of the lesions has been elegantly demonstrated by using duck antibodies to basement membrane antigen of the rabbit. Duck antibodies do not activate

Fig. 13.8. Electron microscopic appearance of glomerular capillaries of a rat. In **a** (control), infiltration by polymorphonuclear leukocytes (*PMN*) is not observed, and the endothelial cells (*end*) are normally distributed over the surface of the basement membrane (*BM*). In **b** is shown a section of kidney obtained from a rat 2.5 h after the injection of nephrotoxic serum. The endothelial cell (*end*) was forced from its position by the polymorphonuclear (*PMN*) cells, leaving the basement membrane denuded. In **c**, the pseudopodia of the polymorphonuclear leukocyte are extended beneath the cytoplasm of the endothelial cell (*end*), entering into intimate contact with the basement membrane. This contact continues for some hours, with disappearance of the leukocytes about 6 h after the injection of the nephrotoxic serum. Cochrane CG et al. (1965) J Exp Med 122:99

mammalian complement: the clinical manifestations and histologic alterations only appear after 7–12 days. The duck antibody combines with the antigen in the basement membrane, yet does not activate complement, and is therefore unable to damage the glomeruli. However, since the duck antibody is foreign, it stimulates the formation of host antibodies, which then, after binding to the duck antibody, activate complement and produce lesions.

The pathogenesis of (isogeneic) basement-membrane antibody-induced glomerulonephritis in humans parallels the ex-perimental disease; however, nothing is known about the cause inducing the formation of auto-antibasement antibodies. It is assumed that cross-reacting antigens of infectious microorganisms (e.g., influenza) and noxious agents such as hydrocarbon solvents (inhaled) may induce the formation of this antibody.

Autoimmune Diseases of the Lung

Goodpasture's syndrome is a disease characterized by focal pulmonary hemorrhages always associated with a rapidly evolving

Fig. 13.9. Histologic appearance of rat lung with acute pulmonary edema produced by injection of nephrotoxic serum

membranous or proliferative glomerulonephritis. Immunofluorescence staining reveals homogeneous deposits of immunoglobulins and of complement along the basement membrane. The auto-antibodies appear to be directed against antigens shared by the lung and kidney. The same syndrome can be induced experimentally when nephrotoxic serum (anti-basement membrane antibodies) is injected into rats (Fig. 13.9).

Autoimmune Diseases of the Heart

Rheumatic fever: Auto-antibodies against antigens of the cardiac muscle appear to be a major pathogenic factor in the pathogenesis of heart disease subsequent to rheumatic fever. The antibody can be detected by complement fixation, antiglobulin consumption test, passive hemagglutination with tanned red blood cells coated with cardiac antigen, and immunofluorescence. With the latter method, it has been demonstrated that IgG and IgM auto-antibodies adhere to the sarcolemma, on the periphery of the sarcoplasm, and on the walls of the heart blood vessels of individuals with rheumatic fever. In addition, the serum of these patients contains antibodies that react with fragments of normal hearts; these antibodies are deposited in the same structures in which they were encountered in the hearts of afflicted individuals. Moreover, these antibodies cross-react with protein antigens in the capsular wall of group A hemolytic streptococci. On the other hand, when rabbits are injected with these streptococci causes them to produce antibodies which cross-react with human heart extract.

These observations suggest that the initial immunogenic stimulus is provided by the antigens of the streptococcus wall and that the progression of these lesions is due to the autoantigens liberated as a consequence of the tissue lesions.

Autoimmune Diseases of the Eye

It is recognized that the eye is the site of two autoimmune processes, one affecting the lens, and the other affecting the uveal tract.

Lens: The human lens contains at least nine or ten organ-specific antigens. Some of these antigens form early on in embryonic development, so that when the immune system is differentiated, these antigens are already isolated from other structures and, therefore, are potential autoantigens.

Endophthalmitis phaco-anaphylactica (greek phakos, lens) results primarily from the liberation of crystalline lens substances due to the rupture of the lens capsule. The inflammatory process is initiated several weeks after the injury and progresses rapidly. The histologic alterations appear around the ruptured lens or its fragments in the form of three characteristic concentric layers: In the center is found the disintegrating crystalline fragment, infiltrated by polymorphonuclear leukocytes; more toward the periphery there is a layer of epithelioid cells with some multinucleated giant cells. Externally, there is granulation tissue of variable thickness, infiltrated by leukocytes and plasma cells. The experimental disease induced in rabbits exhibits, generally, the same sequence of events.

Uveal Tract. Sympathetic ophthalmia is a bilateral ocular disease that appears some weeks after a perforation injury of the eyeball, especially when the iris or the ciliary body is involved. In the beginning, there is infiltration by lymphatic cells that is particularly pronounced around the venules of the uveal tract. Later, epithelioid cells and giant cells appear which extend to the choroid and the iris. Coinciding with the disease – principally during the aggravation phase of the lesions – one observes delayed skin reactions following the injection of uveal-tract extracts. This fact, along with the lack of circulating antibodies during the active state of the disease, suggests that the lesions are mediated by cellular hypersensitivity. This disease can be produced experimentally in the guinea pig by the injection of uveal tract extracts in complete Freund's adjuvant. Studies with albino and pigmented guinea pigs indicate that at least two antigens exist in the uveal tracts that are responsible for sympathetic ophthalmia – one of them probably associated with uveal pigment.

Autoimmune Disease of the Skin

Pemphigus vulgaris is a rare blistering disorder; there is an increased frequency of HLA-A10 and HLA-B13. The etiology is unknown; an almost identical, but less severe disease which is endemic in south central Brazil, Pemphigus foliaceus, is assumed to be caused by an arthropod-borne infection. Histologically, there is an intraepidermal blister formation with acantholysis; electron microscopic studies show a dissolution of intercellular "cement" followed by desmosome destruction. These lesions are caused by an autoantibody with specificity for intercellular substances of the skin and mucosa; the antibody can be detected in the serum of most patients. Immunofluorescence staining reveals deposits of Ig (predominantly IgG) and complement (C1, C4, C3, and properdin factor B) in the skin lesions. Identical lesions can be observed in a culture of epidermis cells to which this antibody is added.

It is assumed that in these patients a T-cell deficiency exists.

Systemic Autoimmune Diseases

Systemic lupus erythematosus (SLE) is characterized by inflammatory and destructive processes in a variety of organs such as skin, joints, kidney, heart, lungs, due to pathologic alterations of arteries and arterioles as a result of multiple immune abnormalities. The disease is more common in females than in males, and has a peak incidence between 25 and 29 years of age. Family studies, particularly of twins, have yielded evidence of a genetic susceptibility to SLE, and there appears to be a slight association of susceptibility to SLE with HLA-D2/D3 types.

The acute condition frequently occurs after exposure to sunlight or drugs. A careful examination almost always reveals autoimmune phenomena which were in existence for some years prior to the time of diagnosis. Clinical manifestations are extremely pleiomorphic: dermatologic lesions such as erythemas (facial butterfly-shaped rash, Fig. 13.10), maculae, bullous and ulcerous lesions; polyserositis causing arthralgia, abdominal and chest pain, myalgia, Raynaud's syndrome due to lesions in arteries and arterioles, lesions of the lacrimal (keratocon-

Fig. 13.10. Cutaneous lesions in SLE. Dermatologic lesions in the areas exposed to the light of a patient with SLE. The involvement of the scalp caused alopecia visible in the photograph. (Courtesy of Dr. Roberto Dias, Hosp. Clinicas, UFMG)

Among the drugs which have been demonstrated to induce autoantibodies and a clinical SLE-like syndrome are procainamide, hydralazine, chloropromazine, isoniazid, hydantoins, trimethadione and α-methyldopa. These substances are able to interact with DNA or nucleoproteins (in vitro), and they induce anti-nuclear antibodies in individuals receiving them.

Sex hormones are important, as already indicated by the female to male ratio; furthermore, during pregnancy, an exacerbation of the disease is common, which extends to the postpartum period.

The most prominent abnormality in patients with SLE is their ability to produce antibodies to a wide array of self-antigens (Table 13.9). Many of these antibodies, particularly anti-nuclear antibodies (ANA), have been implicated in the pathogenesis of the disease, and SLE has been considered as a prototype of immune-complex disorders.

junctivitis sicca) and salivary glands, otitis media, pericarditis, and myocarditis, interstitial pneumonia, vascular lesions of the intestinal tract, glomerulonephritis, hemolytic anemia, thrombocytopenia, and leukopenia.

Histologically, fibrosis, lymphocyto-plasmocytic infiltrations and immune complex depositions prevail.

The etiology of the disease is unknown, but it is assumed that its occurrence is brought about by environmental factors such as UV-light, drugs, and/or viral infections, in genetically predisposed individuals.

Thus, paramyxovirus-like structures have been found in kidney, skin, and circulating lymphocytes of SLE patients; sera from patients contain a high number of antibodies to measles and other RNA and DNA viruses, and antibodies to double-stranded RNA, which is found in viruses but not in mammalian cells. Xenotropic C-type viral antigens (gp 30 and gp 70) in renal and lymphoid tissue have been identified. However, none of these possible agents has been shown to be responsible for the disease in humans.

Table 13.9. Autoantibodies in SLE

To cells (ACA, anti-cell ab):
  Lymphocytes (ALA)
  Erythrocytes
  Platelets
  Neutrophils
To tissue (ATA, anti-tissue ab):
  Heart
  Neurons (brain)
  Collagen
  Muscle
To cytoplasm:
  Ribosomes
  Mitochondria
  Lysosomes
To nuclei:
  Nucleoprotein (NP)
  DNA
  Histones
  Ribonucleoprotein ⎫ ANA
  RNA-nucleoli
To nucleic acid:
  DNA, double- and single-stranded
  RNA, double- and single-stranded ⎭
To others:
  Immunoglobulins (RF)
  Coagulans (prothrombin converter)
  Cardiolipin
  Thyroglobulin

The observation that the antibody response to most microorganisms tested (influenza vaccine, Newcastle disease virus, respiratory syncytial virus, adenovirus, Herpes simplex, cytomegalovirus, papovavirus, hepatitis B virus, rubella; Brucella, proteus OX-2-agglutinins, tetanus toxoid, streptolysin 0) is normal, may indicate that the defect of the immune system in SLE is not a general B-cell hyperactivity, but a failure to make a distinction between self and non-self; the result is a "normal" immune response to everything which comes into contact with immune cells, including, and most prominently, auto-antigens. There appears to be a specific defect to maintain and induce self-tolerance. Indeed, numerous studies have shown that SLE patients exhibit a reduced T-cell response in vivo (delayed-type hypersensitivity reaction to common antigens such as PPD) as well as in vitro (mitogenic and antigen-specific lymphocyte proliferation), and their number of T cells in the circulation is reduced, particularly those with IgG-receptor (Tγ=suppressor T cells). It has been demonstrated that T cells from SLE patients with active disease are unable to suppress the synthesis of immunoglobulins by SLE-B cells (for test, see p. 340). It is not clear whether or not antilymphocytic antibodies (ALA) specifically reacting with T cells and present in SLE patients are responsible for the reduced T-cell number or activity; however, ALA titers correlate positively with disease activity.

In addition to T-lymphocyte impairments, null-(non-T, non-B) and K-cell abnormalities have also been reported to exist during active phases of the disease. Since all of these abnormalities are much less expressed in phases of remission, it might be suspected that the defects are not intrinsic but induced, and once pathogenic antibodies (ANA, ALA, ACA-anti-cellular antibodies-, ATA-anti-tissue antibodies) are formed, which reduce T cells and cause tissue damage, a vicious self-perpetuating cycle is established:

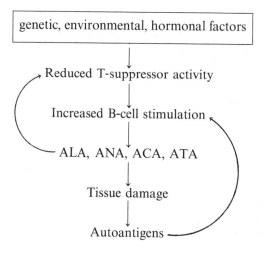

Thus far, there is no evidence for an enhanced cell-mediated reactivity to self-constituents in SLE patients.

For the pathogenesis of the disease, the most important factors appear to be antibodies to DNA (double- and single-stranded), soluble

Fig. 13.11. Blood smear of patient with SLE showing LE cells

and insoluble (iNP) nucleoproteins, saline-extractable nuclear antigens, and RNA (all being anti-nuclear antibodies, ANA). Anti-iNP (also called LE factor) causes the LE phenomenon, in which phagocytic cells ingest nuclear material to which anti-iNP is bound (Fig. 13.11).

ANA and DNA-antigens are found by immunofluorescence technique as immune complexes (without or with fixed complement) deposited in the dermis, serosa, walls of blood vessels, glomeruli, synovia, lung, and heart; in addition, immune complexes formed by tissue-antigen specific antibodies are found in the respective tissue, and usually the kidney. Cell-specific antibodies lyse their target cells in a complement dependent fashion. The immunopathology develops according to type II and III hypersensitivity reactions as described in Chap. 10 (see pp. 281–287).

Experimental systemic lupus erythematosus in New Zealand Black (NZB) mice has been extensively analyzed, and has provided a clear picture of the genesis of the disease.

In NZB mice the disease occurs spontaneously and has a very fixed course: The mice are born with an immune system as mature as that of adults; they produce adult-like levels of antibodies to sheep red blood cells, and they have a very active cellular immunity. By the age of 2 months, they are highly resistant to tolerance induction, and rapidly lose tolerance induced at 3 weeks of age. Suppressor T-cell activity declines simultaneously with a decrease of thymic factors at the age of about 6–8 weeks. Auto-antibodies start to occur concurrently and rise progressively; at the age of 5 months, immune-complex nephritis, Coombs'-positive hemolytic anemia, and lymphocytic tissue infiltrations have developed. Mice which survive these disorders are susceptible to the development of malignant lymphomas, and are profoundly deficient in cell-mediated immune functions, but also in humoral immunity (exhaustion?).

This course of events is less pronounced in males, which do not show an immune-com-plex glomerulonephritis as severely and early as do females. Thymectomy significantly prolongs survival of females, but increases mortality of males as does neonatal splenectomy, which has no effect on female survival. In both instances, the males show the female-type course of the disease. Castration of males gives the same result, whereas females castrated and subsequently treated with androgens produce the male-type of disease.

These findings indicate that sex hormones have a profound influence on the thymus and T-cell maturation, and that T cells are important for the containment of the disease.

NZB mice carry and produce a xenotropic C-type virus in all of their cells, and the destruction (directly or indirectly due to stimulation of cytotoxic T cells specific for virus antigen on T cells) of thymus and T cells concomitant with immune stimulation by viral antigens might be the cause of the disease.

Rheumatoid arthritis is a systemic, chronic inflammatory disease, which manifests itself more dominantly in the joints as synovitis, causing progressive destruction and deformation. Extra articular features are rheumatoid nodules, arteritis, sclerosis, neuropathy, pericarditis, lymphadenopathy, and splenomegaly, which occur rather frequently. The disease occurs more frequently in women than in men; although there is an increasing incidence between 30 and 50 years of age, it also can affect children, usually older than 4 years of age (Still's disease).

Clinically, it is characterized by painful, symmetric, progressive polyarthritis that first affects the smaller, more peripheral joints (hands, wrists, knees, and feet), but later spreads to the larger joints (elbow, shoulder, hips, ankles, cervical articulations). Morning stiffness is highly characteristic of rheumatoid arthritis. The course of the disease is variable with alternating periods of activity and remission.

The pathology is characterized by synovitis, vasculitis, and granuloma formation, desely infiltrated by lymphocytes, plasmacells, mono- and polymorphonuclear cells. The thin synovial membrane thickens and develops to a chronic granulation tissue, pannus. This rheumatoid pannus inflicts severe tissue damage with erosions of the cartilage. The cartilage atrophies and the neighboring bone tissue suffers osteoporosis and erosions, which yield characteristic radiologic images.

Vasculitis involves arteries as well as veins, and is characterized by histiocytic infiltrations that can, at times, assume the appearance of giant cells.

The subcutaneous nodules found in the areas exposed to pressure (elbow, wrists, a. o.) exhibit a central zone of fibrinoid necrosis, surrounded by epithelioid and lymphoid cells.

In 1940, Waaler demonstrated that the sera of patients with rheumatoid arthritis agglutinated sheep erythrocytes coated with rabbit anti-sheep immunoglobulins (Rose-Waaler hemagglutination test). The factor(s) responsible for this agglutination is known as the "rheumatoid factor" (RF). Today, instead of erythrocytes, latex particles coated with human gamma globulin are employed for the agglutination test. The RF has been identified as IgM and/or IgG immunoglobulins reacting with IgG and thus forming IgM/IgG-IgG complexes. Exhaustive studies by many groups have shown that IgG and IgM anti-gammaglobulins with reactivity for IgA, IgE, L-chains, certain genetically determined sites on H-chains of IgG, are produced in rheumatoid arthritis. These anti-Ig antibodies are not only found in sera and synovial fluid of RA patients, but are the predominant or even only kind of immunoglobulins produced by the plasma cells within the inflammatory site (synovia). These findings suggest an intimate association of the production of rheumatoid factor with the pathogenesis of the disease. And indeed there exists a definite correlation between presence and titer of rheumatoid factor and severity of disease. How RF participates in the tissue lesions is not clear. However, RF are capable of complement activation, and thus do enhance inflammatory processes; in addition, immunoglobulin complexes and immunoglobulin-complement complexes (Ig-Ig and Ig-Ig-C) have been demonstrated in vessel walls, synovial fluid and synovia; moreover, it has been shown that immunoglobulin complexes are ingested by phagocytic synovial cells, which then release their lysosomal set of inflammatory digestive substances, including tissue cathepsin, proteases, and collagenase, the latter being able to destroy the skeleton of cartilage.

Most of the lymphocytes detected in synovial tissue inflammatory sites are Tμ cells (T helper cells); this, and the detection of lymphokines in synovial fluid may imply a role for cell-mediated immunity, but might be also a mere reflection of the activity of helper T cells.

The etiology of the disease is unknown as is the cause of the production of the anti-gamma antibodies. It is conceivable that the whole process starts with an infection, and that the initial antigens elicit the formation of antibodies which happen to cross-react with immunoglobulins. It has been indeed been shown that rabbits hyperimmunized with streptococcal peptidoglycan antigens occasionally produce monoclonal IgG rheumatoid factor which shows specificity to the immunizing antigen as well. One frequently observed characteristic of cross-reactive antibodies is that they have a low association constant for the cross-reacting antigen; most rheumatoid factor antibodies have, indeed, a low affinity to Ig compared to anti-Ig antibodies produced against Ig. One may even conceive the increased formation of allotype (and idiotype?) specific antibodies to be a sign of decontrolled immune response or "frustrated allotype suppression."

In support of an infectious cause as etiology of the disease is the fact that rheumatoid factors are found in other chronic infections (see Table 13.4).

Progressive systemic sclerosis (PSS, sclero-derma) is a generalized disorder of connective tissue of vessels with fibrosis and degenerative changes in the skin, synovia, digital arteries, and the parenchyma and small arteries of internal organs.

The etiology is unknown; familial association is evident, and a prevalence of the HLA-B8 type exists. Women are more often affected than men.

The most striking feature of PSS is the widespread overgrowth of collagenous connective tissue, and often consider able inflammatory and vascular changes with lymphocyte and plasma cell infiltrates.

Most patients show hypergammaglobulinemia, predominantly IgG, small amounts of immune complexes, and about one-third have rheumatoid factors in their serum; anti-nuclear antibodies (and LE cell phenomenon), but no antibodies against native DNA are observed.

The number of T cells is reduced in the peripheral blood; however, the lymphocytes in tissue infiltrates are predominantly T cells. Patients' lymphocytes are sensitized against skin antigens, particularly human collagen type I, as measured in the migration inhibition assay. There is an increased production of lymphokines in tissue lesions, which may account for the observed significantly increased activity of fibroblasts, with an accumulation of collagen. The stimulating antigen is, however, not known.

References

Cohen S, Ward PA, McCluskey RT (1979) Mechanisms of immunopathology. John Wiley and Sons, New York

Cunningham AJ (1976) Self-tolerance maintained by active suppressor mechanisms. Transplant Rev 31:23

Gell PGH, Coombs RRA, Lachman PJ (eds) (1975) Clinical aspects of immunology. Blackwell, Oxford, England

Gershon RK, Kondo K (1971) Immunology 21:903

Grabar P (1975) Hypothesis: Auto-antibodies and immunological theories: an analytical review. Clin Immunol Immunopathol 4:453

Hughes GRU (1976) Connective Tissue diseases. Blackwell, Oxford, England

Miescher PA, Müller-Eberhard H (eds) (1976) Textbook of immunopathology. Grune and Stratton, New York

Möller G (1978) Role of macrophages in the immune response. Immunol Rev 40:3. Munksgaard, Copenhagen

Nossal GJV, Pike BL, Teale JM, Layton JE, Kay TW, Battey FL (1979) Immunol Rev 43:18

Parker CW (ed) (1980) Clinical immunology. WB Saunders, Philadelphia

Rose NR, Witebsky E (1956) Studies on organ specificity. V. Changes in the thyroid glands of rabbits following active immunization with rabbit thyroid extracts. J Immunol 76:417

Rosen NR, Bigazzi PE, Warner NL (eds) (1978) Genetic control of autoimmune diseases. Elsevier-North-Holland, New York

Stuart FP, Fitch FW (eds) (1979) Immunologic tolerance and enhancement. MTP Press, Falcon House, Lancaster, England

Talal N (ed) (1977) Autoimmunity: Genetic, immunologic, virologic, and clinical aspects. Academic, New York

Williams jr RC (1980) Immune complexes in clinical and experimental medicine. Harvard University Press, Cambridge, Mass.

Chapter 14 Immunosuppression

WILMAR DIAS DA SILVA

Contents

The different modalities of tissue damage produced by immunologic mechanisms are, generally speaking, chronically progressive, sometimes disfiguring, and frequently lethal. Control of their clinical manifestations has been attempted with corticosteroids, but therapy with these hormones has limitations arising from their nonspecificity, the irregularity with which they act in certain immunologic diseases – for example, in chronic glomerulonephritides – and in the production of undesirable side effects when used for long periods of time.

The difficulties encountered in the therapy of autoimmune diseases in the control of tissue or organ graft rejection (graft rejection, graft-versus-host reaction) have stimulated the search for new immunosuppressives. The success of these efforts depends upon a better conceptual grasp of what occurs at the molecular level and at the cellular level during the sequence of events of the immune response. Specific blockage at some point of this sequence represents the final goal of immunosuppression.

The cellular modifications that occur in the peripheral lymphatic organs following the introduction of an antigen, as well as the biochemical events induced, have been analyzed in the different chapters of this book. This sequence of events is represented schematically in Fig. 14.1 to indicate the most vulnerable sites of the immune response, upon which the various immunosuppressives are believed to act.

For greater ease in describing the different immunosuppressive agents and the possible mechanisms involved, the immune response is divided into the following steps:

Step A. Formation of precursor cells of the lymphocytes and their migration to the central lymphoid organs (thymus, and bursa of Fabricius in birds or corresponding structure in mammals)

**Cytogenetic immunocompetent cells and sequential cell reactions
in the immune response**

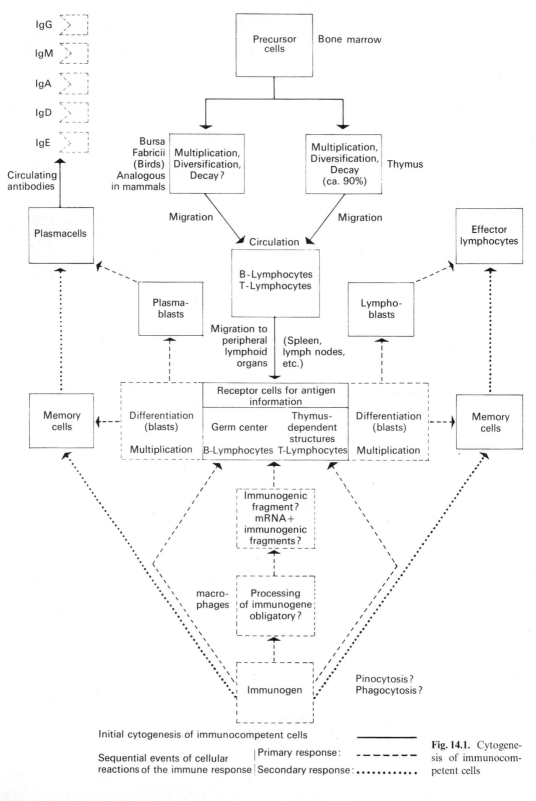

Fig. 14.1. Cytogenesis of immunocompetent cells

Step B. Acquisition of immunologic responsiveness in the central lymphoid organs through differentiation and specialization, terminating in the formation of immunocompetent lymphcytes that migrate to specified regions of the peripheral lymphoid organs (thymus-dependent and thymus-independent structures)

Step C. Recognition of immunogenic stimuli by receptor cells and transfer of the immune information to the immunocompetent lymphocytes (T lymphocytes and B lymphocytes)

Step D. Induction of the immune response, followed by cellular proliferation and differentiation, with the formation of "blast" or "pyroninophilic" cells and of immunologic memory cells. This apparently is the phase most vulnerable to immunosuppressive agents

Step E. Maturation of the "blast cells" into plasma cells and sensitized lymphocytes (effector-cytotoxic T cells)

Step F. Restimulation of memory cells by a secondary immunologic stimulus (secondary response).

General Operative Mechanisms of Immunosuppressives

The immunosuppressive agents listed in Table 14.1 can act upon the immune response in one of the following ways:

1) *Inhibition of formation of precursor cells* (stem-cell toxicity, step A).
2) *Repression of the production of the immunocompetent cells:* thymectomy and bursectomy, either pre- or neonatal, which may or may not be associated with sublethal irradiation. These immunosuppressive measures block the immune response by impeding the formation of B and T lymphocytes (step B).

3) *Destroying or blocking the immunocompetent cells:* irradiation with γ- or x-rays, treatment with antilymphocytic serum (ALS) and alkylating agents. These immunosuppressives act in different steps of the immune response.
4) *Preventing effective contact* between the antigenic determinants of the immunogens and the immunocompetent cells: blockage of antigens by passively transferred specific antibodies, repression of recognition of antigens through receptor blockade with anti-idiotypic antibodies (step C).
5) *Blocking the phagocytic functions* to inhibit the "processing" of antigens: irradiation and corticosteroid hormones (step C).
6) *Inhibiting the biosynthesis of nucleic acids* (DNA and RNA) and of proteins that respond to stimulation of the immunocompetent cells by the immunogen: antimetabolites, analogs of amino acids; antibiotics, antagonists of folic acid and some plant alkaloids. The blockage occurs principally at the level of steps D and E.
7) *Blocking the multiplication and differentiation* of cells already stimulated to impede the formation of sensitized lymphocytes (effector cells), plasma cells, and memory cells: irradiation, alkylating agents, and antimetabolites. Such blockage occurs in steps D, E, and F.
8) *Specific paralysis:* The induction of a state of specific tolerance for the antigenic determinant – an alternative form of the immunocompetent cells (Chap. 9, p. 245).

The activity of immunosuppressive agents is evaluated primarily by assays similar to those employed in experimental chemotherapy. The laboratory animals and the antigens are chosen according to the type of immune response for which the effects of a particular immunosuppressive are to be investigated. For example, if one wishes to study the effect of an agent on the production of reaginic antibodies, the preferred animals are the mouse and the rat; the antigen is injected in small quantities together with an appropriate adjuvant such as aluminum hydroxide or *B. pertussis* suspension. The im-

Group	Immunosuppressive agents
Surgical	Neonatal thymectomy Hormonal Bursectomy Neonatal surgical bursectomy Ductus-thoracicus drainage of lymphocytes
Irradiation	X-rays Gamma rays
Hormone	Adrenocorticotropic hormone Corticosteroids (cortisone, hydrocortisone, prednisone, prednisolone, etc.)

Antimetabolites	Purine analogs:
	    6-Mercaptopurine
	    Azathioprine (Imurel)
	    6-Thioguanine
	Pyrimidine analogs:
	    5-Fluoruracil
	Folic acid analogs:
	    Aminopterine
	    Methotrexate

Plant alkaloids	Vinblastine Vincristine Colchicine
Antibiotics	Actinomycin D Mitomycin C Puromycin Chloramphenicol Azaserine
Amino-acid antagonists	Glutamine Diazomycin A Asparagine L-Asparaginase[a]

Table 14.1. Classification of the most frequently used immunosuppressive agents

[a] Works via the catalytic hydrolysis of L-asparagine, which is split into
   L-asparaginic acid and ammonia

mune response can be evaluated either by testing for cutaneous anaphylaxis or for the liberation of histamine from tissue in vitro. The rabbit is the animal of choice for analysis of the effects upon the production of precipitating antibodies, and the antigen injected should be in Freund's adjuvant. In contrast, the guinea pig is often used to study effects upon delayed hypersensitivity of the tuberculin type; and allogeneic strains of mice are used when the test system is that of skin-graft rejection. The immunosuppressive agents included in Table 14.1 have been or are being tested in almost all forms of immune response.

Inhibition of Cytogenesis of Immunocompetent Cells

Thymectomy and Bursectomy

Pre- or neonatal thymectomy produces a clear reduction in the number of circulating lymphocytes, along with a depopulation of the paracortical regions of the lymph nodes and the periarteriolar sheaths of the spleen (thymus-dependent areas). The lymph follicles and the germinal centers (thymus-independent areas) are not affected, their populations of plasma cells remaining intact. Thymectomy essentially affects specific cellular immunity; depending upon the antigen, it produces only slight alterations in humoral immunity. The extent to which it influences the immune response depends upon the developmental state which the lymphoid system has attained up to birth. In such terms, the less developed the lymphoid system, the more intense are the effects. Mice thymectomized in the first days of life accept skin transplants from donors that differ in strong histocompatibility antigens.

The effects of thymectomy in adult animals are observed only when sufficient time has passed for the disappearance of "long-lived lymphocytes" located in the thymus-dependent areas. Immediate effects are obtained by accompanying thymectomy with total-body irradiation of the animal. Bursectomy (in birds), unlike thymectomy, does not reduce the circulating lymphocyte population, nor does it modify the thymus-dependent structures. The principal modifications are encountered in the thymus-independent regions of the lymph nodes and spleen, which do not exhibit germinal centers and in which there are practically no plasma cells. The level of circulating immunoglobulins is low, and the animal's capacity to produce antibodies is diminished considerably.

"Hormonal bursectomy," performed by inoculating chicken eggs with 19-nortestosterone, is much more efficient than surgical bursectomy. Thymectomy and bursectomy have been important in experimental immunology for the resolution of problems related to the cytophysiology of immunocompetent cells. However, the use of the thymectomy in clinical immunology is limited: It is restricted to situations in which the immune disease is primarily dependent on thymus hyperplasia or to those in which thymus hyperplasia leads to secondary clinical events.

Destruction or Inactivation of Immunocompetent Cells

Irradiation

The intensity of the immunosuppressive effects produced by irradiation depends principally on the X-ray dosage used. Doses of the order of 900–1,200 R (supralethal irradiation) produce almost complete destruction of the lymphoid and myeloid tissues with total suppression of immunologic capacity. When doses of this magnitude are used, the animal does not spontaneously recover its immunologic activity.

When lasting, but not permanent, immunosuppressive effects are sought, smaller doses of the order of 300 R (sublethal irradiation) are used. In the first hours following irradiation, inhibition of mitoses and intense destruction of the lymphocytes are observed, followed by a period of immunologic inactivity. After this period, the lymphocytes begin to proliferate and to repopulate the peripheral lymphoid organs, and the animal partially or even totally recovers its immunologic capacity. The modification in immunologic capacity can be summarized as follows:

1) *The primary immune response is depressed*, possibly even abolished, if the antigen is administered 12 h to 50 days after irradiation. The alterations in immunologic activity are manifested by a delay in the appearance of circulating antibodies; moreover, these never attain the levels normally reached in nonirradiated control animals.

2) *When the antigen is administered* a little before the irradiation, the appearance of the antibodies is slightly retarded, yet they do reach normal levels.

3) *If the immunization is performed in the period of restoration of the lymphoid system*, when the cells are proliferating actively, the circulating antibodies can reach higher than normal response levels. This phenomenon can be explained either as a nonspecific compensatory stimulation, or by the existence, in the lymphoid tissue under reconstruction, of more available space for the stimulated cellular clones. It is probable that the same reasons apply to the situation in which small doses of irradiation, of the order of 10–25 R, actually stimulate rather than inhibit the production of antibodies.

4) *Irradiation only slightly affects the secondary response*. This apparent paradox can be explained by the observation that in the secondary response there is differentiation of cells already stimulated (primed) by the antigen, a situation resembling that described when an animal is irradiated after stimulation by the antigen. Experiments suggest that the X rays affect primarily a population of lymphoid-cells of thymic origin, which regulate the proliferation and maturation of other lymphoid cell populations. The X rays act upon the immune response through their effect upon DNA; they modify its molecular arrangement with the formation of bonds between the chains of the double helix that impede the separation of the chromosomes in the anaphase. These disturbances can occur by deamination of the nitrogenized bases, by rupture of the pentose-base bonds, or by oxidation of the deoxyribose and rupture of the nucleotide chains. Consequently, there is interference with the DNA-dependent protein synthesis and blockage of cellular division. Two substances exist that under experimental conditions protect against the immunosuppressive effects of X rays: mercaptamine and B-mercaptoethylamine.

Antilymphocytic Sera

Antilymphocytic sera (ALS) are prepared by injecting into the appropriate animals – generally rabbits or horses – preparations of lymphoid cells from the thymus, spleen, lymph nodes, or even from the lymph obtained by canulation of the thoracic duct. The lymphoid cell suspension usually is injected intravenously, without Freund's adjuvant. Additional injections are administered either intravenously or subcutaneously. The antisera obtained are absorbed with washed red cells to remove traces of antierythrocytic antibodies; then the γ-globulin fractions are isolated from the absorbed serum. The antilymphocytic immunoglobulins (ALG) can agglutinate lymphocytes or lyse them in the presence of complement.

ALG contain almost exclusively antibodies for antigens of the cell surface.

Effect of ALG on Circulating Lymphocytes and Lymphoid Organs. The injection of a moderate dose of ALG is followed by an abrupt but transitory drop in the number of circulating lymphocytes. In the rat and the dog, lymphopenia is most intense after 4 h; it slowly recedes during the next 24 h until the number of lymphocytes reaches a normal level. The polymorphonuclear leukocytes are practically not affected. The prolonged administration of ALG to guinea pigs produces a more or less persistent reduction in numbers of lymphoid cells that normally populate the thymus-dependent areas of the peripheral lymphoid organs, at the same time hardly affecting the cell populations of the germinal centers of the lymph follicles (thymus-independent areas).

Antilymphocytic serum prevents or prolongs the rejection of grafts in various species of laboratory animals; it can even block second-set reactions to mouse skin grafts. Other manifestations of cellular hypersensitivity, such as hypersensitivity to dinitrochlorobenzene, may also be inhibited.

The use of ALG in clinical immunology is increasing, principally in immunosuppression in transplantation and in the treatment of severe forms of autoimmune disease. In such procedures, ALG is always used together with other immunosuppressive agents, such as corticoids, azathioprine (Imuran), and cyclophosphamide (Endoxan), with the object of reducing the doses of each to levels as far as possible below toxic limits.

Mechanisms of Immunosuppression with ALG. The mechanisms by which ALG suppresses the immune response are not yet completely understood. One such mechanism may be its cytolytic action upon the lymphocytes. Numerous investigations have shown, however, that the immunosuppressive potency of ALG is not entirely dependent upon lysing of lymphocytes, a fact that suggests the participation of other mechanisms. Among these, an antigen-receptor blockade could play a role. The principal objection to this hypothesis is that the immunosuppressive effects upon the lymphocytes are permanent, being transmitted to the descendant cells even beyond two generations. It is thus possible that we are dealing with biochemical alterations much more complicated than those of simple blockage of chemical groupings on the cellular surface. Observations suggest that the ALG acts upon the auxiliary cells of the immune response, blocking them and facilitating the action of the suppressor cells.

Prevention of Contact Between the Antigen Determinants and Receptors of Immunologically Competent Cells.
The prior injection of antibodies specific for a particular antigen can impede the production of antibodies against this antigen. A possible mechanism is that of blockage of antigenic determinants, thus preventing them from contacting the receptors localized on the membranes of immunocompetent cells. This type of immunosuppression is used for the prophylaxis of fetal erythoblastosis induced by Rh incompatibility.

Corticosteroids

Blockage of the Phagocytic Function of Macrophages, or Inhibition of "Processing" of the Antigen.
Corticosteroids (cortisone, dehydrocorticosterone, and similar agents) have been used extensively as immunosuppressive agents. These hormones inhibit even the proliferative nonspecific response in various tissues and possess lymphocytolytic activity – particularly with respect to the T lymphocytes.

Investigations of the operative mechanism of the corticosteroids have disclosed that they possess two biochemical properties particularly significant for their immunosuppressive activity: They have a stabilizing effect upon the cellular membrane and upon the lysosome membranes, along with those of other cellular organelles. In addition, they are capable of inducing the formation of adaptive enzymes. Despite the fact that little is known about the biochemical mechanisms involved in the operation of the corticosteroids, it appears that the primary site of action is glucose metabolism.

Effect on the Production of Circulating Antibodies.
The effect of the corticosteroids upon the production of circulating antibodies depends upon the dose, the species of animal, and the time at which the antigen is injected in relation to administration of cortisone. Large doses of corticosteroids (4 mg/100 g body weight), administered prior to the antigen, inhibit the production of antibodies in the rat. However, man, the monkey, and the guinea pig are much more resistant to the immunosuppressive action of corticosteroids, requiring much larger doses administered over longer periods.

Effect on Antibody-Mediated Hypersensitivities.
Corticosteroids can modify the immediate (humoral) hypersensitivity reactions either by affecting the production of immunoglobulins or by modification of the reaction resulting from the union of these immunoglobulins with the specific antigen. In both cases, the intensity of the reaction depends upon various factors, among them the animal species, the dose used, and the method of administration. Thus, the systemic anaphylactic reaction in the mouse is particularly susceptible to the suppressive action of corticosteroids, whereas in the guinea pig and in the rabbit results have been contradictory. It appears that this discrepancy in relation to the species depends, in part, upon the origin and the susceptibility of the different mediators of the anaphylactic reaction in each species. For example, in systemic anaphylaxis in the mouse, the symptoms and lesions appear to depend upon mediators localized in the lysosomes, whose membranes are stabilized by corticosteroids. Yet the same cannot be said of the guinea pig, a species extremely sensitive to the action of histamine liberated by the mastocytes during the anaphylactic reaction, a process that is

not influenced – at least not markedly so – by the corticosteroids. Corticosteroids also inhibit the production of vascular lesions in the Arthus reaction, attributed to the action of hydrolytic enzymes liberated by the lysosomes of polymorphonuclear leukocytes.

Effect on Phagocytic Activity. Although the influence of the corticosteroids upon phagocytic activity is not yet completely understood, from all indications these hormones affect the capacity of the macrophage system to eliminate particulate substances. Here again, the corticosteroids may stabilize the lysosome membranes and impede the liberation of hydrolytic enzymes into the vacuoles containing the phagocytized particles. This possible depressive action upon the phagocytic activity of macrophages could affect the induction of the immune response in at least two ways: (1) It could act through the blockage of reactions dependent upon phagocytosis or upon liberation of enzymes of lysosomal origin (Arthus reaction); or (2) it could act by affecting the "processing" of the antigen with effects on the induction phase of the immune response.

Effect on Delayed-Type Hypersensitivity Reactions. Cortisone and adrenocorticotropic hormone (ACTH) suppress the development of delayed-type reactions in previously sensitized individuals. In addition, the administration of cortisone, in elevated doses, at the time of the first injection of the immunogen or immediately thereafter, can modify the sensitization process itself. It should be pointed out, however, that doses of cortisone adequate to suppress the clinical symptomatology of eczema do not inhibit the development of the immune mechanisms presumably involved in establishing this disease.

Effect on Autoimmune Diseases. Cortisone and its analog inhibit the development of some forms of autoimmune diseases, for example that of experimental autoimmune encephalitis and that of autoimmune arthritis produced in the rat by Freund's adjuvant.

The corticosteroids are frequently used in the control of autoimmune diseases (e.g., lupus erythematosus and rheumatoid arthritis), usually in association with other immunosuppressives.

Effect on Graft-Rejection Reactions. Administration of cortisone prolongs the time required for skin or kidney graft rejection in animal species including the mouse, the guinea pig, the rabbit, and the dog; in man, high doses can suppress the rejection reaction.

Inhibition of Biosynthesis of Nucleic Acids (RNA and DNA) and of Proteins

Antigenic stimulation induces cellular multiplication and differentiation processes that involve the syntheses of nucleic acids (DNA, RNA) and proteins, and involve the participation of different enzymatic systems. At each stage of the synthesis process, intermediate products are formed, some of fundamental importance for the continuation of these same processes of synthesis. Consequently, numerous facets of the metabolic process are exposed, thus making the cells much more vulnerable to the blocking action of numerous drugs. As a result of the search for substances capable of inhibiting the growth of neoplasms (especially leukemias), a great variety of substances have been investigated for properties inhibitive of the synthesis of DNA, RNA, or proteins. Most of the substances tested are selectively toxic for cells in the process of multiplication. Since the immune response exhibits stages during which intense mitotic activity is observed – principally just after induction by the immunogen – many of these substances have been tested in relation to this response. It should be emphasized that the results, though encouraging, vary depending upon the animal species utilized for testing; this has hindered the formation of definitive conclusions regarding the operative modes of the individual substances tested.

An empirical classification of the immuno-suppressive drugs is given in Table 13.1, whereas Fig. 14.2 presents the chemical reaction steps at which these substances might act. It is beyond the scope of this book to describe all the numerous immunosuppressive drugs that have been tested thus far; however, an important example from each group is described in some detail.

Alkylating Agents. Alkylating agents have been used in experimental immunology for more than 40 years, but only since an association was established between their immunosuppressive properties and their properties toxic for cancerous cells have they been more intensely investigated.

Alkylating agents probably act upon DNA, blocking cellular mitosis. These agents have

Inhibition point
Inhibition point and incorporation of analogs

6-MP = 6-Mercaptopurine	FUDR = 5-Fluordesoxyuridine
6-TG = 6-Thioguanine	5BRU = 5-Bromuracil
AZT = Azathioprine	BUDR = 5-Bromdesoxyuridine
AZS = Azaserine	IUDR = Idoxuridine
DON = 6-Diazo-5-oxo-L-norleucine	MTX = Methotrexate
5-FU = 5-Fluoruracil	FH4 = Tetrahydrofolic acid
	FH2 = Dihydrofolic acid
	VINCA = Vincaleukoblastine

Fig. 14.2. Effect of immunosuppressive agents on biochemical reaction paths

Fig. 14.3. Mechanism of alkylating substances

high affinity for negatively charged proteins of DNA molecules, establishing bonds between the chromatids and inhibiting separation of the DNA strands in mitosis (Fig. 14.3). Guanine is the primary base for such action, which leads to (1) an altered transcription of DNA to mRNA, and (2) rupture of the glycosidic linkages of deoxyribose liberating alkylated guanine. The fact that these agents can also act upon other cellular constituents cannot be excluded; for example, they can alkylate RNA or certain proteins important for cellular multiplication (mitotic fusion proteins). These agents act selectively upon the cells that are in the process of rapid multiplication, as occurs with the T and B lymphocytes stimulated by the antigens.

The compounds called nitrogen mustards (mechlorethamine) suppress the production of antibodies for a series of antigens in various animal species when administered prior to, or at least simultaneously with, injection of the antigen. They have only a weak effect on the secondary response.

Cyclophosphamide is the transport form of nitrogen mustard. The active molecule is liberated after its enzymatic degradation in the liver. It is much more active upon the production of antibodies and upon graft rejection than are other nitrogen mustards, having the additional capability of blocking an immune response that has already been initiated.

Interesting information about the effects of cyclophosphamide at the cellular level has been obtained through comparative studies of this drug and methotrexate. It has been verified that these two drugs inhibit the development of hypersensitivity to oxazolone in guinea pigs, but that they act upon different segments of the immune response. Histologic preparations of regional lymph nodes of guinea pigs sensitized with oxazolone 2 days after the initiation of treatment with cyclophosphamide in daily 10-mg doses reveal that there is no formation of so-called large pyroninophilic cells or lymphoblasts; in contrast, in animals treated with methotrexate, blockage of the immune response appears to occur in the maturation phase of the small lymphocytes. Nitrogen mustards have an inhibitory effect on the cellular elements of bone marrow (inhibition of the formation of polymorphonuclear leukocytes). Cyclophosphamide is usually used in a dose of 5 mg/kg body weight, with its toxic effect upon the bone marrow being controlled by periodic counts of polymorphonuclear leukocytes.

Antimetabolites. The diagrams in Fig. 14.2 show the possible biochemical sites for the action of the antimetabolites cited in Table 14.1. Generally speaking, the antimetabolites are more efficient as immunosuppressives when applied after the injection of the antigen (after about 2 weeks), probably because in this period the antigen-

Azathioprine
(Imurel)

6-Mercaptopurine
(active form)

Fig. 14.4. Conversion of azathioprine to 6-mercaptopurine

induced cellular proliferation already has begun.

6-Mercaptopurine (6-MP). This purine analog blocks the formation of circulating antibodies for a series of antigens in the rabbit, the dog, the mouse, and in man. Doses effective in blocking the primary immune response are about 6 mg/kg of body weight, administered daily and intravenously; larger doses, 12–15 mg/kg body weight, usually are necessary to block the secondary response. Doses of this order also are efficient in prolonging the time required for rejection of skin transplants in the rabbit and kidney transplants in the dog. However, at this level the doses are much more toxic, which prevents more prolonged treatment.

The injection of an antigen such as bovine serum albumin into an animal under treatment with 6-MP can induce tolerance to this antigen. In experiments of this type, the proportion of animals that become tolerant rises with increasing doses of the antigen.

The immunosuppressive activities of 6-MP are due to its antimetabolic action upon purines. This can occur at various biochemical levels, including that of competitive inhibition and, probably, that of being incorporated into the nucleic acid molecules, thus being able to form, for example, a messenger RNA with an incomplete or distorted message.

Azathioprine (Imuran) is an imidazole derivative of 6-MP that is less toxic for the intestinal epithelium and for the bone marrow than the original compound, yet somehow retains its original immunosuppressive properties. Azathioprine is transformed in the liver into its active immunosuppressive form (Fig. 14.4); currently it is included in the majority of immunosuppressive protocols for the treatment of autoimmune diseases and the prevention of graft rejection. This drug must be administered in several daily doses to facilitate the regular liberation of the active form (6-MP) by the liver. Despite its low toxicity in relation to 6-MP, azathioprine can produce collateral effects such as gastrointestinal disturbances and leukopenia.

6-Thioguanine (6-TG). 6-Thioguanine is similar to 6-MP, but it acts more directly through the formation of abnormal DNA. As is the case with its congener, 6-TG also blocks the formation of circulating antibodies and has been used with relative success in the treatment of some autoimmune diseases, including hemolytic anemia, lupus erythematosus, chronic hepatitis, and hyperglobulinemic purpura. This drug has the drawback of cumulative toxic side effects, which to some extent limit its use in the prolonged immunosuppressive protocols usual in transplantation.

5-Fluorouracil (5-FU) and Analogs. Analogs of the pyrimidine bases are not often used in immunosuppression because doses that are effective in vivo are poorly tolerated. However, they have frequently been used in studies in vitro on the production of antibodie, and have given rise to important observations clarifying the cellular processes that occur during the secondary response. These compounds inhibit the production of antibodies. The fact that their effects are reversed by thymidine indicates that they are acting upon the DNA.

C1-Units for { DNA, RNA biosynthesis
               specific co-enzymes

Fig. 14.5. Mechanism of folic acid antagonists

Antagonists of Folic Acid. Aminopterin, and particularly its methylated analog methotrexate, are highly potent immunosuppressive agents that act on cellular metabolism, interfering with the conversion of folic acid to its active form, tetrahydrofolic acid (Fig. 14.5). Despite the fact that this conversion of folic acid is an essential step for many biochemical processes, including the synthesis of DNA and RNA and that of coenzymes containing purines, it still is not known whether or not this is the exclusive means by which antagonists of folic acid block the immune response. It appears, however, that the principal site of inhibition is in the interphase during the synthesis of DNA. Methotrexate acts by inhibiting the formation of large pyrininophilic cells into plasma cells or into sensitized lymphocytes (see Fig. 14.1). As usually occurs with immunosuppressive drugs, the antagonists of folic acid exhibit greater efficiency in blocking the primary response and the production of IgG. Because of its high toxicity, the use of methotrexate is severely restricted in clinical immunology.

Plant Alkaloids. Some plant alkaloids are being investigated in immunosuppression experiments. Notable, among others, are colchicine (from *Colchicum autumnale*) and the vinca alkaloids, vincristine and vinblastine (from *Vinca rosacea* and *Vinca rosea*, respectively). These three alkaloids are mitotic inhibitors that block the formation of the mitotic spindle, paralyzing cell division in metaphase. In addition, they possess lymphotoxic activity: Colchicine acts as a powerful inhibitor of phagocytosis. These pharmacologic properties could explain their immunosuppressive activities upon delayed-type hypersensitivity reactions as well as upon the production of circulating antibodies.

Antibiotics. Almost all antibiotics, even the more common ones, interfere to a lesser or greater extent with the immune response; here we consider briefly those five cited in Table 14.1. Actinomycins C and D are used principally in the study of the production of antibodies in vitro; however, due to their excessive toxicity, their use in vivo is limited. Studies of the operative mechanism of the actinomycins indicate that they form complexes with the guanine residues of the DNA molecules, impeding the subsequent formation of RNA molecules. This inhibition includes not only the formation of ribosomal RNA, but also the synthesis of messenger and transfer RNA; thus such inhibition obviously affects the synthesis of proteins.

Studies of the effects of actinomycin D upon the formation of antibodies have shown that the production of 19 S immunoglobulins is much more affected than is the production of 7 S immunoglobulins. These observations suggest that the RNA destined for 19 S antibody synthesis is especially susceptible to the action of actinomycin.

Puromycin. Puromycin was isolated from *Streptomyces alboniger* and appears to act in cellular metabolism, inhibiting the transfer of amino acids of soluble RNA to the ribosomal protein. Whereas its use in vivo is limited because of its high toxicity, it has been used in some systems in vitro, behaving as a powerful blocker of antibody production. Puromycin is also efficacious in systems in which the formation of antibodies is underway, having the further advantage of not killing the cells.

Chloramphenicol. Chloramphenicol was originally isolated from *Stréptomyces venezuelae;* later it became the first antibiotic to be synthesized. It impedes the transfer of amino acids to the ribosomes by competing, preferentially, for the sites that receive the amino acids.

In relatively high doses, chloramphenicol inhibits the primary response in vivo. Used in cell cultures, it also impedes the secondary response when it has been placed in the culture medium together with the immunogen, but little or no effect is observed if the cells have already begun producing immunoglobulins.

Azaserine. Azaserine is an antibiotic produced by *Streptomyces fragilis* that functions as an analog of glutamine for bacteria and probably as an alkylating agent for animal cells. When used alone, it has almost no immunosuppressive effect, but it has been often used in transplants in association with azathioprine.

Amino Acid Antagonists. The antagonists of amino acids have only recently been used in immunosuppression. L-Asparaginase, for example, catalyzes the hydrolysis of the L-asparagine in aspartic acid and ammonia, thereby indirectly inhibiting the production of antibodies in the mouse for antigens on the surfaces of sheep erythrocytes, blocking the blastogenic response of the lymphocytes to phytohemagglutinin. In doses of 25,000–50,000 IU per day, it suppresses in man the production of antibodies against hemocyanin.

Specific Tolerance

Suppression of the immune response by a feedback mechanism and by induction of tolerance represent two specific immunosuppressive courses of action. By these methods, one can determine which antibodies can be inhibited. The basic mechanism involved in these forms of immunosuppression is not yet understood.

The immunosuppressive agents described thus far act, as we have seen, indiscriminately, blocking or damaging all the cells that happen to be in mitosis, i.e., also normally functioning cells that are particularly important to the organism's survival.

The immune response, characterized at the cellular level by a sequence of divisions and by specifically oriented cellular differentiations, must possess some strategically located mechanism that brings the cell either to a state of immunologic activity (production of antibodies, development of sensitized lymphocytes), or to a state of specific non-reactivity (tolerance). It is probable that, once the biochemical mechanisms involved in this mechanism are understood, agents will be developed that can specifically paralyze it or cause it to induce tolerance.

Rules for Immunosuppression

Immunosuppressive experiments in laboratory animals have permitted the formulation of generalizations that can provide an orientation for the use of immunosuppressive agents in clinical immunology:

1) When the proper doses of the immunosuppressive agent are used and applied at the optimum time with respect to the introduction of the antigen, one can obtain
a) Prevention of the primary and secondary humoral immune responses
b) Induction of immunologic tolerance
c) Prolongation of the period of IgM production, thereby inhibiting the formation of IgG
d) An increase in the formation of antibodies
e) Suppression of delayed-type hypersensitivity.
2) The nearer the dosage of the drug comes to its toxic limit, the greater its immunosuppressive action becomes.
3) Antimetabolites are more active when employed in the induction period of the immune response. Whereas alkylating substances function better in the preinduction phase.

4) After the formation of antibodies has begun, much higher immunosuppressive doses, generally toxic, are required for its suppression.
5) The primary response is more sensitive to the action of immunosuppressive drugs than is the secondary response.
6) It is much easier to block the development of a delayed immune response than it is to alter the manifestation of an already established lesion.
7) Any time the administration of the immunosuppressive is stopped before the antigen is totally catabolized, a subsequent immune response can occur.

References

Bach JF (1975) The mode of action of immunosuppressive agents. North Holland Amsterdam
Cortesini R (ed) (1979) Modulation of immunologic responsiveness. Transplant Proc 11:839
Fauci AS, Dale DC, Balow JE (1976) Glucocorticosteroid therapy: Mechanisms of action and clinical considerations. Ann Intern Med 84:304
Gerber NL, Steinberg AD (1976) Clinical use of immunosuppressive drugs (2 parts). Drugs 11:14, 90
Kaplan SR, Calabresi P (1973) Immunosuppressive agents (2 parts). N Engl J Med 289:952, 1234
Lance EM, Medawar PB, Taub RN (1973) Antilymphocytic serum. Adv Immunol 17:2
Parker CW, Vaura JD (1974) Immunosuppression. Prog Hematol 6:1
Schein PS, Winokur SH (1975) Immunosuppressive and cytotoxic chemotherapy: Long term complications. Ann Intern Med 82:84
Winkelstein A (1977) Effects of immunosuppressive drugs on T and B lymphocytes. Blood 50:81

Brief History of Important Immunologic Discoveries and Developments

Year	Event	Author(s)
1798	Cowpox vaccination	Edward Jenner
1866	Wound disinfection	Joseph Lister
1876	Discovery of *B. antracis*, foundation of bacteriology	Robert Koch
1880	Discovery of attenuated vaccine by invitro passages	Louis Pasteur
1883	Phagocytosis, cellular immunity theory	Elie I. I. Metchnikoff
1888	Discovery of bacterial toxins	P. P. Emile Roux and Alexandre E. J. Yersin
1890	Discovery of antitoxins, foundation of serotherapy	Emil A. von Behring and Shibasaburo Kitasato
1894	Immunologic bacteriolysis	Richard F. J. Pfeiffer and Vasily I. Isaeff
1894	Discovery of antibody and complement activity as the active factors in bacteriolysis	Jules J. B. V. Bordet
1896	Discovery of specific agglutination	Herbert E. Durham and Max von Gruber
1896	Agglutination test for the diagnosis of typhoid (Widal test)	Georges F. I. Widal and Arthur Sicard
1900	Formulation of side-chain theory of antibody formation	Paul Ehrlich
1900	Discovery of A, B, 0 blood groups	Karl Landsteiner
1900	Development of complement fixation reaction	Jules J. B. V. Bordet and Octave Gengou
1902	Discovery of anaphylaxis	Charles R. Richet and Paul Portier
1903	Local anaphylaxis due to antibody-antigen complex: Arthus reaction	Nicholas M. Arthus
1903	Discovery of opsonization	Almroth E. Wright and Steward R. Douglas

Year	Event	Author(s)
1905	Description of serum sickness	Clemens von Pirquet and Bela Schick
1910	Introduction of salvarsan, later neo-salvarsan, foundation of chemotherapy of infections	Paul Ehrlich and Sahachiro Hata
1910	Development of anaphylaxis test (Schultz-Dale)	William Schultz
1914	Formulation of genetic theory of tumor transplantation	Clarence C. Little
1921	Experimental trial with BCG vaccine	Albert L. C. Calmette and Camille Guérin
1921	Development of cutaneous anaphylactic reaction	Carl W. Prausnitz and Heinz Küstner
1923	Production of anatoxin (toxoid) by formaldehyde treatment	Ramon Gaston
1928	Discovery of penicillin, the first antibiotic	Alexander Fleming
1935	Discovery of sulfonamides for chemotherapy of infections	Gerhard Domagk
1935	Discovery of local immunity; oral vaccination	Alexandre Besredka
1935–36	Purification of antibodies, quantitative precipitation reaction	Michael Heidelberger and Forrest E. Kendall
1937	Evidence for identity of the gene for blood group antigen II with one gene for tumor resistance in the mouse (*H–2*)	Peter A. Gorer
1938	Evidence that antibodies are γ-globulins	Arne Tiselius and Elvin A. Kabat
1942	Discovery of cellular transfer of delayed type hypersensitivity in guinea pigs	Karl Landsteiner and Merrill W. Chase
1942	Fluorescence labeling of antibodies and antigens	Albert H. Coons
1942	Introduction of adjuvants	Jules T. Freund
1943–44	Establishment of immunologic basis of rejection of normal tissue transplants	Peter B. Medawar
1944	Theory of acquired immunologic tolerance	Peter B. Medawar and Frank M. Burnet
1946–48	Theory of congenic mouse lines formulated, first congenic lines initiated, and the term histocompatibility introduced	George D. Snell

Year	Event	Author(s)
1945	Development of antiglobulin test for incomplete Rh antibodies	Robin R. A. Coombs, R. R. Race, and A. E. Mourant
1945	Description of tolerance (chimerism) in dizygotic cattle twins	R. D. Owen
1946	Development of precipitin test in gels	Jaques Oudin
1947	Immunoglobulins as "transporteurs"	Pierre Grabar
1948	Development of double immunodiffusion test in gels	Örjan Ouchterlony and Stephen D. Elek
1948	Discovery of plasma cells as antibody producing cells	Astrid E. Fagraeus
1949	Elucidation of the structure of A, B, 0 blood group antigens	Elvin A. Kabat, W. T. J. Morgan, and W. M. Watkins
1952	Description of agammaglobulinemia in human	Ogdon Carr Bruton
1952	Discovery of histamine in mast cells	James F. Riley and Geoffrey B. West
1953	Development of immunoelectrophoresis	Pierre Grabar
1953	Experimental evidence of acquired immunologic tolerance	Milan Hašek
1956	Major histocompatibility (H–2) complex in the mouse defined	George D. Snell
1956	Discovery of human leukocyte antigen, later be shown to belong to the major histocompatibility complex of man (HLA)	Jean Dausset
1956	Experimental induction of autoimmunity	Ernest Witebsky and Noel R. Rose
1956	Discovery of allotypes	Rune Grubb and Jaques Oudin
1957	Discovery of interferon	Jean Lindemann and Alick Isaacs
1957	Discovery of macroglobulins with anti-body activity	H. Hugh Fudenberg and Henry G. Kunkel
1957	Discovery of Australia antigen, later shown to be Hepatitis B antigen	Baruch Blumberg
1957	Discovery of human slow virus infection (Kuru)	Carleton Gajdusek
1959	Introduction of the radioimmune assay	Rosalyn Yalow and Solomon A. Berson
1960	Antibody structure	Alfred Nisonoff, Gerald Edelman, Rodney P. Porter, Henry G. Kunkel

Year	Event	Author(s)
1961	Discovery of the thymus as part of the immune system	Jaques F. A. P. Miller, Robert A. Good
1963	Development of the plaque formation test	Nils K. Jerne, Richard J. Henry, Albert A. Nordin
1963	Ss Locus in the H–2 complex discovered coding for the C4-complement component	Donald C. Shreffler
1964	Development of rosette-test	G. Biozzi
1965	Discovery of the variable region of antibody molecules	Norbert Hilschmann
1965	Linkage of MLR reactivity to the HLA complex discovered	Fritz Bach, Kurt Hirschhorn
1965	Immune response-1 (Ir-1) locus in the mouse discovered	Hugh O. McDevitt and Michael Sela
1966	Enzyme labeling of antibodies and antigens	S. Avremeas
1966	Discovery of IgE as reaginic antibody	Kimishige Ishizaka
1969	Thymus function defined, dichotomy of the immune system discovered	Jaques F. A. P. Miller and Graham Mitchell
1969	H–2 antigen isolated	Stanley G. Nathenson and Akira Shimada
1969	T helper function in antibody formation described (T-B Collaboration)	N. Avrion Mitchison
1969	B lymphocytes as cells with surface-bound Ig discovered	Benvenuto Pernis
1969	Discovery of idiotypes	Jaques Oudin
1971–72	Cytotoxic T cells described	Jean-Charles Cerrotini, K. Theodor Brunner, Peter Perlmann, Hermann Wagner
1971	Discovery of *MLR* locus linked to *HLA* in man	Edmond J. Yunis and Bernhard Amos
1971	Two-locus model of the mouse *MHC* (*H–2*) formulated	George D. Snell, Jan Klein, Donald C. Shreffler, Jack Stimpfling
1971	T and B cell tolerance defined	Jaques Chiller
1972	T suppressor cells described	Richard K. Gershon
1972	Discovery of *MHC*-restriction of T cell dependent immune responses	Berenice Kindred and Donald C. Shreffler
1973	Discovery of Ia antigens	Chella S. David, Donald C. Shreffler, Jan Klein, Dietrich Götze, David H. Sachs

Year	Event	Author(s)
1973	T-B cell collaboration *I* region restricted	David H. Katz and Baruch Benacerraf
1974	Idiotypic network theory formulated	Nils K. Jerne
1974	K,D-restriction of cytotoxic T cells discovered	Peter Doherty and Rolf Zinkernagel
1975	Fusion of myeloma cells with normal, specific antibody-producing plasma cells (hybridoma)	George Köhler and Cesar Milstein
1978	Structure of MHC (H–2 and HLA) antigens defined	Stanley G. Nathenson, Jack Strominger
1978	Macrophage-T cell collaboration *I*-region restricted	Jonathan Sprent
1978–80	Elucidation of immunoglobulin genes; generation of diversity is (almost) solved	Suzuma Tonegawa
1980	Smallpox worldwide eradicated	World Health Organization (WHO)

Glossary of Immunologic Terms

Accessory cells. Lymphoid cells predominantly of the monocyte and macrophage lineage which cooperate with T and B lymphocytes in immune reactions

Acquired immunity. Immunity that develops as a result of exposure to a foreigne substrate

Activated lymphocytes. Lymphocytes that have been stimulated by specific antigen or nonspecific mitogen

Adoptive transfer. Transfer of immunity by immunocompetent cells from one animal to another

Affinity. Binding strength between antibody and antigen in an antibody-antigen reaction

Agglutination. An antibody-antigen reaction in which a solid or particulate antigen forms a lattice with a soluble antibody

Allelic exclusion. The phenotypic expression of a single allele in cells containing 2 different alleles for that genetic locus

Allergens. Antigens which give rise to allergic sensitization by IgE antibodies

Allergy. An overshouting hypersensitivity reaction

Allogeneic. Denotes the relationship which exists between genetically dissimilar members of the same species

Allograft. A tissue or organ graft between two genetically dissimilar members of the same species

Allotype. The genetically determined antigenic difference on molecules, varying in different members of the same species

Anamnesis (immunologic memory). A heightened responsiveness to the second or subsequent administration of antigen to an immune animal

Anaphylatoxin. A substance produced by complement activation which causes an increased vascular permeability through the release of pharmacologically active mediators from mast cells

Anaphylaxis. A reaction of immediate hypersensitivity present in nearly all vertebrates which results from sensitization of tissue-fixed mast cells by cytotropic antibodies following exposure to antigen

Anergy. The inability to react to an antigen (microorganism)

Antibody. A protein that is produced as a result of the introduction of an antigen and which has the ability to combine with the antigen that stimulated its production

Antibody combining site. That configuration present on an antibody molecule which links with a corresponding antigenic determinant

Antibody-dependent cell-mediated cytotoxicity (ADCC). A form of lymphocyte-mediated cytotoxicity in which an effector cell kills an antibody-coated target cell

Anticomplementarity. Unspecific complement activation, i.e., not due to antibody-antigen reaction

Antigen. A substance which can induce a detectable immune response when introduced into an animal

Antigenic determinant (epitope). That area of an antigen which determines the specificity of the antigen-antibody reaction

Antigenicity. Property of a substance to react with an antibody, but not necessarily to induce its formation

Antigen processing. The series of events which occurs following antigen administration until antibody production

Antiglobulin test (Coombs' test). A technic to detect cell-bound immunoglobulin. In the direct Coombs' test, red blood cells taken directly from a sensitized individual are agglutinated by antigammaglobulin antibodies. In the indirect Coombs' test, a patient's serum is incubated with test red blood cells and the sensitized cells are then agglutinated with an anti-immunoglobulin or with Coombs reagent

Antitoxins. Protective antibodies which inactivate soluble toxic proteins of bacteria

Atopy. A genetically determined abnormal state of hypersensitivity as distinguished from hypersensitivity responses in normal individuals

Attenuated. Rendered less virulent

Autoantibody. Antibody to self antigen

Autoantigens. Self antigens

Autograft. A tissue graft between genetically identical members of the same species

Avidity. Refers broadly to the ability of antibodies to bind to antigens. (Affinity is a more precisely used term referring to activity per antibody-combining site)

Basement membrane. A sheet of material up to $0.2\,\mu$ thick lying immediately below epithelial (and endothelial) cells and supporting them. Contains glycoproteins and collagen and to some extent acts as a diffusion barrier for microorganisms. Thickness and structure varies in different parts of the body

B cell (B lymphocyte). Strictly a bursa-derived cell in avian species and, by analogy, bursa-equivalent derived cells in nonavian species. B cells are the precursors of plasma cells that produce antibody

BCG (bacillus Calmette-Guérin). A viable attenuated strain of *Mycobacterium bovis* which has been obtained by progressive reduction of virulence and which confers immunitiy to mycobacterial infection and possibly possesses anticancer activity in selected diseases

Bence-Jones proteins. Monoclonal light chains present in the urine of patients with paraproteinemic disorders

Blast cell. A large lymphocyte or other immature cell containing a nucleus with loosely packed chromatin, a large nucleolus, and a large amount of cytoplasm with numerous polyribosomes

Blocking factors (antibody). Substances that are present in the serum of tumor-bearing animals and are capable of blocking the ability of immune lymphocytes to kill tumor cells

Blood groups. Antigens present at the surface of red blood cells which may vary between individuals of the same species. The most important blood groups in man are the ABO and the Rh blood groups

Bone marrow. Soft connective tissue located in the cavities of the bones

Bone marrow-derived cell. A lymphoid cell present in one of the lymphoid organs which originated in the bone marrow and escaped the influence of the thymus

Bursa of Fabricius. The hindgut organ located in the cloaca of birds which controls the ontogeny of B lymphocytes

Bursal equivalent. Hypothetical organ or organs analogous to the bursa of Fabricius in nonavian species

C. The abbreviation for serum complement

Capping. The movement of cell surface antigens toward one pole of a cell after the antigens are cross-linked by specific antibody

Cardiolipin. A substance derived from beef heart, probably a component of mitochondrial membranes, which serves as an antigenic substrate for reagin or antitreponemal antibody

Carrier. An immunogenic substance which, when coupled to a hapten, renders the hapten immunogenic

Cell-mediated immunity. Immunity in which the participation of lymphocytes and macrophages is predominant

Cell-mediated lymphocytolysis. An in vitro assay for cellular immunity in which a standard mixed lymphocyte reaction is followed by destruction of target cells which are used to sensitize allogeneic cells during the MLC

CH_{50} unit. The quantity or dilution of serum required to lyse 50% of the red blood cells in a standard hemolytic complement assay

Chemotaxis. A process whereby phagocytic cells are attracted to the vicinity of invading pathogens

Classical complement pathway. A series of enzyme-substrate and protein-protein interactions which ultimately leads to biologically active complement enzymes. It proceeds sequentially C 1, 423, 567, 89

Clonal selection theory. The theory of antibody synthesis proposed by Burnet which predicts that the individual carries a complement of clones of lymphoid cells which are capable of reacting with all possible antigenic determinants. The antigens which actually come in contact with the organism select "their" clones; these clones differentiate and expand

Clone. A group of cells all of which are the progeny of a single cell

Cold agglutinins. Antibodies which agglutinate bacteria or erythrocytes more efficiently at temperatures below 37 °C than at 37 °C

Committed cell. Antigen-specifically sensitized lymphocytes

Complement. A system of serum proteins which is the primary humoral mediator of antigen-antibody reactions

Complement fixation. A standard serologic assay used for the detection of an antigen-antibody reaction in which complement is fixed as a result of the formation of an immune complex. The subsequent failure of lysis of sensitized red blood cells by complement which has been fixed indicates the degree of antigen-antibody reaction

Concanavalin A (ConA). A lectin which is derived from the jack bean and which stimulates predominantly T lymphocytes

Congenic. (originally called **congenic resistant**) Denotes a line of mice identical or nearly identical with other inbred strains except for the substitution at one locus of a foreign allele introduced by appropriate crosses with a second inbred strain

Coombs' test. See antiglobulin test

C region (constant region). The carboxyl terminal portion of the H or L chain which is identical in immunoglobulin molecules of a given class and subclass apart from genetic polymorphisms

Cross-reaction. The reaction of an antibody with an antigen other than the one which induced its formation

Cytotoxic antibody. Antibody which reacts with antigens present on a cell surface and which produces damage to that cell or its surface

Cytotoxic T lymphocytes (CTL). Thymus-derived lymphocytes with the ability to lyse complement-independently target cells against which they have been specifically sensitized

Cytotropic antibodies. Antibodies of the IgG and IgE classes which sensitize cells for subsequent anaphylaxis

Defective virus replication. Incomplete virus replication, with production only of viral nucleic acid, proteins or non-infectious virus particles

Degranulation. A process whereby cytoplasmic granules of phagocytic cells fuse with phagosomes and discharge their contents into the phagolysosome thus formed

Delayed hypersensitivity. A cell-mediated immune reaction which can be elicited by subcutaneous injection of antigen, with a subsequent cellular infiltrate and edema which are maximal between 24 and 28 h after antigen challenge

Diapedesis. The outward passage of cells through intact vessel walls

Direct immunofluorescence. The detection of antigens by fluorescently labeled antibody

Diversity. Multitude of different antigen-specific combining sites (V_H and V_L regions)

Domains. Segments of H or L chains that are folded 3-dimensionally and stabilized with disulfide bonds

EAC rosette. Formation of a cluster of red cells (*e*rythrocytes) sensitized with *a*ntibody and *c*omplement around human B lymphocytes

Eczema. A skin eruption common to atopic persons, with characteristic itching, inflammation and swelling

Effector cells. Usually denotes T cells capable of mediating cytotoxicity, suppression, or helper function

Encapsulation. A quasi-immunologic phenomenon in which foreign material is walled off within the tissues of invertebrates

Endocytosis. The process whereby material external to a cell is internalized within a particular cell. It consists of pinocytosis and phagocytosis

Endotoxins. Lipopolysaccharides which are derived from the cell walls of gram-negative microorganisms and have toxic and pyrogenic effects when injected in vivo

Enhancement. Improved survival of tumor cells in animals which have been previously immunized to the antigens of a given tumor

Epitope. The simplest form of an antigenic determinant present on a complex antigenic molecule

Equivalence. A ratio of antigen-antibody concentration where maximal precipitation occurs

E rosette. Formation of a cluster (rosette) of cells consisting of sheep erythrocytes surrounded by bound human T lymphocytes

Erythroblastosis fetalis. The medical term for Rh incompatibility disease of the newborn

Euglobulin. Class of globulins which are insoluble in water, but soluble in salt solution

Exotoxins. Diffusible toxins produced by certain gram-positive and gram-negative microorganisms

Fab. Antigen-binding fragment produced by enzymatic digestion of an IgG molecule with papain

F(ab')$_2$. Fragment obtained by pepsin digestion of immunoglobulin molecules containing the 2 H and 2 L chains linked by disulfide bonds. It contains antigen-binding activity. An F(ab')$_2$ fragment and an Fc fragment comprise an entire monomeric immunoglobulin molecule

Fc fragment. Crystallizable fragment obtained by papain digestion of IgG molecules. Fc fragment consists of the C-terminal half of 2 H chains linked by disulfide bonds. Contains no antigen-binding capability but determines important biologic characteristics of the intact molecule

Fc receptor. A receptor present on various subclasses of lymphocytes for the Fc fragment of immunoglobulins

F_1 generation. The first generation of offspring after a designated mating

F_2 generation. The second generation of offspring after a designated mating

Fluorescence. The emission of light of one color while a substance is irradiated with a light of a different color

Forssman-antigen, -antibody. So-called heterophil antigen that can be demonstrated on tissue cells of different species, e.g., horse, sheep, mouse a.o., but is absent from tissue of human and rabbit. Forssman-antibodies are present as "natural antibodies" in the serum of man, and agglutinate red blood cells, e.g., of sheep

Freund's complete adjuvant (FCA). An oil-water emulsion which contains killed mycobacteria and enhances immune responses when mixed in an emulsion with antigen

Freund's incomplete adjuvant. Contains all of the elements of Freund's complete adjuvant with the exception of killed mycobacteria

Gamma globulins. Serum proteins with gamma mobility in electrophoresis which comprise the majority of immunoglobulins

Gammopathy. Paraprotein disorder involving abnormalities of immunoglobulins

Genetic switch hypothesis. A hypothesis which postulates that there is a switch in the gene controlling heavy chain synthesis in plasma cells during the development of an immune response

Germinal centers. A collection of metabolically active lymphoblasts, macrophages, and plasma cells which appears within the primary follicle of lymphoid tissues following antigenic stimulation

Glomerulonephritis. An autoimmune disease in which the major damage is to the glomeruli of the kidney

Gm marker. Allotypic determinant on the heavy chain of human IgG

Graft rejection. A cell-mediated immune reaction elicited by the grafting of genetically dissimilar tissue onto a recipient. The reaction leads to destruction and ultimate rejection of the transplanted tissue

Graft-versus-host (GVH reaction). The clinical and phatologic sequelae of the reactions of immunocompetent cells in a graft against the cells of the histoincompatible and immunodeficient recipient

Gram-negative. Losing the primary violet or blue during decolorization in Gram's staining method

Gram-positive. Retaining the primary violet or blue stain in Gram's method

Granuloma. A local accumulation of densely packed macrophages, often fusing to form giant cells and sometimes together with lymphocytes and plasma cells. Seen in chronic infections such as tuberculosis and syphilis

Granulopoietin (Colony-stimulating factor). A glycoprotein with a molecular weight of 45,000 derived from monocytes which controls the production of granulocytes by the bone marrow

H-2 locus. The major histocompatibility complex (MHC) in the mouse

Haplotype. That portion of the phenotype determined by closely linked genes of a single chromosome inherited from one parent

Hapten. A substance which is not immunogenic but can react with an antibody of appropriate specificity

Hassall's corpuscles. Whorls of thymic epithelial cells whose function is unknown

HB antigen. Hepatitis B virus antigen detectable in serum of infected though not necessarily sick individuals

Hay fever. A seasonal allergic disease causing inflammation of the eyes and nasal passages

H chain (heavy chain). One pair of identical polypeptide chains making up an immunoglobulin molecule. The heavy chain contains approximately twice the number of amino acids and is twice the molecular weight of the light chain

Heavy chain diseases. A heterogeneous group of paraprotein disorders characterized by the presence of monoclonal but incomplete heavy chains without light chains in serum or urine

Helper T cells. A subtype of T lymphocytes which cooperate with B cells in antibody formation

Hemagglutination inhibition. A technic for detecting small amounts of antigen in which homologous antigen inhibits the agglutination of red cells or other particles coated with antigen by specific antibody

Hematopoietic system. All tissues responsible for production of the cellular elements of peripheral blood

Hemolysin. Antibody or other substance capable of lysing red blood cells

Heterocytotropic antibodies. Antibody which can passively sensitize tissues of species other than those in which the antibody is present

Heterologous antigen. An antigen which participates in a cross-reaction

High dose (high zone) tolerance. Classical immunologic unresponsiveness produced by repeated injections of large amounts of antigen

Hinge region. The area of the H chains in the C region between the first and second C region domains. It is the site of enzymatic cleavage into $F(ab')_2$ and Fc fragments

Histocompatible. Sharing transplantation antigens

HLA (human leukocyte antigen). The major histocompatibility complex in man

Homocytotropic antibody. Antibody which attaches to cells of animals of the same species

Homologous antigen. An antigen which induces an antibody and reacts specifically with it

Homozygous typing cells (HTC). Cells that carry the same allele at their two HLA-D loci (homozygous) which are used as stimulating cells in mixed lymphocyte cultures for the typing of HLA-D phenotypes

Horizontal transmission. The transmission of infection from individual to individual in a population rather than from parent to offspring

Hot antigen suicide. A technic in which an antigen is labeled with high-specific-activity radioisotope (^{131}I). Used either in vivo or in vitro to inhibit specific lymphocyte function by attachment to an antigen-binding lymphocyte, subsequently killing it by radiolysis

Humoral. Pertaining to molecules in solution in a body fluid, particularly antibody and complement

Hybridoma. Specific antibodies secreting *hybrid* cells obtained by fusion of plasma cells with mye*loma* cells

Hypersensitivity. The state, existing in a previously immunized individual, in which tissue damage results from the immune reaction to a further dose of antigen. If tissue damage is severe, the condition may be referred to as one form of allergy

Hypervariable regions. At least 4 regions of extreme variability which occur throughout the V region of H and L chains and which determine the antibody combining site of an antibody molecule

Hypogammaglobulinemia (agammaglobulinemia). Deficiency of all major classes of serum immunoglobulins

Ia antigens (I region-associated antigens). Antigens which are controlled by Ir genes and are present on lymphocytes and macrophages

Idiotope. An epitope of the antigen-binding site of an antibody

Idiotype. Unique antigenic determinants present on homogeneous antibody or myeloma protein. The idiotype appears to represent the antigenicity of the antigen-binding site of an antibody and is therefore located in the V region

IgA. Predominant immunoglobulin class present in secretions

IgD. Predominant immunoglobulin class present on human B lymphocytes

IgE. Reaginic antibody involved in immediate hypersensitivity reactions

IgG. Predominant immunoglobulin class present in human serum

IgM. A pentameric immunoglobulin comprising approximately 10% of normal human serum immunoglobulins, with a molecular weight of 900,000 and a sedimentation coefficient of 19 S

7S IgM. A monomeric IgM consisting of one monomer of 5 identical subunits

Immediate hypersensitivity. An immunologic sensitivity to antigens that manifests itself by tissue reactions occurring within minutes after the antigen combines with its appropriate antibody

Immune complexes. Antigen-antibody complexes

Immune elimination. The enhanced clearance of an injected antigen from the circulation as a result of immunity to that antigen brought about by enhanced phagocytosis of the reticuloendothelial system

Immune response genes (Ir genes). Genes which control immune responses to specific antigens

Immune surveillance. A theory which holds that the immune system destroys tumor cells, which are constantly arising during the life of the individual

Immunodominant. That antigenic determinant of an antigen which is dominant in eliciting antibody formation

Immunoelectrophoresis. A technic combining an initial electrophoretic separation of proteins followed by immunodiffusion with resultant precipitation arcs

Immunofluorescence. A histo- or cytochemical technic for the detection and localization of antigens in which specific antibody is conjugated with fluorescent compounds, resulting in a sensitive tracer which can be detected by fluorometric measurements

Immunogen. A substance which, when introduced into an animal, stimulates the immune response

Immunogenicity. Property of a substance making it capable of inducing a detectable immune response

Immunoglobulin. A glycoprotein composed of H and L chains which functions as antibody. All antibodies are immunoglobulins, but it is not certain that all immunoglobulins have antibody function

Imunoglobulin class. A subdivision of immunoglobulin molecules based on structural and unique antigenic differences in the C regions of the H chains. In man there are 5 classes of immunoglobulins designated IgG, IgA, IgM, IgD, and IgE

Immunoglobulin subclass. A subdivision of the classes of immunoglobulins based on structural and antigenic differences in the H chains. For human IgG there are 4 subclasses: IgG 1, IgG 2, IgG 3, and IgG 4

Immunopathology. Pathological changes partly or completely caused by the immune response

Immunosuppression. Suppression of immune responsiveness by irradiation, drugs, or microbial toxins

Immune tolerance. An immunologically specific reduction in immune responsiveness to a given antigen

Interferon. A heterogeneous group of low-molecular-weight proteins elaborated by infected host cells which protect noninfected cells from viral infection

Inv marker. See Km marker

I region. That portion of the major histocompatibility complex which contains genes that control immune responses

Ir genes. See Immune response genes

J chain. A glycopeptide chain which is normally found in polymeric immunoglobulins, particularly IgA and IgM

Joining. Linking together DNA segments (introns) of genes in somatic cells which are separated by non-translated DNA sequences (exons) in the germ line

Kappa (κ) chains. One of 2 major types of L chains

K cell. Killer cell responsible for antibody-dependent cell-mediated cytotoxicity

K and D regions. Genetic loci in the major histocompatibility complex of the mouse, coding for H-2 molecules which are the restricting elements of cytotoxic T cells

Kinin. A peptide that increases vascular permeability and is formed by the action of esterases on kallikreins, which then act as vasodilators

Km marker (also called **Inv**). Allotypic marker on the κ L chain of human immunoglobulins

Koch phenomenon. Delayed hypersensitivity reaction by tuberculin in the skin of a guinea pig following infection with *Mycobacterium tuberculosis*

Kupffer cells. Fixed mononuclear phagocytes of the reticuloendothelial system that are present within the sinusoids of the liver

Lambda (λ) chain. One of 2 major types of L chains

Latency. Stage of persistent infection in which microorganism causes no disease, but remains capable of activation and disease production

Latex fixation test. An agglutination reaction in which latex particles are used to passively adsorb soluble protein and polysaccharide antigens

LATS (long-acting thyroid stimulator). An antibody reacting with the thyroid stimulating hormone (TSH) receptor in the thyroid gland; this antibody is present in about 45% of patients with hyperthyroidism and causes delayed uptake of iodine in an animal assay system

LE cell phenomenon. Phagocytic leukocytes that have engulfed DNA, immunoglobulin, and complement and are present as a large homogeneous mass which is extruded from a damaged lymphocyte in systemic lupus erythematosus and other rheumatoid diseases

Lectin. A substance that is derived from a plant and has panagglutinating activity for red blood cells. Lectins are commonly mitogens as well

Leishmaniasis. Disease caused by protozoa of genus *Leishmania*, e.g. cutaneous leishmaniasis (oriental sore) or generalized leishmaniasis (kala-azar)

Leukocyte inhibitory factor (LIF). A lymphokine which inhibits the migration of polymorphonuclear leukocytes

Leukocyte mitogenic factor (LMF). A lymphokine that will induce normal lymphocytes to undergo blast transformation and DNA synthesis

Leucocytes. Circulating white blood cells. There are about 9,000/mm³ in human blood, divided into granulocytes (polymorphs 68%–70% eosinophils 3% basophils 0.5%) and mononuclear cells (monocytes 4% lymphocytes 23–25%)

Light chain (L chain). Polypeptide chain present in all immunoglobulin molecules. Two types exist in most species and are termed kappa (κ) and lambda (λ)

Linkage disequilibrium. When alleles of two closely linked loci are found together more frequently than predicted by their individual gene frequencies

Lipopolysaccharide (also called endotoxin). A compound derived from a variety of gram-negative enteric bacteria which have various biologic functions including mitogenic activity for B lymphocytes

Low dose (low zone) tolerance. A state of tolerance induced with small subimmunogenic doses of soluble antigen

Lupus erythematosus. A fatal autoimmune disease, characterized by certain antinuclear antibodies

Ly antigens. Differentiation antigens present on thymocytes and peripheral T cells

Lymph nodes. Small pea-sized organs distributed widely throughout the body which are composed mostly of lymphoid cells

Lymphocyte. A mononuclear cell 7–12 μm in diameter containing a nucleus with densely packed chromatin and a small rim of cytoplasm

Lymphocyte activation (lymphocyte stimulation, lymphocyte transformation, or blastogenesis). An in vitro technic in which lymphocytes are stimulatedto become metabolically active by antigen or mitogen

Lymphocyte defined (LD) antigens. A series of histocompatibility antigens that are present on the majority of mammalian cells and detectable primarily by reactivity in the mixed lymphocyte reaction (MLR)

Lymphokine. Soluble factor released by primed lymphocyte on contact with specific antigen

Lysosome. Cytoplasmic sac present in many cells, bounded by a lipoprotein membrane and containing various enzymes. Plays an important part in intracellular digestion

Lysostrip. Removal of one kind of surface antigen by capping with subsequent reaction of the same cells with antibodies and complement to another kind of surface antigen. Employed for the demonstration of antigenic determinants on the same or different molecules

Lysozyme. An enzyme present in the granules of polymorphs, in macrophages, in tears, mucus and saliva. It lyses certain bacteria, especially gram-positive cocci, splitting the muramic acid-β (1-4)-N-acetylglucosamine linkage in the bacterial cell wall. It potentiates the action of complement on these bacteria

Macrophage activation factor (MAF). A lymphokine which will activate macrophages to become avid phagocytic cells

Macrophage chemotactic factor (MCF). A lymphokine which selectively attracts monocytes or macrophages to the area of its release

Macrophages. Phagocytic mononuclear cells that derive from bone marrow monocytes and subserve accessory roles in cellular immunity

Macrophage processing. Uptake of antigens by macrophages, especially in the form of large particles or microorganisms, and preparation of antigen or antigens for delivery to adjacent immunocompetent lymphoytes

Major histocompatibility complex (MHC). An as yet undetermined number of genes located in close proximity which determine histocompatibility antigens of members of a species

Mast cell. A tissue cell which resembles a peripheral blood basophil and contains granules with serotonin and histamine present

Memory cells. Sensitized cells generated during an immune response, and surviving in large enough numbers to give an accelerated immune response on challenge

β_2 Microglobulin. A protein (MW 11,600) that is associated with the outer membrane of many cells, including lymphocytes, and which may function as a structural part of the histocompatibility antigens on cells

Migration inhibitory factor (MIF). A lymphokine which is capable of inhibiting the migration of macrophages

Mitogens (also called **phytomitogens**). Substances which cause DNA synthesis, blast transformation, and ultimately division of lymphocytes

Mixed lymphocyte culture (mixed leukocyte culture) (MLC). An in vitro test for cellular immunity in which lymphocytes or leukocytes from different individuals are mixed and mutually stimulate DNA synthesis

Mixed lymphocyte reaction (MLR). See Mixed lymphocyte culture

Monoclonal immunoglobulin molecules. Identical copies of antibody which consist of one H chain class and one L chain type

Monoclonal protein. A protein produced from the progeny of a single cell called a clone

Monokines. Soluble factors released by activated macrophages/monocytes

Multiple myeloma. A paraproteinemic disorder consisting typically of the presence of serum paraprotein, anemia, and lytic bone lesions

Myeloma protein. Either an intact monoclonal immunoglobulin molecule or a portion of one produced by malignant plasma cells

Myeloperoxidase. An enzyme that is present within granules of phagocytic cells and catalyzes peroxidation of a variety of microorganisms

Natural antibody. Antibody present in the serum produced against unknown antigens, primarily antigenic structures of the intestinal microorganism flora

Neutralization. The process by which antibody or antibody and complement neutralizes the infectivity of microorganisms, particularly viruses

NK cells (natural killer cells). Cytotoxic cells of undefined lineage, responsible for cellular cytotoxicity without prior sensitization

Nonresponder. An animal unable to respond to an antigen, usually because of genetic factors

Nude mouse. A hairless mouse which congenitally lacks a thymus and has a marked deficiency of thymus-derived lymphocytes

Null cells. Cells lacking the specific identifying surface markers for either T or B lymphocytes

NZB mouse. A genetically inbred strain of mice in which autoimmune disease resembling systemic lupus erythematosus develops spontaneously

Ontogeny. The developmental history of an individual organism within a group of animals

Opsonin. A substance capable of enhancing phagocytosis. Antibodies and complement are the 2 main opsonins

Paralysis. The pseudotolerant condition in which an ongoing immune response is masked by the presence of overwhelming amounts of antigen

Paraproteinemia. A heterogeneous group of diseases characterized by the presence in serum or urine of a monoclonal immunoglobulin

Paratope. An antibody combining site for epitope, the simplest form of an antigenic determinant

Passive cutaneous anaphylaxis (PCA). An in vivo passive transfer test for recognizing cytotropic antibody responsible for immediate hypersensitivity reactions

Passive immunity. Transfer of preformed antibodies to non-immune individual by means of blood, serum components, etc. e.g. maternal antibodies transferred to fetus via placenta or milk, or immunoglobulins injected to prevent or modify infections

Patching. The reorganization of a cell surface membrane component into discrete patches over the entire cell surface

Pathogenic. Producing disease or pathological changes

Persistent infection. An infection in which the microorganism persists in the body, not necessarily in a fully infectious form, but often for long periods or throughout life

Peyer's patches. Collections of lymphoid tissue in the submucosa of the small intestine which contain lymphocytes, plasma cells, germinal centers, and T cell-dependent areas

Pfeiffer phenomenon. Demonstration that cholera vibrios introduced into the peritoneal cavity of an immune guinea pig lose their mobility and are lysed regardless of the presence of cells

Phagocytes. Cells which are capable of ingesting particulate matter

Phagocytosis. The engulfment of microorganisms or other particles by leukocytes

Phagolysosome. A cellular organelle which is the product of the fusion of a phagosome and a lysosome

Phagosome. A phagocytic vesicle bounded by inverted plasma membrane

Phylogeny. The developmental and evolutionary history of a group of animals

Phytohemagglutinin (PHA). A lectin which is derived from the red kidney bean (*Phaseolus vulgaris*) and which stimulates predominantly T lymphocytes

Pinocytosis. The ingestion of soluble materials by cells

Plaque-forming cells (PFC). Antibody producing cell capable of forming a hemolytic plaque in the presence of complement and antigenic erythrocytes

Plasma cells. Fully differentiated antibody-synthesizing cells which are derived from B lymphocytes

Pokeweed mitogen (PWM). A lectin that is derived from pokeweed *(Phytolacca americana)* and stimulates both B and T lymphocytes

Polyclonal mitogens. Mitogens which activate large subpopulations of lymphocytes

Polyethylenglycol (PEG). Substance used as fusion reagent for the production of somatic cell hybrids

Pre-B cells. Large immature lymphoid cells with diffuse cytoplasmic IgM which eventually develop into cells

Precipitation. A reaction between a soluble antigen and soluble antibody in which a complex lattice of interlocking aggregates forms

Primary follicles. Tightly packed aggregates of lymphocytes found in the cortex of the lymph node or in the white pulp of the spleen after antigenic stimulation. Primary follicles develop into germinal centers

Primary lymphoid organs. Lymphoid organs that are essential to the development of the immune response, i.e., the thymus and the bursa of Fabricius

Private antigen. A composition of antigenic determinants on MHC molecules characteristic of an allele

Properdin system (or alternate pathway of complement activation). A group of proteins which after activation by microbial substances (e.g. zymosan, complex polysaccharides a. o.) activate C 3 of the classical complement pathway independently of antibody-antigen reactions

Prostaglandins. A variety of naturally occurring aliphatic acids with various biologic activities, including increased vascular permeability, smooth muscle contraction, bronchial constriction, and alteration in the pain threshold

Prothymocytes. Immature precursors of mature thymocytes which develop within the thymus gland

Prozone phenomenon. Suboptimal immune reaction in vitro (precipitation, cytolysis, agglutination) which occurs in the region of antibody excess during immune reactions

Pyogenicmicroorganisms. Microorganisms whose presence in tissues stimulates an outpouring of polymorphonuclear leukocytes

Pyrogens. Substances released either endogenously from leukocytes or administered exogenously, usually from bacteria, and which produce fever in susceptible hosts

Reagin. Synonymous with IgE antibody. Also denotes a complement-fixing antibody which reacts in the Wassermann reaction with cardiolipin

Receptor. A chemical structure on the surface of any immunologically competent cell

Recombinant. An animal which has experienced a recombinational event during meiosis, consisting of cross-over and recombination of parts of 2 chromosomes

Rejection response. Immune response with both humoral and cellular components directed against transplanted tissue

Reservoir. Animal (bird, mammal, mosquito, etc.) or animals in which microorganism maintains itself independently of human infection

Restriction. Stimulation and activation of cooperating cells in the immune response occurs only if the reacting cells share either K, D molecules (cytotoxic T cells) or Ia molecules (helper/suppressor T cells), i.e. the recognition of antigens is restricted to the concomitant presence of antigen and the own MHC molecules

Reticuloendothelial system. A system of cells that take up particles and certain dyes injected into the body. Comprises Kupffer cells of liver, tissue, histocytes, monocytes, and the lymph node, splenic, alveolar, peritoneal, and pleural macrophages

Rh incompatibility. Incompatibility between certain blood group antigens of a mother and her baby or between donor and recipient in blood transfusions

Rheumatoid factor (RF). An anti-immunoglobulin antibody directed against denatured IgG present in the serum of patients with rheumatoid arthritis and other rheumatoid diseases

Rocket electrophoresis (Laurell technic). An electroimmunodiffusion technic in which antigen is electrophoresed into agar containing specific antibody and precipitates in a tapered rocket-shaped pattern. This technic is used for quantitation of antigens

Rose-Waaler test. A type of passive hemagglutination test for the detection of rheumatoid factor which employs tanned red blood cells coated with rabbit 7S IgG antibodies specific for sheep red blood cells

Schistosomiasis (=bilharzia). Disease with urinary symptoms common in many parts of Africa. Caused by the fluke (trematode) *Schistosoma haematobium;* larvae from infected snails enter water and penetrate human skin

Secondary lymphoid organs. Lymphoid organs not essential to the ontogeny of immune responses, i.e., the spleen, lymph nodes, tonsils, and Peyer's patches

Secretory IgA. A dimer of IgA molecules with a sedimentation coefficient of 11 S, linked by J chain and secretory component

Secretory immune system. A distinct immune system that is common to external secretions and consists predominantly of IgA

Secretory piece (T piece). A molecule of MW 70,000 produced in epithelial cells and associated with secretory immunoglobulins, particularly IgA and IgM

Self-recognition. Recognition of self-antigens by one's own immunologic system

Sensitized. Synonymous with immunized

Serologically defined (SD) antigens. Antigens that are present on membranes of nearly all mammalian cells and are controlled by genes present in the major histocompatibility complex. They can be easily detected with antibodies

Serology. Literally, the study of serum. Refers to the determination of antibodies to infectious agents important in clinical medicine

Serum (pl. sera). The liquid part of the blood remaining after cells and fibrin have been removed

Serum sickness. An adverse immunologic response to a foreign antigen, usually a heterologous protein

Shedding. The liberation of microorganisms from the infected host

Side chain theory. Theory of antibody synthesis proposed by Ehrlich in 1900 suggesting that specific side chains which form antigen receptors are present on the surface membranes of antibody-producing cells

Slow virus. A virus which produces disease with a greatly delayed onset and protracted course

Specificity. A term referring to the selective reaction which occurs between an antigen and its corresponding antibody or lymphocyte

Spleen. An organ in the abdominal cavity, composed largely of lymphocytes and macrophages. It is an important site of antibody production

S region. The chromosomal region in the H-2 complex containing the gene for a serum β-globulin (C4 complement component)

Streptococci. Classified into groups A–H by antigenic properties of carbohydrate extracted from cell wall. Important human pathogens belong to Group A ($=$ *Streptococcus pyogenes*), which is divided into 47 types according to antigenic properties of M protein present on outermost surface of bacteria

Streptolysin O. Exotoxin produced by *Streptococcus pyogenes*. Oxygen-labile, haemolytic, and a powerful antigen

Streptolysin S. Exotoxin produced by *Streptococcus pyogenes*. Oxygen-stable, causing β haemolysis on blood agar plates, but not demonstrably antigenic

Suppressor T cells. A subset of T lymphocytes which suppress antibody synthesis by B cells or inhibit other cellular immune reactions by effector T cells

Surveillance. The process by which an intact immune system monitors both self and foreign antigens

S value. Svedberg unit. Denotes the sedimentation coefficient of a protein, determined usually by analytic ultracentrifugation

Syngeneic. Denotes the relationship which exists between genetically identical members of the same species

Systemic infection. Infection that spreads throughout the body

T cell (T lymphocyte). A thymus-derived cell which participates in a variety of cell-mediated immune reactions

T cell rosette. See E rosette

Teleology. Doctrine that biological phenomena generally have a purpose, serving some function

Thy-1 antigen (theta antigen). An alloantigen present on the surface of most thymocytes and peripheral T lymphocytes

Thymopoietin (originally termed thymin). A protein of MW 7,000 that is dervied originally from the thymus of animals with autoimmune thymitis and myasthenia gravis and which can impair neuromuscular transmission

Thymosin. A thymic hormone protein of MW 12,000 which can restore T cell immunity in rhymectomized animals

Thymus. The central lymphoid organ which is present in the thorax and controls the ontogeny of T lymphocytes

Thymus-dependent antigen. Antigen which depends on T cell interaction with B cells for antibody synthesis, e.g., erythrocytes, serum proteins, and hapten-carrier complexes

Thymus-derived lymphocytes (T lymphocyte). Small lymphocytes which on (or after) residence in the thymus attain new immunologic capabilities

Thymus-independent antigen. Antigen which can induce an immune response without the apparent participation of T lymphocytes

Tissue typing. The processes of identifying and matching antigens on prospective donor and recipient tissues

Titre (1). A measure of units of antibody per unit volume of serum, usually quoted as reciprocal of last serum dilution giving antibody-mediated reaction e.g. 120. (2) Measure of units of virus per unit volume of fluid or tissue. Usually given in log 10 units per ml or G e.g. $10^{5.5}$ pfu/ml

TL antigen. A membrane antigen that is present on prothymocytes in mice with a TL+ gene, but which is lost during thymic maturation

Tolerance. Traditionally denotes that condition in which responsive cell clones have been inactivated by prior contact with antigen, with the result that no immune response occurs on administration of antigen

Toxoids. Antigenic but nontoxic derivatives of toxins

T piece. See Secretory piece

Transfer factor. A dialyzable extract of immune lymphocytes that is capable of transferring cell-mediated immunity in humans and possibly in other animal species

Translocon. Stretch of chromosome containing gene sequences coding for heavy, kappa or lambda polypeptide chains of immunoglobulins

Transplantation antigens. Those antigens which are expressed on the surface of virtually all cells and which induce rejection of tissues transplanted from one individual to a genetically disparate individual

Tuberculin test. A skin test for delayed hypersensitivity to antigens from *Mycobacterium tuberculosis*. In man the antigen is introduced into the skin by intradermal injection (Mantoux test)

Tuftsin. A γ-globulin which is capable of stimulating endocytosis by neutrophils

Vaccination. Immunization with antigens administered for the prevention of infectious diseases (term originally coined to denote immunization against vaccinia or cowpox virus)

V antigens. Virally induced antigens which are expressed on viruses and virus-infected cells

Vertical transmission. The transmission of infection directly from parent to offspring. This can take place *in utero* via egg, sperm, placenta, or postnatally via milk, blood, contact, etc.

Viremia. Presence of virus in blood stream. Virus may be associated with leucocytes (leucocyte viraemia), or free in the plasma (plasma viraemia), or occasionally associated with erythrocytes or platelets

Virion. The complete virus particle

V (variable) region. The amino terminal portion of the H or L chain of an immunoglobulin molecule, containing considerable heterogeneity in the amino acid residues compared to the constant region

V region subgroups. Subdivisions of V regions of kappa chains based on substantial homology in sequences of amino acids

Wasting disease (runt disease). A chronic, ultimately fatal illness associated with lymphoid atrophy in mice who are neonatally thymectomized

Xenogeneic. Denotes the relationship which exists between members of genetically different species

Xenograft. A tissue or organ graft between members of 2 distinct or different species

References

Fudenberg HH, Stites DP, Caldwell JL, Wells JV (1980) Basic and clinical immunology, 4th ed. Lange Medical Publications, Los Altos/Calif.

Mims CA (1977) The pathogenesis of infectious diseases. Academic Press, New York

Amos DB (ed) (1976) Immunology: Its role in disease and health. US DHEW publication No. (NIH) 75–940

Subject and Author Index

Page numbers in *italics* refer to the principle discussion of each subject.

J. C. Cawley, G. F. Burns, F. G. J. Hayhoe

Hairy-Cell Leukaemia

1980. 64 figures, 4 tables. IX, 123 pages
(Recent Results in Cancer Research, Vol. 72)
ISBN 3-540-09920-4

Current Topics
in Microbiology and Immunology

Editors: W. Arber, S. Falkow, W. Henle, P. H. Hofschneider,
J. H. Humphrey, J. Klein, P. Koldovský, H. Koprowski,
O. Maaløe, F. Melchers, R. Rott, H. G. Schweiger, L. Syruček,
P. K. Vogt

Volume 86
1979. 29 figures, 22 tables. III, 168 pages
ISBN 3-540-09432-6

Contents: Genetic Potential of Bunyaviruses. – Defective
Interfering Particles of Togaviruses. – The Fv-1 Gene of
Mouse and its Control of Murine Leukemia Virus Repli-
cation. – Defective Interfering Particles of Rhabdoviruses.

Immune Deficiency

Editors: M. D. Cooper, A. R. Lawton, P. A. Miescher,
H. J. Müller-Eberhard

1979. 10 figures, 22 tables. IV, 184 pages
ISBN 3-540-09490-3

Immunodermatology

Editors: I. N. Gigli, P. A. Miescher, H. J. Müller-Eberhard
1983. 34 figures, 37 tables. VI, 183 pages
ISBN 3-540-11738-5
(Monograph edition of the international journal "Springer
Seminars in Immunopathology, Vol. 4, Nos. 1 and 3)

Springer-Verlag
Berlin
Heidelberg
New York
Tokyo

Immunodiagnosis and Immunotherapy
of Malignant Tumors

Relevance to Surgery

Editors: H.-D. Flad, C. Herfarth, M. Betzler
1979. 101 figures, 109 tables. X, 329 pages
ISBN 3-540-09161-0

Immunological Aspects of Liver Disease

Editors: H. C. Thomas, P. A. Miescher,
H. J. Müller-Eberhard

1982. 22 figures, 20 tables. VI, 208 pages
ISBN 3-540-11310-X
(Monograph edition of the international journal "Springer
Seminars in Immunopathology", Vol. 3, Nos. 3 and 4)

Immunostimulation

Editors: L. Chedid, P. A. Miescher, H. J. Müller-Eberhard
1980. 44 figures, 39 tables. VIII, 236 pages
ISBN 3-540-10354-6

J. Klein
Biology of the Mouse Histocompatibility-2 Complex

Principles of Immunogenetics Applied to a Single System
1975. 58 figures, 90 tables. XII, 620 pages
ISBN 3-540-06733-7

Lymphocyte Hybridomas

Second Workshop on "Functional Properties of Tumors
of T and B Lymphocytes" Sponsored by the National
Cancer Institute (NIH) April 3–5, 1978 Bethesda,
Maryland, USA

Editors: F. Melchers, M. Potter, N. L. Warner

Reprint. 1979. 85 figures, 86 tables. XXI, 246 pages
ISBN 3-540-09670-1

The Major Histocompatibility System in Man and Animals

Editor: D. Götze

With contributions by numerous experts

1977. 23 figures. X, 404 pages
ISBN 3-540-08097-X

W. E. Stewart II
The Interferon System

Second, enlarged edition. 1981. 23 figures. XII, 493 pages
ISBN 3-211-81634-8

Springer-Verlag
Berlin
Heidelberg
New York
Tokyo